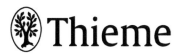

Anatomy for Dental Medicine
Third Edition

Edited by
Eric W. Baker, MA, MPhil
Department of Basic Science and Craniofacial Biology
New York University College of Dentistry
New York, New York

Associate Editor
Elisabeth K. N. Lopez, PhD
Department of Basic Science and Craniofacial Biology
New York University College of Dentistry
New York, New York

Based on the work of
Michael Schuenke, MD, PhD
Institute of Anatomy
Christian Albrecht University, Kiel

Erik Schulte, MD
Institute of Functional and Clinical Anatomy
Johannes Gutenberg University, Mainz

Udo Schumacher, MD, FRCPath, CBiol, FRSB, DSc
Center for Experimental Medicine
Institute of Anatomy and Experimental Morphology
University Medical Center, Hamburg-Eppendorf

Illustrations by
Markus Voll
Karl Wesker

Thieme
New York • Stuttgart • Delhi • Rio de Janeiro

Illustrators: Markus Voll and Karl Wesker
Production Editor: Barbara Chernow
Compositor: Carol Pierson, Chernow Editorial Services, Inc.

Library of Congress Cataloging-in-Publication Data
    Names: Baker, Eric W. (Eric William), 1961- editor. | Lopez, Elisabeth K. N., editor. | Schünke, Michael. | Schulte, Erik. | Schumacher, Udo.
    Title: Anatomy for dental medicine / editor, Eric W. Baker ; associate editor, Elisabeth K.N. Lopez ; based on the work of Michael Schuenke, Erik Schulte, Udo Schumacher ; illustrations by Markus Voll, Karl Wesker.
Description: Third edition. | New York : Thieme, [2020] | Includes index. | Summary: "Dental students/residents and other allied health students who deal with anatomy in the area of the head and neck need to master anatomy of those regions. Most of the atlases that are on the market cover whole body anatomy without the focus and additional details that these students require. Anatomy for Dental Medicine strikes an optimal balance between systemic and regional approaches to this complex anatomy, which suits both first-time student learner as well as anatomy review for the boards or specialty courses. The new edition continues to combine our award-winning, full-color illustrations with explanatory text and summary tables. The clinical correlations, multiple choice questions and explanations as well as an appendix on the anatomy of common dental anesthetic injections specifically support dental students. The new edition is updated with radiology images, new factual and clinical questions, and a general revision of content"— Provided by publisher.
    Identifiers: LCCN 2019053817 | ISBN 9781684200467 (paperback) | ISBN 9781684200474 (ebook)
    Subjects: MESH: Head—anatomy & histology | Dentistry | Neck—anatomy & histology | Atlas
    Classification: LCC QM535 | NLM WE 17 | DDC 611/.910223—dc23
    LC record available at https://lccn.loc.gov/2019053817

Thieme Publishers New York
333 Seventh Avenue, New York, NY 10001 USA
+1 800 782 3488, customerservice@thieme.com

Thieme Publishers Stuttgart
Rüdigerstrasse 14, 70469 Stuttgart, Germany
+49 [0]711 8931 421, customerservice@thieme.de

Thieme Publishers Delhi
A-12, Second Floor, Sector-2, Noida-201301
Uttar Pradesh, India
+91 120 45 566 00, customerservice@thieme.in

Thieme Revinter Publicações Ltda.
Rua do Matoso, 170 – Tijuca
Rio de Janeiro RJ 20270-135 - Brasil
+55 21 2563-9702, www.thiemerevinter.com.br

Printed in Germany by CPI books GmbH, Leck   5 4 3 2 1

ISBN 978-1-68420-046-7

Also available as an e-book:
eISBN 978-1-68420-047-4

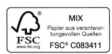

To my wonderful wife, Amy Curran Baker,
and my awe-inspiring daughters, Phoebe and Claire. — E.W.B.

To my loving and supportive family, Leonardo,
Penelope, and Ariadne, who never cease to inspire me. — E.K.N.L.

Contents

Head

1 Embryology of the Head & Neck

2 Cranial Bones

3 Vasculature & Lymphatics of the Head & Neck

Contents

Regions of the Head

7   Nose & Nasal Cavity

8   Oral Cavity & Pharynx

9   Orbit & Eye

Contents

Neck

11 Bones, Ligaments, & Muscles of the Neck

12 Neurovascular Topography of the Neck

13 Larynx & Thyroid Gland

Sectional Anatomy

14 Sectional Anatomy of the Head & Neck

Rest of Body Anatomy

15 Rest of Body Anatomy

Contents

Appendices

Index

Preface

The third edition of *Anatomy for Dental Medicine* keeps the key features of the first and second editions:

- A user-friendly format in which each two-page spread is a self-contained guide to a specific topic.

- An intuitive approach to each region, in which bones and joints are discussed first, followed by muscles, vasculature, and nerves, before showing an integrated neurovasculature topography.

- Detailed artwork supplemented with descriptive captions, simplified schematics, and tables of key information.

- Chapter dedicated to sectional anatomy, comparing such images to clinical imagery, to demonstrate how students will see anatomical structures in a clinical setting.

- Systemic anatomy at the start of the book, followed by a regional approach that allows this atlas to be used in conjunction with many lecture- and dissection-based courses.

- Information on embryology, histology, neuroanatomy, and anatomy of the body below the head, which allows students to integrate anatomy with different topics and makes this atlas a good companion for combined courses, as well as courses that only cover anatomy of the head and neck.

- An appendix that explains the anatomical basis of local anesthesia techniques used in dentistry.

- Two appendices with practice questions and explanations.

In preparing the third edition, we included additional radiology images to enhance the clinical relevance of the anatomy depicted in the artwork. We also added discussions of several structures that are commonly used as landmarks, both in learning the anatomy as a student and in the clinical setting. We reorganized the neuroanatomy sections to be in a more logical progression. And finally, we added additional practice questions, including some in the style of the Integrated National Board Dental Examination (INBDE).

Acknowledgments

First, we would like to thank our New York University dentistry students for their feedback on the second edition. We would also like to thank our colleagues at NYU for their assistance with this third edition (as well as previous editions): Dr. Richard Cotty, Dr. Johanna Warshaw, Dr. Jessica Manser, Dr. Julie O'Meara, Dr. Elena Cunningham, and Professor Joshua Johnson. Special thanks are due to Dr. Louis Terracio and Dr. Nicola Partridge for their support of all things related to anatomical education at NYU Dentistry.

For their invaluable input and advise in preparing the third edition, thanks to:

- Michelle Singleton, PhD, Professor of Anatomy, College of Graduate Studies, Midwestern University, Downers Grove, Illinois
- Earlanda L. Williams, PhD, University of the Incarnate Word, School of Osteopathic Medicine, San Antonio, Texas
- Alison F. Doubleday, PhD, Associate Professor, Department of Oral Medicine and Diagnostic Sciences, University of Illinois at Chicago, College of Dentistry, Chicago, Illinois
- Jessica M. Manser, PhD, Adjunct Assistant Professor, Department of Basic Science and Craniofacial Biology, New York University, College of Dentistry, New York, New York
- Claire A. Kirchhoff, PhD, Department of Biomedical Sciences, Marquette University, Milwaukee, Wisconsin
- Anita Joy-Thomas, BDS, PhD, Professor, Anatomical Sciences, Department of Diagnostic and Biomedical Sciences, University of Texas Health Science Center at Houston, School of Dentistry, Houston, Texas

We thank those who helped shape the second edition of this atlas: Dr. Roger A. Dashner, Clinical Anatomist and CEO, Advanced Anatomical Services, Columbus, Ohio; Dr. Dorothy Burk, Associate Professor of Biomedical Sciences, University of the Pacific Arthur A. Dugoni School of Dentistry, San Francisco, California; Douglas Gould, PhD, Professor, Oakland University William Beaumont School of Medicine, Rochester, Michigan; Dr. Stanley P. Freeman, DDS, FACD, FICD, Course Director and Professor of Dental Anatomy, Columbia School of Dentistry, New York; Dr. Bob Hutchins, Professor of Biomedical Sciences, TX A&M University, Baylor College of Dentistry, Dallas, TX (recently retired); Dr. Geoffroy Noel, Assistant Professor and Director of Division of Anatomical Sciences, McGill University, Montreal, Quebec, Canada; Justin Gorgi PhD, Associate Professor, Midwestern University, Glendale, Arizona; Michelle Singleton, PhD, Professor of Anatomy, Chicago College of Osteopathic Medicine, Midwestern University, Downers Grove, Illinois; Dr. Nicole Herring, Assistant Professor of Anatomical Sciences and Neurobiology, University of Louisville, Louisville, Kentucky; Dr. Rita Hardiman, Lecturer in Oro-facial and Head and Neck Anatomy, Melbourne Dental School, University of Melbourne, Parkville, Australia; Brian R. MacPherson, PhD, Professor and Vice-Chair, Department of Anatomy and Neurobiology, University of Kentucky College of Medicine, Lexington, Kentucky; Henry Edinger, PhD, Director of Educational Programs, Department of Pharmacology & Physiology, Rutgers-New Jersey Medical School, Newark, New Jersey.

For the clinical vignette-style questions and the factual-type questions, respectively, thanks to:

- Dr. Lawrence C. Zoller, Professor of Biomedical Sciences, UNLV School of Dental Medicine, Las Vegas, Nevada
- Frank J. Daly, PhD, Associate Professor of Anatomy, University of New England College of Osteopathic Medicine, Biddeford, Maine

For their contribution to photographic coverage of the anatomy of dental local anesthesia, thanks to:

- Dr. Stanley P. Freeman, Dr. Brian S. Duchan, Alison Smith, Jazmin Smith, and Bridget Bieler of Westport Dental Associates.

Thank you to our colleagues at New York University who contributed to the second edition: Dr. Jean-Pierre Saint-Jeannet for his expert opinions related to the expanded neuroanatomy coverage in this edition; Dr. Kenneth Allen for his review of the coverage of the anatomy of local anesthesia; and Dr. Kenneth Fleisher for his assistance with the photographic coverage of the anatomy of dental local anesthesia.

We thank those who helped shape the original edition of this atlas: Susana Tejada, class of 2010, Boston University School of Dental Medicine; Dr. Norman F. Capra, Department of Neural and Pain Sciences, University of Maryland Dental School, Baltimore, Maryland; Dr. Bob Hutchins, Associate Professor, Department of Biomedical Sciences, Baylor College of Dentistry, Dallas, Texas; Dr. Brian R. MacPherson, Professor and Vice-Chair, Department of Anatomy and Neurobiology, University of Kentucky, Lexington, Kentucky; and Dr. Nicholas Peter Piesco, Associate Professor, Department of Oral Medicine, University of Pittsburgh, Pittsburgh, Pennsylvania.

We would once again like to thank everyone at Thieme Publishers who so professionally facilitated the production of this atlas: Dr. Cathrin Weinstein, Bridget Queenan, Dr. Julie O'Meara, Elsie Starbecker, Anne T. Vinnicombe, Huvie Weinreich, Dr. Barbara Chernow, Sarah Landis, and Delia DeTurris.

Finally, we thank the authors of the original Prometheus text, Michael Schuenke, MD, PhD, Erik Schulte, MD, and Udo Schumacher, MD, FRCPath, CBiol, FRSB, DSc, as well as the illustrators, Markus Voll and Karl Wesker.

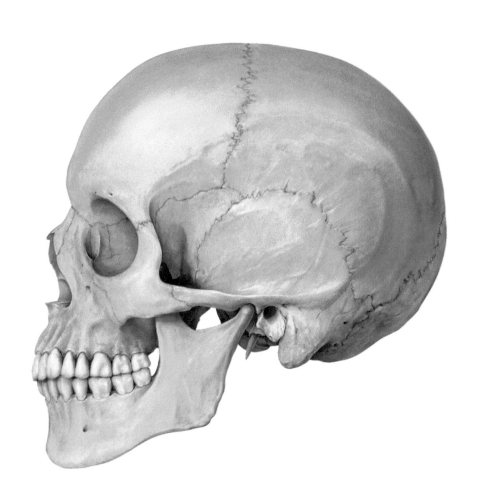

Head

Germ Layers & the Developing Embryo

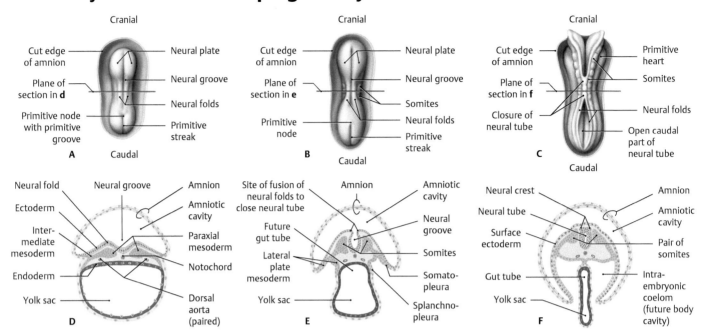

Fig. 1.1 Embryonic development (after Sadler)
Age in postovulatory days.
A–C Posterior (dorsal) view after removal of the amnion.
D–E Schematic cross sections of the corresponding stages at the horizontal planes of section marked in **A** to **C**. Gastrulation occurs in week 3 of human embryonic development. It produces three germ layers in the embryonic disk: ectoderm (light grey), mesoderm (red), and endoderm (dark grey).
A, D Day 19, the three layers are visible in the embryonic disk. The amnion forms the amniotic cavity dorsally, and the endoderm encloses the yolk sac. The neural tube is developing in the area of the neural plate.
B, E Day 20, the first somites have formed, and the neural groove is beginning to close to form the neural tube, with initial folding of the embryo.
C, F Day 22, eight pairs of somites flank the partially closed neural tube, which has sunk below the ectoderm. The yolk sac elongates ventrally to form the gut tube and yolk sac. At the sites where the neural folds fuse to close the neural tube, cells form a bilateral neural crest that detaches from the surface and migrates into the mesoderm.

Table 1.1 Differentiation of germ layers

Germ layer	Embryonic structure		Adult derivative
Ectoderm	Neural tube		Brain, retina, spinal cord
	Neural crest	Neural crest of the head	Sensory and parasympathetic ganglia; parafollicular cells; pigment cells; carotid body; cartilage, bone, dermis, subcutaneous tissue, and other connective tissues in the head; part of cardiac septum
		Neural crest of the trunk	Sensory, sympathetic, and parasympathetic ganglia; peripheral glia; pigment cells; adrenal medulla; intramural plexuses and enteric nervous system
	Surface ectoderm	Placodes	Anterior pituitary, cranial sensory ganglia, olfactory epithelium, inner ear, lens
			Epithelium of the oral cavity, salivary glands, nasal cavities, paranasal sinuses, lacrimal passages, external auditory canal, epidermis, hair, nails, cutaneous glands
Mesoderm	Paraxial	Somites	Dermis of skin (from dermatome), musculature (from myotome), vertebral column (from sclerotome)
	Axial	Notochord	Nucleus pulposus
		Prechordal mesoderm	Extraocular muscles
	Intermediate		Kidneys, gonads, renal and genital excretory ducts
	Lateral plates	Visceral (splanchnic)	Heart, blood vessels, smooth muscle, bowel wall, blood, adrenal cortex, visceral serosa
		Parietal (somatic)	Sternum, limbs without muscles (muscles develop from the myotomes), dermis and subcutaneous tissue of the anterolateral body wall, smooth muscle, connective tissue, parietal serosa
Endoderm	Intestinal tube		Epithelium of the bowel, respiratory tract, digestive glands, pharyngeal glands, pharyngotympanic (auditory) tube, tympanic cavity, urinary bladder, parathyroid glands, thyroid gland

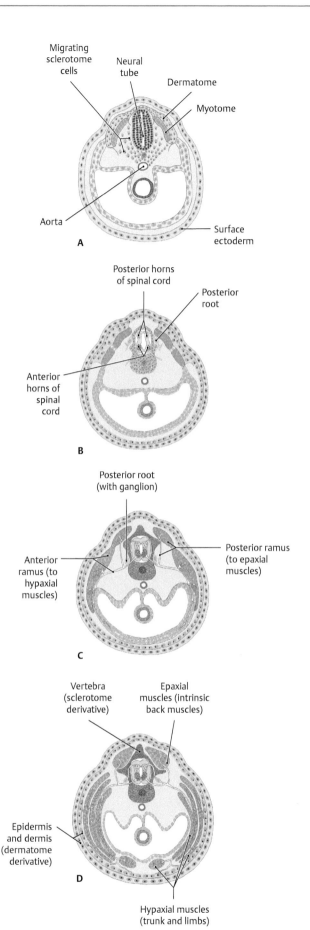

A

Migrating sclerotome cells
Neural tube
Dermatome
Myotome
Aorta
Surface ectoderm

B

Posterior horns of spinal cord
Posterior root
Anterior horns of spinal cord

C

Posterior root (with ganglion)
Anterior ramus (to hypaxial muscles)
Posterior ramus (to epaxial muscles)

D

Vertebra (sclerotome derivative)
Epaxial muscles (intrinsic back muscles)
Epidermis and dermis (dermatome derivative)
Hypaxial muscles (trunk and limbs)

Fig. 1.2 Somatic muscle development
Age in postovulatory days. Each somite divides into a dermatome (cutaneous), myotome (muscular), and sclerotome (vertebral) at around day 22 (see **Fig. 1.1**).

A Day 28, sclerotomes migrate to form the vertebral column around the notochord (primitive spinal cord).

B Day 30, all 34 or 35 somite pairs have formed. The neural tube differentiates into a primitive spinal cord. Motor and sensory neurons differentiate in the anterior and posterior horns of the spinal cord, respectively.

C By day 40, the posterior and anterior roots form the mixed spinal nerve. The posterior branch supplies the epiaxial muscles (future intrinsic back muscles); the anterior branch supplies the hypaxial muscles (anterior muscles, including all muscles except the intrinsic back muscles).

D Week 8, the epiaxial and hypaxial muscles have differentiated into the skeletal muscles of the trunk. Cells from the sclerotomes also migrate into the limbs. During this migration, the spinal nerves form the plexuses (cervical, branchial, and lumbosacral), which innervate the muscles of the neck, upper limb, and lower limb, respectively.

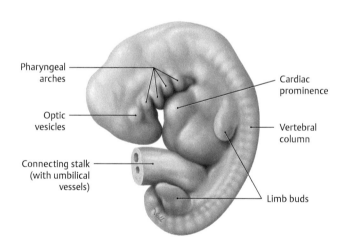

Pharyngeal arches
Optic vesicles
Connecting stalk (with umbilical vessels)
Cardiac prominence
Vertebral column
Limb buds

Fig. 1.3 5-week-old embryo
The human embryo at 5 weeks has a crown-rump length of approximately 5 to 7 mm. The umbilical cord, which attaches the embryo to the mother, is seen. The future cerebral hemispheres form along with the eye, ear, pharyngeal arches (which form a large portion of the structures of the head and neck), heart, neural tube, and limb buds.

Development of the Brain & Spinal Cord

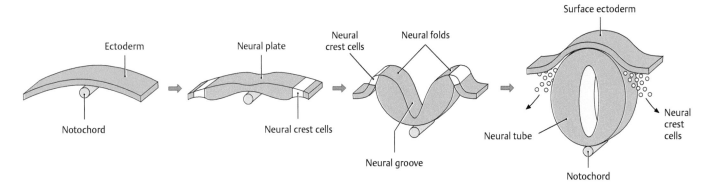

Fig. 1.4 Development of the neural tube and neural crest (after Wolpert)

The tissues of the nervous system orginate embryonically from the posterior surface ectoderm. The notochord in the midline of the body induces the formation of the neural plate, which lies dorsal to the notochord, and of the neural crests, which are lateral to the notochord. With further development, the neural plate deepens at the center to form the neural groove, which is flanked on each side by the neural folds. Later the groove deepens and closes to form the neural tube, which sinks below the ectoderm. The neural tube is the structure from which the central nervous system (CNS) – the brain and spinal cord –

develops (further development of the spinal cord is shown in **Fig. 1.5**, further brain development in **Fig. 1.7**). Failure of the neural folds to fuse completely in the caudal region will leave an anomalous cleft in the vertebral column known as spina bifida. In the cranial region, this will lead to a defect known as anencephaly. The administration of folic acid to potential mothers around the time of conception can significantly reduce the incidence of spina bifida and other neural tube defects. Cells that migrate from the neural crest develop into various structures, including cells of the peripheral nervous system (PNS), such as Schwann cells, and the pseudounipolar cells of the spinal ganglion (see **Fig. 1.6**).

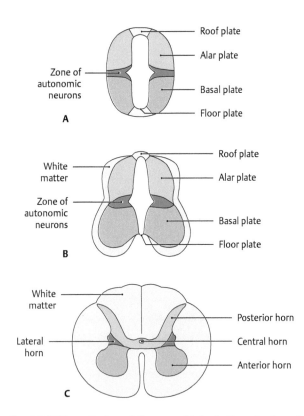

Fig. 1.5 Differentiation of the neural tube in the spinal cord during development

Cross-section, superior view.
A Early neural tube. **B** Intermediate Stage. **C** Adult spinal cord.
The neurons that form the basal plate are efferent (motor neurons), while the neurons that form the alar plate are afferent (sensory neurons). In the future thoracic, lumbar, and sacral spinal cord, there is another zone between them that gives rise to autonomic neurons. The roof plate and the floor plate do not form neurons.

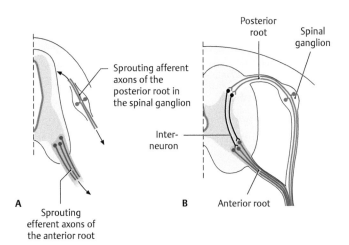

Fig. 1.6 Development of a peripheral nerve

Afferent (sensory) axons (blue) and efferent (motor) axons (red) sprout from the neuronal cell bodies during early embryonic development.
A Primary afferent neurons develop in the spinal ganglion, and alpha motor neurons develop from the basal plate of the spinal cord.
B The interneurons (black), which functionally interconnect the afferent and efferent neurons, develop at a later stage.

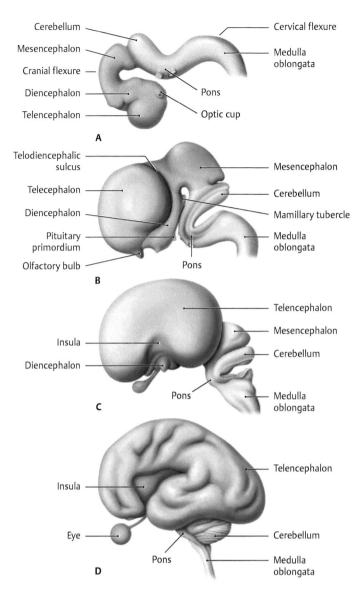

Cerebellum
Mesencephalon
Cranial flexure
Diencephalon
Telencephalon
Cervical flexure
Medulla oblongata
Pons
Optic cup

A

Telodiencephalic sulcus
Telecephalon
Diencephalon
Pituitary primordium
Olfactory bulb
Mesencephalon
Cerebellum
Mamillary tubercle
Medulla oblongata
Pons

B

Insula
Diencephalon
Telencephalon
Mesencephalon
Cerebellum
Pons
Medulla oblongata

C

Insula
Eye
Telencephalon
Cerebellum
Pons
Medulla oblongata

D

Fig. 1.7 **Development of the brain**
A Embryo with the greatest length (GL) of 10 mm at the beginning of the 2nd month of development. Even at this stage, we can see the differentiation of the neural tube into segments that will generate various brain regions.

- Red: telencephalon (cerebrum)
- Yellow: diencephalon
- Dark blue: mesencephalon (midbrain)
- Light blue: cerebellum
- Gray: pons and medulla oblongata

Note: The telencephalon outgrows all of the other brain structures as development proceeds.
B Embryo with a GL of 27 mm near the end of the 2nd month of development (end of the embryonic period). The telencephalon and the diencephalon have enlarged. The olfactory bulb is developing from the telencephalon, and the primordium of the pituitary gland is developing from the diencephalon.
C Fetus with a GL of 53 mm in approximately the 3rd month of development. By this stage the telencephalon has begun to cover the other brain areas. The insula is still on the brain surface but will subsequently be covered by the hemispheres (compare with **D**).
D Fetus with GL of 27 cm (270 mm) in approximately the 7th month of development. The cerebrum (telencephalon) has begun to develop well-defined gyri and sulci.

Table 1.2 Development of the brain

Primary vesicle		Region		Structure
Neural tube	Prosencephalon (forebrain)	Telencephalon		Cerebral cortex, white matter, basal ganglia
		Diencephalon		Epithalamus (pineal gland), thalamus, subthalamus, hypothalamus
	Mesencephalon (midbrain)*			Tectum, tegmentum, cerebral peduncles
	Rhombencephalon (hindbrain)	Metencephalon	Cerebellum	Cerebellar cortex, nuclei, peduncles
			Pons*	Nuclei, fiber tracts
		Myelencephalon	Medulla oblongata*	Nuclei, fiber tracts

*The mesencephalon, pons, and medulla oblongata are collectively known as the brainstem.

5

Development & Derivatives of the Pharyngeal (Branchial) Arches

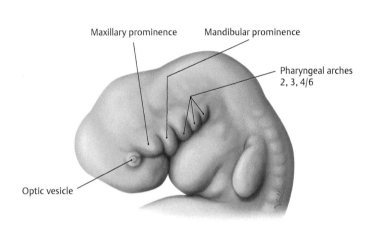

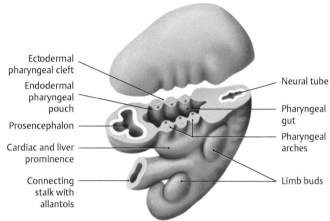

Fig. 1.8 Head and neck region of a 5-week-old embryo, showing the pharyngeal (branchial) arches and clefts
Left lateral view. The pharyngeal arches are instrumental in the development of the face, neck, larynx, and pharynx. Development of the pharyngeal arches begins in the 4th week of embryonic life as cells migrate from the neural crest to the future head and neck region. Within 1 week, a series of four oblique ridges (first through sixth pharyngeal arches, with the fifth arch only rudamentary in humans and the sixth arch not visible on the surface) form that are located at the level of the cranial segment of the foregut and are separated externally by four deep grooves (pharyngeal clefts). The pharyngeal arches and clefts are prominent features of the embryo at this stage.

Fig. 1.9 Cross section through an embryo at the level of the pharyngeal gut (after Drews)
Left superior oblique view. Due to the craniocaudal curvature of the embryo, the cross section passes through the pharyngeal arches and pharyngeal gut as well as the prosencephalon and spinal cord. The pharyngeal gut is bounded on both sides by the pharyngeal arches, which contain the mesodermal core. They are covered externally by ectoderm and internally by endoderm. Ectodermal pharyngeal clefts and endodermal pharyngeal pouches lie directly opposite one another. Because the embryo is curved craniocaudally, the pharyngeal gut and pharyngeal arches overlie the prominence of the rudimentary heart and liver.

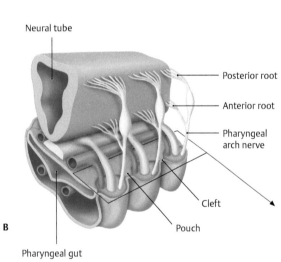

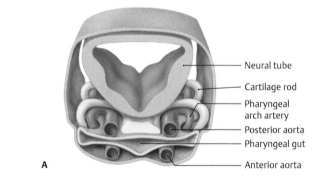

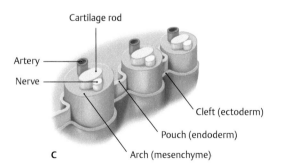

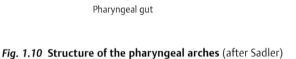

Fig. 1.10 Structure of the pharyngeal arches (after Sadler)
A Cross section through a pharyngeal arch and the neural tube, showing the pharyngeal arch cartilage and artery. **B** Oblique cross section through a pharyngeal arch and the neural tube, showing the pharyngeal arch nerves. **C** Blow up of section in **B**, showing the relationship of pharyngeal arch cartilage, artery, and nerve in the pharyngeal arches. The pharyngeal arches are covered externally by ectoderm (blue) and internally by endoderm (green). Each pharyngeal arch contains an arch artery, an arch nerve, and a cartilaginous skeletal element, all of which are surrounded by mesenchyme and muscular tissue. The external grooves are called the pharyngeal clefts, and the internal grooves are called the pharyngeal pouches.

Fig. 1.11 The arrangement and derivatives of the pharyngeal arches (after Sadler and Drews)
A The pharyngeal arches with the associated pharyngeal arch nerves
B The mandibular nerve (CN V₃), facial nerve (CN VII), glossopharyngeal nerve (CN IX), and vagus nerve (CN X) derived from the pharyngeal arch nerves
C Muscles derived from the pharyngeal arches
D Skeletal and ligamentous elements derived from the pharyngeal arches

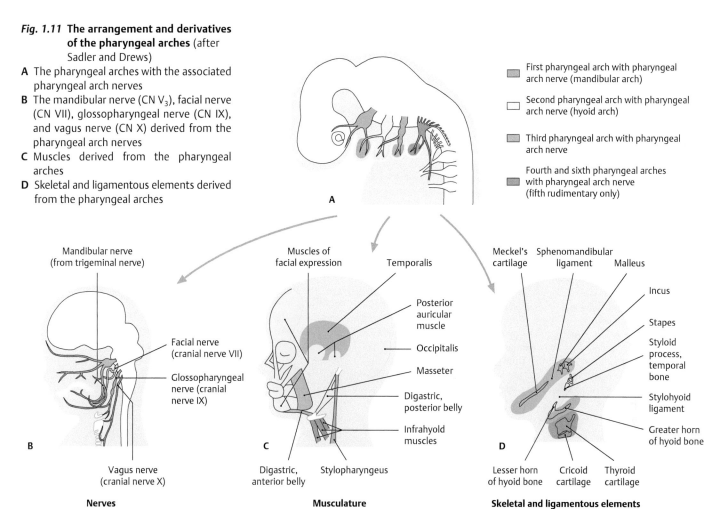

Nerves | **Musculature** | **Skeletal and ligamentous elements**

Pharyngeal arch	Muscles*		Skeletal and ligamentous elements	Nerve accompanying arch
1	Muscles of mastication • Temporalis • Masseter • Lateral ptyergoid • Medial pterygoid Mylohyoid Digastric, anterior belly Tensor tympani Tensor veli palatini		Maxilla Mandible Malleus and incus Meckel's cartilage Sphenomandibular ligament Anterior ligament of malleus	Mandibular n. (CN V₃)
2	Muscles of facial expression Stylohyoid Digastric, posterior belly Stapedius		Stapes Styloid process, temporal bone Lesser horn, hyoid bone Upper part, hyoid bone Stylohyoid ligament	Facial n. (CN VII)
3	Stylopharyngeus		Greater horn, hyoid bone Lower part, hyoid bone	Glossopharyngeal n. (CN IX)
4 and 6	Pharyngeal muscles • Levator veli palatini • Uvular muscle • Palatoglossus • Salpingopharyngeus • Palatopharyngeus • Pharyngeal constrictors	Laryngeal muscles • Thyroarytenoid • Vocalis • Lateral cricoarytenoid • Cricothyroid • Oblique arytenoids • Transverse arytenoids • Posterior arytenoids • Aryepiglottic folds • Thyroepiglottic	Laryngeal skeleton • Thyroid cartilage • Cricoid cartilage • Arytenoid cartilage • Corniculate cartilage • Cuneiform cartilage	Vagus n. (CN X)

Table 1.3 Derivatives of the pharyngeal arches

Abbreviation: CN, cranial nerve.
*All branchial skeletal muscles

Development & Derivatives of the Pharyngeal Pouches, Membranes, & Clefts

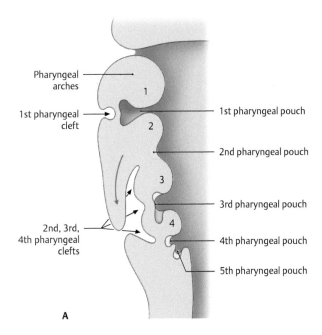

A

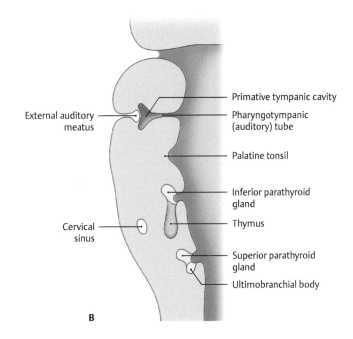

B

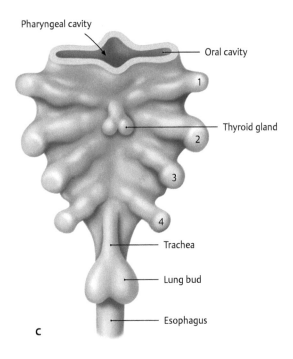

C

Fig. 1.12 Development of the pharyngeal pouches, membranes, and clefts

A Schematic view of developing pharyngeal pouches and clefts.
B Schematic view of adult structures formed by pharyngeal pouches.
C Three-dimensional representation of the pharyngeal pouches and their relationship to the oral cavity, pharyngeal cavity, and structures of the neck.

The pharyngeal pouches are paired, diverticula-like outpouchings of the endodermal pharyngeal gut. A total of four distinct pharyngeal pouches develop on each side; the fifth is often absent or rudimentary. The pharyngeal pouches develop into the tympanic cavity and the endocrine glands in the neck.

The first pharyngeal cleft develops into the external acoustic meatus. The second pharyngeal arch grows over the third and fourth pharyngeal arches and as it does so it buries the second, third, and fourth pharyngeal clefts. Remnants of these clefts form the cervical sinus, which is normally obliterated.

The pharyngeal membranes separate the pharyngeal pouches from the pharyngeal clefts in the developing embryo. The first pharyngeal membrane develops into the tympanic membrane.

Fig. 1.13 Pharyngeal pouches and the aortic arches (after Sadler)
The aortic arches (pharyngeal arch arteries) arise from the paired embryonic anterior aorta and run between the pharyngeal pouches. They open posteriorly into the posterior aorta, which is also paired. The definitive aortic arch develops from the fourth aortic arch on the left side. Note: The pouch protruding from the roof of the oral cavity is called Rathke's pouch (precursor of the anterior pituitary). Note also the lung bud extending anteriorly from the pharyngeal gut, and the primordial (anlage) of the thyroid gland.

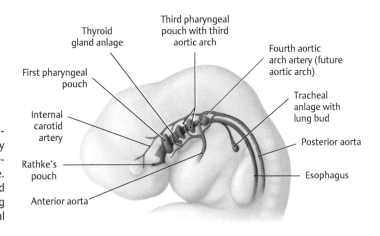

Table 1.4 Derivatives of the pharyngeal pouches

Pouch	Germ layer	Embryonic structure	Adult structure
1	Endoderm	Tubotympanic recess	Epithelium of the pharyngotympanic (auditory) tube Tympanic cavity
2		Primitive palatine tonsils	Tonsillar fossa Epithelium of the palatine tonsil
3		Divides into a posterior and an anterior part at its distal end	Inferior parathyroid gland (from posterior part) Thymus (from anterior part)
4		Divides into a posterior and an anterior part at its distal end	Superior parathyroid gland (from posterior part) Ultimobranchial body (from anterior part). This is later incorporated in thyroid gland and gives rise to the parafollicular or C cells, which secrete calcitonin.

Table 1.5 Derviative of the pharyngeal membranes

Membranes	Germ layers	Adult structure
1	Composed externally of ectoderm and internally of endoderm. The intervening core consists of mesoderm and neural crest cells.	Tympanic membrane
2 to 4		The 2nd to 4th membranes disappear when the 2nd arch grows over the cleft

Table 1.6 Derivatives of the pharyngeal clefts

Cleft	Germ layer	Adult structure
1	Ectoderm	External acoustic meatus
2 to 4		Cervical sinus, which is rapidly obliterated by the 2nd pharyngeal arch, which grows over clefts 2 to 4

Treacher Collins syndrome is a rare autosomal dominant craniofacial defect involving the structures derived from the first pharyngeal arch. It is characterized by malar hypoplasia (underdevelopment or incomplete development of the cheek), mandibular hypoplasia, downslanting eyes, eyelid coloboma (notching of the lower eyelids), and malformed external ears. It may also be associated with cleft palate, hearing loss (due to defects in the ossicles), vision loss, and difficulty breathing (dyspnea). Treatment will depend on the severity of the defects but will involve a multidisciplinary team of clinicians.

Pierre-Robin syndrome is characterized by an abnormally small mandible (micrognathia). As a result, the tongue musculature is unsupported by the mandible, allowing it to displace posteriorly, partially obstructing the airway, resulting in dyspnea (shortness of breath). This posterior displacement of the tongue (glossoptosis) is also responsible for cleft palate because it prevents the palatal shelves from fusing (see **Figs. 1.21** and **1.22**). Initial treatment involves surgery to repair the cleft palate to improve feeding and speech development.

Development of the Tongue & Thyroid Gland

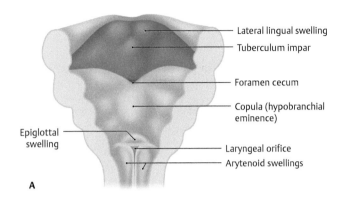

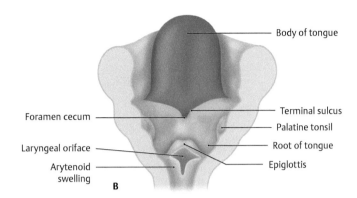

Fig. 1.14 Development of the tongue
A Early tongue development, around week 4. **B** Late tongue development, around week 8.

The tongue develops within the pharynx. While the musculature of the tongue is derived from somites, the tongue develops from the four pharyngeal (lingual) swellings. Three swellings are associated with the 1st arch and one, with the 3rd, 4th, and 6th arches. The two lateral and one midline swelling (the tuberculum impar) from the 1st pharyngeal arch contribute to the development of the anterior two thirds of the tongue. The single midline swelling (the hypobranchial eminence [copula]) from the 3rd, 4th, and 6th arches contributes to the development of the posterior one third of the tongue. A U-shaped sulcus develops around the tongue allowing it to move freely, except in one area, which is the lingual frenulum, which anchors the tongue to the floor of the oral cavity.

The lingual mucosa derived from the 1st arch swelling that covers the anterior two thirds of the tongue is innervated by the mandibular division of the trigeminal nerve (GSA) and the chorda tympani branch of

the facial nerve (SVA); the lingual mucosa derived from the 3rd, 4th, and 6th arch swellings receives sensory innervation from both CN IX (glossopharyngeal nerve) and CN X (vagus nerve).

The V-shaped terminal sulcus (sulcus terminalis) separates the anterior two thirds of the tongue from the posterior one third. Located at the vertex of the terminal sulcus, between the tuberculum impar and the hypobranchial eminence, the foramen cecum marks the site of exit for the thyroid gland from the floor of the inside of the pharynx to an extrapharyngeal location.

Ankyloglossia (tongue-tie) is a congenital anomaly in which the lingual frenulum is unusually short or thick, thereby tethering the ventral surface of the tip of the tongue to the floor of the mouth. Clinical features include restricted elevation, protrusion, and side-to-side movement of the tongue, and demonstration of a heart-shaped tongue on protrusion. It may be noticed as difficulty feeding in infants. Treatment, when required, involves a frenectomy, where the frenulum is incised, releasing the tongue.

Table 1.7 Derivation of the tongue

Pharyngeal arch	Embryonic structure(s)	Adult structure	Innervation
1	Two lateral lingual swellings Tuberculum impar	Anterior two thirds of the tongue	GSA: lingual branch of the mandibular division of the trigeminal n. (CN V₃)
2	Is obliterated by the 3rd arch and therefore does not contribute to the adult tongue Hypobranchial eminence (minor involvement)	-	SVA: chorda tympani branch of the facial n. (CN VII) (it carries sensation from the anterior 2/3 of the tongue)
3	Hypobranchial eminence	Posterior one third of the tongue	GSA: glossopharyngeal n. (CN IX) SVA: glossopharyngeal n. (CN IX)
4	Hypobranchial eminence Epiglottic swelling Arytenoid swelling Laryngotracheal groove	Root of the tongue	GSA: internal laryngeal branch of the vagus n. (CN X) SVA: internal laryngeal branch of the vagus n. (CN X)

Abbreviations: GSA, general somatic afferent; SVA, special visceral afferent.

Table 1.8 Derivation of the skeletal muscles of the tongue

Muscle origin	Muscles	Cranial nerves
Somites (from myotomes)	Intrinsic muscles of the tongue Extrinsic muscles of the tongue (genioglossus, styloglossus, and hyoglossus; ***not*** palatoglossus)	Hypoglossal n. (CN XII)

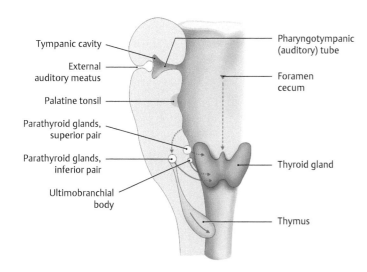

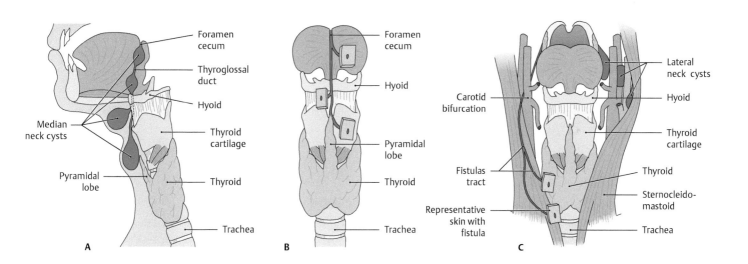

Fig. 1.15 **Migration of the pharyngeal arch tissues** (after Sadler)
Anterior view. During embryonic development, the epithelium from which the thyroid gland forms migrates from its site of origin on the basal midline of the tongue to the level of the first tracheal cartilage, where the thyroid gland is located in postnatal life. As the thyroid tissue buds off from the tongue base, it leaves a vestigial depression on the dorsum of the tongue, the foramen cecum. The parathyroid glands are derived from the 4th pharyngeal pouch (superior pair) or the 3rd pharyngeal pouch (inferior pair), which also gives rise to the thymus. The ultimobranchial body, whose cells migrate into the thyroid gland to form the calcitonin-producing C cells, or parafollicular cells, is derived from the 5th pharyngeal pouch. The external auditory meatus is derived from the 1st pharyngeal cleft, the tympanic cavity and pharyngotympanic tube from the 1st pharyngeal pouch, and the palatine tonsil from the 2nd pharyngeal pouch.

Ectopic thyroid is a rare condition in which the entire thyroid gland or thyroid tissues are not found in their normal position in the neck, i.e., inferolateral to the thyroid cartilage. Dentists may encounter this as a firm midline mass, which may appear as light pink to bright red, and may be regular or irregular on the dorsal tongue, just posterior to the foramen cecum (the embryonic origin of the thyroid gland). This is known as a lingual thyroid and represents approximately 90% of ectopic thyroid cases. Symptoms of lingual thyroid may include cough, pain, difficulty swallowing (dysphagia), difficulty speaking (dysphonia), and difficulty breathing (dyspnea).

Fig. 1.16 **Location of cysts and fistulas in the neck**
A Median cysts. **B** Median fistulas. **C** Lateral fistulas and cysts.

A, B Median cysts and fistulas in the neck are remnants of the thyroglossal duct. Failure of this duct to regress completely may lead to the formation of a mucus-filled cavity (cyst), which presents clinically as a palpable, fluctuant, midline swelling in the neck at around the level of the hyoid bone. It is seen to move upward on swallowing or protrusion of the tongue due to the connection of the tongue with the duct. Symptoms may include dyspnea (difficulty breathing), dysphagia (difficulty swallowing), and pain (only if the cyst becomes infected).

C Lateral cysts and fistulas in the neck are anomalous remnants of the ductal portions of the cervical sinus, which forms as a result of tissue migrations during embryonic development.

If epithelium-lined remnants persist, neck cysts (right) or fistulas (an abnormal communication between structures; left) may appear in postnatal life. A complete fistula opens into the pharynx and onto the surface of the skin, whereas an incomplete (blind) fistula is open at one end only. The external orifice of a lateral cervical fistula is typically located at the anterior border of the sternocleidomastoid muscle.

Development of the Face

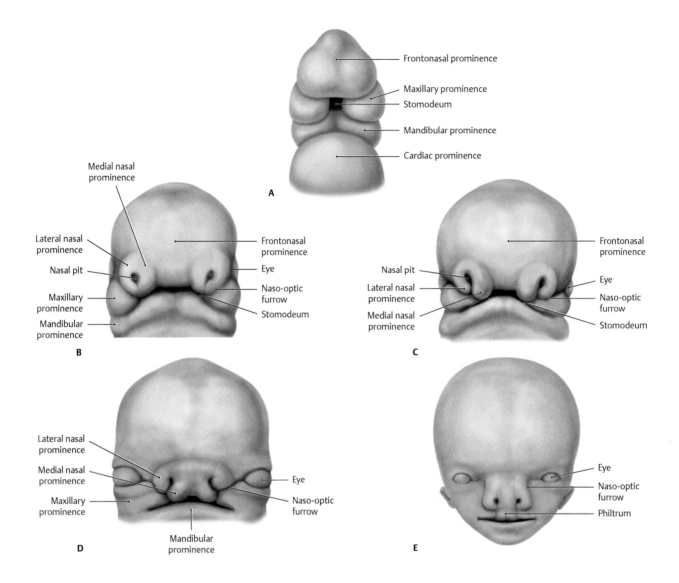

Fig. 1.17 Development of the face (after Sadler)
A Anterior view at 24 days. The surface ectoderm of the 1st pharyngeal arch invaginates to form the *stomodeum*, which is a depression between the forebrain and the pericardium in the embryo. It is the precursor of the mouth, oral cavity, and the anterior pituitary gland. At this stage, the stomodeum is separated from the primitive pharynx by the buccopharyngeal (oropharyngeal) membrane. This membrane later breaks down and the stomodeum become continuous with the pharynx.

The stomodeum is surrounded by five neural-crest-cell–derived mesenchymal swellings, known as *prominences*, which contribute to the development of the face.
B Anterior view at 5 weeks. Nasal placodes, ectodermal thickenings, form on each side of the frontonasal prominence. Invagination of the nasal placodes into the frontonasal prominence leads to the formation of the lateral and medial nasal prominences. The placodes now lie in the floor of a depression known as the *nasal pit*. The maxillary prominences continue to increase in size and merge laterally with the mandibular prominences to form the cheek. Medially, the maxillary prominences compress the medial nasal prominences toward the midline. A furrow (the naso-optic furrow) separates the nasal processes from the maxillary process. Ectoderm from the floor of the nasolacrimal groove (naso-optic furrow) will give rise to the nasolacrimal duct that connects the orbit with the nasal cavity; the two prominences will join to close the groove and create the nasolacrimal canal.

C Anterior view at 6 weeks. The medial nasal swellings enlarge, grow medially, and merge with each other to form the intermaxillary segment.
D Anterior view at 7 weeks. The medial nasal processes have fused with each other along the midline and with the maxillary processes and their lateral margins.
E Anterior view at 10 weeks. Cell migration is complete.

Table 1.9 Prominences contributing to facial structures	
Prominence	**Facial structure**
Frontonasal prominence*	Forehead, nose, medial and lateral nasal prominences
Maxillary prominences	Cheeks, lateral parts of the upper lip
Medial nasal prominences	Philtrum of the upper lip, crest and tip of nose
Lateral nasal prominences	Alae of nose
Mandibular prominences	Lower lip

*The frontonasal prominence is a single unpaired structure; all other prominences listed are paired.

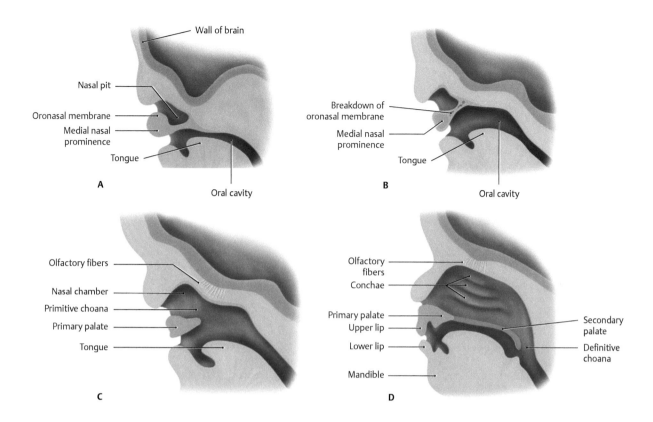

Fig. 1.18 Development of the nasal cavity
Sagittal section of embryo. At week 6, the primitive nasal cavity is separated from the oral cavity by the oronasal membrane **(A)**, which then breaks down **(B)**, leaving the nasal and oral cavities in open connection by week 7 **(C)**. In week 9, the nasal cavity and oral cavity are in their definitive arrangement **(D)**, separated by the primary and secondary palate with choanae at their junction in the pharynx. The lateral walls of the nasal cavity develop the superior, middle, and inferior conchae. The ectodermal epithelium in the roof of the nasal cavity becomes the specialized olfactory epithelium. The olfactory cells within the olfactory epithelium give rise to the olfactory nerve fibers (CN I) that grow into the olfactory bulb. The nasal septum (not shown) develops as a downgrowth of the merged medial nasal prominences. It fuses with the palatine process by weeks 9 to 12.

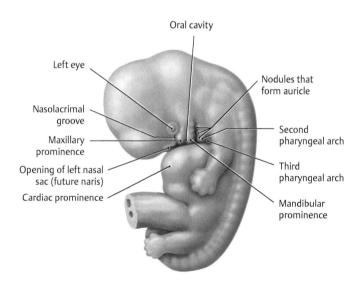

Fig. 1.19 Development of the eyes and ears
At about 22 days, the eyes and ears begin to develop. The eyes develop laterally in the embryo but during growth move medially to occupy their familiar position on the face. The auricle of the ear is formed from six swellings, known as *auricular hillocks*, from the first and second pharyngeal pouches. The germ layers that contribute to the eyes and ears are listed in **Table 1.10**.

Table 1.10 Derivation of the structures of the eye and ear		
Germ layer	**Structure**	
Eye		
Surface ectoderm	Corneal and conjunctival epithelium, lens, lacrimal glands, tarsal glands	
Neural crest cell ectoderm (neuroectoderm)	Retina, optic nerve (CN II), iris	
Mesenchyme	Corneal stroma, sclera, choroid, iris, parts of vitrous, ciliary muscle, muscles lining the anterior chamber	
Ear		
Ectoderm	Otic placode	Vestibulocochlear organ
	1st pharyngeal cleft	External acoustic meatus
Mesoderm	Cartilaginous otic capsule	Bony labryrinth
	Auricular hillocks	Auricle
Endoderm	1st pharyngeal pouch	Middle ear and auditory tube

Development of the Palate

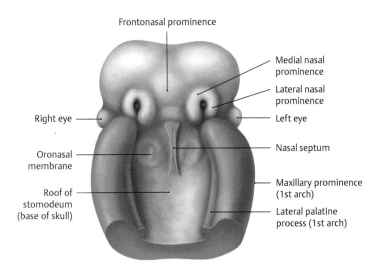

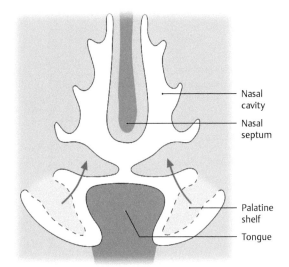

Fig. 1.20 Palate formation, 7- to 8-week-old embryo
Inferior view. Before the palate has formed, the oral cavity is open to the nasal cavity. The nasal septum can be seen as well as the oronasal membrane, which will ultimately form the choana. Development of the palate begins during week 5, but fusion of its parts is not complete until week 12. The most critical period for palate development is between the end of week 6 and the beginning of week 9. The palate forms from two major parts, the primary and secondary palates. The primary palate is derived from the wedge-shaped intermaxillary segment, which is formed by the merging of the two medial nasal prominences. The secondary palate is derived from two shelf-like outgrowths of the maxillary prominence, which, at this stage, are directed downward beside the tongue (removed).

Fig. 1.21 Elevation of the palatine shelves
The palatine shelves, which form the secondary palate, are seen at around 6 weeks and are directed obliquely downward on each side of the tongue. At around 7 weeks, the palatine shelves ascend to a horizontal position above the tongue and fuse.

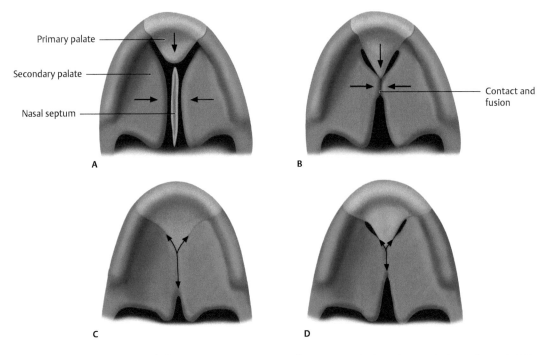

Fig. 1.22 Fusion and merging of the palatine shelves
Fusion of the palate begins at around 9 weeks and is completed posteriorly by week 12. **(A)** The primary palate and both halves of the secondary palate migrate toward each other as indicated by the arrows. **(B)** They contact and fuse at a point (marked by the incisive foramen) and merge anteriorly and posteriorly, as shown in **(C)** and **(D)**. The primary and secondary palates ossify, forming the hard palate. The posterior portions of the palatine shelves do not become ossified but extend beyond the nasal septum to form the soft palate and uvula.

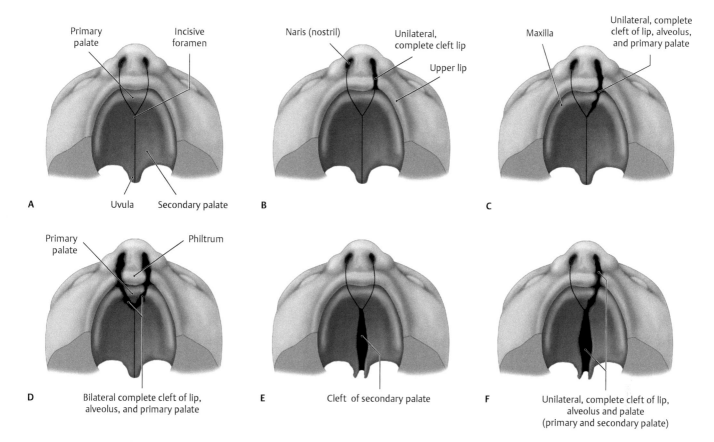

A Primary palate — Incisive foramen — Uvula — Secondary palate

B Naris (nostril) — Unilateral, complete cleft lip — Upper lip

C Maxilla — Unilateral, complete cleft of lip, alveolus, and primary palate

D Primary palate — Philtrum — Bilateral complete cleft of lip, alveolus, and primary palate

E Cleft of secondary palate

F Unilateral, complete cleft of lip, alveolus and palate (primary and secondary palate)

***Fig. 1.23* Formation of facial clefts** (after Sadler)
Inferior view.
Clefts (fissures or openings) can involve the lips and/or the palate. Clefts are classified as isolated (cleft lip or cleft palate), unilateral or bilateral, and as complete (when they extend to the nose) or incomplete (if they do not extend to the nose).
A Normal lips and palate, in which the maxillary prominences and medial nasal prominences have merged to form the upper lip and primary palate. The primary palate has also fused with the palatine processes of the maxillary prominences (secondary palate) to form the complete, unified, hard palate. The posterior portion of the secondary palate is unossified and forms the soft palate and uvula.
B Unilateral, complete cleft lip results from failure of fusion of the maxillary prominence with the medial nasal prominence on the affected side.
C Unilateral, complete cleft lip, alveolus, and primary palate (part of palate anterior to the incisive foramen) results from failure of fusion of the maxillary prominence with the medial nasal prominence on the affected side.
D Bilateral, complete cleft lip, alveolus, and primary palate result from failure of the maxillary prominences to fuse with the medial nasal prominences on both sides.
E Cleft of secondary palate (part of palate posterior to the incisive foramen) results from incomplete fusion of the two lateral palatine processes.
F Unilateral, complete cleft lip and complete cleft palate (involving both primary and secondary palate) result from failure of fusion of the maxillary prominence with the medial nasal prominence and failure of fusion of the two lateral palatine processes on the affected side.
Cleft lip and palate can cause difficulty in eating and speaking, and result in failure to thrive in infants. Treatment by a multidisciplinary team of healthcare professionals principally involves corrective surgery, which is usually performed between 6 and 12 months of age, often followed by surgical revisions, speech therapy, and orthodontic therapy.

Development of the Cranial Bones

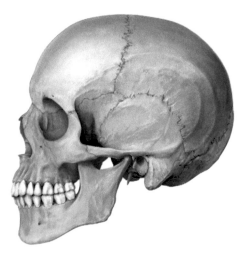

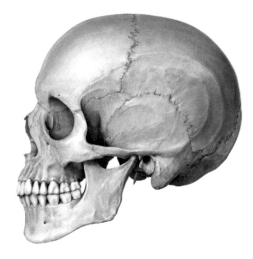

Fig. 2.1 Bones of the skull
Left lateral view. The skull forms a bony capsule that encloses the brain and viscera of the head. The bones of the skull are divided into two parts. The viscerocranium (orange), the facial skeleton, is formed primarily from the pharyngeal (branchial) arches (see pp. 6 and 7). The neurocranium (gray), the cranial vault, is the bony capsule enclosing the brain. It is divided into two parts based on ossification (see **Fig. 2.2**). The *cartilaginous* neurocranium undergoes endochondral ossification to form the base of the skull. The *membranous* neurocranium undergoes intramembranous ossification.

Fig. 2.2 Ossification of the cranial bones
Left lateral view. The bones of the skull develop either directly or indirectly from mesenchymal connective tissue. The bones of the desmocranium (gray) develop directly via intramembranous ossification of mesenchymal connective tissue. The bones of the chondrocranium (blue) develop indirectly via endochondral ossification of hyaline cartilage. *Note:* The skull base is formed exclusively by the chondrocranium. Elements formed via intramembranous and endochondral ossification may fuse to form a single bone (e.g., the elements of the occipital, temporal, and sphenoid bones contributing to the skull base are cartilaginous, while the rest of the bone is membranous).

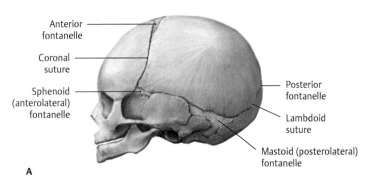

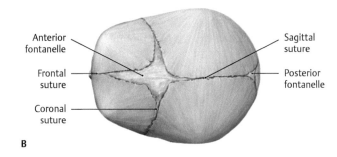

Fig. 2.3 Cranial sutures (craniosynostoses) and fontanelles
A Left lateral view of neonatal skull.
B Superior view of neonatal skull.
The flat cranial bones grow as the brain expands; thus the sutures between them remain open after birth. In the neonate, there are six areas (fontanelles) between the still-growing cranial bones that are occupied by unossified fibrous membrane. The posterior fontanelle provides a reference point for describing the position of the fetal head during childbirth. The anterior fontanelle provides access for drawing cerebrospinal fluid (CSF) samples in infants (e.g., in suspected meningitis).

Table 2.1 Closure of sutures and fontanelles			
Fontanelle	**Age at closure**	**Suture**	**Age at ossification**
1 Posterior fontanelle	2–3 months (lambda)	Frontal suture	Childhood
2 Sphenoid (anterolateral) fontanelles	6 months (pterion)	Sagittal suture	20–30 years old
2 Mastoid (posterolateral) fontanelles	18 months (asterion)	Coronal suture	30–40 years old
1 Anterior fontanelle	36 months (bregma)	Lambdoid suture	40–50 years old

Table 2.2 Development of the skull

Bone	Ossification	Arch	Embryological tissue
Viscerocranium			
Maxilla (premaxilla)	I	Frontonasal process	Neural crest
Nasal bone	I	Frontonasal process	Neural crest
Lacrimal bone	I	Frontonasal process	Neural crest
Vomer	I	Frontonasal process	Neural crest
Ethmoid (part)	E	Frontonasal process	Neural crest
Inferior nasal concha	E	Frontonasal process	Neural crest
Maxilla	I	1st arch	Neural crest
Zygomatic bone	I	1st arch	Neural crest
Mandible	I	1st arch	Neural crest
Palatine bone	I	1st arch	Neural crest
Temporal bone (tympanic ring)	I	1st arch	Neural crest
Sphenoid (pterygoid)	I	1st arch	Neural crest
Malleus	E	1st arch	Neural crest
Incus	E	1st arch	Neural crest
Hyoid (superior body, lesser horn)	E	2nd arch	Neural crest
Temporal (styloid)	E	2nd arch	Neural crest
Stapes	E	2nd arch	Neural crest
Hyoid (inferior body, greater horn)	E	3rd arch	Neural crest
Membranous neurocranium			
Greater wings of sphenoid (lateral)	I		Neural crest
Frontal	I		Neural crest
Squamous temporal	I		Neural crest
Parietal	I		Paraxial mesoderm
Supranuchal squamous occipital	I		Paraxial mesoderm
Cartilaginous neurocranium			
Ethmoid (part)	E		Neural crest
Sphenoid (lesser wing)	E		Neural crest
Sphenoid (body)	E		Paraxial mesoderm
Occipital (base)	E		Paraxial mesoderm
Temporal	E		Paraxial mesoderm
Sphenoid (greater wing, medial)	E		Neural crest
Infranuchal squamous occipital	E		Paraxial mesoderm

Abbreviations: I, intramembranous; E, endochondral.
Note: Tubular (long) bones undergo endochondral ossification. The clavicle is the only exception. Congenital defects of intramembranous ossification therefore affect both the skull and clavicle (cleidocranial dysostosis).

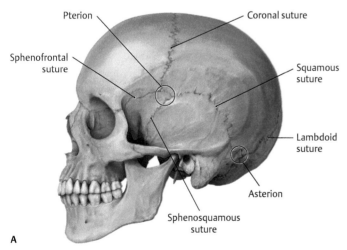

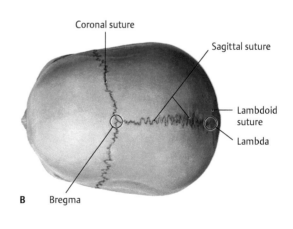

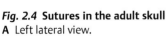

Fig. 2.4 Sutures in the adult skull
A Left lateral view.
B Superior view.
Synostosis (the fusion of the cranial bones along the sutures) occurs during adulthood. Although the exact times of closure vary, the order (sagittal, coronal, lambdoid) does not. Closure of each fontanelle yields a particular junction (see **Table 2.1**). Premature closure of the cranial sutures produces characteristic deformities (see **Fig. 2.11**, p. 22).

Skull: Lateral View

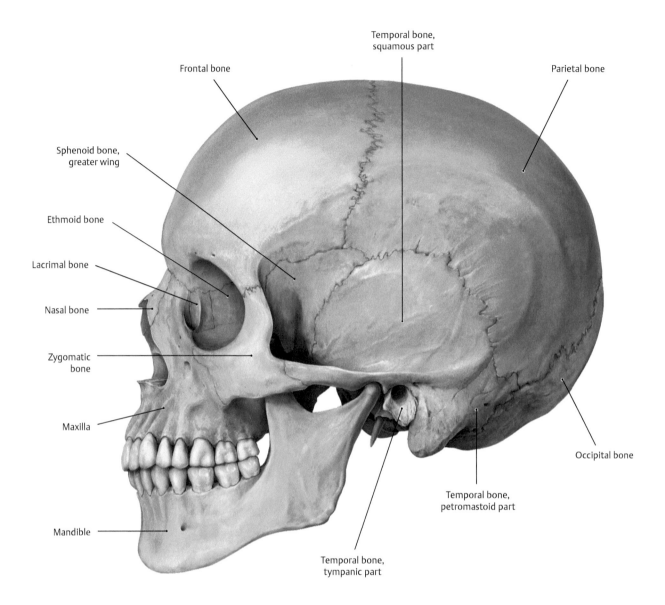

Temporal bone,
squamous part

Frontal bone

Parietal bone

Sphenoid bone,
greater wing

Ethmoid bone

Lacrimal bone

Nasal bone

Zygomatic
bone

Maxilla

Occipital bone

Mandible

Temporal bone,
petromastoid part

Temporal bone,
tympanic part

***Fig. 2.5* Cranial bones**
Left lateral view.

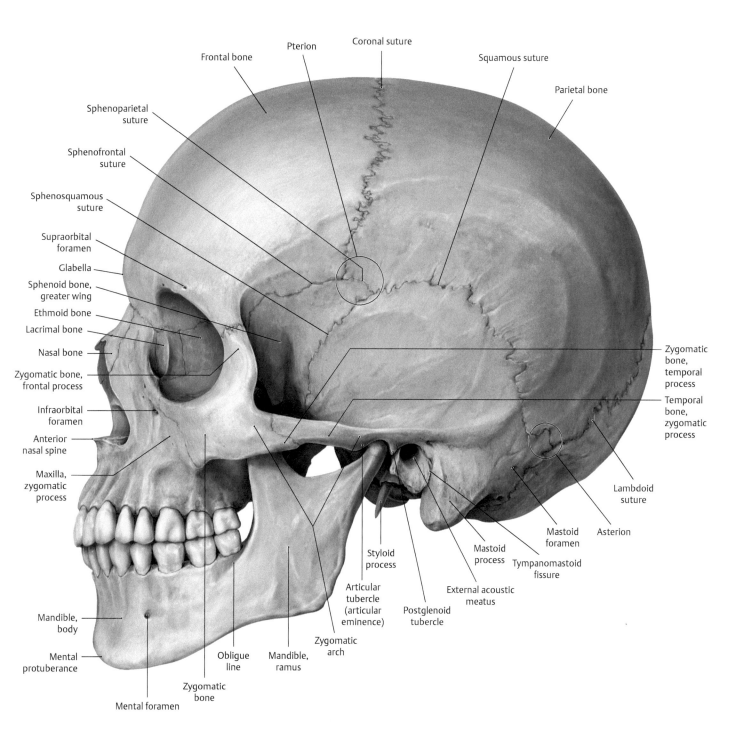

Fig. 2.6 Skull (cranium)
Left lateral view. This view displays the greatest number of cranial bones (indicated by different colors in **Fig. 2.5**). The zygomatic arch is formed by the zygomatic process of the temporal bone and the temporal process of the zygomatic bone, which are united by an oblique suture.

Skull: Anterior View

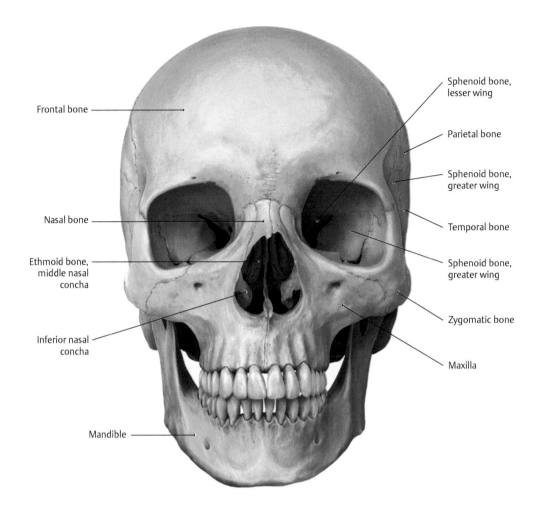

Frontal bone

Nasal bone

Ethmoid bone,
middle nasal
concha

Inferior nasal
concha

Mandible

Sphenoid bone,
lesser wing

Parietal bone

Sphenoid bone,
greater wing

Temporal bone

Sphenoid bone,
greater wing

Zygomatic bone

Maxilla

Fig. 2.7 Cranial bones.
Anterior view.

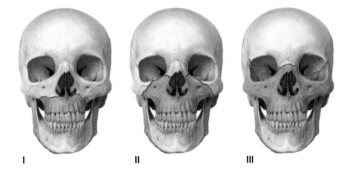

I   II   III

Fig. 2.8 Le Fort classification of midfacial fractures
The framelike construction of the facial skeleton leads to characteristic patterns of fracture lines in the midfacial region (Le Fort I, II, and III).
Le Fort I: This fracture line runs across the maxilla and above the hard palate. The maxilla is separated from the upper facial skeleton, disrupting the integrity of the maxillary sinus (*low transverse fracture*).
Le Fort II: The fracture line passes across the nasal root, ethmoid bone, maxilla, and zygomatic bone, creating a *pyramid fracture* that disrupts the integrity of the orbit.
Le Fort III: The facial skeleton is separated from the base of the skull. The main fracture line passes through the orbits, and the fracture may additionally involve the ethmoid bones, frontal sinuses, sphenoid sinuses, and zygomatic bones.

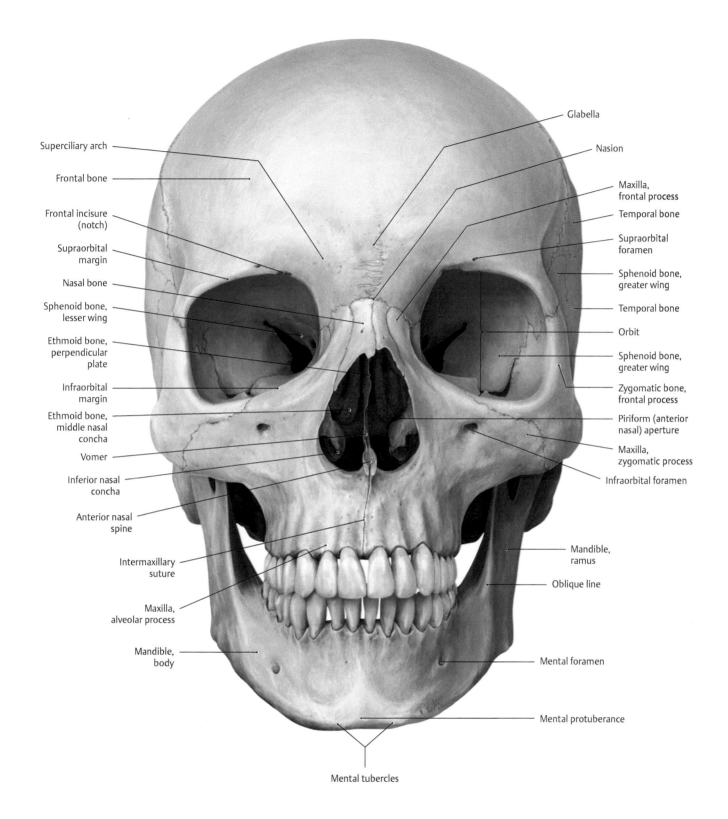

Fig. 2.9 Skull

Anterior view. The boundaries of the facial skeleton (viscerocranium) can be clearly appreciated in this view. The bony margins of the anterior nasal aperture mark the start of the respiratory tract in the skull. The nasal cavity, like the orbits, contains a sensory organ (the olfac-

tory mucosa). The *paranasal sinuses* are shown schematically in **Fig. 7.8**, p. 187. The anterior view of the skull also displays the three clinically important openings through which sensory nerves pass to supply the face: the supraorbital foramen, infraorbital foramen, and mental foramen.

Skull: Posterior View

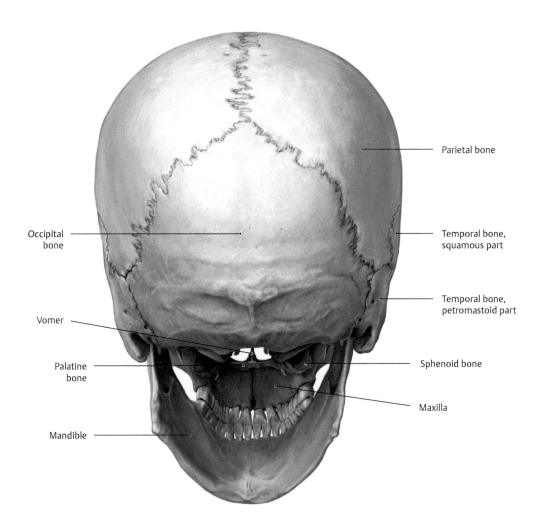

Parietal bone

Occipital bone

Temporal bone, squamous part

Temporal bone, petromastoid part

Vomer

Palatine bone

Sphenoid bone

Maxilla

Mandible

***Fig. 2.10* Cranial bones.**
Posterior view.

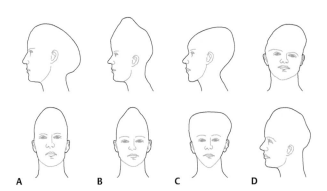

A   B   C   D

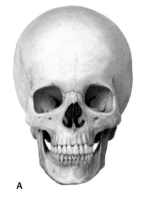

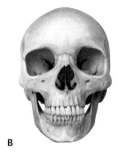

A   B

***Fig. 2.11* Premature closure of cranial sutures**
The premature closure of a cranial suture (craniosynostosis) may lead to characteristic cranial deformities:

A Sagittal suture: scaphocephaly (long, narrow skull).
B Coronal suture: oxycephaly (pointed skull).
C Frontal suture: trigonocephaly (triangular skull).
D Asymmetrical suture closure, usually involving the coronal suture: plagiocephaly (asymmetric skull).

***Fig. 2.12* Hydrocephalus and microcephaly**
A Hydrocephalus: When the ventricles become dilated due to cerebrospinal fluid (CSF) accumulation *before* the cranial sutures ossify, the neurocranium will expand, whereas the facial skeleton remains unchanged.
B Microcephaly: Premature closure of the cranial sutures or decreased growth of brain results in a small neurocranium with relatively large orbits.

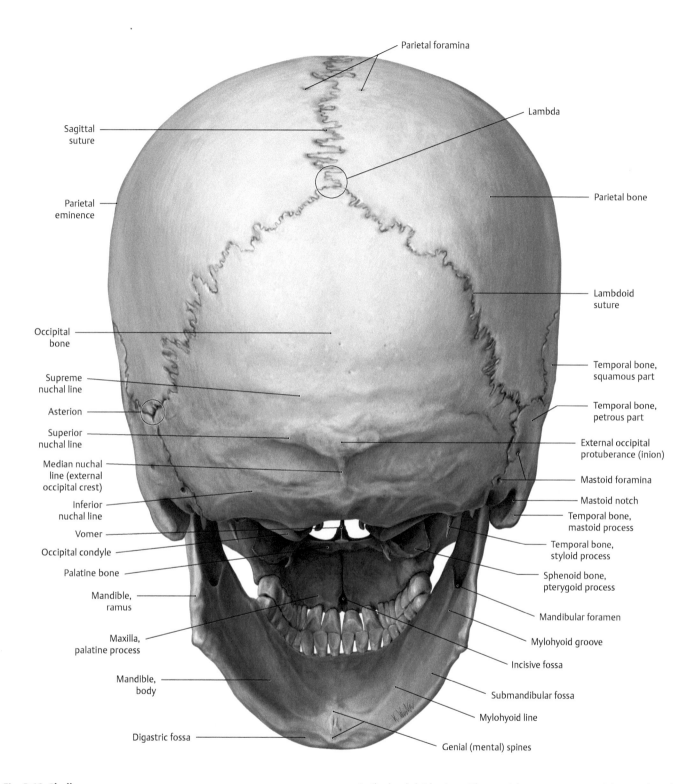

Parietal foramina

Lambda

Sagittal
suture

Parietal bone

Parietal
eminence

Lambdoid
suture

Occipital
bone

Temporal bone,
squamous part

Supreme
nuchal line

Asterion

Temporal bone,
petrous part

Superior
nuchal line

External occipital
protuberance (inion)

Median nuchal
line (external
occipital crest)

Mastoid foramina

Mastoid notch

Inferior
nuchal line

Temporal bone,
mastoid process

Vomer

Temporal bone,
styloid process

Occipital condyle

Sphenoid bone,
pterygoid process

Palatine bone

Mandible,
ramus

Mandibular foramen

Mylohyoid groove

Maxilla,
palatine process

Incisive fossa

Mandible,
body

Submandibular fossa

Mylohyoid line

Digastric fossa

Genial (mental) spines

Fig. 2.13 Skull

Posterior view. The occipital bone, which is dominant in this view, articulates with the parietal bones, to which it is connected by the lambdoid
suture. Wormian (sutural) bones are isolated bone plates often found
in the lambdoid suture. The cranial sutures are a special type of syndes-
mosis (i.e., ligamentous attachments that ossify with age). The outer
surface of the occipital bone is contoured by muscular origins and insertions: the inferior, superior, median, and supreme nuchal lines.

Calvaria

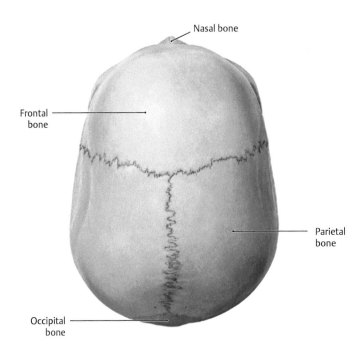

Fig. 2.14 Bones of the calvaria
External surface, superior view.

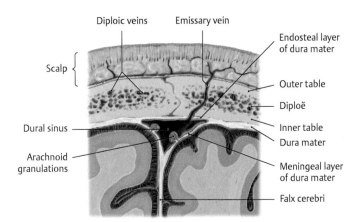

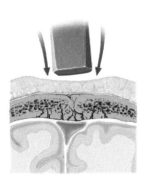

Fig. 2.15 The scalp and calvaria
The three-layered calvaria consists of the outer table, the diploë, and the inner table. The diploë has a spongy structure and contains red (blood-forming) bone marrow. With a plasmacytoma (malignant transformation of certain white blood cells), many small nests of tumor cells may destroy the surrounding bony trabeculae, and radiographs will demonstrate multiple lucent areas ("punched-out lesions") in the skull.

Fig. 2.16 Sensitivity of the inner table to trauma
The inner table of the calvaria is very sensitive to external trauma and may fracture even when the outer table remains intact.

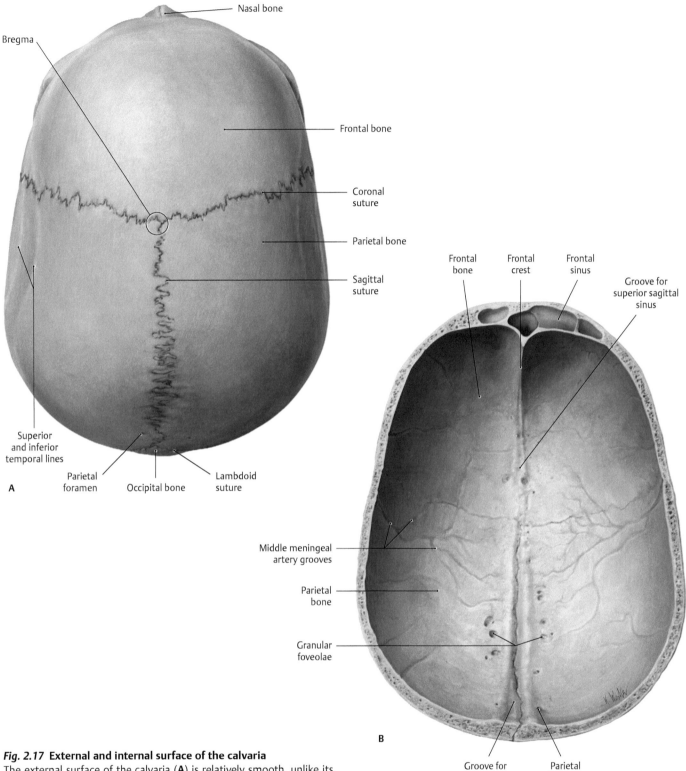

A

Bregma

Nasal bone

Frontal bone

Coronal suture

Parietal bone

Sagittal suture

Superior and inferior temporal lines

Parietal foramen

Occipital bone

Lambdoid suture

Frontal bone

Frontal crest

Frontal sinus

Groove for superior sagittal sinus

Middle meningeal artery grooves

Parietal bone

Granular foveolae

Groove for superior sagittal sinus

Parietal foramen

B

***Fig. 2.17* External and internal surface of the calvaria**

The external surface of the calvaria (**A**) is relatively smooth, unlike its internal surface (**B**). It is defined by the frontal, parietal, and occipital bones, which are interconnected by the coronal, sagittal, and lambdoid sutures. The smooth external surface is interrupted by the parietal foramina, which gives passage to the parietal emissary veins (see **Fig. 3.24**, p. 71). The internal surface of the calvaria bears a number of pits and grooves:

- Granular foveolae (small pits in the inner surface of the skull caused by saccular protrusions of the arachnoid membrane [arachnoid granulations] covering the brain)
- Groove for the superior sagittal sinus (a dural venous sinus of the brain, see **Fig. 3.22**, p. 70)

- Arterial grooves (which mark the positions of the arterial vessels of the dura mater, such as the middle meningeal artery, which supplies most of the dura mater and overlying bone)
- Frontal crest (which gives attachment to the falx cerebri, a sickle-shaped fold of dura mater between the cerebral hemispheres).

25

Skull Base: Exterior

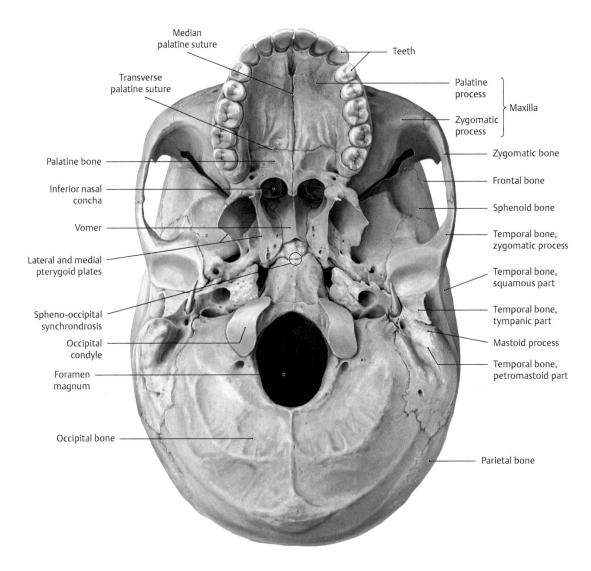

Fig. 2.18 Bones of the skull base
External surface, inferior view. The base of the skull is composed of a mosaic-like assembly of various bones.

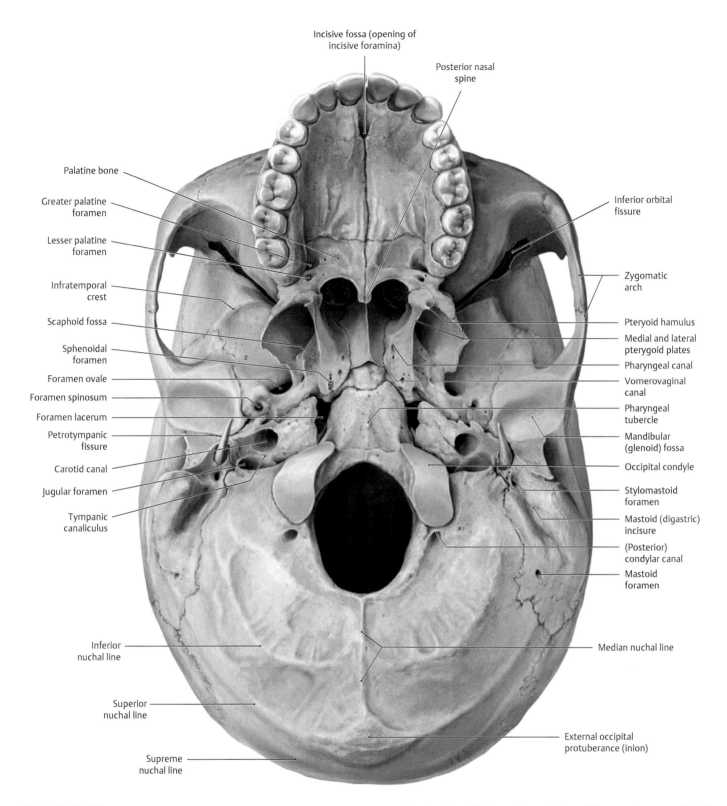

Incisive fossa (opening of incisive foramina)

Posterior nasal spine

Palatine bone

Greater palatine foramen

Lesser palatine foramen

Infratemporal crest

Scaphoid fossa

Sphenoidal foramen

Foramen ovale

Foramen spinosum

Foramen lacerum

Petrotympanic fissure

Carotid canal

Jugular foramen

Tympanic canaliculus

Inferior nuchal line

Superior nuchal line

Supreme nuchal line

Inferior orbital fissure

Zygomatic arch

Pteryoid hamulus

Medial and lateral pterygoid plates

Pharyngeal canal

Vomerovaginal canal

Pharyngeal tubercle

Mandibular (glenoid) fossa

Occipital condyle

Stylomastoid foramen

Mastoid (digastric) incisure

(Posterior) condylar canal

Mastoid foramen

Median nuchal line

External occipital protuberance (inion)

Fig. 2.19 Skull base

External surface, inferior view. Note the openings that transmit nerves and vessels. With abnormalities of bone growth, these openings may remain too small or may become narrowed, compressing the neuro-vascular structures that pass through them. The symptoms associated with these lesions depend on the affected opening. All of the structures depicted here will be considered in more detail in subsequent pages.

Skull Base: Interior

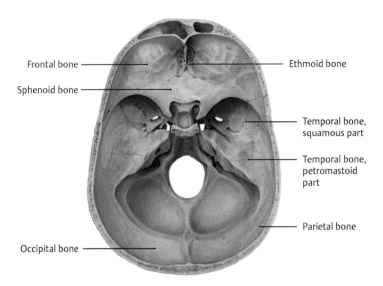

Fig. 2.20 Bones of the skull base
Internal surface, superior view.

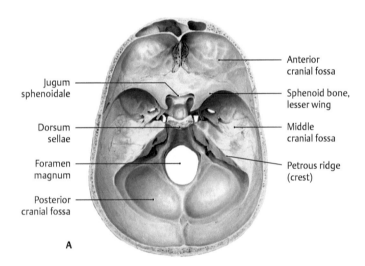

A

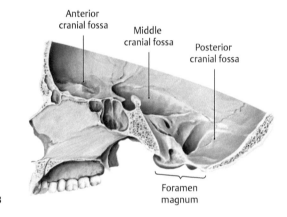

B

Fig. 2.21 The cranial fossae
A Skull base, internal surface, superior view. **B** Skull base, midsagittal section. The interior of the skull base is deepened to form three successive fossae: the anterior, middle, and posterior cranial fossae. These depressions become progressively deeper in the frontal-to-occipital direction, forming a terraced arrangement that is displayed most clearly in **B**.

The cranial fossae are bounded by the following structures:

- Anterior to middle: lesser wings of the sphenoid bone and the jugum sphenoidale
- Middle to posterior: superior border (ridge) of the petrous part of the temporal bone and the dorsum sellae

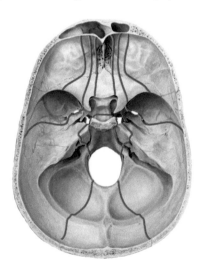

Fig. 2.22 Common fracture lines of skull base
Internal surface, superior view. In response to masticatory pressures and other mechanical stresses, the bones of the skull base are thickened to form "pillars" along the principal lines of force. The intervening areas that are not thickened are sites of predilection for bone fractures, resulting in the typical patterns of skull base fracture lines shown here in red. An analogous phenomenon of typical fracture lines is found in the midfacial region (see the anterior views of Le Fort fractures on p. 20).

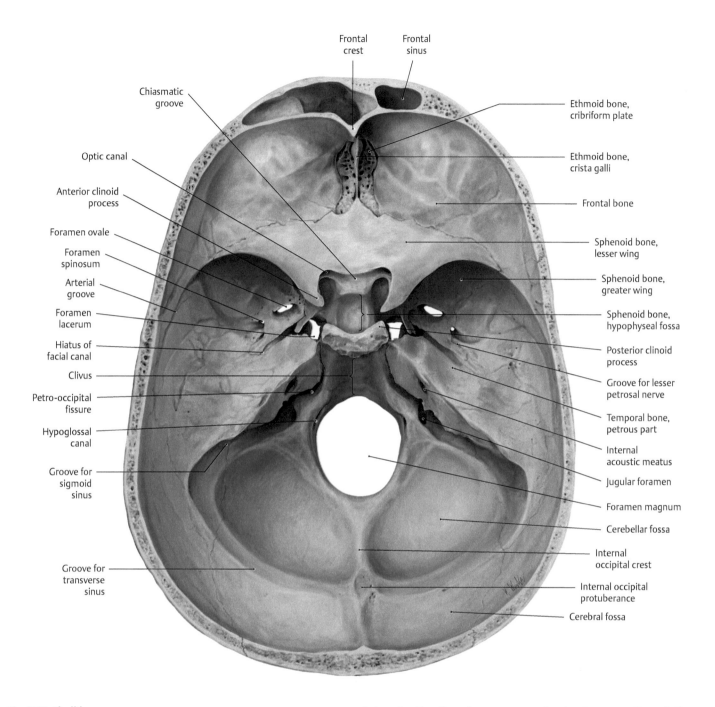

Fig. 2.23 Skull base

Internal surface, superior view. The openings in the interior of the base of the skull do not always coincide with the openings visible on the exterior because some neurovascular structures change direction when passing through the bone or pursue a relatively long intraosseous course. An example of this is the internal acoustic meatus, through which the facial nerve, among other structures, passes from the interior of the skull into the petrous part of the temporal bone. Most of its fibers then leave the petrous bone through the stylomastoid foramen, which is visible from the external aspect (see **Fig. 4.87**, p. 137, and **Fig. 2.45**, p. 44, for further details).

In learning the sites where neurovascular structures pass through the base of the skull, it is helpful initially to note whether these sites are located in the anterior, middle, or posterior cranial fossa. The arrangement of the cranial fossae is shown in **Fig. 2.21** (page 28).

The cribriform plate of the ethmoid bone connects the nasal cavity with the anterior cranial fossa and is perforated by numerous foramina for the passage of the olfactory fibers (see **Fig. 7.22**, p. 192). *Note:* Because the bone is so thin in this area, a frontal head injury may easily fracture the cribriform plate and lacerate the dura mater, allowing cerebrospinal fluid (CSF) to enter the nose. This poses a risk of meningitis, as bacteria from the nonsterile nasal cavity may enter the sterile CSF.

Sphenoid Bone

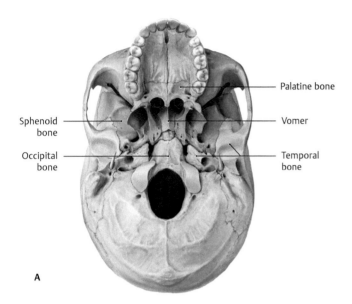

A

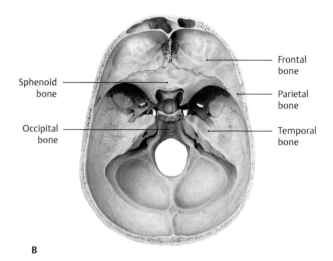

B

Fig. 2.24 Position of the sphenoid bone in the skull
The sphenoid bone is the most structurally complex bone in the human body. It must be viewed from various aspects in order to appreciate all its features (see also **Fig. 2.25**):

A **Skull base, exterior.** The sphenoid bone combines with the occipital bone to form the load-bearing midline structure of the skull base.
B **Skull base, interior.** The lesser wing of the sphenoid bone forms the boundary between the anterior and middle cranial fossae. The openings for the passage of nerves and vessels are clearly displayed (see details in **Fig. 2.45**).
C **Left lateral view.** Portions of the greater wing of the sphenoid bone can be seen above the zygomatic arch, and portions of the pterygoid process can be seen below the zygomatic arch.

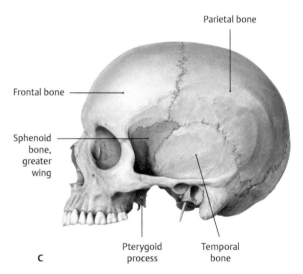

C

Fig. 2.25 Isolated sphenoid bone
A **Inferior view** (its position in situ is shown in **Fig. 2.24**). This view demonstrates the medial and lateral plates of the pterygoid process. Between them is the pterygoid fossa, which is occupied by the medial pterygoid muscle. The foramen spinosum and foramen ovale provide pathways through the base of the skull (see also in **C**).
B **Anterior view.** This view illustrates why the sphenoid bone was originally called the sphecoid bone ("wasp bone") before a transcription error turned it into the sphenoid ("wedge-shaped") bone. The apertures of the sphenoid sinus on each side resemble the eyes of the wasp, and the pterygoid processes of the sphenoid bone form its dangling legs, between which are the pterygoid fossae. This view also displays the superior orbital fissure, which connects the middle cranial fossa with the orbit on each side. The two sphenoid sinuses are separated by an internal septum (see **Fig. 7.11**, p. 187).

C **Superior view.** The superior view displays the sella turcica, whose central depression, the hypophyseal fossa, contains the pituitary gland. The foramen spinosum, foramen ovale, and foramen rotundum can be identified.
D **Posterior view.** The superior orbital fissure is seen clearly in this view, whereas the optic canal is almost completely obscured by the anterior clinoid process. The foramen rotundum is open from the middle cranial fossa to the pterygopalatine fossa of the skull (the foramen spinosum is not visible in this view; compare with **A**). Because the sphenoid and occipital bones fuse together during puberty ("tribasilar bone"), a suture is no longer present between the two bones. The cancellous trabeculae are exposed and have a porous appearance.

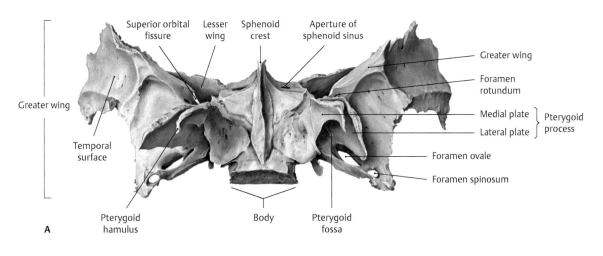

A

Greater wing

Superior orbital fissure
Lesser wing
Sphenoid crest
Aperture of sphenoid sinus
Greater wing
Foramen rotundum
Medial plate | Pterygoid process
Lateral plate
Foramen ovale
Foramen spinosum
Temporal surface
Pterygoid hamulus
Body
Pterygoid fossa

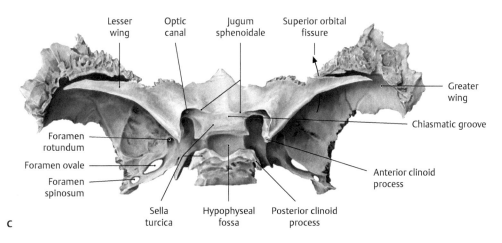

B

Greater wing

Lesser wing
Sphenoid crest
Aperture of sphenoid sinus
Orbital surface
Temporal surface
Superior orbital fissure
Foramen rotundum
Pterygoid canal
Medial plate | Pterygoid process
Lateral plate
Pterygoid fossa
Pterygoid hamulus

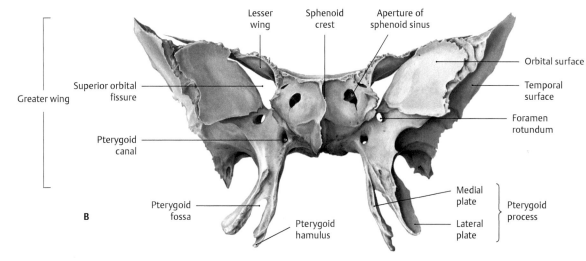

C

Lesser wing
Optic canal
Jugum sphenoidale
Superior orbital fissure
Greater wing
Chiasmatic groove
Foramen rotundum
Foramen ovale
Foramen spinosum
Anterior clinoid process
Sella turcica
Hypophyseal fossa
Posterior clinoid process

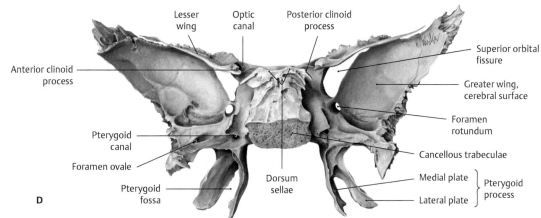

D

Lesser wing
Optic canal
Posterior clinoid process
Superior orbital fissure
Anterior clinoid process
Greater wing, cerebral surface
Foramen rotundum
Pterygoid canal
Cancellous trabeculae
Foramen ovale
Medial plate | Pterygoid process
Lateral plate
Pterygoid fossa
Dorsum sellae

Temporal Bone

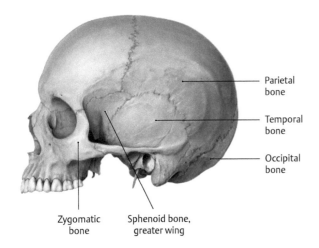

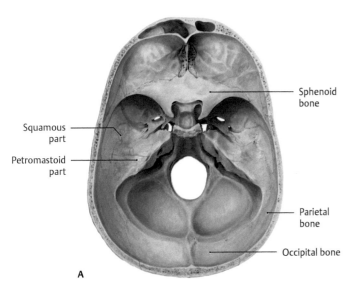

A

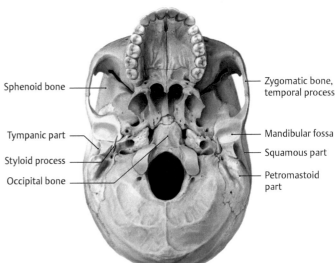

B

Fig. 2.26 Position of the temporal bone in the skull
Left lateral view. The temporal bone is a major component of the base of the skull. It forms the capsule for the auditory and vestibular apparatus and bears the articular fossa of the temporomandibular joint (TMJ).

Fig. 2.27 Temporal bone in the skull
A Internal view. **B** Inferior view.
The temporal bone, develops from four centers that fuse to form a single bone:

- The *squamous part* (light green) includes the articular fossa (mandibular [glenoid] fossa) of the temporomandibular joint (TMJ).

- The *petromastoid part* (pale green) contains the auditory and vestibular apparatus.
- The *tympanic part* (darker green) forms large portions of the external auditory canal.
- The *styloid process* develops from cartilage derived from the second pharyngeal arch and is a site of muscle attachment.

Fig. 2.28 Projection of clinically important structures onto the left temporal bone
The tympanic membrane is shown translucent in this lateral view. Because the petrous bone contains the middle and inner ear and the tympanic membrane, a knowledge of its anatomy is of key importance in otological surgery. The internal surface of the petrous bone has openings (see **Fig. 2.29**) for the passage of the facial nerve, internal carotid artery, and internal jugular vein. A fine nerve, the chorda tympani, passes through the tympanic cavity and lies medial to the tympanic membrane. The chorda tympani arises from the facial nerve, which is susceptible to injury during surgical procedures. The mastoid process of the petrous bone forms air-filled chambers, the mastoid cells, that vary greatly in size. Because these chambers communicate with the middle ear, which in turn communicates with the nasopharynx via the pharyngotympanic (auditory or Eustachian) tube, bacteria in the nasopharynx may pass up the pharyngotympanic tube and gain access to the middle ear. From there they may pass to the mastoid air cells and finally enter the cranial cavity, causing meningitis.

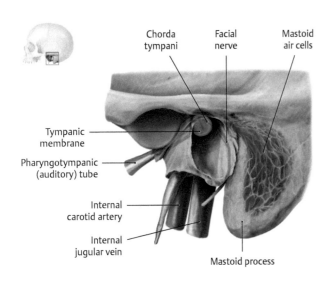

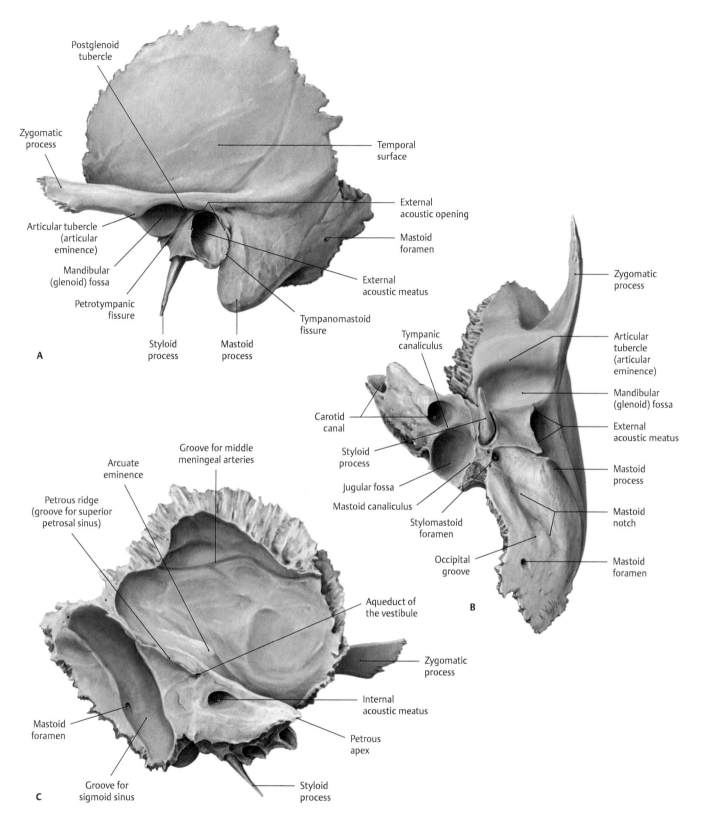

Fig. 2.29 Left temporal bone

A Lateral view. An emissary vein passes through the mastoid foramen (external orifice shown in **A**, internal orifice in **C**), and the chorda tympani passes through the medial part of the petrotympanic fissure. The mastoid process develops gradually in life due to traction from the sternocleidomastoid muscle and is pneumatized from the inside (see **Fig. 2.28**).

B Inferior view. The shallow articular fossa of the temporomandibular joint, the mandibular (glenoid) fossa, is clearly seen from the inferior view. The facial nerve emerges from the base of the skull through

the stylomastoid foramen. The initial part of the superior jugular bulb is adherent to the jugular fossa, and the internal carotid artery passes through the carotid canal to enter the skull.

C Medial view. This view displays the internal orifice of the mastoid foramen and the internal acoustic meatus. The facial nerve and vestibulocochlear nerve are among the structures that pass through the internal meatus to enter the petrous bone. The part of the petrous bone shown here is also called the *petrous pyramid*, whose apex (often called the "petrous apex") lies on the interior of the base of the skull.

33

Occipital Bone & Ethmoid Bone

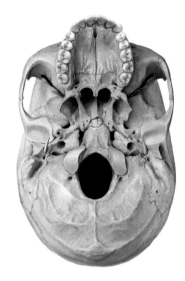

Fig. 2.30 Position of the occipital bone in the exterior skull base
Inferior view.

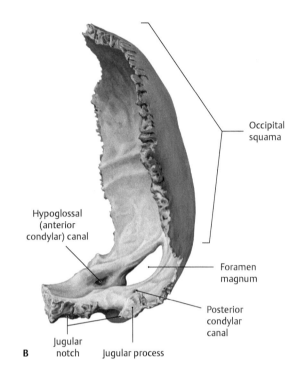

B Jugular notch   Jugular process

Labels: Occipital squama; Hypoglossal (anterior condylar) canal; Foramen magnum; Posterior condylar canal

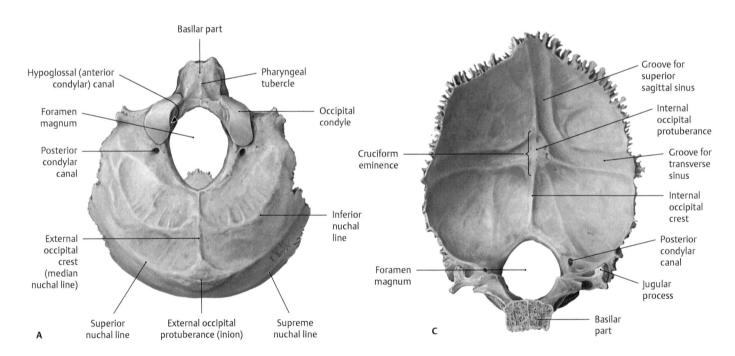

A labels: Basilar part; Hypoglossal (anterior condylar) canal; Pharyngeal tubercle; Foramen magnum; Occipital condyle; Posterior condylar canal; External occipital crest (median nuchal line); Inferior nuchal line; Superior nuchal line; External occipital protuberance (inion); Supreme nuchal line

C labels: Groove for superior sagittal sinus; Internal occipital protuberance; Cruciform eminence; Groove for transverse sinus; Internal occipital crest; Posterior condylar canal; Jugular process; Foramen magnum; Basilar part

Fig. 2.31 Isolated occipital bone

A Inferior view. This view shows the basilar part of the occipital bone, whose anterior portion is fused to the sphenoid bone. The condylar canal terminates posterior to the occipital condyles, and the hypoglossal canal passes superior and opens anterior to the occipital condyles. The condylar canal is a venous channel that begins in the sigmoid sinus and ends in the occipital vein. The hypoglossal canal contains a venous plexus in addition to the hypoglossal nerve (CN XII). The pharyngeal tubercle gives attachment to the pharyngeal raphe, and the external occipital protuberance provides a palpable bony landmark on the occiput.

B Left lateral view. The extent of the occipital squama, which lies above the foramen magnum, is clearly appreciated in this view. The internal openings of the condylar canal and hypoglossal canal are visible along with the jugular process, which forms part of the wall of the jugular foramen (see p. 27).

C Internal surface. The grooves for the dural venous sinuses of the brain can be identified in this view. The cruciform eminence overlies the confluence of the superior sagittal sinus and transverse sinuses. The configuration of the eminence shows that in some cases the sagittal sinus drains predominantly into the left transverse sinus.

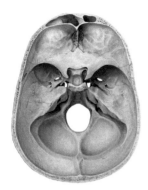 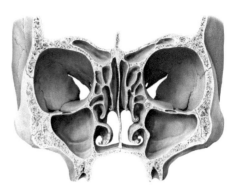

Fig. 2.32 Position of the ethmoid bone in the interior skull base
Superior view. The superior part of the ethmoid bone forms part of the anterior cranial fossa, and its inferior portions contribute structurally to the nasal cavities and orbit. The ethmoid bone is bordered by the frontal and sphenoid bones.

Fig. 2.33 Position of the ethmoid bone in the facial skeleton
Anterior view. The ethmoid bone is the central bone of the nose and paranasal sinuses. It also forms the medial wall of each orbit.

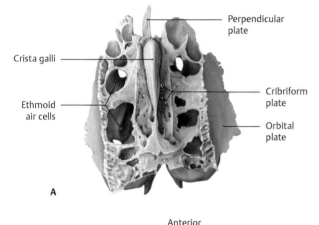

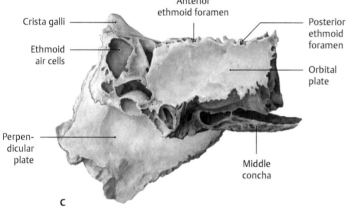 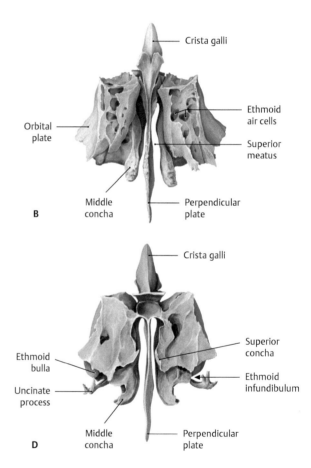

Fig. 2.34 Isolated ethmoid bone

A Superior view. This view demonstrates the crista galli, which gives attachment to the falx cerebri and the horizontally directed cribriform plate. The cribriform plate is perforated by foramina through which the olfactory fibers pass from the nasal cavity into the anterior cranial fossa (see **Fig. 7.22**, p. 192). With its numerous foramina, the cribriform plate is a mechanically weak structure that fractures easily in response to trauma. This type of fracture is manifested clinically by CSF leakage from the nose ("runny nose" in a patient with head injury).

B Anterior view. The anterior view displays the midline structure that separates the two nasal cavities: the perpendicular plate. Note also the middle nasal concha, which is part of the ethmoid bone (of the conchae, only the inferior nasal concha is a separate bone), and the ethmoid cells, which are clustered on both sides of the middle conchae.

C Left lateral view. Viewing the bone from the left side, we observe the perpendicular plate and the opened anterior ethmoid cells. The orbit is separated from the ethmoid cells by a thin sheet of bone called the orbital plate.

D Posterior view. This is the only view that displays the uncinate process, which is almost completely covered by the middle concha when in situ. It partially occludes the entrance to the maxillary sinus, the semilunar hiatus, and it is an important landmark during endoscopic surgery of the maxillary sinus. The narrow depression between the middle concha and uncinate process is called the ethmoid infundibulum. The frontal sinus, maxillary sinus, and anterior ethmoid air cells open into this "funnel." The superior concha is located at the posterior end of the ethmoid bone.

Zygomatic (Malar) Bone & Nasal Bone

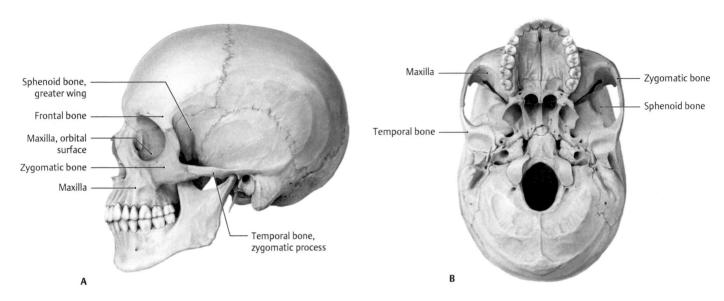

Fig. 2.35 Zygomatic bone in the skull
A Left lateral view. **B** Inferior view.
The zygomatic (malar) bone, or zygoma, is important in determining the width and morphology of the face and is a major buttress between the maxilla and the skull. In addition, it forms a significant portion of the floor and lateral walls of the orbit. The zygoma contains foramina that transmit the zygomaticofacial and zygomaticotemporal arteries and the corresponding nerves (from the maxillary nerve [CN V_2]) . Muscles that attach along the zygomatic arch include the masseter, zygomaticus major, and some fibers of the temporalis fascia. The Whitnall tubercle, which is the attachment site for the lateral canthal tendon, is located on the zygoma. This tendon is crucial in maintaining the contour of the eye.

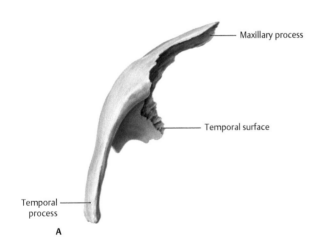

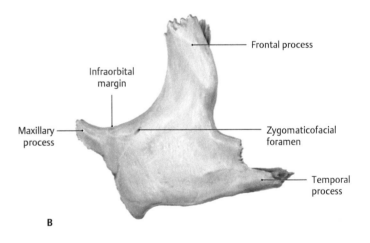

Fig. 2.36 Isolated zygomatic bone
A Inferior view. **B** Left lateral view.
The zygoma is a substantial bone but its prominent position on the face leaves it vulnerable to fracture following trauma. Trauma that transmits minimal force to the zygoma may cause a non-displaced fracture at the suture lines. Greater force, for example, following a motor vehicle accident, will result in displacement of the bone and involvement of the orbital rim and floor, the zygomaticofrontal suture, the zygomaticomaxillary buttress, and the zygomatic arch. Symptoms of zygoma fracture include pain, facial bruising and swelling, a flattened malar eminence, diplopia (double vision), trismus (lock jaw), and altered mastication (due to masseteric spasm or interference of the normal mechanism of the coronoid process by bony fragments), loss of sensation below the orbit (due to infraorbital nerve involvement), and ipsilateral epistaxis (nosebleed) (due to laceration of the mucosa of the maxillary sinus). Nondisplaced fractures do not require treatment. Displaced fractures commonly require open reduction and fixation, with reconstruction of the orbit. Displacement of the zygomatic arch may be reduced by the Gillies technique, in which an incision is made over the temporalis muscle and an instrument is slid under the arch and hooked and the arch is elevated into its normal position.

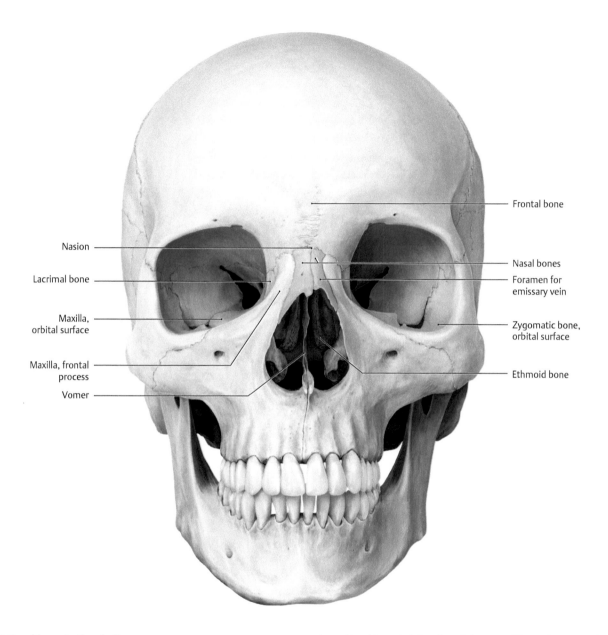

Nasion

Lacrimal bone

Maxilla, orbital surface

Maxilla, frontal process

Vomer

Frontal bone

Nasal bones

Foramen for emissary vein

Zygomatic bone, orbital surface

Ethmoid bone

***Fig. 2.37* Nasal bone in the skull**
Anterior view.
Fractures of the nasal bones are common following facial trauma, for example, motor vehicle accidents, sports injuries, or fights. This is due both to the prominence of the nose and the fragility of the nasal bones. Symptoms of nasal fractures include pain, bruising, swelling, epistaxis (nosebleeds), and deformity of the nose. The patient may also experience difficulty breathing. Minor nasal fractures require no treatment while those that cause deformity will require manual realignment. More severe nasal fractures, for example, those involving the nasal septum or other facial bones will require surgery.

Maxilla & Hard Palate

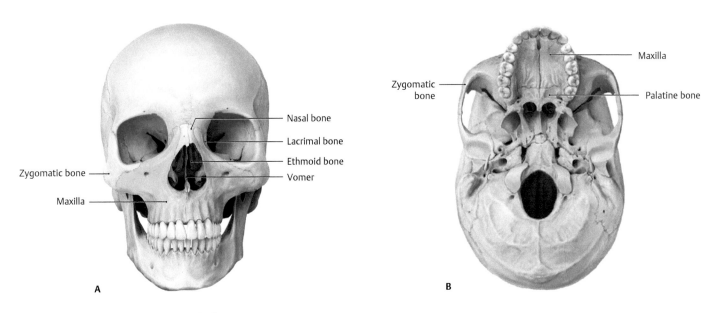

Fig. 2.38 Maxilla and hard palate in skull
A Anterior view. **B** Exterior of skull base, inferior view.

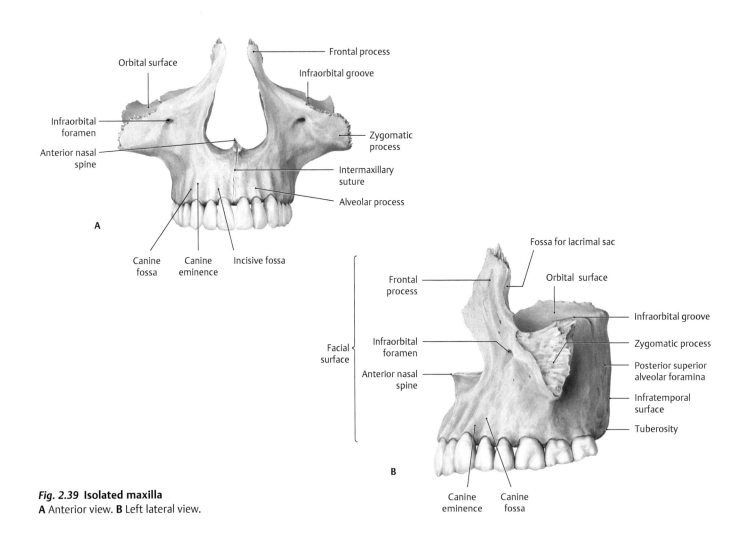

Fig. 2.39 Isolated maxilla
A Anterior view. **B** Left lateral view.

Fig. 2.40 Bones of the hard palate

A Superior view. The upper part of the maxilla is removed. The floor of the nasal cavity shown here and the roof of the oral cavity (B) are formed by the union of the palatine processes of the two maxillary bones with the horizontal plates of the two palatine bones. Cleft palate results from a failed fusion of the palatine processes at the median palatine suture (see p. 15).

B Inferior view. The nasal cavity communicates with the nasopharynx via the choanae, which begin at the posterior border of the hard palate. The two nasal cavities communicate with the oral cavity via the incisive canals (A), which combine and emerge at the incisive foramen.

C Oblique posterior view. This view illustrates the close anatomic relationship between the oral and nasal cavities. Note: The pyramidal process of the palatine bone is integrated into the lateral pterygoid plate of the sphenoid bone. The palatine margin of the vomer articulates with the hard palate along the nasal crest.

Tori are bony exostoses (lumps) that can be found on both jaws. Torus palatinus occurs in the center of the hard palate; torus mandibularis occurs in the lingual premolar or molar region of the mandible. Tori are completely benign but may cause problems for denture retention, in which case they can be surgically excised.

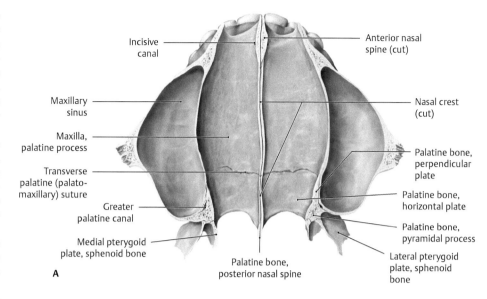

A

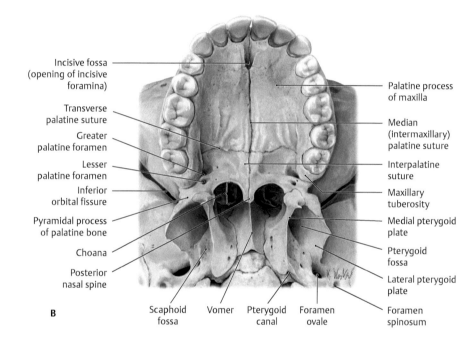

B

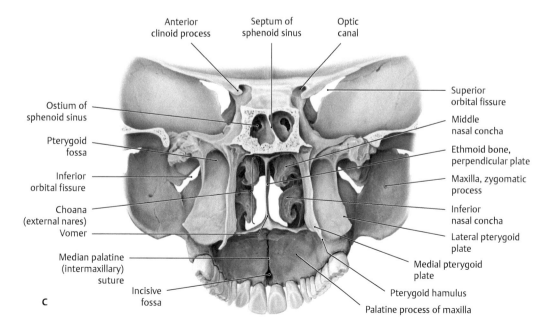

C

Mandible & Hyoid Bone

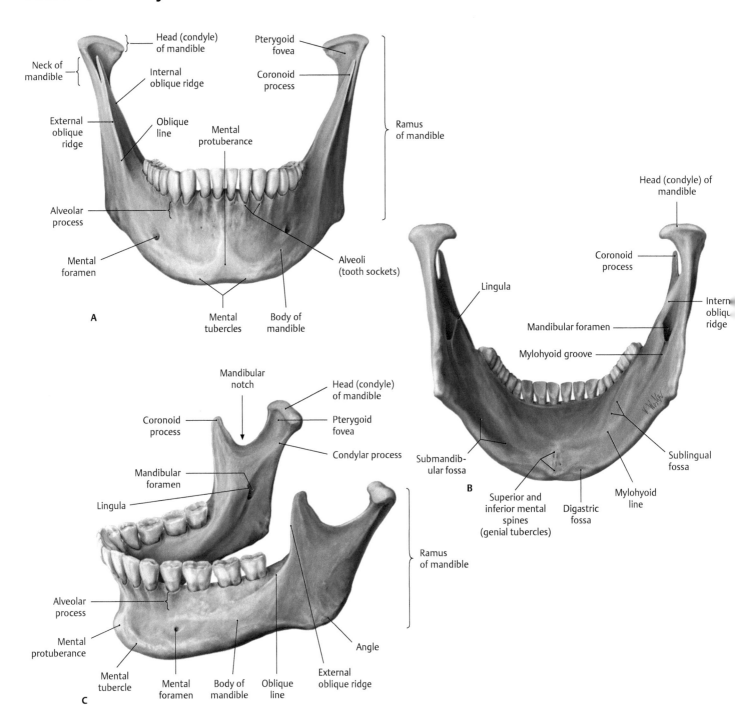

Fig. 2.41 Mandible

A Anterior view. The mandible is connected to the viscerocranium at the temporomandibular joint, whose convex surface is the head of the mandibular condyle. This "head of the mandible" is situated atop the vertical (ascending) ramus of the mandible, which joins with the body of the mandible at the mandibular angle. The teeth are set in the alveolar processes (alveolar part) along the upper border of the mandibular body. This part of the mandible is subject to typical age-related changes as a result of dental development (see **Fig. 2.43**). The mental branch of the trigeminal nerve exits through the mental foramen. The location of this foramen is important in clinical examinations, as the tenderness of the nerve to pressure can be tested at that location.

B Posterior view. The mandibular foramen is particularly well displayed in this view. It transmits the inferior alveolar nerve, which supplies sensory innervation to the mandibular teeth. Its terminal

branch emerges from the mental foramen. The mandibular foramen and the mental foramen are interconnected by the mandibular canal.

C Oblique left lateral view. This view displays the coronoid process, the condylar process, and the mandibular notch between them. The coronoid process is a site for muscular attachments, and the condylar process bears the head of the mandible, which articulates with the articular disk in the mandibular (glenoid) fossa of the temporal bone. A depression on the medial side of the condylar process, the pterygoid fovea, gives attachment to portions of the lateral pterygoid muscle.

D Superior view. This view displays the retromolar fossa, retromolar triangle, and buccal shelf. The retromolar fossa is the insertion point for some fibers of the temporalis muscle. Lower dentures should be designed to avoid this area so that they are not dislodged during mastication. The buccal shelf (as a primary bearer of stress) and the retromolar triangle are areas that are utilized to provide support for lower dentures.

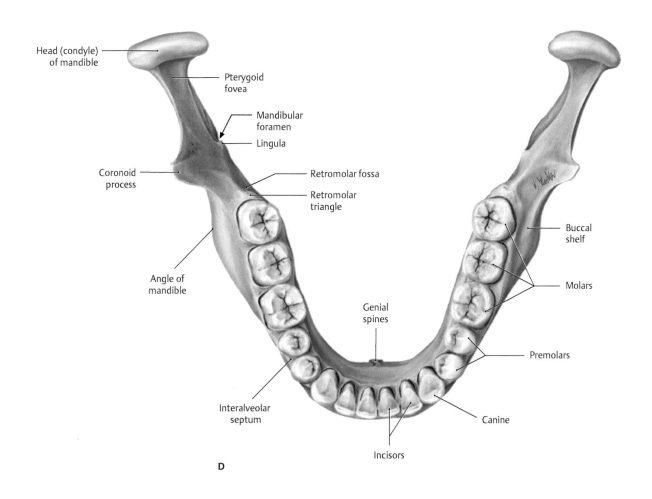

D

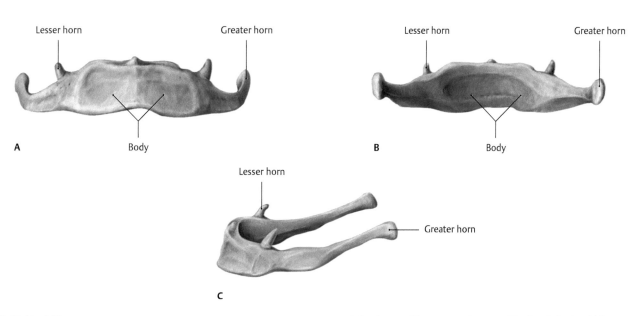

Fig. 2.42 Hyoid bone
A Anterior view. **B** Posterior view. **C** Oblique left lateral view. The hyoid bone is suspended by muscles and ligaments between the oral floor and the larynx. The greater horn and body of the hyoid bone are palpable in the neck. The physiological movement of the hyoid bone can be palpated during swallowing.

Mandible: Age-related Changes & Mandibular Fractures

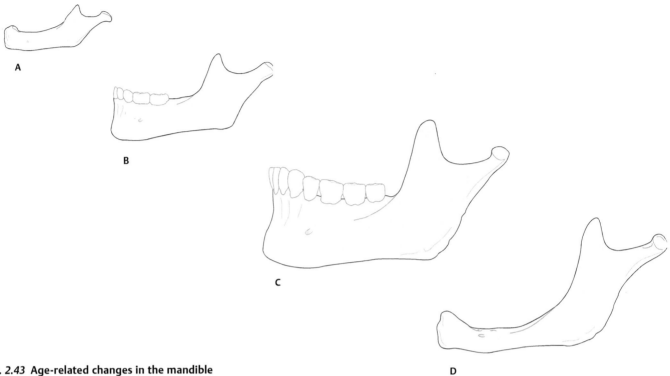

Fig. 2.43 Age-related changes in the mandible

The structure of the mandible is greatly influenced by the alveolar process the teeth. Because the angle of the mandible adapts to changes in the alveolar process, the angle between the body and ramus also varies with age-related changes in the dentition. The angle measures approximately 150 degrees at birth and approximately 120 to 130 degrees in adults, decreasing to 140 degrees in the edentulous mandible of old age.

A At birth the mandible is without teeth, and the alveolar process has not yet formed.

B In children the mandible bears the deciduous teeth. The alveolar process is still relatively poorly developed because the deciduous teeth are considerably smaller than the permanent teeth.

C In adults the mandible bears the permanent teeth, and the alveolar process is fully developed.

D In old age, the mandible can be edentulous (toothless), with accompanying resorption of the alveolar process.

Note: The resorption of the alveolar process with age leads to a change in the position of the mental foramen (which is normally located below the second premolar tooth, as in **C**). This change must be taken into account in surgery or dissections involving the mental nerve. The alveolar process is the portion of the maxilla and mandible that supports the roots of the teeth. It is composed of two parts, the alveolar bone proper and the supporting bone. The alveolar bone proper lines the tooth sockets (alveoli). Supporting bone consists of cortical plates of compact bone on the inner and outer surfaces of the maxilla and mandible and the intervening spongy bone between the cortical plates and alveolar bone proper. Alveolar bone is subject to resorption following tooth loss (a normal physiological process) and in certain disease states (e.g., abscess formation, cysts, osteoporosis). Basal bone is that portion of the maxilla and mandible deep to the alveolar bone. It is not subject to resorption.

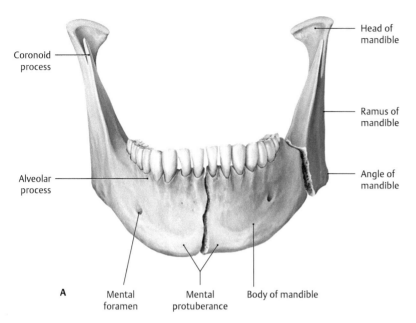

Coronoid process

Alveolar process

A

Mental foramen

Mental protuberance

Body of mandible

Head of mandible

Ramus of mandible

Angle of mandible

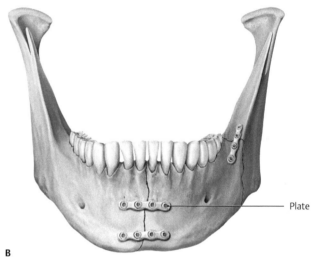

B

Plate

Fig. 2.44 Mandibular fracture

Anterior view. **A** Mandibular fracture. **B** Reduction and fixation of mandibular fracture. Mandibular fracture is a common injury, for example, following motor vehicle accidents, fights, or sporting accidents, due to the prominence of the mandible and its relative lack of support. Most fractures occur in the body (~30%), condyle (~25%), angle (~25%), and symphysis (~17%). To avoid misdiagnosis of the injury, the history should include not just information about the current injury but information about previous mandibular trauma or temporomandibular joint (TMJ) dysfunction. Determine the patency of the airway and the presence of other injuries (facial lacerations, swellings, or hematomas). Inspect intraoral tissuesa for bruising, which, if present, is suggestive of a fracture of the body or symphysis. Palpate the mandible from the symphysis to the angle, noting any swelling, tenderness, or step deformities. Next palpate the condyle through the external acoustic meatus; tenderness may indicate a fracture at this site. Note any deviation on opening the mouth. With condylar fractures, the mandible deviates toward the side of the fracture. Note also any obstruction to

mouth opening, e.g., trismus (lock jaw due to spasm of the muscles of mastication) or impaction of the coronoid process. Now evaluate the occlusion. If the teeth do not occlude as normal, this is highly suggestive of mandibular fracture, although this can also occur following tooth subluxation (loosening) or TMJ injury. Note any areas of altered sensation (paresthesia, dysesthesia, or anesthesia). The latter is suggestive of a fracture distal to the mandibular foramen. Following this, the mandible should be grasped at either side of the suspected fracture and gently manipulated to assess mobility. Confirm the diagnosis via either radiography or CT scans. Treat with antibiotics to prevent infection, followed by reduction (to the patient's normal occlusion) and surgical fixation of the fracture. The fixation method depends on many factors including the type and site of fracture and may involve the use of bars, wires, or plates for intermaxillary fixation.

The double mandibular fracture shown here is treated in a two-step process. First, the fracture at the midline is fixated with metal plates followed by the angle fracture. Note that two plates provide much more stability than a single plate.

Neurovascular Pathways through the Skull Base

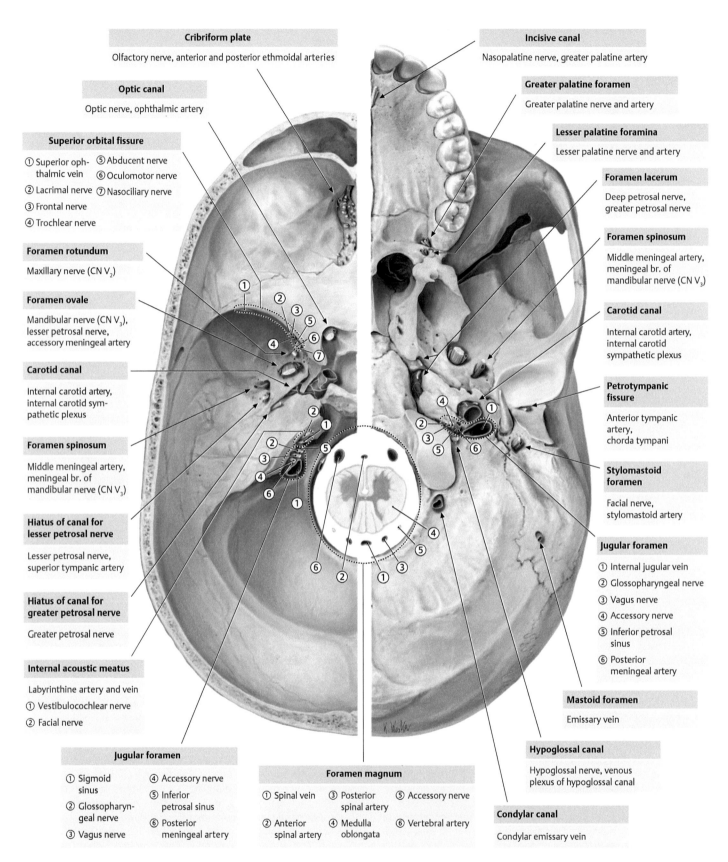

Cribriform plate

Olfactory nerve, anterior and posterior ethmoidal arteries

Optic canal

Optic nerve, ophthalmic artery

Superior orbital fissure

① Superior oph- ⑤ Abducent nerve
   thalmic vein   ⑥ Oculomotor nerve
② Lacrimal nerve ⑦ Nasociliary nerve
③ Frontal nerve
④ Trochlear nerve

Foramen rotundum

Maxillary nerve (CN V₂)

Foramen ovale

Mandibular nerve (CN V₃), lesser petrosal nerve, accessory meningeal artery

Carotid canal

Internal carotid artery, internal carotid sympathetic plexus

Foramen spinosum

Middle meningeal artery, meningeal br. of mandibular nerve (CN V₃)

Hiatus of canal for lesser petrosal nerve

Lesser petrosal nerve, superior tympanic artery

Hiatus of canal for greater petrosal nerve

Greater petrosal nerve

Internal acoustic meatus

Labyrinthine artery and vein
① Vestibulocochlear nerve
② Facial nerve

Jugular foramen

① Sigmoid sinus   ④ Accessory nerve
② Glossopharyngeal nerve ⑤ Inferior petrosal sinus
③ Vagus nerve   ⑥ Posterior meningeal artery

Foramen magnum

① Spinal vein   ③ Posterior spinal artery   ⑤ Accessory nerve
② Anterior spinal artery ④ Medulla oblongata   ⑥ Vertebral artery

Incisive canal

Nasopalatine nerve, greater palatine artery

Greater palatine foramen

Greater palatine nerve and artery

Lesser palatine foramina

Lesser palatine nerve and artery

Foramen lacerum

Deep petrosal nerve, greater petrosal nerve

Foramen spinosum

Middle meningeal artery, meningeal br. of mandibular nerve (CN V₃)

Carotid canal

Internal carotid artery, internal carotid sympathetic plexus

Petrotympanic fissure

Anterior tympanic artery, chorda tympani

Stylomastoid foramen

Facial nerve, stylomastoid artery

Jugular foramen

① Internal jugular vein
② Glossopharyngeal nerve
③ Vagus nerve
④ Accessory nerve
⑤ Inferior petrosal sinus
⑥ Posterior meningeal artery

Mastoid foramen

Emissary vein

Hypoglossal canal

Hypoglossal nerve, venous plexus of hypoglossal canal

Condylar canal

Condylar emissary vein

Fig. 2.45 Passage of neurovascular structures through the skull base
A Cranial cavity (interior of skull base), superior view.
B Exterior of skull base, inferior view.
This image and the corresponding table only address structures entering and exiting the skull. Many neurovascular structures pass through bony canals within the skull (to pterygopalatine fossa, infratemporal fossa, etc.).
Note: The deep petrosal nerve and greater petrosal nerve travel over the surface of foramen lacerum but not through it.

Table 2.3 Openings in the skull base

Cranial cavity	Opening	Transmitted structures	
		Nerves	**Arteries and veins**
Internal view, base of the skull			
Anterior cranial fossa	Cribriform plate	• CN I (olfactory fibers collected to form olfactory n.)	• Anterior and posterior ethmoidal aa. (from ophthalmic a.) • Ethmoidal vv. (to superior ophthalmic v.)
Middle cranial fossa	Optic canal	• CN II (optic n.)	• Ophthalmic a. (from internal carotid a.)
	Superior orbital fissure	• CN III (oculomotor n.) • CN IV (trochlear n.) • CN VI (abducent n.) • CN V_1 (ophthalmic n.) divisions (lacrimal, frontal, and nasociliary nn.)	• Superior and inferior ophthalmic vv. (to cavernous sinus) (*Note:* The inferior ophthalmic v. also drains through the inferior orbital fissure to the pterygoid plexus.)
	Foramen rotundum*	• CN V_2 (maxillary n.)	
	Foramen ovale	• CN V_3 (mandibular n.) • Lesser petrosal n. (CN IX)	• Accessory meningeal a. (from mandibular part of maxillary a.)
	Foramen spinosum	• CN V_3, recurrent meningeal branch	• Middle meningeal a. (from mandibular part of maxillary a.)
	Carotid canal	• Carotid plexus (postganglionic sympathetics from superior cervical ganglion)	• Internal carotid a.
	Hiatus of canal for greater petrosal n.	• Greater petrosal n. (CN VII)	• Superficial petrosal a. (from middle meningeal a.)
	Hiatus of canal for lesser petrosal n.	• Lesser petrosal n. (CN IX)	• Superior tympanic a. (from middle meningeal a.)
Posterior cranial fossa	Internal acoustic meatus	• CN VII (facial n.) • CN VIII (vestibulocochlear n.)	• Labyrinthine a. (from vertebral a.) • Labyrinthine vv. (to superior petrosal or transverse sinus)
	Jugular foramen	• CN IX (glossopharyngeal n.) • CN X (vagus n.) • CN XI (accessory n., cranial root)	• Internal jugular v. (bulb) • Sigmoid sinus (to bulb of internal jugular v.) • Posterior meningeal a. (from ascending pharyngeal a.) • Inferior petrosal sinus
	Hypoglossal canal	• CN XII (hypoglossal n.)	• Venous plexus of hypoglossal canal
	Foramen magnum	• Medulla oblongata with meningeal coverings • CN XI (accessory n.)	• Vertebral aa. • Anterior and posterior spinal aa. (from vertebral a.) • Emissary vv.
External aspect, base of the skull (where different from internal aspect)			
	Incisive canal	• Nasopalatine n. (from CN V_2)	• Branch of greater palatine a.
	Greater palatine foramen	• Greater palatine n. (from CN V_2)	• Greater palatine a. (from pterygopalatine part of maxillary a. or descending palatine a.)
	Lesser palatine foramen	• Lesser palatine n. (from CN V_2)	• Lesser palatine aa. (from pterygopalatine part of maxillary a. or as branch of greater palatine a. or descending palatine a.)
	Foramen lacerum**	• Deep petrosal n. (from superior cervical ganglion via carotid plexus) • Greater petrosal n. (from CN VII)	
	Petrotympanic fissure	• Chorda tympani (from CN VII)	• Anterior tympanic a. (from mandibular part of maxillary a.)
	Stylomastoid foramen	• Facial n. (CN VII)	• Stylomastoid a. (from posterior auricular a.)
	(Posterior) condylar canal		• Condylar emissary v. (to sigmoid sinus)
	Mastoid foramen		• Mastoid emissary v. (to sigmoid sinus)

*The external opening of the foramen rotundum is located in the pterygopalatine fossa, which is located deep on the lateral surface of the base of the skull and is not visible here.

**Structures travel over the superior surface of the foramen lacerum, not through it, from external to internal (with the exception of lymphatic vessels and emissary veins).

Muscles of the Head: Origins & Insertions

The bony origins and insertions of the muscles are indicated by color shading: origins (red) and insertions (blue).

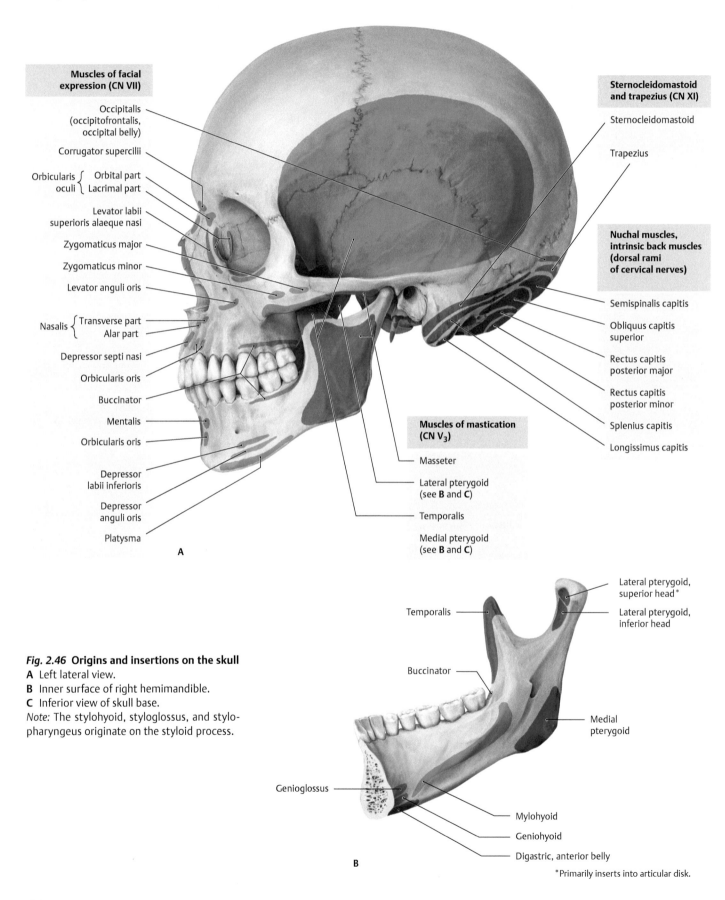

Muscles of facial expression (CN VII)

Occipitalis (occipitofrontalis, occipital belly)

Corrugator supercilii

Orbicularis oculi { Orbital part / Lacrimal part

Levator labii superioris alaeque nasi

Zygomaticus major

Zygomaticus minor

Levator anguli oris

Nasalis { Transverse part / Alar part

Depressor septi nasi

Orbicularis oris

Buccinator

Mentalis

Orbicularis oris

Depressor labii inferioris

Depressor anguli oris

Platysma

A

Sternocleidomastoid and trapezius (CN XI)

Sternocleidomastoid

Trapezius

Nuchal muscles, intrinsic back muscles (dorsal rami of cervical nerves)

Semispinalis capitis

Obliquus capitis superior

Rectus capitis posterior major

Rectus capitis posterior minor

Splenius capitis

Longissimus capitis

Muscles of mastication (CN V₃)

Masseter

Lateral pterygoid (see **B** and **C**)

Temporalis

Medial pterygoid (see **B** and **C**)

Temporalis

Buccinator

Genioglossus

Lateral pterygoid, superior head*

Lateral pterygoid, inferior head

Medial pterygoid

Mylohyoid

Geniohyoid

Digastric, anterior belly

B

*Primarily inserts into articular disk.

Fig. 2.46 **Origins and insertions on the skull**
A Left lateral view.
B Inner surface of right hemimandible.
C Inferior view of skull base.
Note: The stylohyoid, styloglossus, and stylopharyngeus originate on the styloid process.

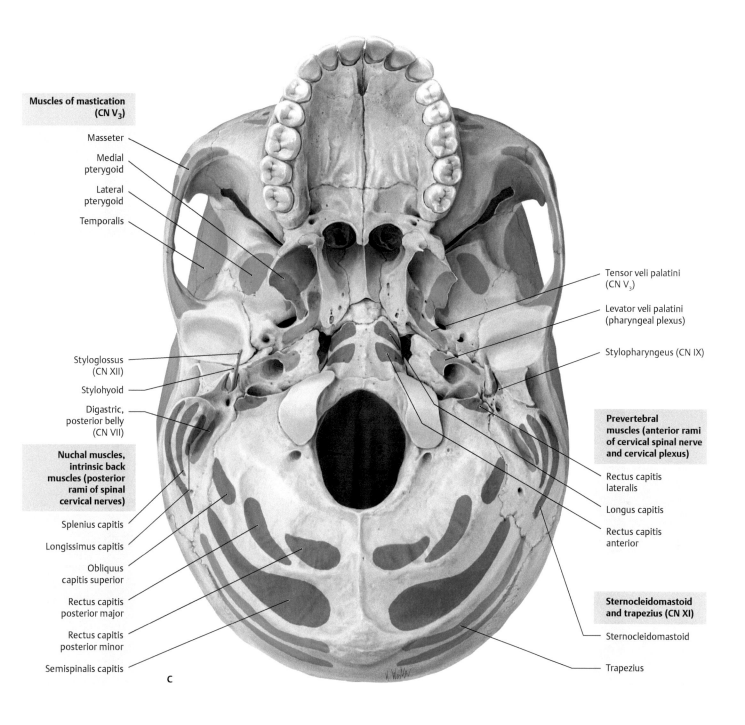

Muscles of mastication (CN V₃)

Masseter

Medial pterygoid

Lateral pterygoid

Temporalis

Styloglossus (CN XII)

Stylohyoid

Digastric, posterior belly (CN VII)

Nuchal muscles, intrinsic back muscles (posterior rami of spinal cervical nerves)

Splenius capitis

Longissimus capitis

Obliquus capitis superior

Rectus capitis posterior major

Rectus capitis posterior minor

Semispinalis capitis

Tensor veli palatini (CN V₃)

Levator veli palatini (pharyngeal plexus)

Stylopharyngeus (CN IX)

Prevertebral muscles (anterior rami of cervical spinal nerve and cervical plexus)

Rectus capitis lateralis

Longus capitis

Rectus capitis anterior

Sternocleidomastoid and trapezius (CN XI)

Sternocleidomastoid

Trapezius

C

Radiographs of the Skull

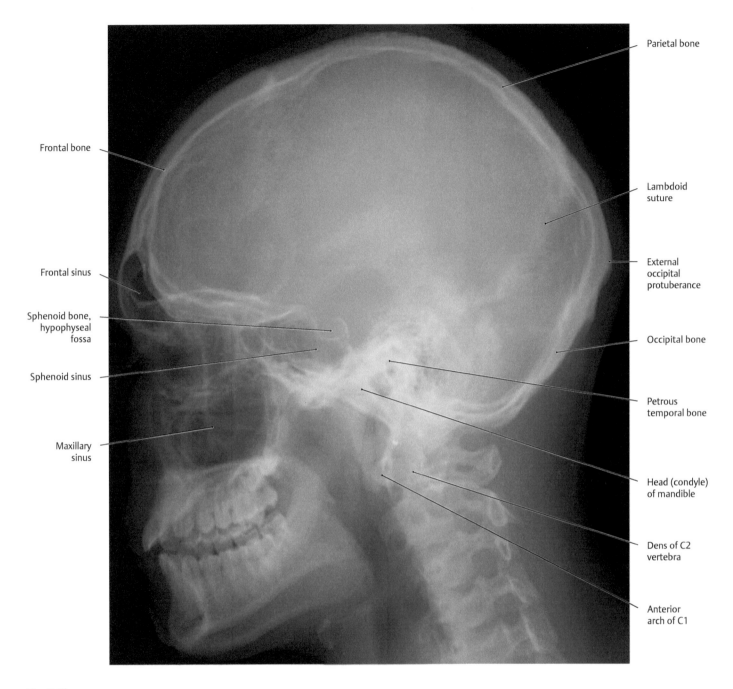

Frontal bone

Frontal sinus

Sphenoid bone, hypophyseal fossa

Sphenoid sinus

Maxillary sinus

Parietal bone

Lambdoid suture

External occipital protuberance

Occipital bone

Petrous temporal bone

Head (condyle) of mandible

Dens of C2 vertebra

Anterior arch of C1

Fig. 2.47
A lateral radiograph of the skull highlights the maxillary sinuses and their relationship to the orbits and oral cavity. The frontal and sphenoid sinuses can also be seen in this view.

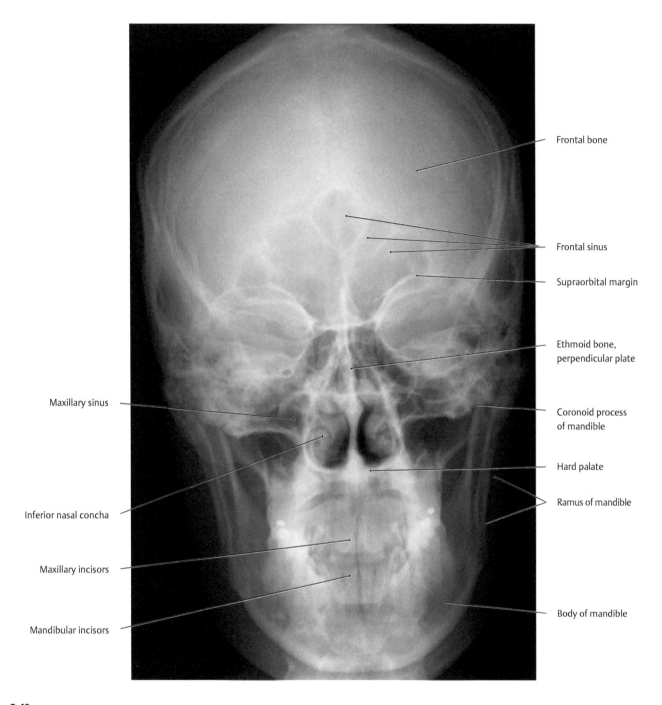

Frontal bone

Frontal sinus

Supraorbital margin

Ethmoid bone,
perpendicular plate

Coronoid process
of mandible

Hard palate

Ramus of mandible

Body of mandible

Maxillary sinus

Inferior nasal concha

Maxillary incisors

Mandibular incisors

Fig. 2.48
An anteroposterior radiograph of the skull displays the paranasal sinuses, nasal conchae, and boundaries of the orbits.

Radiographs of the Sphenoid Bone

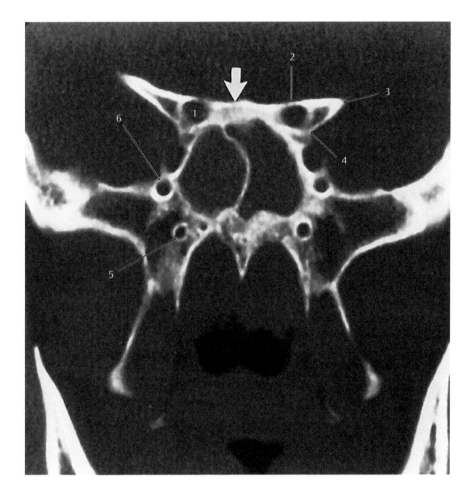

Fig. 2.49
Coronal CT scan shows the optic canal (1), superior (posterior) root of lesser wing of the sphenoid (2), anterior clinoid (3), inferior (anterior) root of lesser wing of the sphenoid (4), pterygoid (vidian) canal (5), foramen rotundum (6), and planum sphenoidale (arrow).

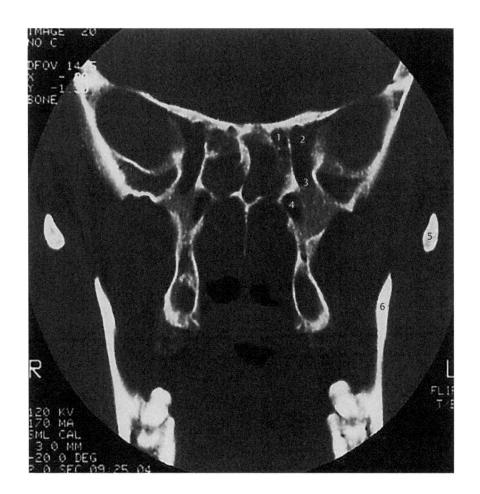

Fig. 2.50
Coronal CT scan 6 mm anterior to a, showing the optic canal (1), superior (2) and inferior (3) orbital fissures, pterygopalatine fossa (4), zygomatic arch (5), and mandible (6). Note prominent adenoidal tissue.

Arteries of the Head & Neck: Overview & Subclavian Artery

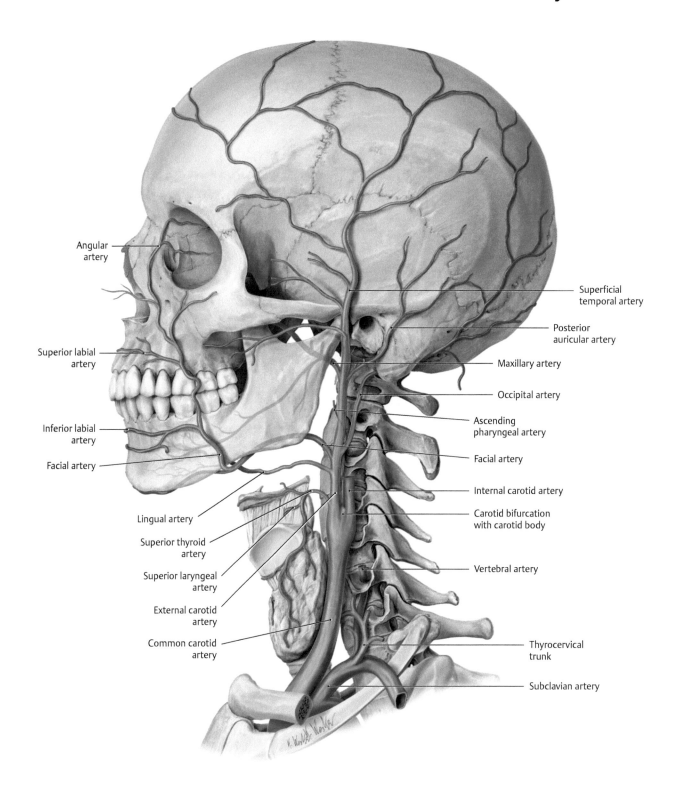

Fig. 3.1 Overview of the arteries of the head and neck
Left lateral view. The left common carotid artery arises from the aortic arch; the right common carotid artery from the brachiocephalic trunk. Each common carotid artery divides into an internal carotid artery and an external carotid artery at the carotid bifurcation, which is at the approximate level of the fourth cervical vertebra. The carotid body is located at the carotid bifurcation. It contains the chemoreceptors that respond to oxygen deficiency in the blood (hypoxia) and to changes in pH (both are important in the regulation of breathing). The internal carotid artery does not branch further before entering the skull, where it mainly supplies blood to the brain. It also gives off branches that supply areas of the facial skeleton that emerge from the cranium.

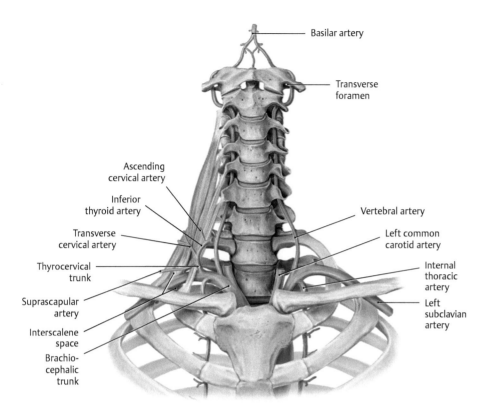

Basilar artery

Transverse foramen

Ascending cervical artery

Inferior thyroid artery

Vertebral artery

Transverse cervical artery

Left common carotid artery

Thyrocervical trunk

Internal thoracic artery

Suprascapular artery

Left subclavian artery

Interscalene space

Brachio-cephalic trunk

***Fig. 3.2* Subclavian artery and its branches**

Anterior view. The subclavian artery distributes a number of branches to structures located at the base of the neck and in the region of the thoracic inlet. Note that the branches of the subclavian artery may arise in a variable sequence. After emerging from the thoracic inlet, the subclavian artery passes through the interscalene space (between the anterior scalene and middle scalene) and on into the axilla as the axillary artery. Each *vertebral artery* arises from the posterior aspect of the subclavian artery on each side and ascends through the foramina in the transverse processes of the cervical vertebrae (C6–C1). After entering the skull through the foramen magnum, the vertebral arteries unite to form the basilar artery and contribute to the formation of both the cerebral arteries, forming anastomoses (circle of Willis) that have major clinical importance in supplying the blood to the brain.

Table 3.1 Branches of the subclavian artery

Artery	Branch	Further branches	Regions supplied
Subclavian a.	Internal thoracic a.		Internal anterior chest wall
	Vertebral a.	Meningeal branches	Falx cerebelli
		Posterior spinal a.	Posterior spinal cord, especially the posterior columns; medulla oblongata (nucleus coneatus and nucleus gracilis)
		Anterior spinal a.	Meninges; anterior spinal cord; medulla oblongata (dorsal motor nucleus of CN X, nucleus ambiguus, spinal accessory nucleus and hypoglossal nucleus)
		Posterior inferior cerebellar a.	Cerebellum, medulla oblongata (cochlear nucleus, vestibular nucleus, dorsal motor nucleus of CN X, nucleus ambiguous)
	Thyrocervical trunk	Inferior thyroid a.	Inferior portion of thyroid gland and larynx, upper trachea, upper esophagus, deep neck muscles
		Suprascapular a.	Supraspinatus and infraspinatus muscles, shoulder joint
		Transverse cervical a.	Trapezius muscle and surrounding tissues
	Costocervical trunk	Deep cervical a.	Muscles at the root of the neck
		Supreme intercostal a.	Posterior part of the 1st and 2nd intercostals spaces
	Dorsal scapular a. (descending scapular a.)*		Levator scapulae, rhomboid and trapezius muscles

* Arises from the subclavian a. in around two thirds of individuals and from the transverse cervical a. in the remaining one third.

External & Internal Carotid Arteries: Overview

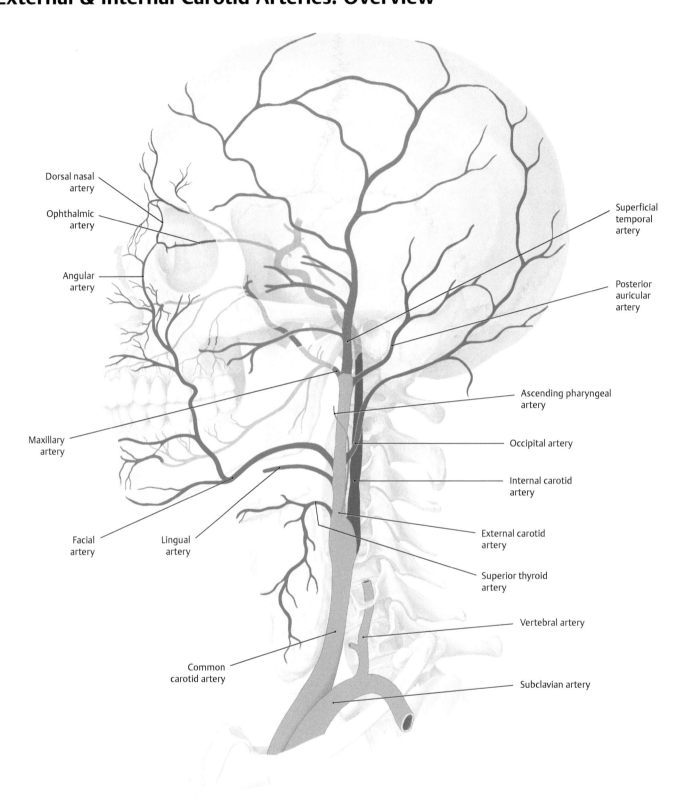

Fig. 3.3 Arteries of the head

Left lateral view. The common carotid artery divides into the internal carotid artery (purple) and the external carotid artery (gray) at the carotid bifurcation (at the level of the C4 Vertebra, between the thyroid cartilage and hyoid bone). The external carotid artery divides into eight major branches that supply the scalp, face, and structures of the head and neck. These eight branches can be arranged into four groups: anterior (red), medial (blue), posterior (green), and terminal (yellow). The internal carotid artery does not branch before entering the skull. It gives off branches within the cranial cavity.

The ophthalmic branch of the internal carotid artery provides branches that will anastomose with branches of the facial artery on the face (see **Fig. 3.12**).

A carotid bruit is a noise ("swooshing" sound) caused by turbulent blood flow in the carotid artery. It is suggestive of carotid artery stenosis (narrowing) due to atherosclerosis (hardening of the arteries). It is best heard with the stethoscope placed over the carotid bifurcation (at the upper border of the thyroid cartilage). Surgical intervention is necessary for those with >60% lumen stenosis, which is indicated by imaging.

Table 3.2 **Branches of the external carotid and internal carotid arteries**

Artery	Branch	Regions supplied
External carotid a.*(gray)	Superior thyroid a. (red)	Larynx, thyroid gland, pharynx, sternocleidomastoid muscle
	Ascending pharyngeal a. (blue)	Muscles of the pharyngeal wall, mucosa of the middle ear, dura, posterior cranial fossa
	Lingual a. (red)	Floor of the oral cavity, tongue, sublingual gland, epiglottis, suprahyoid muscles
	Facial a. (red)	Superficial face, submandibular gland, pharyngeal wall, soft palate, palatine tonsils, anterior belly of digastric, mylohyoid, nose and nasal septum
	Occipital a. (green)	Scalp in occipital region; posterior neck muscles
	Posterior auricular a. (green)	Tympanic cavity, posterior auricle, parotid gland, posterior scalp
	Maxillary a. (yellow)	Mandibular and maxillary dentition, muscles of mastication, posteromedial facial skeleton, nasal cavity, face, and meninges
	Superficial temporal a. (yellow)	Scalp of forehead and vertex, soft tissue below zygomatic arch, masseter, parotid gland, external orbital wall, orbicularis oculi
Internal carotid a. (purple)	Caroticotympanic arteries	Pharyngotympanic (auditory) tube and anterior wall of tympanic cavity
	Artery of pterygoid canal	Anastomosis with external carotid a.
	Superior and inferior hypophyseal aa.	Pituitary gland
	Cavernous sinus branch	Anastomosis with external carotid a.
	Anterior meningeal branch	Meninges of the anterior cranial fossa
	Ganglionic branch	Trigeminal ganglion
	Ophthalmic a.	Optic n., optic chiasm, optic tract, retina, extraocular muscles, eyelids, lacrimal gland, forehead, ethmoidal air cells, frontal sinus, lateral nasal wall, dorsum of the nose, and meninges
	Anterior cerebral a.	Medial aspect of frontal and parietal lobes, corpus callosum
	Middle cerebral a.	Frontal, parietal, and temporal lobes
	Posterior communicating a.	Anastomosis with cerebral aa. as part of Circle of Willis
	Anterior choroidal a.	Choroid plexus of the lateral and 3rd ventricle, optic chiasm and optic tract, internal capsule, lateral geniculate body, globus pallidus, caudate nucleus, hippocampus, amygdale, substantia nigra, red nucleus, crus cerebelli

* Anterior branches of external carotid artery are red; medial branches are blue; posterior branches are green; and terminal branches are yellow

External Carotid Artery: Anterior & Medial Branches

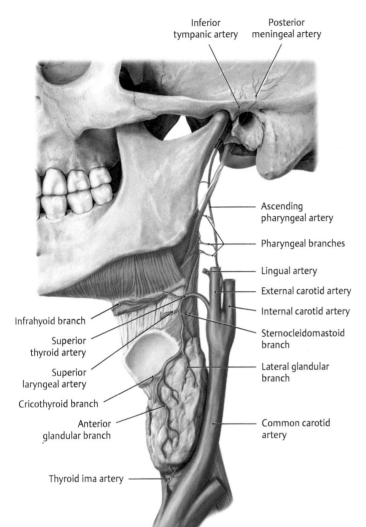

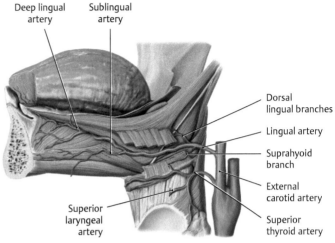

Fig. 3.5 Lingual artery and its branches
Left lateral view. The lingual artery is the second anterior branch of the external carotid artery. It has a relatively large caliber, providing the tongue and oral cavity with its rich blood supply. It also gives off branches to the tonsils.

Fig. 3.4 Superior thyroid and ascending pharyngeal arteries
Left lateral view. The superior thyroid artery is typically the first branch to arise from the external carotid artery. One of the anterior branches, it supplies the larynx (via the superior laryngeal branch) and thyroid gland. The ascending pharyngeal artery springs from the medial side of the external carotid artery, usually arising above the level of the superior thyroid artery.

Table 3.3 Branches of the superior thyroid, lingual, and ascending pharyngeal arteries		
Branch of external carotid a.	**Further branches**	**Region supplied**
Superior thyroid a.	Superior laryngeal a.	Larynx
	Glandular branches	Thyroid gland
	Sternocleidomastoid branch	Sternocleidomastoid muscle
	Muscular branches	Pharynx
	Infrahyoid branch	Region of thyrohoid membrane
	Cricothyroid branch	Region of the cricothyroid membrane
Lingual a.	Suprahyoid branch	Suprahyoid muscles
	Dorsal lingual branches	Base of tongue, epiglottis
	Sublingual a.	Sublingual gland, tongue, floor of the oral cavity
	Deep lingual a.	Tongue
Ascending pharyngeal a.	Pharyngeal branches	Muscles of the pharyngeal wall
	Inferior tympanic a.	Mucosa of middle ear
	Posterior meningeal a.	Dura of the posterior cranial fossa

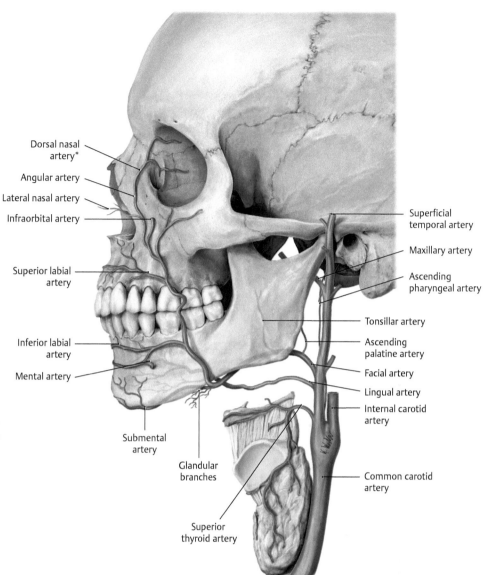

Dorsal nasal artery*

Angular artery

Lateral nasal artery

Infraorbital artery

Superficial temporal artery

Maxillary artery

Ascending pharyngeal artery

Superior labial artery

Tonsillar artery

Inferior labial artery

Ascending palatine artery

Mental artery

Facial artery

Lingual artery

Internal carotid artery

Submental artery

Glandular branches

Common carotid artery

Superior thyroid artery

*Branch of ophthalmic artery

Fig. 3.6 Facial artery and its branches
Left lateral view. The facial artery has four cervical and four facial branches. The four cervical branches (ascending palatine, tonsillar, glandular, and submental arteries) arise in the neck before the facial artery crosses the mandible to reach the face. The four facial branches (inferior and superior labial, lateral nasal, and angular arteries) supply the superficial face. Branches of the facial artery anastomose with branches of the internal carotid artery as well as other branches derived from the external carotid artery (see **Fig. 3.12**, p. 63).

Table 3.4 Branches of the facial artery	
Course: The facial artery arises from the external carotid artery in the carotid triangle of the neck. It then passes superiorly immediately deep to the posterior belly of digastric and the stylohyoid. It runs along the submandibular gland then loops under and over the body of the mandible at the anterior border of the masseter. It then runs anterosuperiorly across the cheek to the angle of the mouth and then continues superiorly along the side of the nose. It terminates as the angular artery along the medial aspect of the orbit. At its termination, the angular artery anastomoses with the dorsal nasal artery.	
Branch	**Region supplied**
Cervical branches	
Ascending palatine a.	Pharyngeal wall, soft palate, pharyngotympanic tube, palatine tonsils, pharynx
Tonsillar a.	Palatine tonsils and oropharynx
Glandular branch	Submandibular gland
Submental a.	Anterior belly of digastric, mylohyoid, submandibular gland, sublingual gland
Facial branches	
Inferior labial a.	Lower lip
Superior labial a.	Upper lip; nasal septum (via septal branches)
Lateral nasal a.	Dorsum of the nose
Angular a.	Root of the nose

External Carotid Artery: Posterior Branches

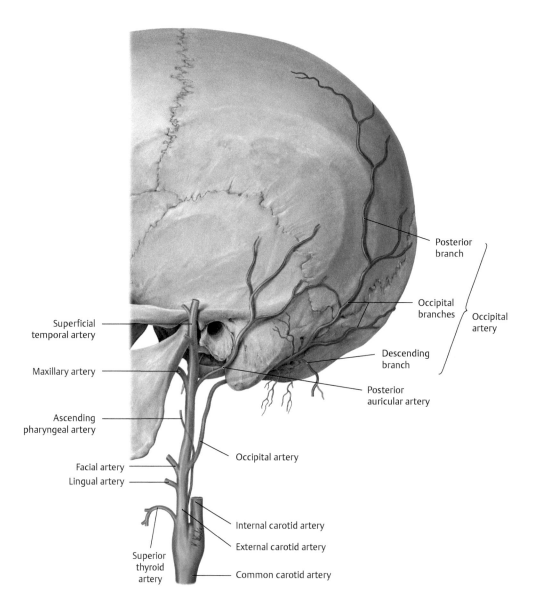

Fig. 3.7 Branches of the occipital artery

The occipital artery generally arises from the external carotid artery, just opposite the origin of the facial artery and just inferior to the posterior belly of the digastric muscle (not shown). The artery passes posteriorly and near its origin is crossed laterally by the hypoglossal nerve (not shown). In its course to the posterior of the occiput, the occipital artery passes lateral to the internal carotid artery (at the same time that it is passing lateral to both the internal jugular vein and cranial nerves CN X and CN XI--not shown). At the base of the skull, the occipital artery passes medial to the mastoid process, travelling in the occipital groove. Branches of the occipital artery anastomose with branches of both the posterior auricular and superficial temporal arteries. On the posterior aspect of the cranium, the artery converges with the greater occipital nerve (not shown). The occipital artery gives rise to eight named branches (see **Table 3.5**).

Fig. 3.8 Branches of the posterior auricular artery

The posterior auricular artery arises from the external carotid artery as the last branch before the origin of its two terminal branches (maxillary and superficial temporal arteries). It arises superior to the posterior belly of digastric. In its course the posterior auricular artery travels deep to the parotid gland and ascends along the lateral aspect of the styloid process of the temporal bone. The artery then passes superiorly between the mastoid process and the posterior aspect of the auricle. It gives rise to 5 named branches (see **Table 3.5**).

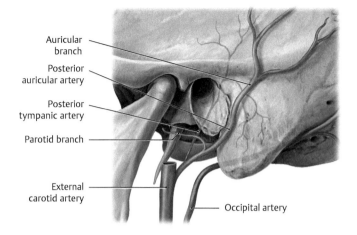

Table 3.5 Branches of the occipital and posterior auricular arteries

Branch	Further branches	Region supplied
Occipital a.	Muscular branch	Regional muscles including posterior belly of digastric and stylohyoid
	Sternocleidomastoid branch	Sternocleidomastoid
	Descending branch	Posterior neck muscles
	Meningeal branch	Structures internal and external to jugular foramen
	Mastoid branch	Mastoid air cells and dura
	Auricular branch	Auricle (medial side)
	Occipital branches	Scalp of occipital region
	Stylomastoid a.*	Facial n. in facial canal; tympanic cavity
Posterior auricular a.	Stylomastoid a.*	Facial n. in facial canal; tympanic cavity
	Occipital branch	Occiput
	Muscular branches	Posterior belly of digastric and stylohyoid
	Parotid branch	Parotid gland
	Auricular branch	Posterior side of auricle

* The stylomastoid a. has a variable origin; it arises from the occipital a. two thirds of the time and the posterior auricular a. one third of the time.

External Carotid Artery: Terminal Branches (I)

The two terminal branches of the external carotid artery are the maxillary artery and the superficial temporal artery. They divide within the substance of the parotid gland. The maxillary artery is the largest of the two terminal branches. It supplies the maxilla and mandible (including the teeth), the muscles of mastication, the palate, the nose, and the dura covering the brain.

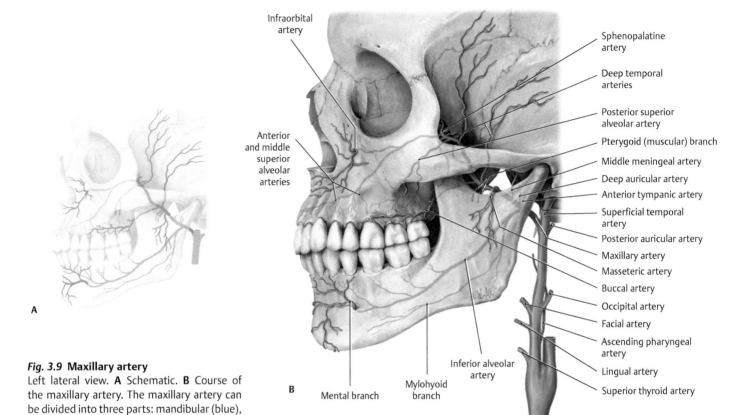

Fig. 3.9 Maxillary artery
Left lateral view. **A** Schematic. **B** Course of the maxillary artery. The maxillary artery can be divided into three parts: mandibular (blue), pterygoid (green), and pterygopalatine (yellow). See **Table 3.6**.

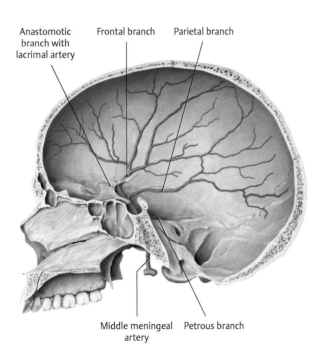

Fig. 3.10 Middle meningeal artery
Medial view of right middle meningeal artery. The middle meningeal artery arises from the mandibular portion of the maxillary artery. It passes through the foramen spinosum into the middle cranial fossa. Despite its name, it supplies blood not just to the meninges, but also to the overlying calvaria. Rupture of the middle meningeal artery by head trauma results in an epidural hematoma (see **Fig. 4.58**, p. 109).

Table 3.6 Branches of the maxillary artery

Branch	Course	Distribution
Mandibular part (blue): Also known as the bony part or 1st part, this portion runs medial to the neck of the mandible and gives off 5 major branches, all of which enter bone.		
Inferior alveolar a.	Gives off a lingual and a mylohyoid branch before entering the mandibular foramen to travel along the mandibular canal; it splits into 2 terminal branches (incisive and mental)	Mandibular molars and premolars with associated gingiva, mandible
	• Lingual branch	Lingual mucous membrane
	• Mylohyoid branch	Mylohyoid
	• Incisive branch	Mandibular incisors
	• Mental branch	Chin
Anterior tympanic a.	Runs through the petrotympanic fissure along with the chorda tympani	Middle ear
Deep auricular a.	Travels through the wall of the external acoustic meatus	Lateral tympanic membrane, skin of external acoustic meatus
	• Branch to temporomandibular joint	Temporomandibular joint
Middle meningeal a.	Runs through the foramen spinosum to the middle cranial cavity	Bones of the cranial vault, dura of anterior and middle cranial fossae
Accessory meningeal a.	Runs through the foramen ovale to the middle cranial fossa	Medial and lateral pterygoid, tensor veli palatini, sphenoid bone, dura, trigeminal ganglion
Pterygoid part (green): Also known as the muscular part or 2nd part, this portion runs between the temporalis and lateral pterygoid. It gives off 5 major branches, all of which supply muscle.		
Masseteric a.	Runs through the mandibular incisure (notch)	Masseter, temporomandibular joint
Deep temporal aa.	Consist of anterior, middle, and posterior branches, which course deep to the temporalis	Temporalis
Lateral pterygoid a.	Runs directly to the lateral pterygoid muscle	Lateral pterygoid
Medial pterygoid a.	Runs directly to the medial pterygoid muscle	Medial pterygoid
Buccal a.	Accompanies the buccal n.	Buccal mucosa and skin, buccinator
Pterygopalatine part or 3rd part (yellow): This portion runs through the pterygomaxillary fissure to enter the pterygopalatine fossa. It gives off 6 major branches, which accompany the branches of the maxillary nerve (CN V$_2$).*		
Posterior superior alveolar a.	Runs through the pterygomaxillary fissure; may arise from the infraorbital a.	Maxillary molars and premolars, with associated gingiva; maxillary sinus
Infraorbital a.	Runs through the inferior orbital fissure into the orbit, where it runs along the infraorbital groove and canal, exiting onto the face via the infraorbital foramen	Cheek, upper lip, nose, lower eyelid
	• Anterior and middle superior alveolar aa.	Maxillary teeth and maxillary sinus
Descending palatine a.	• Greater palatine a.: runs via the greater (anterior) palatine canal; in the canal it gives off several lesser palatine aa.; continues through greater palatine foramen onto hard palate	Roof of hard palate, nasal cavity (inferior meatus), maxillary gingiva
	• Lesser palatine aa.: runs via the lesser palatine foramen	Soft palate
	• Anastomosing branch: runs via the incisive canal; joins with the sphenopalatine a.	Nasal septum
Sphenopalatine a.	Runs via the sphenopalatine foramen to the nasal cavity; gives off posterior lateral nasal branches, then travels to the nasal septum, where it terminates as posterior septal branches	
	• Posterior lateral nasal aa.: anastomose with the ethmoidal aa. and nasal branches of the greater palatine a.	Nasal air sinuses (frontal, maxillary, ethmoidal, and sphenoidal)
	• Posterior septal branches: anastomose with the ethmoidal arteries on the nasal septum	Nasal conchae and nasal septum
A. of the pterygoid canal	Runs through the pterygoid canal	Pharyngotympanic tube, tympanic cavity, upper pharynx
Pharyngeal a.	Runs through the palatovaginal canal	Nasopharynx, sphenoidal sinus, and pharyngotympanic tube; mucosa of nasal cavity

*All branches are named for the nerve they travel with except for the sphenopalatine artery, which travels with the nasopalatine nerve.

External Carotid Artery: Terminal Branches (II) & Anastomoses

***Fig. 3.11* Superficial temporal artery**
Left lateral view. The superficial temporal artery is the second of the two terminal branches of the external carotid artery. Particularly in elderly or cachectic patients, the often tortuous course of the frontal branch of this vessel can be easily traced across the temple. Temporal arteritis (giant cell arteritis, cranial arteritis) is an inflammatory condition affecting the medium-sized arteries that supply the temple region, scalp, eyes, and optic nerves. The average age of onset of this condition is 70 years and it affects women twice as commonly as men. Symptoms may begin as general malaise and progress rapidly to headaches, tenderness of the scalp, severe pain in the temple region, transient blurred vision, diplopia (double vision), ptosis (drooping eyelid), neck pain, and jaw claudication (pain on jaw manipulation, e.g., during eating, due to ischemia of the masseter muscle). It is diagnosed by blood tests that indicate an inflammatory process is ongoing and by biopsy of the temporal artery (definitive test). If not treated promptly (usually before biopsy results confirm the condition), then it may cause painless loss of vision in the affected eye that is usually permanent. Having temporal arteritis also increases the risk of stroke and aortic aneurysm. Treatment is with corticosteroids, often long-term.

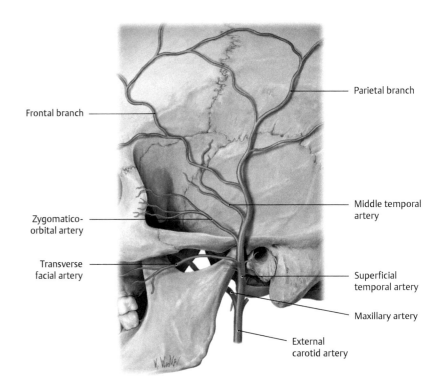

Table 3.7 Branches of the superficial temporal artery		
Branch	**Further branches**	**Region supplied**
Superficial temporal a.	Transverse facial a.	Soft tissues below zygomatic arch, parotid gland, masseter muscle
	Anterior auricular a.	External auditory meatus, anterior area of auricle
	Middle temporal a.	Temporalis
	Zygomatico-orbital a.	Lateral external orbital wall and obicularis oculi
	Frontal (anterior) branches	Scalp of forehead
	Parietal (posterior) branches	Scalp of vertex

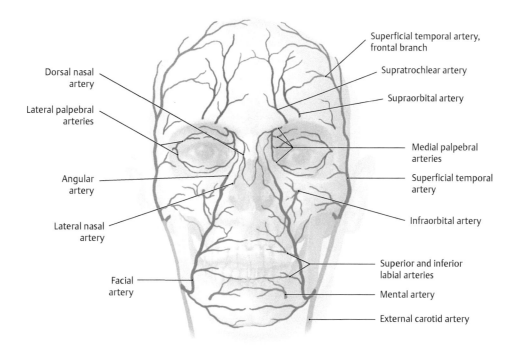

Fig. 3.12 Anastomoses of the external carotid and internal carotid arteries

Branches of the external carotid artery (e.g., facial artery [red], superficial temporal artery [yellow], and infraorbital arteries [yellow]) and the internal carotid artery (e.g., dorsal nasal and supraorbital arteries [purple]) anastomose in certain facial regions to ensure blood flow to the face and head. Anastomoses occur between the angular artery and dorsal nasal artery and between the superficial temporal artery and supraorbital artery. Due to the extensive arterial anastomoses, facial injuries tend to bleed profusely but also heal quickly.

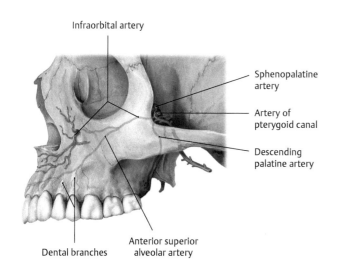

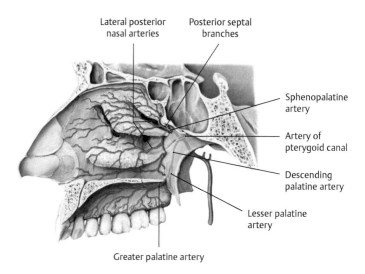

Fig. 3.13 Infraorbital artery

Left lateral view. The infraorbital artery arises from the pterygopalatine part of the maxillary artery (a terminal branch of the external carotid artery), and the supraorbital artery (not shown) arises from the internal carotid artery (via the ophthalmic branch). These vessels therefore provide a path for potential anastomosis between the internal and external carotid arteries on the face.

Fig. 3.14 Sphenopalatine artery

Medial view of right nasal wall and right sphenopalatine artery. The sphenopalatine artery enters the nasal cavity through the sphenopalatine foramen. The anterior portion of the nasal septum contains a highly vascularized region (Kiesselbach's area), which is supplied by both the posterior septal branches of the sphenopalatine artery (external carotid artery) and the anterior septal branches of the anterior ethmoidal artery (internal carotid artery via ophthalmic artery). When severe nasopharyngeal bleeding occurs, it may be necessary to ligate the maxillary artery in the pterygopalatine fossa.

Internal Carotid Artery

Fig. 3.15 Overview of the internal carotid artery

The internal carotid artery branches from the common carotid artery at the level of the carotid bifurcation (C4 vertebral level). Its extracranial part gives off no branches. The internal part has four anatomical parts that supply blood to the brainstem and brain (see **Fig. 3.16**).

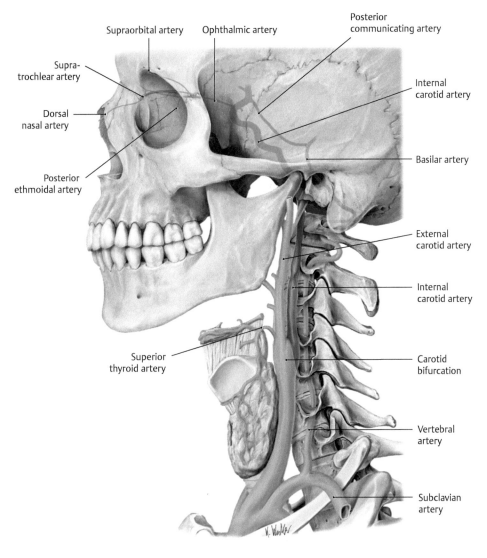

Fig. 3.16 Subdivisions of the internal carotid artery

Anatomical segments of the internal carotid artery and their branches. The internal carotid artery is distributed chiefly to the brain but also supplies extracerebral regions of the head. It consists of four parts (listed from bottom to top):

- Cervical part
- Petrous part
- Cavernous part
- Cerebral part

The petrous part of the internal carotid artery (traversing the carotid canal) and the cavernous part (traversing the cavernous sinus) have a role in supplying extracerebral structures of the head. They give off additional small branches that supply local structures and are usually named for the areas they supply. Of the branches not supplying the brain, of special importance is the ophthalmic artery, which arises from the cerebral part of the internal carotid artery. *Note:* The ophthalmic artery forms an anastomosis with the artery of the pterygoid canal derived from the maxillary artery.

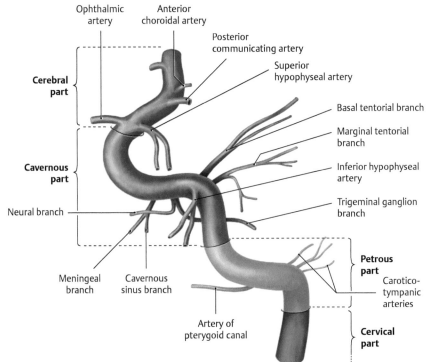

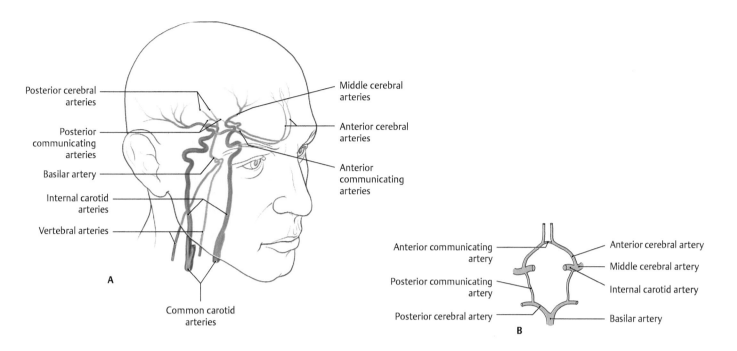

Fig. 3.17 Blood supply to the brain
A Schematic of circle of Willis in situ. **B** Schematic of isolated circle of Willis.
The brain is supplied by four arteries that leave the root of the neck separately, the left and right internal carotid arteries and the left and right vertebral arteries. However, the vertebral arteries converge to form the basilar artery and so only three arteries reach the base of the brain, where they form the circle of Willis. The circle of Willis is a means by which the brain can receive blood when one or more of its major arterial contributors becomes narrowed or blocked, for example, by an emboli, possibly preventing ischemic stroke.

Table 3.8 Contribution of the internal carotid artery to the blood supply of the eye, nose, face, and surrounding areas

Course: The ophthalmic artery branches from the internal carotid artery (ICA) just after the ICA passes through the cavernous sinus. It runs along the medial side of the anterior clinoid process passing anteriorly through the optic canal with the optic nerve. It then courses in the medial wall of the orbit. The two terminal branches of the ophthalmic artery are the dorsal nasal and supratrochlear arteries.

Origin	Artery	Region supplied
Ophthalmic a. (branch of internal carotid artery)	*Ocular branches*	
	Central artery of the retina	Retina
	Anterior ciliary a.	Eyeball
	Long and short posterior ciliary aa.	Eyeball
	Orbital branches	
	Lacrimal a.	Lacrimal glands, eyelids, and conjunctiva
	Muscular aa.	Extraocular muscles
	Middle palpebral a.	Eyelids
	Posterior ethmoidal a.	Ethmoidal air cells, posterosuperior nasal septum, part of sphenoid sinus and meninges
	Anterior ethmoidal a.	Ethmoidal air cells, anterosuperior nasal septum, lateral nasal wall, and anterior cranial fossa
	Supratrochlear a.	Muscles and skin of the medial forehead, and frontal sinus
	Supraorbital a.	Muscles and skin of the forehead, and frontal sinus
	Meningeal a.	Middle cranial fossa
	Dorsal nasal a.	Region along the bridge of the nose

Veins of the Head & Neck: Overview

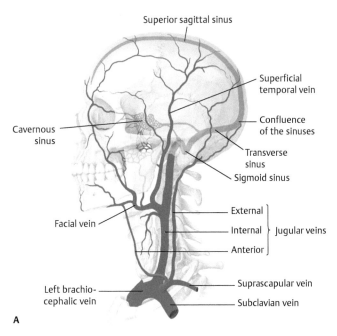

A

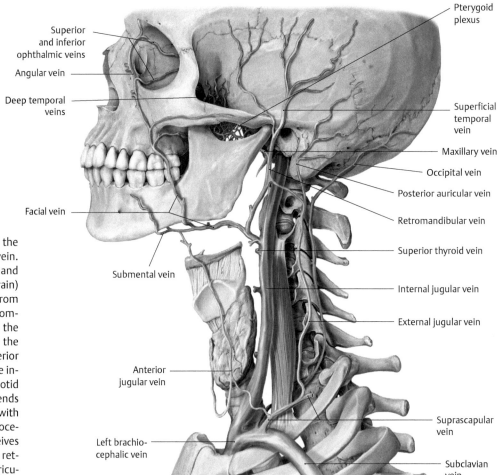

Fig. 3.18 Veins of the head and neck

Left lateral view. The principal vein of the head and neck is the internal jugular vein. This drains blood from both the exterior and the interior of the skull (including the brain) in addition to receiving venous blood from the neck. It receives blood from the common facial vein (formed by the union of the facial vein and the anterior division of the retromandibular vein), the lingual, superior thyroid, and middle thyroid veins, and the inferior petrosal sinus. Enclosed in the carotid sheath, the internal jugular vein descends from the jugular foramen to its union with the subclavian vein to form the brachiocephalic vein. The external jugular vein receives blood from the posterior division of the retromandibular vein and the posterior auricular vein. The occipital vein normally drains to the deep cervical veins. The subclavian vein in the thorax can be catheterized in acutely ill or chronically ill patients to provide a fast and stable route for administering medication, fluids, and nutrition, and for measuring central oxygen saturation and central venous pressure (to quantify their fluid status). This is called *central venous catheterization* or a "central line." Other large veins in the neck (e.g., the internal jugular vein), thorax (e.g., the axillary vein), or the groin (e.g., the femoral vein) can also be catheterized in this way.

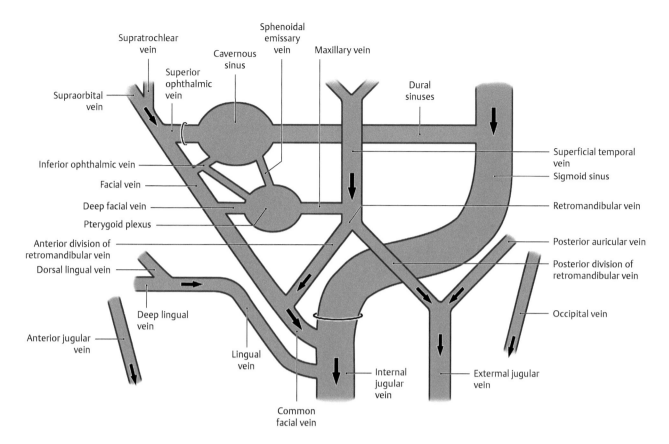

Fig. 3.19 Veins of the head: overview
The superficial veins of the head communicate with each other and with the dural sinuses via the deep veins of the head (pterygoid plexus and cavernous sinus). The pterygoid plexus connects the facial vein and the retromandibular vein (via the deep facial vein and maxillary vein, respectively). The cavernous sinus connects the facial vein to the sigmoid sinus (via the ophthalmic veins and the petrosal sinuses, respectively). Cavernous sinus thrombosis is the formation of a thrombus (blood clot) in the cavernous sinuses. It usually occurs secondary to an infection in the nasal sinuses, teeth, ears, eyes, or the skin of the face. The infective organism is typically Staphlococcus aureus, but it can also be caused by streptococci, pneumococci, and fungi. Signs and symptoms include headache, eye pain, exophthalmos (bulging eyeball), ptosis (drooping eyelid), vision loss, sluggish pupillary responses, and limitation of movement of the eye due to paralysis of the oculomotor, trochelar and abducent nerves. It may progress to meningitis or sepsis.

Table 3.9 Venous drainage of the head and neck

Vein	Location	Tributaries	Region drained
Internal jugular v.	Within carotid sheath	Common facial v. — Facial v. — Retromandibular v., anterior division Pharyngeal vv. Lingual v. Superior and middle thyroid vv.	Skull, anterior and lateral face, oral cavity, external pharynx, neck
		Sigmoid sinus and inferior petrosal sinuses	Interior of skull (including brain)
External jugular v.	Within superficial cervical fascia	Retromandibular v., posterior division	Lateral skull
		Posterior auricular v.	Occiput
Anterior jugular v.		Superficial veins in submandibular region	Anterior neck

Superficial Veins of the Head

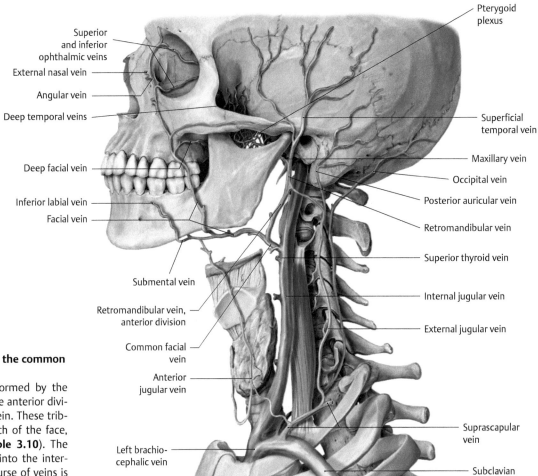

Fig. 3.20 **Venous drainage to the common facial vein**

The common facial vein is formed by the union of the facial vein and the anterior division of the retromandibular vein. These tributaries combine to drain much of the face, eye, and oral cavity (see **Table 3.10**). The common facial vein empties into the internal jugular vein. *Note:* The course of veins is highly variable.

Table 3.10 Tributaries of the common facial vein		
Course: tributaries of the common facial vein course parallel to the branches of the maxillary a.		
Tributary	**Further tributaries**	**Region drained**
Facial v.	Angular v.*	Anterior scalp, forehead, upper and lower eyelids, conjunctiva, root of the nose, cavernous sinus (via communication with ophthalmic vein)
	External nasal v.	External nose
	Superior labial v.	Upper lip
	Inferior labial v.	Lower lip
	Deep facial vein (from pterygoid plexus)	Contributes to drainage from pterygoid plexus (see maxillary vein below)
	Parotid vv.	Parotid region
	External palatine (paratonsillar) v.	Soft palate and tonsils
	Submental v.	Mylohyoid region
	Submandibular v.	Submandibular gland
Retromandibular v., anterior division	Maxillary v. (from pterygoid plexus)	Orbit and eye, muscles of mastication, muscles of facial expression, buccal mucosa and skin, hard palate, soft palate, teeth nend their associated gingival, submandibular, sublingual, and parotid glands, temporomandibular joint, chin, nasal air sinuses (frontal, maxillary, ethmoidal, and sphenoidal), nasal conchae, nasal septum, external acoustic meatus, tympanic membrane
	Superficial temporal v.	Anterior auricle, temple region, and scalp
* The angular vein is formed by the confluence of the supratrochlear and subraorbital vv.		

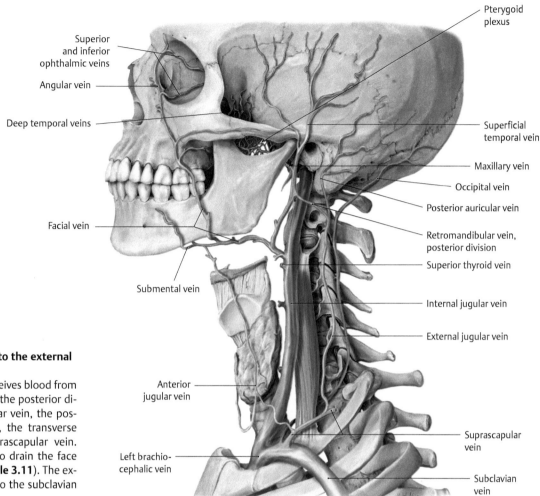

Superior and inferior ophthalmic veins

Angular vein

Deep temporal veins

Facial vein

Submental vein

Anterior jugular vein

Left brachio-cephalic vein

Pterygoid plexus

Superficial temporal vein

Maxillary vein

Occipital vein

Posterior auricular vein

Retromandibular vein, posterior division

Superior thyroid vein

Internal jugular vein

External jugular vein

Suprascapular vein

Subclavian vein

Fig. 3.21 Venous drainage to the external jugular vein

The external jugular vein receives blood from the posterior auricular vein, the posterior division of the retromandibular vein, the posterior external jugular vein, the transverse cervical vein, and the suprascapular vein. These tributaries combine to drain the face and superficial neck (see **Table 3.11**). The external jugular vein drains into the subclavian vein.

Table 3.11 Tributaries of the external jugular vein

Course: Arises at the confluence of posterior auricular vein and the posterior division of the retromandibular vein within the substance of the parotid gland, at the level of the angle of the mandible. It travels inferiorly within superficial cervical fascia to drain into the subclavian vein.

Tributary	Further tributaries	Region drained
Posterior auricular v.		Posterior auricle, external acoustic meatus, tympanic membrane, posterior scalp, parotid gland
Retromandibular v., posterior division	Maxillary v.	Orbit and eye, muscles of mastication, muscles of facial expression, buccal mucosa and skin, hard palate, soft palate, teeth and their associated gingival, submandibular, sublingual, and parotid glands, temporomandibular joint, chin, nasal air sinuses (frontal, maxillary, ethmoidal, and sphenoidal), nasal conchae, nasal septum, external acoustic meatus, tympanic membrane
	Superficial temporal v.	Anterior auricle, superficial face
Posterior external jugular v.		Skin and superficial muscles in the upper and back part of the neck
Transverse cervical v.		Trapezius muscle and surrounding tissue
Suprascapular v.		Supraspinatus and infraspinatus muscles; shoulder joint
Anterior jugular v.		Superficial parts of the anterior neck

Deep Veins of the Head

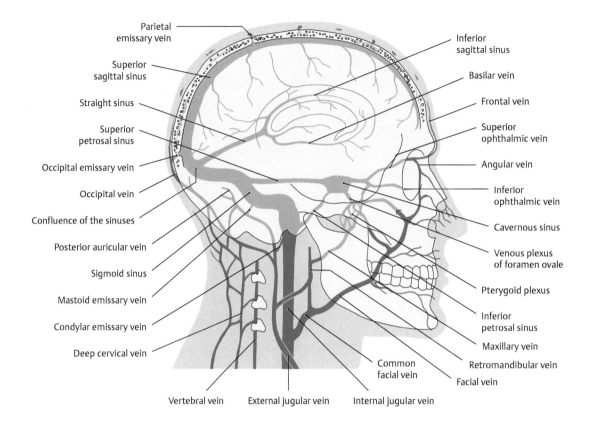

Fig. 3.22 Venous drainage of the head
The superficial veins of the head have extensive connections with the deep veins of the head and the dural sinuses. The meninges and brain are drained by the dural sinuses, which lie within the skull. Emissary veins connect the superficial veins of the skull directly to the dural sinuses. In addition, the deep veins of the head (e.g., pterygoid plexus) are intermediaries between the superficial veins of the face and the dural venous sinuses.

Table 3.12 Venous anastomoses as portals of infection		
The extracranial veins of the head are connected to the deep veins and dural sinuses. Patients who sustain midfacial fractures may bleed profusely due to the extensive venous anastomoses. Because the veins are generally valveless, extracranial bacteria may migrate to the deep veins, causing infections (e.g., bacteria from boils on the upper lip or nose may enter the angular vein and travel to the cavernous sinus). Bacteria in the cavernous sinus may cause thrombosis.		
Extracranial vein	**Connecting vein**	**Venous sinus**
Angular v.	Superior ophthalmic v.	Cavernous sinus
Vv. of palatine tonsil	Pterygoid plexus, inferior ophthalmic v.	
Superficial temporal v.	Parietal emissary v.	Superior sagittal sinus
Occipital v.	Occipital emissary v.	Transverse sinus, confluence of the sinuses
Posterior auricular v.	Mastoid emissary v.	Sigmoid sinus
External vertebral venous plexus	Condylar emissary v.	

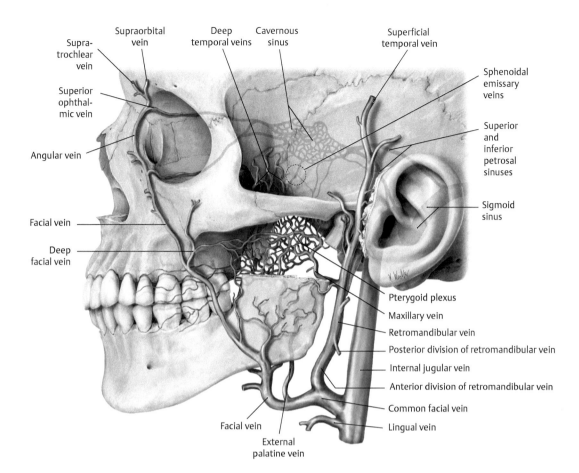

Fig. 3.23 Deep veins of the head

Left lateral view. The pterygoid plexus is a venous network situated behind the mandibular ramus and embedded in the pterygoid muscles. Because the veins of the face have no valves (small valves may be present but are generally nonfunctional), the movement of the pterygoid muscles forces blood from the pterygoid plexus into the jugular veins.

The pterygoid plexus is linked to the facial vein via the deep facial vein and to the retromandibular vein via the maxillary vein. The plexus is also linked to the cavernous sinus via the sphenoidal emissary vein. The cavernous sinus receives blood from the superior and inferior ophthalmic veins.

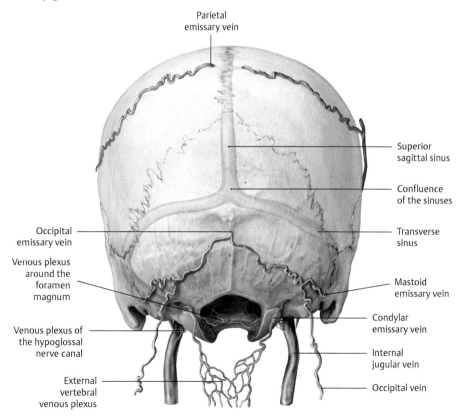

Fig. 3.24 Veins of the occiput

Posterior view. The dural sinuses are the series of venous channels that drain the brain. The superficial veins of the occiput communicate with the dural sinuses by way of the emissary veins. The emissary veins enter a similarly named foramen to communicate with the dural sinuses.

Lymphatics of the Head & Neck (I)

A distinction is made between regional lymph nodes, which are associated with a particular organ or region and constitute their primary filtering stations, and collecting lymph nodes, which usually receive lymph from multiple regional lymph node groups. Lymph from the head and neck region, gathered in scattered regional nodes, flows through its system of deep cervical collecting lymph nodes into the right and left

jugular trunks, each closely associated with its corresponding internal jugular vein. The jugular trunk on the right side drains into the right lymphatic duct, which terminates at the right jugulosubclavian junction. The jugular trunk on the left side terminates at the thoracic duct, which empties into the left jugulosubclavian junction (see **Fig. 12.16**).

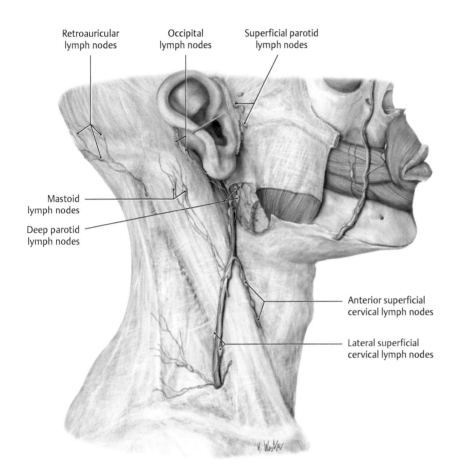

Fig. 3.25 Superficial cervical lymph nodes
Right lateral view. Enlarged cervical lymph nodes are a common finding at physical examination. The enlargement of cervical lymph nodes may be caused by inflammation (usually a *painful* enlargement) or neoplasia (usually a *painless* enlargement) in the area drained by the nodes. The superficial cervical lymph nodes are primary drainage locations for lymph from adjacent areas or organs.

Fig. 3.26 Deep cervical lymph nodes
Right lateral view. The deep lymph nodes in the neck consist mainly of collecting nodes. They have major clinical importance as potential sites of metastasis from head and neck tumors. Affected deep cervical lymph nodes may be surgically removed (neck dissection) or may be treated by regional irradiation. For this purpose, the American Academy of Otolaryngology—Head and Neck Surgery has grouped the deep cervical lymph nodes into six levels (Robbins 1991):

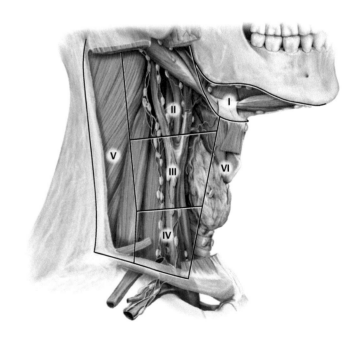

I   Submental and submandibular lymph nodes
II–IV Deep cervical lymph nodes along the internal jugular vein (lateral jugular lymph nodes):
    – II   Deep cervical lymph nodes (upper lateral group)
    – III Deep cervical lymph nodes (middle lateral group)
    – IV   Deep cervical lymph nodes (lower lateral group)
V   Lymph nodes in the posterior cervical triangle
VI   Anterior cervical lymph nodes

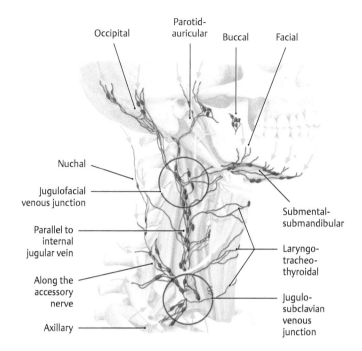

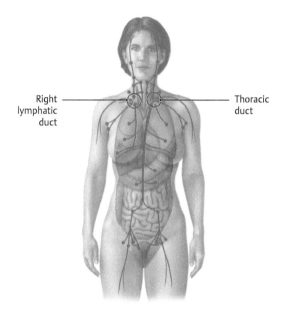

Fig. 3.27 Directions of lymphatic drainage in the neck
Right lateral view. Understanding this pattern of lymphatic flow is critical to identifying the location of a potential cause of enlarged cervical lymph nodes. There are two main sites in the neck where the lymphatic pathways intersect:

- Jugulofacial venous junction: Lymphatics from the head pass obliquely downward to this site, where the lymph is redirected vertically downward in the neck.
- Jugulosubclavian venous junction: The main lymphatic trunk, the thoracic duct, terminates at this central location, where lymph collected from the left side of the head and neck region is combined with lymph draining from the rest of the body.

If only peripheral nodal groups are affected, this suggests a localized disease process. If the central groups (e.g., those at the venous junctions) are affected, this usually signifies an extensive disease process. Central lymph nodes can be obtained for diagnostic evaluation by prescalene biopsy.

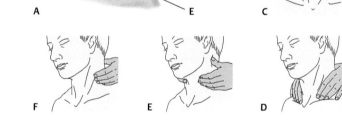

Fig. 3.28 Relationship of the cervical nodes to the systemic lymphatic circulation
Anterior view. The cervical lymph nodes may be involved by diseases that are not primary to the head and neck region, because lymph from the entire body is channeled to the left and right jugulosubclavian junctions (red circles). This can lead to retrograde involvement of the cervical nodes. The *right lymphatic duct* terminates at the right jugulosubclavian junction, the *thoracic duct* at the left jugulosubclavian junction. Besides cranial and cervical tributaries, the lymph from thoracic lymph nodes (mediastinal and tracheobronchial) and from abdominal and caudal lymph nodes may reach the cervical nodes by way of the thoracic duct. As a result, diseases in those organs may lead to cervical lymph node enlargement.
For example, gastric carcinoma may metastasize to the left supraclavicular group of lymph nodes, producing an enlarged *sentinel node* that suggests an abdominal tumor. Systemic lymphomas may also spread to the cervical lymph nodes by this pathway.

Fig. 3.29 Systematic palpation of the cervical lymph nodes
The cervical lymph nodes are systematically palpated during the physical examination to ensure the detection of any enlarged nodes.
Panel **A** shows the sequence in which the various nodal groups are successively palpated. The examiner usually palpates the submental-submandibular group first (**B**), including the mandibular angle (**C**), then proceeds along the anterior border of the sternocleidomastoid muscle (**D**). The supraclavicular lymph nodes are palpated next (**E**), followed by the lymph nodes along the accessory nerve and the nuchal group of nodes (**F**).
If lymph nodes are palpable, the following characteristics should be noted and described: size (<1 cm in diameter is normal), pain/tenderness (suggestive of inflammation), consistency (soft nodes suggest inflammation; firm, rubbery nodes suggest lymphoma; stony-hard nodes may be a sign of cancer), location of lymphadenopathy, and whether it is localized or generalized as this may help aid diagnosis.

Lymphatics of the Head & Neck (II)

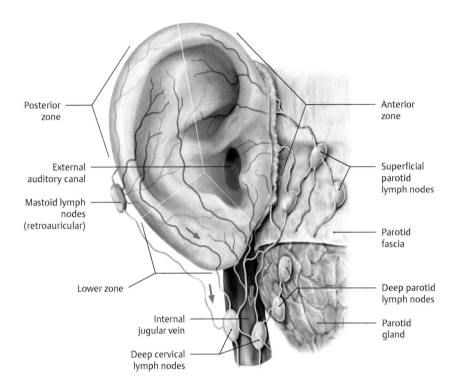

Posterior zone

External auditory canal

Mastoid lymph nodes (retroauricular)

Lower zone

Anterior zone

Superficial parotid lymph nodes

Parotid fascia

Deep parotid lymph nodes

Parotid gland

Internal jugular vein

Deep cervical lymph nodes

Fig. 3.30 **Auricle and external auditory canal: lymphatic drainage**
Right ear, oblique lateral view. The lymphatic drainage of the ear is divided into three zones, all of which drain directly or indirectly into the deep cervical lymph nodes along the internal jugular vein. The lower zone drains directly into the deep cervical lymph nodes. The anterior zone first drains into the parotid lymph nodes, the posterior zone into the mastoid lymph nodes.

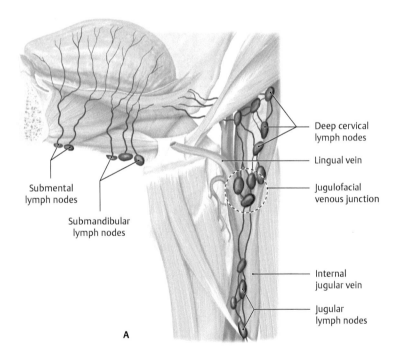

Deep cervical lymph nodes

Lingual vein

Jugulofacial venous junction

Submental lymph nodes

Submandibular lymph nodes

Internal jugular vein

Jugular lymph nodes

A

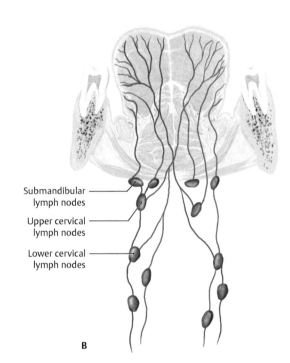

Submandibular lymph nodes

Upper cervical lymph nodes

Lower cervical lymph nodes

B

Fig. 3.31 **Lymphatic drainage of the tongue and oral floor**
A Left lateral view. **B** Anterior view.
The lymphatic drainage of the tongue and oral floor is mediated by submental and submandibular groups of lymph nodes that ultimately drain into the lymph nodes along the internal jugular vein (**A**, jugular lymph nodes). Because the lymph nodes receive drainage from both the ipsilateral and contralateral sides (**B**), tumor cells may become widely disseminated in this region (e.g., metastatic squamous cell carcinoma, especially on the lateral border of the tongue, frequently metastasizes to the opposite side).

Table 3.13 Lymphatic drainage of the head and neck

Note: Lymphatic drainage of the oral cavity is in bold.

Region	Node(s)	Secondary node(s)
Occipital region of the scalp and upper neck	Occipital nodes	Superficial cervical nodes
Scalp in temporoparietal region, posterior surface of the ear, and skin in mastoid region	Mastoid nodes (retroauricular)	Superficial and deep cervical nodes
Anterior parietal region of the scalp, anterior surface of the ear, external acoustic meatus, face, and **buccal mucosa**	**Superficial parotid nodes (preauricular)**	**Deep parotid and deep cervical nodes**
External acoustic meatus, pharyngotympranic (auditory) tube, middle ear	Deep parotid nodes	Deep cervical nodes
Nasal cavity, paranasal sinuses, **hard palate (rarely), soft palate**, nasopharynx, oropharynx, and auditory tubes	**Retropharyngeal nodes**	**Deep cervical nodes**
Superficial face and cheek	**Buccal nodes**	**Submandibular nodes**
Upper lip, lateral part of the lower lip, cheek, nasal vestibule, anterior nasal cavity, **gingivae, teeth, medial canthus, hard palate, soft palate, anterior pillar, anterior part of the tongue, submandibular and sublingual glands, and floor of mouth**	**Submandibular nodes**	**Deep cervical nodes**
Chin, middle part of the lower lip, **anterior gingivae, tip of tongue, and anterior floor of mouth**	**Submental nodes**	**Submandibular and deep cervical nodes**
Oral cavity, oropharynx, nasopharynx, laryngopharynx, larynx, and parotid	**Jugulodigastric nodes**	**Deep cervical nodes**
Submental region, head and neck above this level	Jugulo-omohyoid nodes	Deep cervical nodes
Esophagus, larynx, trachea, and thyroid gland	Juxtavisceral nodes (prelaryngeal, pretracheal, and paratracheal)	Deep cervical nodes
Skin and muscles of the anterior infrahyoid region of the neck	Anterior jugular nodes	Deep cervical nodes
Inferior part of the ear and parotid region	External jugular nodes Tracheal nodes	Deep cervical nodes
Lungs, upper esophagus, part of the larynx below the vocal folds	Tracheal nodes	Bronchomediastinal trunk
Lateral part of the neck, anterior thoracic wall, mammary gland	Transverse cervical nodes	Jugular lymphatic trunk, or right lymphatic trunk, or thoracic duct

Most of the lymph from the head and neck ultimately drains to the superficial or deep cervical nodes then into the jugular lymphatic trunk. Some lymph also drains into the bronchomediastinal trunk. These trunks both empty into either the thoracic duct or right lymphatic duct and into the venous system.

Radiographs of the Head & Neck

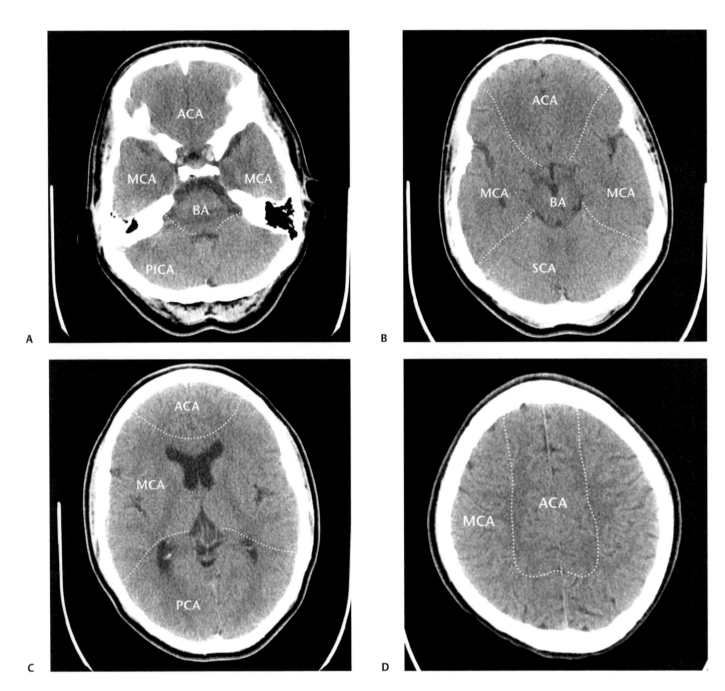

Fig. 3.32
Cerebral vascular territories and anatomy. ACA: Anterior cerebral artery. PCA: Posterior cerebral artery. MCA: Middle cerebral artery. Ach: Anterior choroidal artery. CCA: Common carotid artery. ICA: Internal carotid artery. ECA: External carotid artery. SThA: Superior thyroid artery. LA: Lingual artery. FA: Facial artery. PA: Posterior auricular artery. OC: Occipital artery. MA: Maxillary artery. STA: Superficial temporal artery. BA: Basilar artery. SCA: Superior cerebellar artery. PICA: Posterior inferior cerebellar artery. AICA: Anterior inferior cerebellar artery. PCom: Posterior communicating artery.

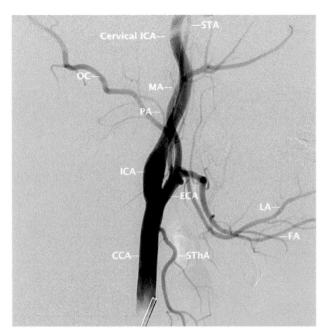

E

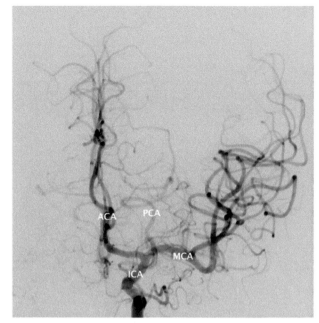

F

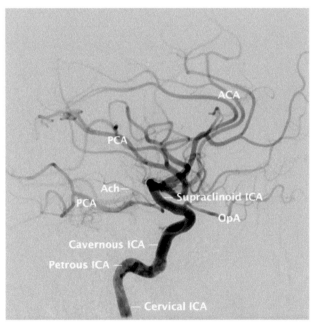

G

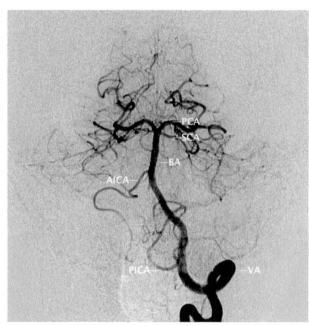

H

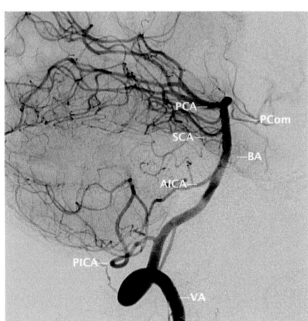

I

Organization of the Nervous System

Fig. 4.1 Nervous system

A Anterior view. **B** Posterior view. The nervous system is a collection of neurons that can be divided anatomically into two groups:

- **Central nervous system** (CNS, pink): Brain and spinal cord.
- **Peripheral nervous system** (PNS, yellow): Nerves emerging from the CNS. These are divided into two types depending on their site of emergence:
  - **Cranial nerves:** 12 pairs of nerves emerge from the brain (telencephalon, diencephalon, and brainstem only). These nerves may contain sensory and/or motor fibers.
  - **Spinal nerves:** 31 pairs of nerves emerge from the spinal cord. Spinal nerves contain both sensory and motor fibers that emerge from the spinal cord as separate roots and unite to form the mixed nerve. In certain regions, the spinal nerves may combine to form plexuses (e.g., cervical, brachial, or lumbosacral).

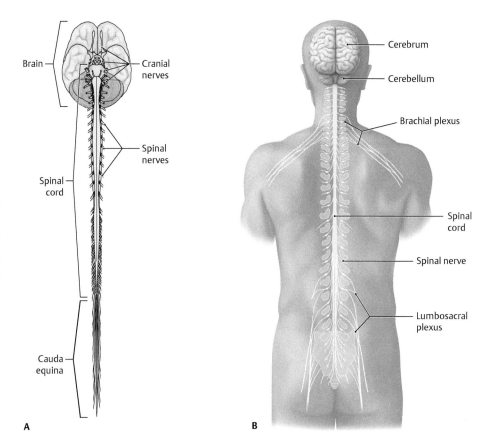

A

B

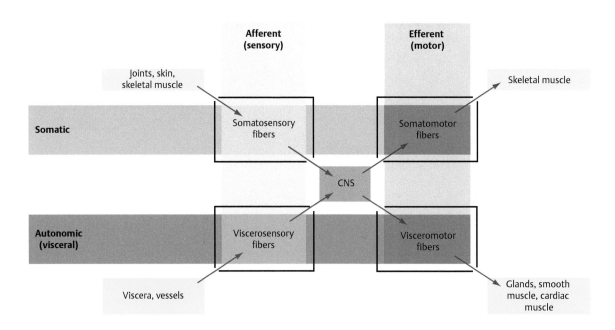

Fig. 4.2 Organization of the nervous system

The nervous system is a vast network that can be divided according to two criteria:

1. Type of information: Afferent (sensory) cells and pathways receive information and transmit it to the CNS. Efferent (motor) cells and pathways convey information from the CNS.

2. Destination/origin: The somatic division of the nervous system primarily mediates interaction with the external environment. These processes are often voluntary. The autonomic (visceral) nervous system primarily mediates regulation of the internal environment. These processes are frequently involuntary.

These two criteria yield four types of nerve fibers addressed above that connect the CNS to the PNS.

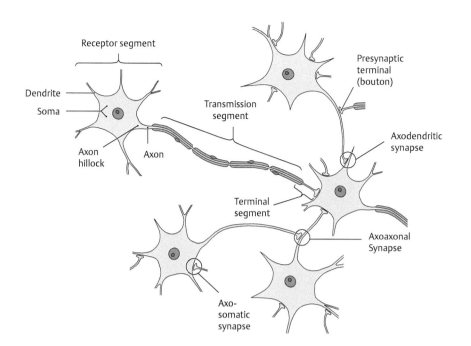

Fig. 4.3 Neurons (nerve cells)

The nervous system is composed of neurons (nerve cells) and supporting neuroglial cells, which vastly outnumber them (10 to 1). Each neuron contains a cell body (soma) with one axon (projecting segment) and one or more dendrites (receptor segments). The release of neurotransmitters at synapses creates an excitatory or inhibitory postsynaptic potential at the target neuron. If this exceeds the depolarization threshold of the neuron, the axon "fires," initiating the release of a transmitter from its presynaptic knob (bouton).

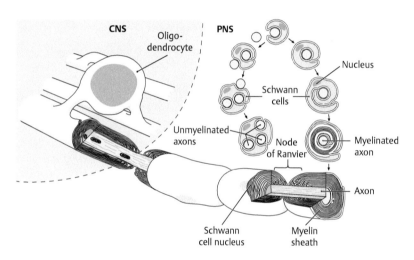

Fig. 4.4 Myelination

Certain glial cells with lipid-rich membranes may myelinate axons (nerve fibers). Myelination electrically insulates axons, thereby increasing impulse conduction speed. In the central nervous system, one oligodendrocyte myelinates one internode on multiple axons; in the peripheral nervous system, one Schwann cell myelinates one internode on a single axon.

Table 4.1 Cells of the central nervous system (CNS) and peripheral nervous system (PNS)	
Cell type	**Function**
Neurons (CNS and PNS)	Impulse formation, impulse conduction, information processing
Glial cells	
Astrocytes (CNS only)	Maintain a constant internal milieu in the CNS, help form the blood brain-barrier, phagocytosis of non-functioning synapses, scar formation in the CNS (e.g., following cerebral infarction [Stroke] or in multiple sclerosis), absorb excess neurotransmitters and K^+
Microglial cells (CNS only)	Cells specialized for phagocytosis and antigen processing; secrete cytokines and growth factors
Oligodendrocytes (CNS only)	Form myelin sheaths in the CNS
Ependymal cells (CNS only)	Line cavities in the CNS
Cells of the choroid plexus (CNS only)	Secrete cerebrospinal fluid (CSF)
Schwann cells (PNS only)	Form myelin sheaths in the PNS
Satellite cells (PNS only)	Modified Schwann cells; surround the cell body of neurons in PNS ganglia

Spinal Cord: Overview

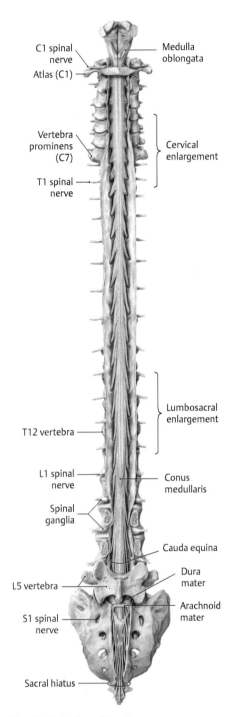

Fig. 4.5 **Spinal cord in situ**
Posterior view with vertebral canal windowed.
The spinal cord is located in the vertebral foramen and extends from the medulla oblongata to around the level of T12/L1. It gives off 31 pairs of spinal nerves. The *cervical enlargement* corresponds with the attachments of the large nerves that supply the upper limbs. It extends from about C3 to T1. Similarly, the *lumbosacral enlargement* corresponds with the attachments of the large nerves that supply the lower limbs. The posterior and anterior spinal nerve roots extending from the lower end of the spinal cord are collectively known as the cauda equina. During lumbar puncture at this level, a needle introduced into the subarachnoid space (lumbar cistern) normally slips past the spinal nerve roots without injuring them (see **Fig. 4.9**).

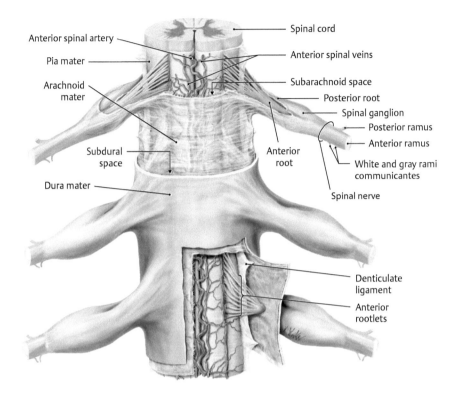

Fig. 4.6 **Spinal cord and its meningeal layers**
Posterior view. The dura mater is opened and the arachnoid is sectioned. The spinal cord, like the brain, is covered by three meninges. The outermost layer, the tough dura mater, extends from the foramen magnum to the sacrum and coccyx. The middle layer, the arachnoid mater, loosely envelopes the spinal cord and extends from foramen magnum to around the S2 vertebral level. The inner layer, the pia mater, closely invests the spinal cord and the anterior spinal artery.

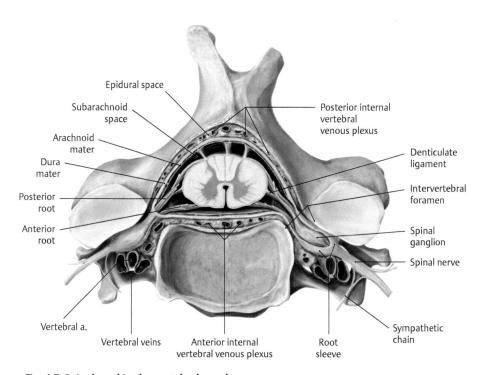

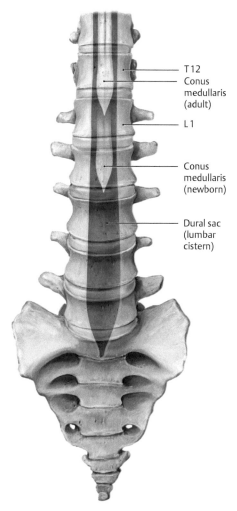

Fig. 4.7 Spinal cord in the vertebral canal

Transverse section at the level of the C4 vertebra, viewed from above. The spinal cord occupies the center of the vertebral foramen and is anchored within the subarachnoid space to the spinal dura mater by the denticulate ligament. The root sleeve, an outpouching of the dura mater in the intravertebral foramen, contains the spinal ganglion and the posterior and anterior roots of the spinal nerve. The spinal dura mater is bounded externally by the epidural space, which contains venous plexuses, fat, and connective tissue. The epidural space extends upward as far as the foramen magnum, where the dura becomes fused to the cranial periosteum.

Fig. 4.8 Age-related changes of spinal cord levels

Anterior view. As an individual grows, the longitudinal growth of the spinal cord increasingly lags behind that of the vertebral column. At birth the distal end of the spinal cord, the conus medullaris, is at the level of the L3 vertebral body (where lumbar puncture is contraindicated). The spinal cord of a tall adult ends at the T12/L1 level, whereas that of a short adult extends to the L2/L3 level. The dural sac always extends into the upper sacrum. It is important to consider these anatomical relationships during lumbar puncture. It is best to introduce the needle at the L3/L4 interspace (see **Fig. 4.9**).

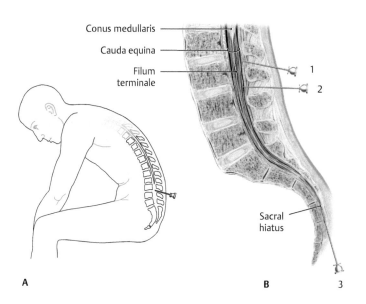

Fig. 4.9 Lumbar puncture, epidural anesthesia, and lumbar anesthesia

In preparation for a **lumbar puncture**, the patient bends far forward to separate the spinous processes of the lumbar spine. The spinal needle is usually introduced between the spinous processes of the L3 and L4 vertebrae. It is advanced through the skin and into the dural sac (lumbar cistern, see **Fig. 4.8**) to obtain a CSF sample. This procedure has numerous applications, including the diagnosis of meningitis. For **epidural anesthesia**, a catheter is placed in the epidural space without penetrating the dural sac (1). **Lumbar anesthesia** is induced by injecting a local anesthetic solution into the dural sac (2). Another option is to pass the needle into the epidural space through the sacral hiatus (3).

Spinal Cord: Circuitry & Spinal Nerves

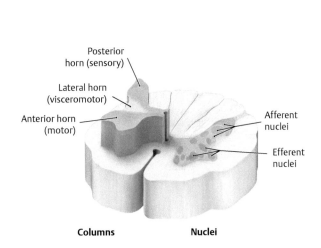

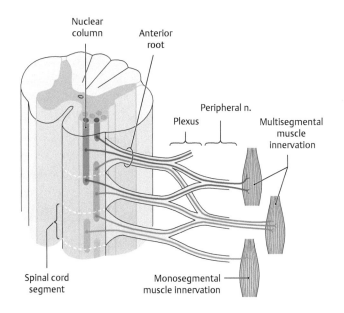

Fig. 4.10 Organization of the gray matter
Left oblique anterosuperior view. The gray matter of the spinal cord is divided into three columns (horns). Afferent (blue) and efferent (red) neurons within these columns are clustered according to function.

Fig. 4.11 Muscle innervation
Indicator muscles are innervated by motor neurons in the anterior horn of one spinal cord segment. Most muscles (multisegmental muscles) receive innervation from a motor column, a vertical arrangement of motor nuclei spanning several segments.

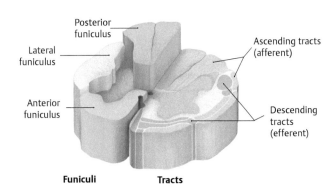

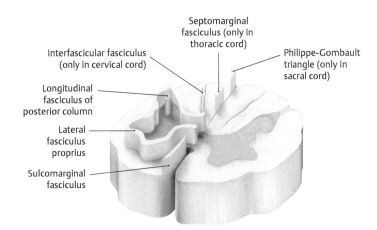

Fig. 4.12 Reflexes
Principal intrinsic fascicles of the spinal cord. Muscular function at the unconscious (reflex) level is controlled by the gray matter of the spinal cord. The intrinsic fascicles are the conduction apparatus of the intrinsic circuits, allowing axons to ascend and descend to coordinate spinal reflexes for multisegmental muscles.

Fig. 4.13 Sensory and motor systems
White matter of the spinal cord. The white matter of the spinal cord contains ascending tracts (afferent tracts) and descending tracts (efferent tracts), which are the CNS equivalent of peripheral nerves. The sensory system (see pp. 110, 111) and motor system (see pp. 114, 115) are so functionally interrelated they may be described as one (sensorimotor system).

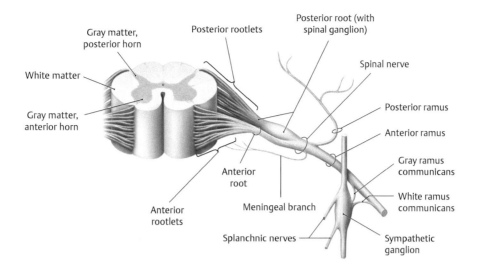

Fig. 4.14 Spinal cord segment

The spinal cord consists of 31 segments, each innervating a specific area of the skin (a dermatome) of the head, trunk, or limbs. Afferent (sensory) posterior rootlets and efferent (motor) anterior rootlets form the posterior and anterior roots of the spinal nerve for that segment. The two roots fuse to form a mixed (motor and sensory) spinal nerve that exits the intervertebral foramen and immediately thereafter divides into an anterior and posterior ramus (or branch).

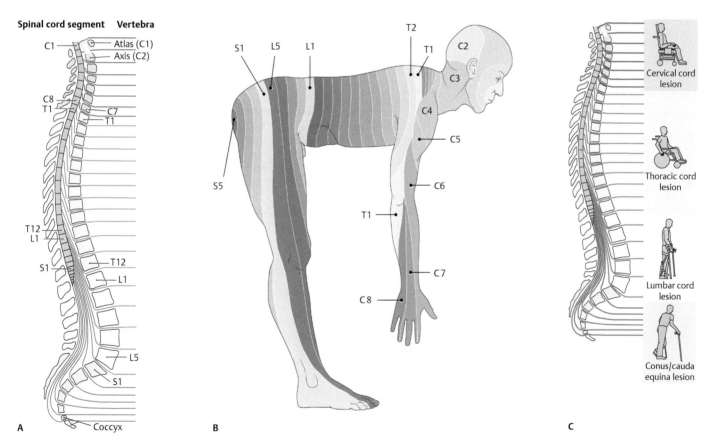

Fig. 4.15 Spinal cord segments, dermatomes, and effects of spinal cord lesions

The spinal cord is divided into four major regions: cervical, thoracic, lumbar, and sacral. The regions of the spinal cord are designated by colors: red, cervical; brown, thoracic; green, lumbar; blue, sacral.

A Spinal cord segments. Initially spinal nerves pass out above the vertebrae for which they are numbered. However, since there is an 8th cervical spinal nerve but no 8th cervical vertebra, C8 passes out above the vertebral level T1, and the spinal nerve for T1 and following pass out below the vertebral level for which they are named.

B Dermatome, bandlike areas of skin receiving sensory innervation from a single pair of spinal nerves (from a single segment of the spinal cord). *Note:* Spinal nerve C1 is purely motor; consequently there is no C1 dermatome.

C Effects of lesions in each region of the spinal cord.

Organization of the Brain & Cerebellum

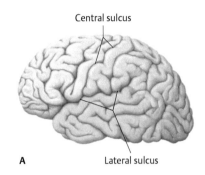

A

Central sulcus

Lateral sulcus

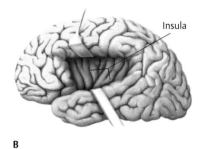

B

Insula

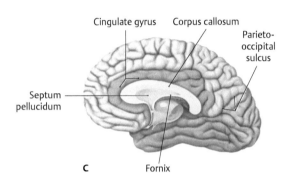

Cingulate gyrus   Corpus callosum

Parieto-occipital sulcus

Septum pellucidum

C   Fornix

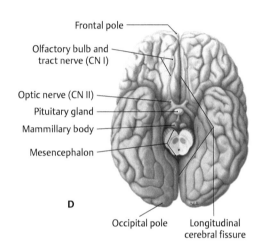

Frontal pole

Olfactory bulb and tract nerve (CN I)

Optic nerve (CN II)

Pituitary gland

Mammillary body

Mesencephalon

D

Occipital pole   Longitudinal cerebral fissure

Fig. 4.16 The brain
A Lateral view of the left hemisphere. **B** Lateral view of the retracted left hemisphere. **C** Lateral view of a sagittal section of the right hemisphere. **D** Basal (inferior) view with the brainstem removed.

The brain is divided in four major parts: telencephalon (cerebrum), diencephalon, brainstem, and cerebellum. The telencephalon (cerebrum) is the large outer portion of the brain, consisting of two hemispheres separated by a longitudinal fissure (see **D**). The telencephalon is divided into five lobes: frontal, parietal, temporal, occipital, and insular. The surface contours of the cerebrum are defined by convolutions (gyri) and depressions (sulci). The central sulcus, an important reference point on the cerebrum, separates the precentral gyrus from the postcentral gyrus. The precentral gyrus mediates voluntary motor activity, and the postcentral gyrus mediates the conscious perception of body sensation. Sulci may be narrowed and compressed in brain edema, due to excessive fluid accumulation in the brain, and are enlarged in brain atrophy (e.g., Alzheimer disease), due to tissue loss from the gyri.

Table 4.2 Functions of the cerebrum (telencephalon)		
Brain structure	**Lobe**	**Function**
Cerebrum (telencephalon)	Frontal	Motor movement; motor aspect of speech (Broca's area); reasoning; personality; problem solving
	Parietal	Sensory perceptions related to pain, temperature, touch, and pressure; spatial orientation and perception; sensory aspect of language (Wernicke's area)
	Temporal	Auditory perceptions; learning; memory; sensory aspect of language (Wernicke's area)
	Occipital	Vision
	Insula	Associated with visceral functions, e.g., taste

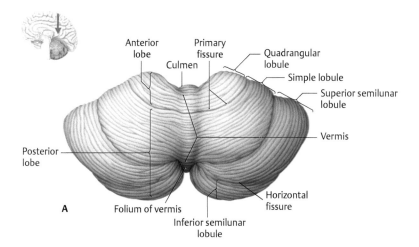

A

Anterior lobe
Primary fissure
Culmen
Quadrangular lobule
Simple lobule
Superior semilunar lobule
Vermis
Posterior lobe
Horizontal fissure
Folium of vermis
Inferior semilunar lobule

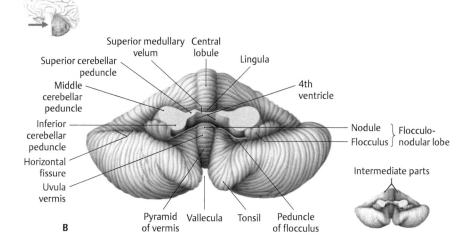

B

Superior medullary velum
Central lobule
Lingula
Superior cerebellar peduncle
Middle cerebellar peduncle
4th ventricle
Inferior cerebellar peduncle
Nodule ⎫ Flocculo-
Flocculus ⎭ nodular lobe
Horizontal fissure
Uvula vermis
Intermediate parts
Pyramid of vermis
Vallecula
Tonsil
Peduncle of flocculus

Fig. 4.17 Cerebellum
A Superior view. **B** Anterior view.
The cerebellum is part of the motor system. It cannot initiate conscious movements by itself but is responsible for unconscious coordination and fine control of muscle actions. Grossly, the cerebellar surface presents a much finer arrangement of gyri and sulci than the cerebrum, providing an even greater expansion of its surface area. Externally the cerebellum consists of two large lateral masses, the cerebellar hemispheres, and a central part, called the vermis. Cerebellar fissures further subdivide the cerebellum into lobes:

- The primary fissure separates the anterior lobe of the cerebellum from the posterior lobe.
- The posterolateral fissure separates the posterior lobe of the cerebellum from the flocculonodular lobe.

The cerebellum is connected to the brainstem by three cerebellar peduncles (superior, middle, and inferior), through which the afferent and efferent tracts enter and leave the cerebellum (see **Fig. 4.18**). The superior medullary velum stretches between the superior cerebellar peduncles and forms part of the roof of the fourth ventricle. The cerebellar tonsils protrude downward near the midline on each side, almost to the foramen magnum at the base of the skull (not shown). Increased intracranial pressure may cause the cerebellar tonsils to herniate into the foramen magnum, impinging on vital centers in the brainstem and posing a threat to life.

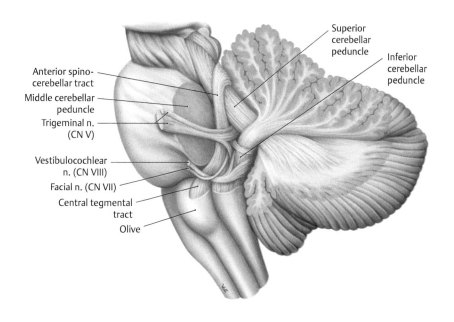

Superior cerebellar peduncle
Inferior cerebellar peduncle
Anterior spinocerebellar tract
Middle cerebellar peduncle
Trigeminal n. (CN V)
Vestibulocochlear n. (CN VIII)
Facial n. (CN VII)
Central tegmental tract
Olive

Fig. 4.18 Cerebellar peduncles
Left lateral view. The substantial mass of the peduncles reflects the extensive neural connections they carry. The cerebellum requires these numerous connections because it is the integrating center for the control of fine movements. It contains and processes vestibular and proprioceptive afferents and modulates motor nuclei in other brain regions and in the spinal cord.

Telencephalon (I): Overview, Basal Ganglia, & Neocortex

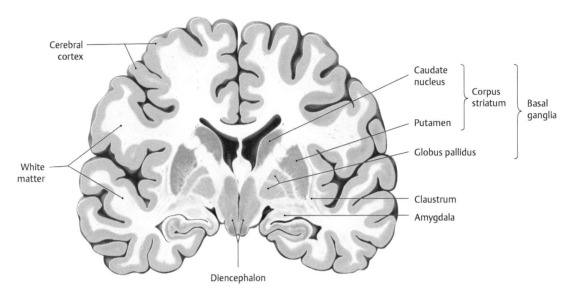

Fig. 4.19 Divisions of the telencephalon
Coronal section, anterior view. The telencephalon is divided into the cerebral cortex, white matter, and basal ganglia. The cerebral cortex is further divided into the allocortex and neocortex. The allocortex consists of the olfactory cortex and hippocampus. The neocortex is remainder and the largest portion of the cerebral cortex.

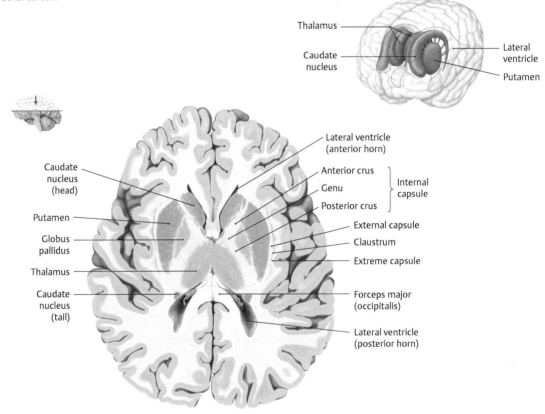

Fig. 4.20 Basal ganglia
Transverse section through the cerebrum at the level of the corpus striatum, superior view. The basal ganglia consists of the caudate nucleus, putamen, and globus pallidus and are an essential component of the extrapyramidal motor system, which controls involuntary movement and reflexes and coordinates complex movements (see p. 114). The caudate nucleus and putamen, which are separated from each other by the fibrous white matter of the internal capsule, together constitute the corpus striatum. Deficiency of dopamine in the basal ganglia is responsible for Parkinson disease.

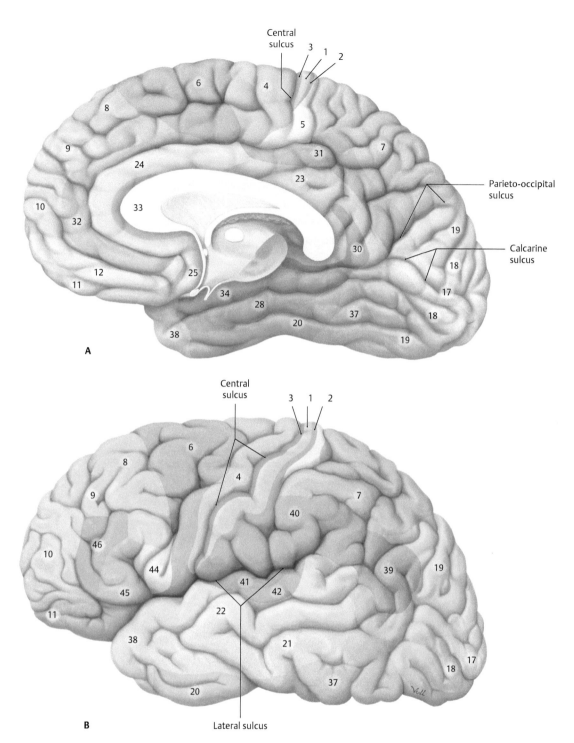

Fig. 4.21 Brodmann areas in the neocortex
A Medial view of midsagittal section of the right cerebral hemisphere; **B** Lateral view of the left cerebral hemisphere.

The surface of the brain consists macroscopically of lobes, gyri, and sulci. Microscopically, however, subtle differences can be found in the distribution of the cortical neurons, and some of these differences do not conform to the gross surface anatomy of the brain. Portions of the cerebral cortex that have the same basic microscopic features are called *cortical areas or cortical fields*. This organization into cortical areas is based on the distribution of neurons in the different layers of the cortex (*cytoarchitectonics*). In the brain map shown above, these areas are indicated by different colors. Although the size of the cortical areas may vary between individuals, the brain map pictured here is still used today as a standard reference chart. It has long been thought that the map (created by Korbinian Brodmann) accurately reflects the functional organization of the cortex, and indeed, modern imaging techniques have shown that many of the cytologically defined areas are associated with specific functions. There is no need, of course, to memorize the location of all the cortical areas, but the following areas are of special interest:

- Areas 1, 2, and 3: primary somatosensory cortex
- Area 4: primary motor cortex
- Area 17: primary visual cortex (striate area, the extent of which is best appreciated in the midsagittal section)
- Areas 41 and 42: auditory cortex

87

Telecephalon (II): Allocortex & Limbic System

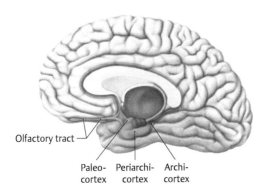

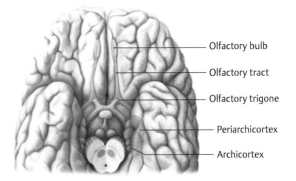

Fig. 4.22 Allocortex
A Left lateral view of the right hemisphere. **B** Basal (inferior) view.
The allocortex consists of the olfactory cortex (blue) and the hippocampus (pink). The olfactory cortex is involved with processing the sense of smell. It receives sensory afferent impulses directly from the olfactory bulb, unlike all other sensory afferent impulses that reach the cerebral cortex via the dorsal thalamus. The hippocampus is an important area for information integration and memory. Damage to the hippocampus, which occurs early in Alzheimer disease, contributes to memory loss and disorientation.

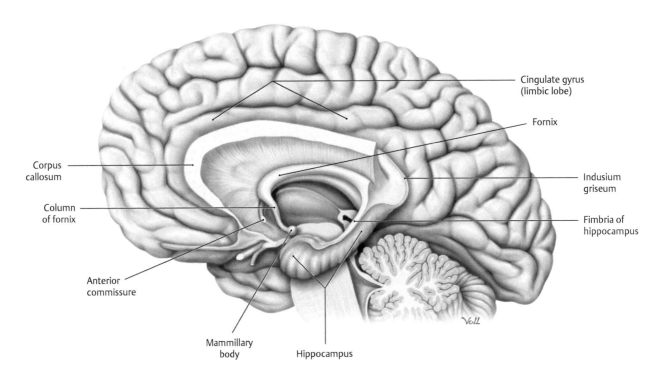

Fig. 4.23 Left hippocampal formation
Lateral view. Most of the left hemisphere has been dissected away, leaving only the corpus callosum, fornix, and hippocampus. The intact right hemisphere is visible in the background.
The hippocampal formation is an important component of the *limbic system* (see **Fig. 4.24**). It consists of three parts:

- subiculum (not shown),
- hippocampus proper, and
- dentate gyrus (not shown).

The fiber tract of the fornix connects the hippocampus to the mammillary body. The hippocampus integrates information from various brain areas and influences endocrine, visceral, and emotional processes via its efferent output. It is particulary associated with the establishment of short-term memory. Lesions of the hippocampus can therefore cause specific deficits in memory formation.

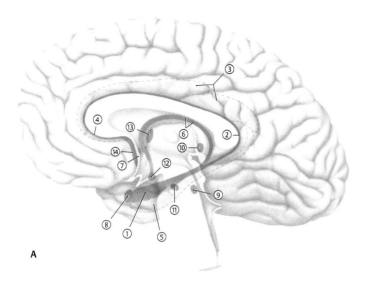

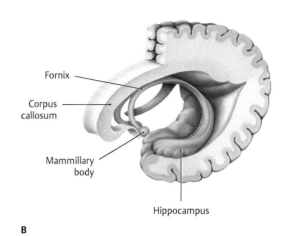

Fornix

Corpus callosum

Mammillary body

Hippocampus

A

B

Fig. 4.24 Limbic system

A Midsagittal section, left lateral view. **B** Hippocampus, left anterior oblique view.

The limbic system, which exchanges and integrates information between the telencephalon, diencephalon, and mesencephalon, regulates drive and affective behavior. It plays a crucial role in memory and learning. The amygdala (⑧, one of the subcortical nuclei) is an important structure for the processing of emotions. It is involved in the flight-or-fight response and in sexual pleasure. Dysfunction of the amygdala has been linked to conditions such as anxiety, depression, post-traumatic stress disorder, and phobias.

Table 4.3 Structures of the limbic system

Outer arc		Inner arc*		Subcortical nuclei	
①	Parahippocampal gyrus	⑤	Hippocampal formation (hippocampus, entorhinal area of parahippocampal gyrus)	⑧	Amygdala
②	Indusium griseum	⑥	Fornix	⑨	Dorsal tegmental nuclei
③	Cingulate (limbic) gyrus	⑦	Septal area (septum)	⑩	Habenular nuclei
				⑪	Interpeduncular nuclei
④	Subcallosal (paraolfactory) area	⑭	Paraterminal gyrus	⑫	Mammillary bodies
				⑬	Anterior thalamic nuclei

* The inner arc also contains the diagonal band of Broca (not shown).

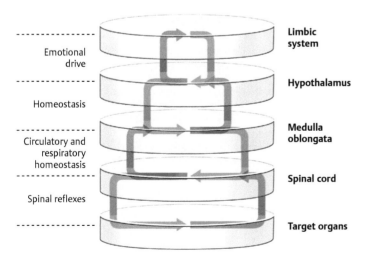

Emotional drive

Limbic system

Homeostasis

Hypothalamus

Circulatory and respiratory homeostasis

Medulla oblongata

Spinal reflexes

Spinal cord

Target organs

Fig. 4.25 Limbic regulation of the peripheral autonomic nervous system

The limbic system receives afferent feedback signals from its target organs. See **Fig. 4.68** for a diagram of the autonomic nervous system.

Diencephalon: Overview & Development

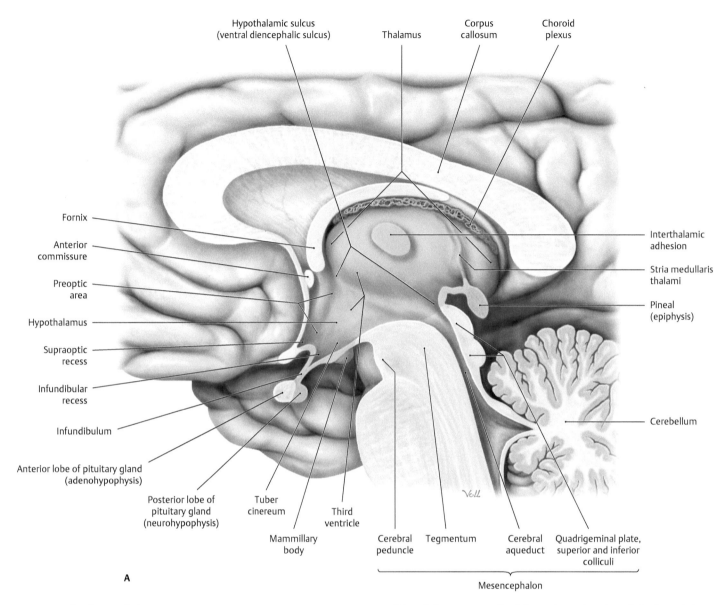

Fig. 4.26 The diencephalon

A Diencephalon and brainstem in situ, midsagittal section of the right hemisphere viewed from the left side.

B Left lateral view with telencephalon removed. The diencephalon is located below the corpus callosum, part of the telencephalon, and above the mesencephalon (midbrain). The lateral wall of the third ventricle, visible here, forms the medial boundary of the diencephalon. The thalamus makes up four fifths of the entire diencephalon, but the only parts of the diencephalon that can be seen externally are the hypothalamus (visible from the basal aspect) and portions of the epithalamus (pineal gland, visible from the occipital aspect). The diencephalon is involved in endocrine functioning and autonomic coordination of the pineal gland, the poste-

rior lobe of the pituitary gland (neurohypophysis), and the hypothalamus. It also acts as a relay station for sensory information and somatic motor control (via the thalamus).

Visible in **B** are the thalamus, the lateral geniculate body, and the optic tract. The lateral geniculate body and optic tract are components of the visual pathway. *Note:* The retina and associated optic nerve form an anterior extension of the diencephalon and therefore are colored blue here, which departs from the convention of yellow for nerves.

The optic tract marks the lateral boundary of the diencephalon. It winds around the cerebral peduncles, which are part of the adjacent mesencephalon (midbrain).

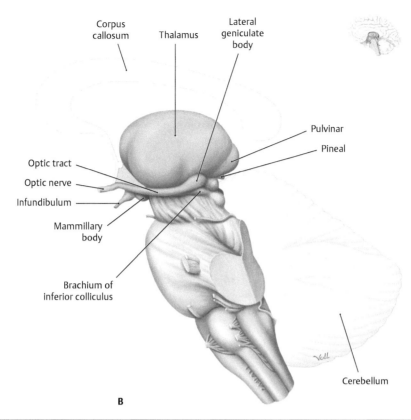

B

Table 4.4 Functions of the diencephalon

Part	Structures	Function
Epithalamus	Pineal gland Habenulae	Regulation of circadian rhythms; linking of olfactory system to brain
Thalamus	Thalamus	Relay center for the somatosensory system and parts of the motor system
Subthalamus	Subthalamic nucleus Zona incerta (not shown) Globus pallidus	Relay of sensory information (somatomotor zone of diencephalon)
Hypothalamus	Optic chiasm, optic tract Tuber cinereum (not shown) Posterior lobe of pituitary gland (neurohypophsis) Mammillary bodies	Coordination of autonomic nervous system with endocrine system; participation in visual pathway

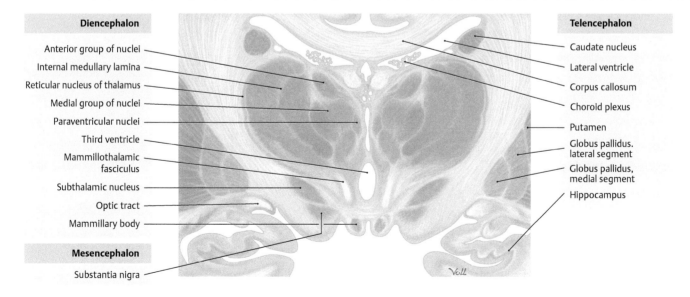

Fig. 4.27 Internal structure of the diencephalon and telecephalon
Coronal section at the level of the mammillary bodies.

Diencephalon: Thalamus & Hypothalamus

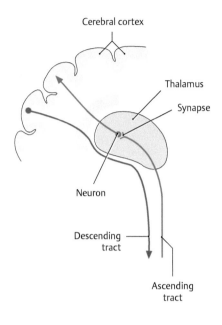

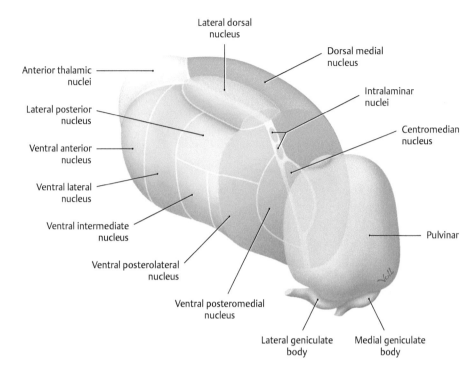

Fig. 4.28 Functional organization of the thalamus

Almost all of the sensory pathways are relayed via the thalamus and project to the cerebral cortex. Consequently, a lesion of the thalamus or its cortical projection fibers caused by a stroke or other disease leads to sensory disturbances. Although a diffuse kind of sensory perception may take place at the thalamic level (especially pain perception), cortical processing (by the telencephalon) is necessary in order to transform unconscious perception into conscious perception. The olfactory system is an exception to this rule, although its olfactory bulb is still an extension of the telencephalon. *Note:* Major descending motor tracts from the cerebral cortex generally bypass the thalamus.

Fig. 4.29 Spatial arrangement of the thalamic nuclear groups

Left thalamus viewed from the lateral and occipital aspect. The thalamus is a collection of approximately 120 nuclei that process sensory information. They are broadly classified as specific or nonspecific:

- Specific nuclei and the fibers arising from them (thalamic radiation) have direct connections with specific areas of the *cerebral cortex.* The specific thalamic nuclei are subdivided into four groups:
  - Anterior nuclei (yellow)
  - Medial nuclei (red)
  - Ventrolateral nuclei (green)
  - Dorsal nuclei (blue).

The dorsal nuclei are in contact with the medial and lateral geniculate bodies. Located beneath the pulvinar, these two nuclear bodies contain the *nuclei of the medial and lateral geniculate bodies,* and are collectively called the *metathalamus.* Like the pulvinar, they belong to the category of specific thalamic nuclei.

- *Nonspecific nuclei* have no direct connections with the cerebral cortex. Part of a general arousal system, they are connected directly to the brainstem. The only nonspecific nuclei shown in this diagram (orange) are the centromedian nucleus and the intralaminar nuclei.

Table 4.5 Clinically important connections of the thalamic nuclei		
Thalamic afferent	**Thalamic nucleus**	**Thalamic efferents**
Mammillary body (mammallothalamic fasciclus)	Anterior nucleus (NA)	Cingulate gyrus (limbic system)
Cerebellum, red nucleus	Ventral lateral nucleus (VL)	Premotor cortex
Posterior funiculus, lateral funiculus (somatosensory input from limbs and trunk)	Ventral posterolateral nucleus (VPL)	Postcentral gyrus (sensory cortex)
Trigeminothalamic tract (somatosensory input from head)	Ventral posteromedial nucleus (VPM)	Postcentral gyrus (sensory cortex)
Inferior brachium (part of auditory pathway)	Medial geniculate nucleus (body) (MGB)	Transverse temporal gyri (auditory cortex)
Optic tract	Lateral geniculate nucleus (body) (LGB)	Striate area (visual cortex)

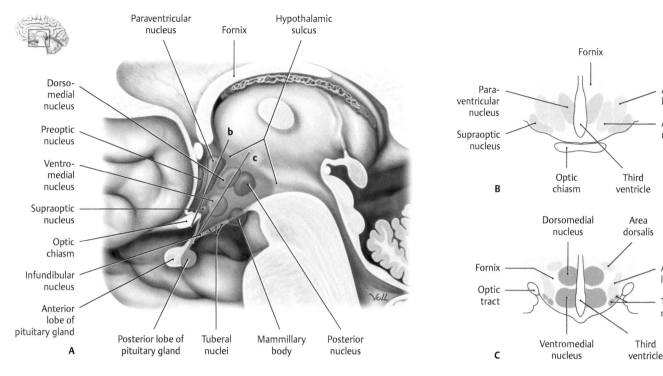

Fig. 4.30 Nuclei in the right hypothalamus
A Midsagittal section of the right hemisphere viewed from the medial side. **B, C** Coronal sections. The hypothalamus is a small nuclear complex located ventral to the thalamus and separated from it by the hypothalamic sulcus. Despite its small size, the hypothalamus is the command center for all autonomic functions in the body. Only a few of the larger, more clinically important hypothalmic nuclei are mentioned in this unit. Three groups of nuclei are listed below in an oral-to-caudal sequence, and their functions are briefly described:

* The anterior (rostral) group of nuclei (green) synthesizes the hormones released from the posterior lobe of the pituitary gland, and consists of the:
  – preoptic nucleus,
  – paraventricular nucleus, and
  – supraoptic nucleus.
* The middle (tuberal) group of nuclei (blue) controls hormone release from the anterior lobe of the pituitary gland, and consists of the:
  – dorsomedial nucleus,

  – ventromedial nucleus, and
  – tuberal nuclei.
* The posterior (mammillary) group of nuclei (red) activates the sympathetic nervous system when stimulated. It consists of the:
  – posterior nucleus and
  – mammillary nuclei located in the mammillary bodies.

The coronal section (**C**) shows the further subdivision of the hypothalamus by the fornix into lateral and medial zones. The three nuclear groups described above are part of the *medial* zone, whereas the nuclei in the *lateral* zone are not subdivided into specific groups (e.g., the area lateralis takes the place of a nucleus). Bilateral lesions of the mammillary bodies and their nuclei are manifested by *Korsakoff syndrome,* which is frequently associated with alcoholism (cause: vitamin B1 [thiamine] deficiency). The memory impairment that occurs in this syndrome mainly affects short-term memory, and the patient may fill in the memory gaps with fabricated information. A major neuropathological finding is the presence of hemorrhages in the mammillary bodies, which are sectioned at autopsy to confirm the diagnosis.

Table 4.6 Functions of the hypothalamus

Region or nucleus	Function	Lesion
Anterior preoptic region	Maintains constant body temperature	Central hypothermia
Posterior region	Responds to temperature changes, e.g., sweating	Hypothermia
Midanterior and posterior regions	Activate sympathetic nervous system	Autonomic dysfunction
Paraventricular and anterior regions	Activate parasympathetic nervous system	Autonomic dysfunction
Supraoptic and paraventricular nuclei	Regulate water balance	Diabetes insipidus Hyponatremia (low Na$^+$)
Anterior nuclei	Regulate appetite and food intake	Lesion of medial part causes obesity Lesion of lateral part causes anorexia and emaciation

Brainstem: Organization & External Structure

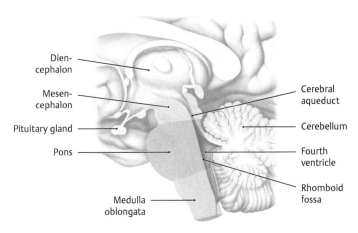

Fig. 4.31 Division of the brainstem into levels
Midsagittal section. The brainstem is divided macroscopically into three levels, with the bulge of the pons marking the boundary lines between the parts:

- Mesencephalon (midbrain)
- Pons
- Medulla oblongata

The three levels are easily distinguished from one another by gross visual inspection, although they are not differentiated in a functional sense. The *functional organization* of the brainstem is determined chiefly by the arrangement of the cranial nerve nuclei (see pp. 122, 123). Given the close proximity of nuclei and large fiber tracts in this region, even a small lesion of the brainstem (e.g., hemorrhage, tumor) may lead to extensive and complex alterations of sensorimotor function.

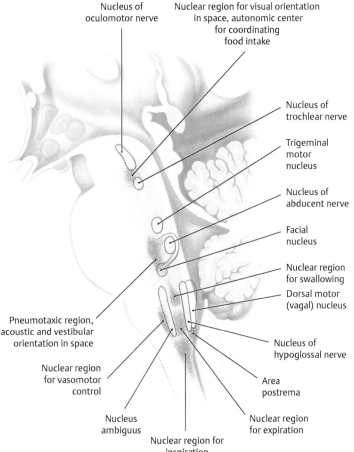

Fig. 4.32 Structural-functional relationships in the reticular formation
Midsagittal section of the brainstem viewed from the left side. While the cranial nerve nuclei, substantia nigra, and red nucleus have well-defined boundaries, as we have seen, the reticular formation (light green) is a relatively diffuse network of nerve cells and fibers in the brainstem, occupying the areas between the cranial nerve nuclei described above. It can be roughly divided into two main groups of nuclei:

- *Medial group* (specific nuclei labeled in the diagram): nuclei containing *large neurons* whose axons form long ascending and descending tracts.
- *Lateral group* (not individually labeled in the diagram): nuclei containing *small neurons* whose axons usually stay within the brainstem. They are therefore called "association areas."

Besides *respiratory and circulatory regulation,* the diffuse neuronal network of the reticular formation performs many other important autonomic functions.

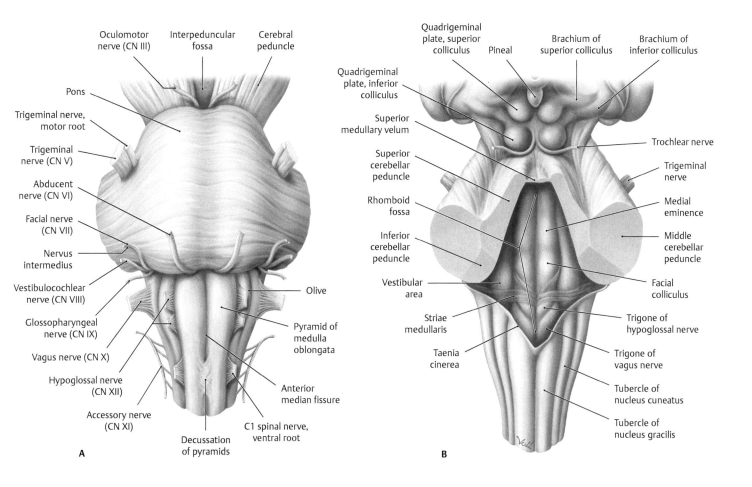

A

Oculomotor nerve (CN III)
Interpeduncular fossa
Cerebral peduncle
Pons
Trigeminal nerve, motor root
Trigeminal nerve (CN V)
Abducent nerve (CN VI)
Facial nerve (CN VII)
Nervus intermedius
Vestibulocochlear nerve (CN VIII)
Glossopharyngeal nerve (CN IX)
Vagus nerve (CN X)
Hypoglossal nerve (CN XII)
Accessory nerve (CN XI)
Decussation of pyramids
C1 spinal nerve, ventral root
Anterior median fissure
Pyramid of medulla oblongata
Olive

B

Quadrigeminal plate, superior colliculus
Pineal
Brachium of superior colliculus
Brachium of inferior colliculus
Quadrigeminal plate, inferior colliculus
Superior medullary velum
Superior cerebellar peduncle
Rhomboid fossa
Inferior cerebellar peduncle
Vestibular area
Striae medullaris
Taenia cinerea
Trochlear nerve
Trigeminal nerve
Medial eminence
Middle cerebellar peduncle
Facial colliculus
Trigone of hypoglossal nerve
Trigone of vagus nerve
Tubercle of nucleus cuneatus
Tubercle of nucleus gracilis

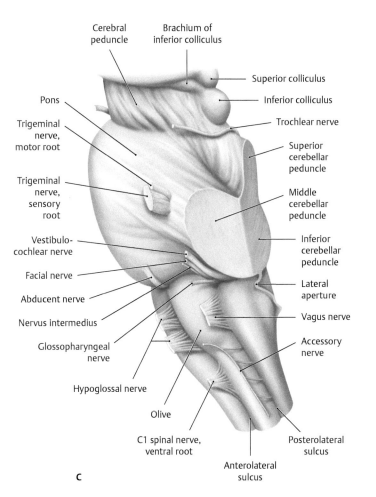

C

Cerebral peduncle
Brachium of inferior colliculus
Pons
Trigeminal nerve, motor root
Trigeminal nerve, sensory root
Vestibulo-cochlear nerve
Facial nerve
Abducent nerve
Nervus intermedius
Glossopharyngeal nerve
Hypoglossal nerve
Olive
C1 spinal nerve, ventral root
Anterolateral sulcus
Superior colliculus
Inferior colliculus
Trochlear nerve
Superior cerebellar peduncle
Middle cerebellar peduncle
Inferior cerebellar peduncle
Lateral aperture
Vagus nerve
Accessory nerve
Posterolateral sulcus

Fig. 4.33 Brainstem

A Anterior view. The sites of entry and emergence of the ten pairs of true cranial nerves (III–XII) are particularly well displayed in this view. *Note*: The ophthalmic nerve (CN I) is a derivative of the telecephalon; the optic nerve (CN II) is a derivative of the diencephalon. Note also the site below the pyramids where the pyramidal fibers cross over the midline from each side (decussation of the pyramids). Most of the axons of the large motor pathway for the trunk and limbs cross to the opposite side at this level. The cranial nerves are discussed in detail on pp. 124 to 151.

B Posterior view. Since the cerebellum has been removed, we can see the rhomboid fossa, which forms the floor of the fourth ventricle. The surface of the fossa is raised by several cranial nerve nuclei, which bulge into the fourth ventricle. The cerebellum is connected to the brainstem by three cerebellar peduncles on each side:

- Superior cerebellar peduncle
- Middle cerebellar peduncle
- Inferior cerebellar peduncle

The superior and inferior cerebellar peduncles border portions of the rhomboid fossa and thus contribute to the boundaries of the fourth ventricle.

C Left lateral view. In addition to the cerebellar peduncles, this view displays the superior and inferior colliculi. Together with their counterparts on the right side, the colliculi form the quadrigeminal plate (see **B**), which is a prominent structure of the mesencephalon. The two superior colliculi are part of the visual pathway, while the inferior colliculi are part of the auditory pathway. The trochlear nerve (CN IV) runs forward below the inferior colliculus, and is the only cranial nerve that emerges from the posterior side of the brainstem. The olive appears as a prominence on the side of the medulla oblongata. The nuclei within the olive function as a relay station for the motor system.

95

Mesencephalon & Pons: Transverse Sections

***Fig. 4.34* Transverse section through the mesencephalon (midbrain)**

Superior view.

Nuclei: The most rostral cranial nerve nucleus is the relatively small *nucleus of the oculomotor nerve*. In the same transverse plane is the *mesencephalic nucleus of the trigeminal nerve*; other trigeminal nuclei can be identified in sections at lower levels (see **Fig. 4.36**). Unique in the CNS, the mesencephalic nucleus of the trigeminal nerve contains displaced pseudounipolar sensory neurons, closely related to the PNS neurons of the trigeminal ganglion (both populations are derived embryonically from the neural crest). The peripheral processes of these mesencephalic neurons are proprioceptors in the muscles of mastication. The *superior collicular nucleus* is part of the visual system. The *red nucleus* and *substantia nigra* are involved in coordination of motor activity. The red nucleus and all of the cranial nerve nuclei are located in the tegmentum of the mesencephalon, the superior colliculus is in the tectum (roof) of the mesencephalon, and the substantia nigra is in the cerebral peduncle. Different parts of the reticular formation, a diffuse aggregation of nuclear groups (see Fig. 4.32, p. 94), are visible here and in sections below.

Tracts: The tracts at this level run anterior to the nuclear regions. Prominent descending

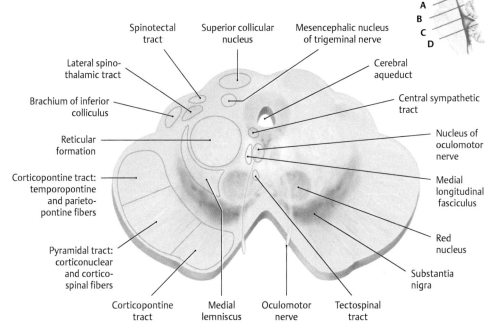

tracts seen at this level include the pyramidal tract and the corticonuclear fibers that branch from it. Ascending tracts visible at this level include the lateral spinothalamic tract and the medial lemniscus, both of which terminate in the thalamus.

***Fig. 4.35* Transverse section through the upper pons**

Superior view.

Nuclei: The only cranial nerve nucleus appearing in this plane of section is the mesencephalic trigeminal nucleus. It can be seen that the fibers from the nucleus of the trochlear nerve (CN IV) cross to the opposite side (decussate) while still within the brainstem.

Tracts: The ascending and descending tract systems are the same as in **Figs. 4.34** and **4.36**. The pyramidal tract appears less compact at this level compared with the previous section due to the presence of intermingled pontine nuclei. This section cuts the tracts (mostly efferent) that exit the cerebellum through the superior cerebellar peduncle. The lateral lemniscus at the posteiror surface of the section is part of the auditory pathway. The relatively large *medial* longitudinal fasciculus extends from the mesencephalon (see **Fig. 4.34**) into the spinal cord. It interconnects the brainstem nuclei and contains a variety of fibers that enter and emerge at various levels (*"highway of the brainstem nuclei"*). The smaller *dorsal* longitudinal fasciculus connects hypothalamic nuclei with the parasympathetic cranial nerve nuclei. The size and location of the nuclei of the reticular formation, which here are shown

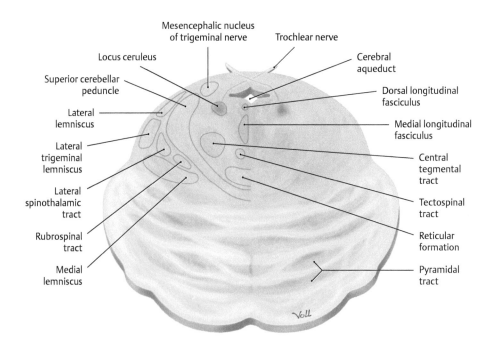

graphically within a compact area, vary with the plane of the section. This diagram indicates only the approximate location of the reticular formation, and other smaller nuclei and fibers may be found within these regions.

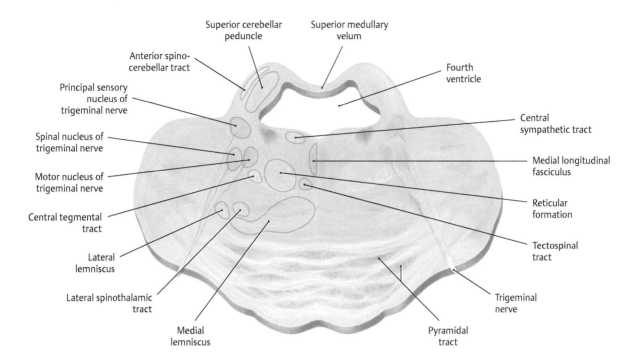

Fig. 4.36 Transverse section through the midportion of the pons
Nuclei: The trigeminal nerve leaves the brainstem at the midlevel of the pons, its various nuclei dominating the pontine tegmentum. The *principal sensory nucleus* of the trigeminal nerve relays afferents for touch and discrimination, while its *spinal nucleus* relays pain and temperature fibers. The trigeminal motor nucleus contains the motor neurons for the muscles of mastication.

Tracts: This section cuts the anterior spinocerebellar tract, which passes to the cerebellum, immediately dorsal to the pons.
CSF space: At this level the cerebral aqueduct has given way to the fourth ventricle, which appears in cross section. It is covered dorsally by the medullary velum.

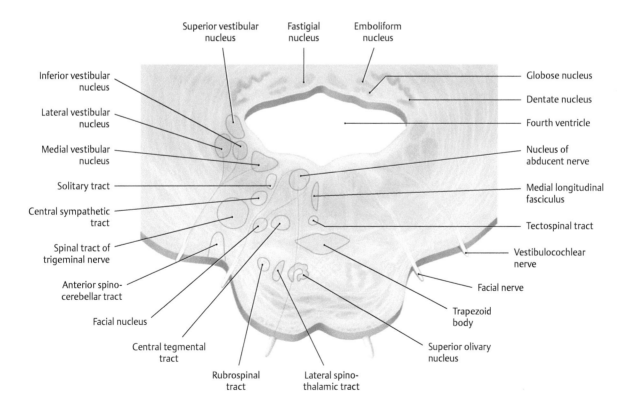

Fig. 4.37 Transverse section through the lower pons (D)
Nuclei: The lower pons contains a number of cranial nerve nuclei including the nuclei of the vestibulocochlear and abducent nerves, and the facial (motor) nucleus. The rhomboid fossa is covered dorsally by the cerebellum, whose nuclei also appear in this section—the fastigial nucleus, emboliform nucleus, globose nucleus, and dentate nucleus.

Tracts: The trapezoid body with its subnuclei is an important relay station and crossing point in the auditory pathway. The central tegmental tract is an important pathway in the motor system.

Medulla Oblongata: Transverse Sections

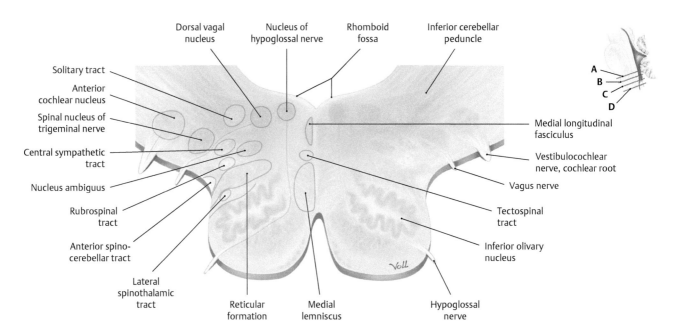

Fig. 4.38 Transverse section through the upper medulla oblongata (A)

Nuclei: The nuclei of the hypoglossal nerve, vagus nerve, vestibulocochlear nerve, and the spinal nucleus of the trigeminal nerve appear in the *posterior* part of the medulla oblongata. The inferior olivary nucleus, which belongs to the motor system, is located in the *anterior* part of the medulla oblongata. The reticular formation is interposed between the cranial nerve nuclei and the inferior olivary nucleus. It appears in all the transverse sections of this section.

Tracts: Most of the ascending and descending tracts are the same as in **Fig. 4.37**. A new structure appearing at this level is the *inferior cerebellar peduncle*, through which afferent tracts pass to the cerebellum.

CSF space: The floor of the fourth ventricle is the rhomboid fossa, which marks the dorsal boundary of this section.

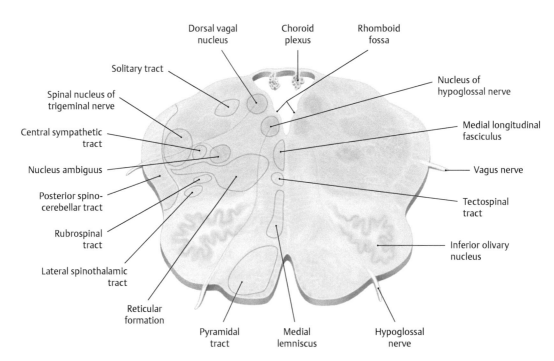

Fig. 4.39 Transverse section just above the middle of the medulla oblongata (B)

Nuclei: The only cranial nerve nuclei visible at this level are those of the hypoglossal nerve, vagus nerve, and trigeminal nerve, appearing in the posterior medulla. The lower portion of the inferior olivary nucleus appears in the anterior medulla.

Tracts: The ascending and descending tracts are the same as in **Fig. 4.37**. Ascending sensory tracts (from nuclei gracilis and cuneatus) decussate in the *medial lemniscus*. The solitary tract carries the gustatory fibers of cranial nerves V, VII, and X. Posterolateral to it is the *nucleus of the solitary tract* (not shown). The *pyramidal tract* again appears as a compact structure at this level due to the absence of interspersed nuclei and decussating fibers.

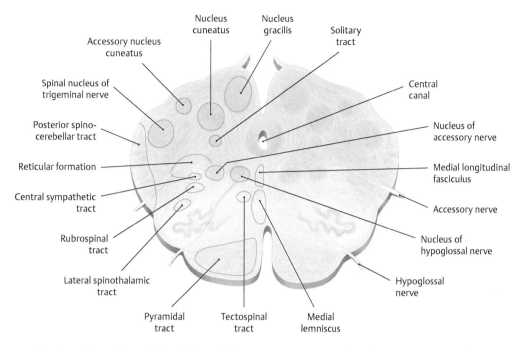

Nucleus cuneatus
Nucleus gracilis
Solitary tract
Accessory nucleus cuneatus
Spinal nucleus of trigeminal nerve
Central canal
Posterior spino-cerebellar tract
Nucleus of accessory nerve
Reticular formation
Medial longitudinal fasciculus
Central sympathetic tract
Accessory nerve
Rubrospinal tract
Nucleus of hypoglossal nerve
Lateral spinothalamic tract
Hypoglossal nerve
Pyramidal tract
Tectospinal tract
Medial lemniscus

Fig. 4.40 Transverse section just below the middle of the medulla oblongata (C)
Nuclei: The nuclei of the hypoglossal, vagus, and trigeminal nerves appear at this level. The irregular outline of the inferior olivary nucleus is still just visible in the anterior medulla. The nuclei that relay signals from the posterior funiculus—the nucleus cuneatus and nucleus gracilis—appear prominently in the posterior part of the section. The tracts that arise from these nuclei decussate in the medial lemniscus (see above).
Tracts: The ascending and descending tracts correspond to those in the previous figures in this section. The rhomboid fossa, which is the floor of the fourth ventricle, has narrowed substantially at this level to become the central canal.

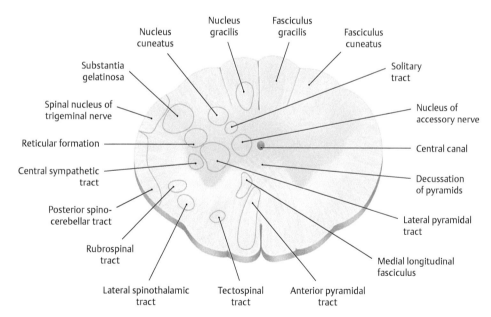

Nucleus cuneatus
Nucleus gracilis
Fasciculus gracilis
Fasciculus cuneatus
Substantia gelatinosa
Solitary tract
Spinal nucleus of trigeminal nerve
Nucleus of accessory nerve
Reticular formation
Central canal
Central sympathetic tract
Decussation of pyramids
Posterior spino-cerebellar tract
Lateral pyramidal tract
Rubrospinal tract
Medial longitudinal fasciculus
Lateral spinothalamic tract
Tectospinal tract
Anterior pyramidal tract

Fig. 4.41 Transverse section through the lower medulla oblongata (D)
The medulla oblongata is continuous with the spinal cord at this level, showing no distinct transition.
Nuclei: The cranial nerve nuclei visible at this level are the spinal part of the trigeminal nerve and the nucleus of the accessory nerve. This section passes through the caudal ends of the nuclei in the relay station of the posterior funiculus—the nucleus cuneatus and nucleus gracilis.
Tracts: The ascending and descending tracts correspond to those in the previous figures in this section. The section passes through the decussation of the pyramids, and we can now distinguish the anterior pyramidal tract (uncrossed) from the lateral pyramidal tract (crossed).
CSF space: This section passes through a portion of the central canal, which is markedly smaller at this level than in **Fig. 4.40**. It may even be obliterated at some sites, but this has no clinical significance.

Cerebrospinal Fluid (CSF) Spaces & Ventricles

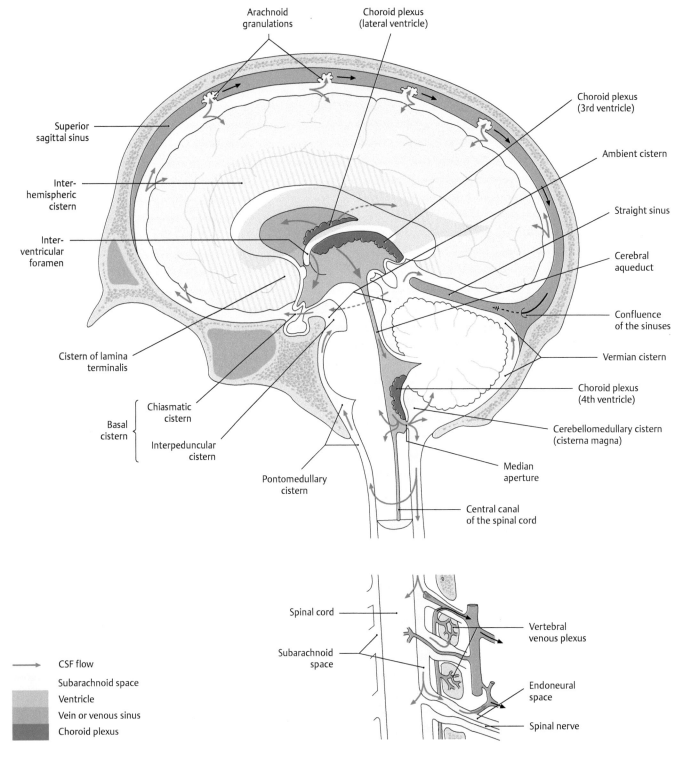

Fig. 4.42 CSF spaces

Schematic midsagittal section. Medial view of right hemisphere. The brain and spinal cord are suspended in CSF. CSF is located in the subarachnoid space enclosed by the meningeal layers surrounding the brain and spinal cord. The cerebral ventricles and subarachnoid space have a combined capacity of approximately 150 mL of CSF (80% in subarachnoid space, 20% in ventricles). This volume is completely replaced two to four times daily. CSF is produced in the choroid plexus (red) and is present in each of the four cerebral ventricles. It flows from the ventricles through the median and lateral apertures (not shown) into the subarachnoid space. Most CSF drains from the subarachnoid space through the arachnoid granulations into the dural venous sinuses. Smaller amounts drain along the proximal portions of the spinal nerves into venous plexuses or lymphatic pathways. Obstruction of CSF drainage will cause a rapid rise in intracranial pressure due to the high rate of CSF turnover.

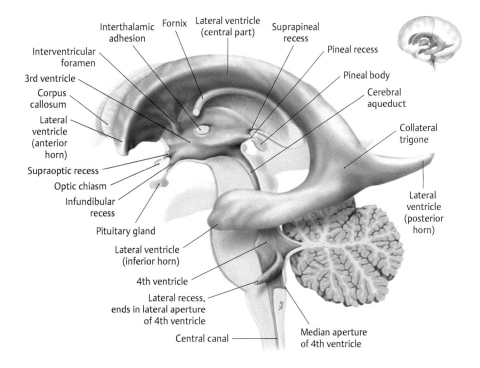

Fig. 4.43 Ventricular system with its neighboring structures
Left lateral view. The ventricular system is a greatly expanded and convoluted tube that represents a continuation of the central spinal canal into the brain. There are *four cerebral ventricles*, or cavities, filled with cerebrospinal fluid and lined by a specialized epithelium, the ependyma. The four ventricles are as follows:

- The *two* lateral ventricles, each of which communicates through an interventricular foramen with the
- third ventricle, which in turn communicates through the cerebral aqueduct with the
- fourth ventricle. This ventricle communicates with the subarachnoid space (see **Fig. 4.42**).

The largest ventricles are the lateral ventricles, each of which consists of an anterior, inferior, and posterior horn and a central part. Certain portions of the ventricular system can be assigned to specific parts of the brain: the anterior (frontal) horn to the frontal lobe of the cerebrum, the inferior (temporal) horn to the temporal lobe, the posterior (occipital) horn to the occipital lobe, the third ventricle to the diencephalon, the aqueduct to the mesencephalon (midbrain), and the fourth ventricle to the rhombencephalon (hindbrain).

Certain diseases (e.g., atrophy of brain tissue in Alzheimer's disease and internal hydrocephalus) are characterized by abnormal enlargement of the ventricular system and are diagnosed from the size of the ventricles in sectional images of the brain.

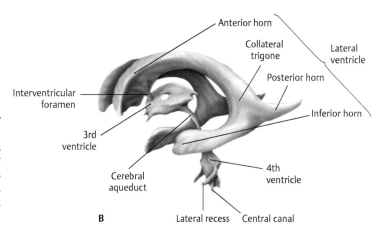

Fig. 4.44 Cast of the ventricular system
A Superior view. B Left lateral view.
These cast specimens demonstrate the four ventricular cavities and their connections.
Hydrocephalus is an excess of cerebrospinal fluid (CSF) in the ventricles of the brain. It usually occurs due to partial obstruction of the flow of CSF between the ventricles or between the ventricles and other parts of the brain. Excess CSF in the ventricles causes them to dilate and exert pressure on the surrounding cortex. In infants, the bones of the calvaria separate giving the characteristic increase in head size.

Arteries of the Brain

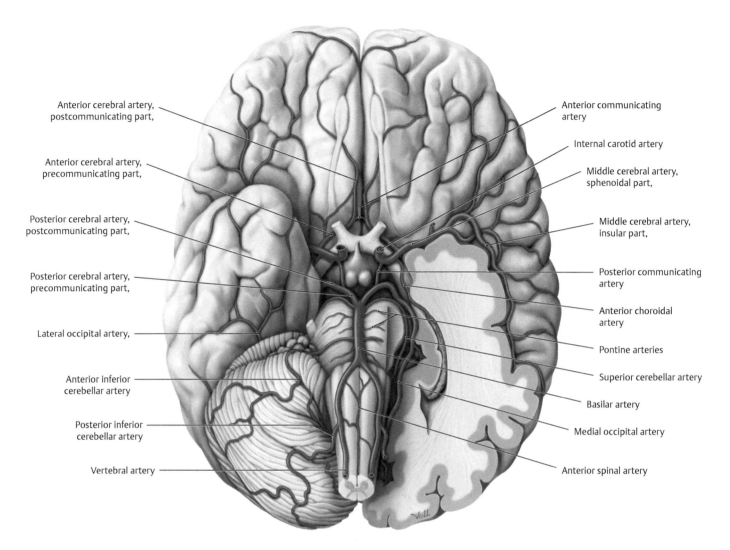

Anterior cerebral artery, postcommunicating part,

Anterior cerebral artery, precommunicating part,

Posterior cerebral artery, postcommunicating part,

Posterior cerebral artery, precommunicating part,

Lateral occipital artery,

Anterior inferior cerebellar artery

Posterior inferior cerebellar artery

Vertebral artery

Anterior communicating artery

Internal carotid artery

Middle cerebral artery, sphenoidal part,

Middle cerebral artery, insular part,

Posterior communicating artery

Anterior choroidal artery

Pontine arteries

Superior cerebellar artery

Basilar artery

Medial occipital artery

Anterior spinal artery

Fig. 4.45 Arteries at the base of the brain
The cerebellum and temporal lobe have been removed on the left side to display the course of the posterior cerebral artery. This view was selected because most of the arteries that supply the brain enter the cerebrum from its basal aspect (also see **Fig. 3.17** for the circle of Willis).
Note: The three principal arteries of the cerebrum, the anterior, middle and posterior cerebral arteries, arise from different sources. The anterior

and middle cerebral arteries are branches of the internal carotid artery, while the posterior cerebral arteries are terminal branches of the basilar artery. The vertebral arteries, which fuse to form the basilar artery, distribute branches to the spinal cord, brainstem, and cerebellum (anterior spinal artery, posterior spinal arteries, superior cerebellar artery, and anterior and posterior inferior cerebellar arteries).

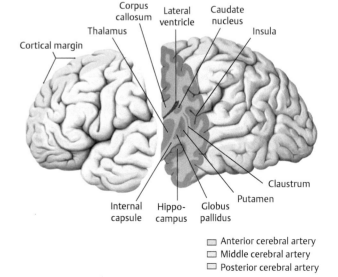

Corpus callosum

Lateral ventricle

Caudate nucleus

Thalamus

Insula

Cortical margin

Claustrum

Putamen

Internal capsule

Hippo-campus

Globus pallidus

□ Anterior cerebral artery
□ Middle cerebral artery
□ Posterior cerebral artery

Fig. 4.46 Cerebral arteries: Distribution areas
Lateral view of the left hemisphere. The central gray and white matter have a complex blood supply (yellow) that includes the anterior choroidal artery.

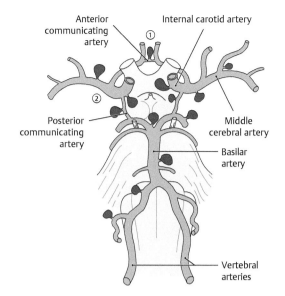

Fig. 4.47 **Sites of berry aneurysms at the base of the brain**
(after Bähr and Frotscher)
The rupture of congenital or acquired arterial aneurysms at the base of the brain is the most frequent cause of subarachnoid hemorrhage and accounts for approximately 5 % of all strokes. These are abnormal saccular dilations of the circle of Willis and are especially common at the site of branching. When one of these thin-walled aneurysms ruptures, arterial blood escapes into the subarachnoid space. The most common site is the junction between the anterior cerebral and anterior communicating arteries (1); the second most likely site is the branching of the posterior communicating artery from the internal carotid artery (2).

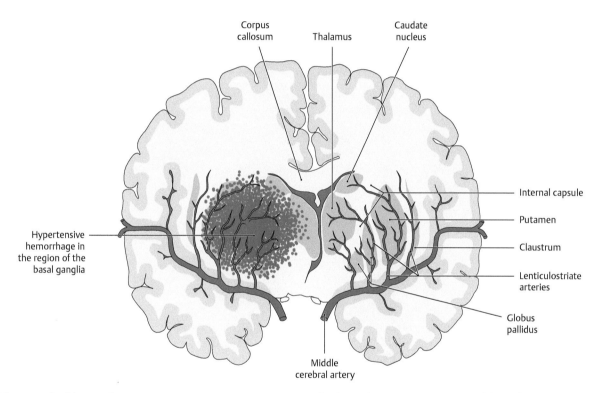

Fig. 4.48 **Intracerebral hemorrhage**
Coronal section at the level of the thalamus. Unlike the *extracerebral* hemorrhages described above, *intracerebral* hemorrhage occurs when damaged arteries bleed directly *into the substance of the brain*. This distinction is of very great clinical importance because extracerebral hemorrhages can be controlled by surgical hemostasis of the bleeding vessel, whereas intracerebral hemorrhages cannot. The most frequent cause of intracerebral hemorrhage (hemorrhagic stroke) is hypertension (high blood pressure). Because the soft brain tissue offers very little resistance, a large hematoma may form within the brain. The most common sources of intracerebral bleeding are specific branches of the middle cerebral artery—

the lenticulostriate arteries pictured here (known also as the "stroke arteries"). The hemorrhage causes a cerebral infarction (death of brain tissue) in the region of the internal capsule, one effect of which is to disrupt the pyramidal tract, which passes through the capsule. The loss of pyramidal tract function below the lesion is manifested clinically by spastic paralysis of the limbs on the side of the body *opposite* to the injury (the pyramidal tracts cross below the level of the lesion). The hemorrhage is not always massive, and smaller bleeds may occur in the territories of the three main cerebral arteries, producing a typical clinical presentation (see **Fig. 4.55**).

Veins of the Brain: Superficial & Deep Veins

Because the veins of the brain do not run parallel to the arteries, marked differences are noted between the regions of arterial supply and venous drainage. While all of the cerebral arteries enter the brain at its base, venous blood is drained from the entire surface of the brain, including the base, and also from the interior of the brain by two groups of veins: *the superficial cerebral veins* and the *deep cerebral veins*. The superficial veins drain blood from the cerebral cortex (via cortical veins) and white matter

(via medullary veins) directly into the dural sinuses. The deep veins drain blood from the deeper portions of the white matter, basal ganglia, corpus callosum, and diencephalon into the great cerebral vein, which enters the straight sinus. The two venous regions (those of the superficial and deep veins) are interconnected by numerous intracerebral anastomoses (see **Fig. 4.52**).

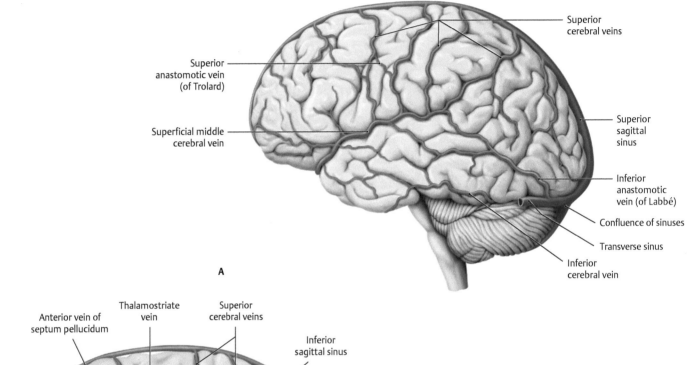

A

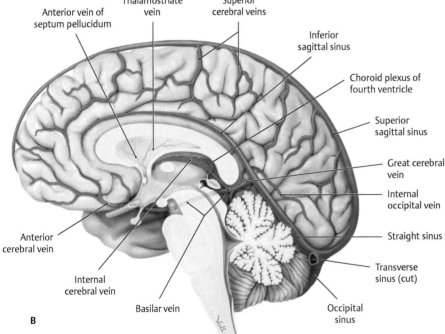

B

Fig. 4.49 Superficial veins of the brain (superficial cerebral veins)
A Left lateral view. **B** Medial view.
A, B The superficial cerebral veins drain blood from the short cortical veins and long medullary veins in the white matter (see **Fig. 4.52**) into the dural sinuses. Their course is extremely variable, and veins in the subarachnoid space do not follow arteries, gyri, or sulci. Consequently, only the most important of these vessels are named here.

Just before terminating in the dural sinuses, the veins leave the subarachnoid space and run a short subdural course between the dura mater and arachnoid. These short subdural venous segments are called *bridging veins*. The bridging veins have great clinical importance because they may be ruptured by head trauma, resulting in a subdural hematoma (see p. 109).

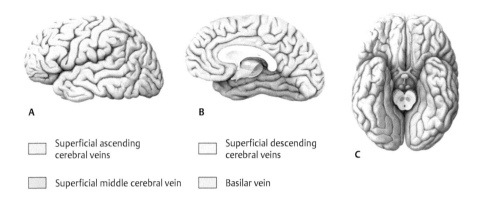

A **B** **C**

☐ Superficial ascending cerebral veins

☐ Superficial descending cerebral veins

▨ Superficial middle cerebral vein

☐ Basilar vein

Fig. 4.50 Regions drained by the superficial cerebral veins
A Left lateral view, **B** view of the medial surface of the right hemisphere, **C** basal view.
The veins on the lateral surface of the brain are classified by their direction of drainage as ascending (draining into the superior sagittal sinus) or descending (draining into the transverse sinus). The superficial middle cerebral vein drains into both the cavernous and transverse sinuses.

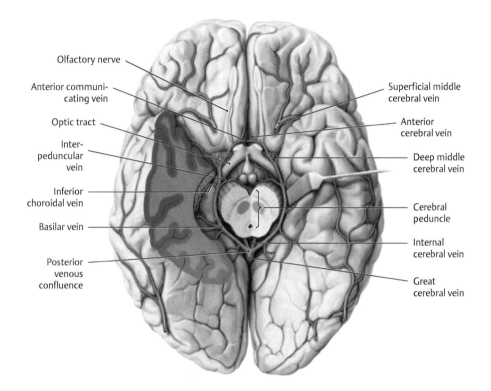

Olfactory nerve

Anterior communicating vein

Optic tract

Interpeduncular vein

Inferior choroidal vein

Basilar vein

Posterior venous confluence

Superficial middle cerebral vein

Anterior cerebral vein

Deep middle cerebral vein

Cerebral peduncle

Internal cerebral vein

Great cerebral vein

Fig. 4.51 Basal cerebral venous system
The basal cerebral venous system drains blood from both superficial and deep cerebral veins. A venous circle formed by the basilar veins (of Rosenthal) exists at the base of the brain, analogous to the arterial circle of Willis. The basilar vein is formed in the anterior perforate substance by the union of the anterior cerebral and deep middle cerebral veins. Following the course of the optic tract, the basilar vein runs posteriorly around the cerebral peduncle and unites with the basilar vein from the opposite side on the dorsal aspect of the mesencephalon. The two internal cerebral veins also terminate at this venous junction, the posterior venous confluence. This junction gives rise to the midline great cerebral vein, which enters the straight sinus. The basilar vein receives tributaries from deep brain regions in its course (e.g., veins from the thalamus and hypothalamus, choroid plexus of the inferior horn, etc.). The two anterior cerebral veins are interconnected by the anterior communicating vein, creating a closed, ring-shaped drainage system.

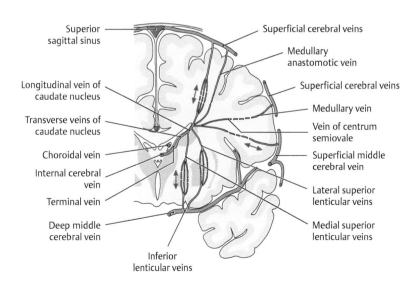

Superior sagittal sinus

Longitudinal vein of caudate nucleus

Transverse veins of caudate nucleus

Choroidal vein

Internal cerebral vein

Terminal vein

Deep middle cerebral vein

Inferior lenticular veins

Superficial cerebral veins

Medullary anastomotic vein

Superficial cerebral veins

Medullary vein

Vein of centrum semiovale

Superficial middle cerebral vein

Lateral superior lenticular veins

Medial superior lenticular veins

Fig. 4.52 Anastomoses between the superficial and deep cerebral veins
Basal cerebral venous system
Transverse section through the left hemisphere, anterior view. The superficial cerebral veins communicate with the deep cerebral veins through the anastomoses shown here. Flow reversal (double arrows) may occur in the boundary zones between two territories.

105

Blood Vessels of the Brain: Cerebrovascular Disease

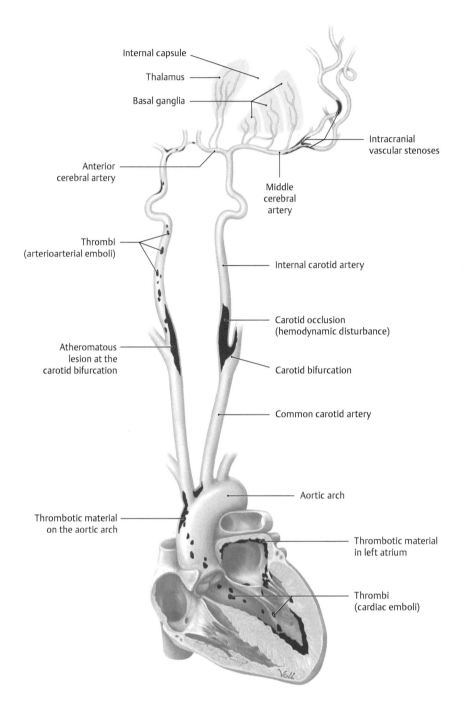

Fig. 4.53 Frequent causes of cerebrovascular disease (after Mumenthaler)

Disturbances of cerebral blood flow that deprive the brain of oxygen (cerebral ischemia) are the most frequent cause of central neurological deficits. The most serious complication is stroke: the vast majority of all strokes are caused by cerebral *ischemic* disease. Stroke has become the third leading cause of death in western industrialized countries (approximately 700,000 strokes occur in the United States each year). Cerebral ischemia is caused by a prolonged diminution or interruption of blood flow and involves *the distribution area of the internal carotid artery* in up to 90 % of cases. Much less commonly, cerebral ischemia is caused by an obstruction of venous outflow due to cerebral venous thrombosis

(see **Fig. 4.54**). A decrease of arterial blood flow in the carotid system most commonly results from an embolic or local thrombotic occlusion. Most emboli originate from atheromatous lesions at the carotid bifurcation (arterioarterial emboli) or from the expulsion of thrombotic material from the left ventricle (cardiac emboli). Blood clots (thrombi) may be dislodged from the heart as a result of valvular disease or atrial fibrillation. This produces emboli that may be carried by the bloodstream to the brain, where they may cause the functional occlusion of an artery supplying the brain. The most common example of this involves all of the distribution region of the middle cerebral artery, which is a direct continuation of the internal carotid artery.

Right 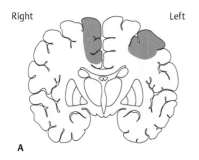 Left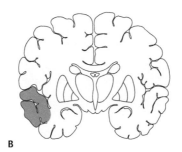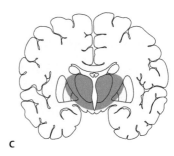

A   B   C

***Fig. 4.54* Cerebral venous thrombosis**
Coronal section, anterior view. The cerebral veins, like the cerebral arteries, serve specific territories (see pp. 102 and 105). Though much less common than decreased arterial flow, the obstruction of venous outflow is an important potential cause of ischemia and infarction. With a thrombotic occlusion, for example, the quantity of blood and thus the venous pressure are increased in the tributary region of the occluded vein. This causes a drop in the capillary pressure gradient, with an increased extravasation of fluid from the capillary bed into the brain tissue (edema). There is a concomitant reduction of arterial inflow into the affected region, depriving it of oxygen. The occlusion of specific cerebral veins (e.g., due to cerebral venous thrombosis) leads to brain infarctions (stroke) at characteristic locations:

A Superior cerebral veins: Thrombosis and infarction in the areas drained by the:

- Medial superior cerebral veins (right, *symptoms:* contralateral lower limb weakness);

- Posterior superior cerebral veins (left, *symptoms:* contralateral hemiparesis).

Motor aphasia occurs if the infarction involves the motor speech center in the dominant hemisphere.

B Inferior cerebral veins: Thrombosis of the right inferior cerebral veins leads to infarction of the right temporal lobe (*symptoms:* sensory aphasia, contralateral hemianopia).

C Internal cerebral veins: Bilateral thrombosis leads to a symmetrical infarction affecting the thalamus and basal ganglia. This is characterized by a rapid deterioration of consciousness ranging to coma.

Because the dural sinuses have extensive anastomoses, a limited occlusion affecting part of a sinus often does not cause pronounced clinical symptoms, unlike the venous thromboses described here.

Vascular territory	Neurological symptoms	
Anterior cerebral artery	Hemiparesis (with or without hemisensory deficit)	Bladder dysfunction
Middle cerebral artery	Hemiparesis (with or without hemisensory deficit) mainly affecting the arm and face (Wernicke-Mann type)	Aphasia
Posterior cerebral artery	Hemisensory losses	Hemianopia

***Fig. 4.55* Cardinal symptoms of occlusion of the three main cerebral arteries** (after Masuhr and Neumann)
When the *anterior, middle* or *posterior cerebral artery* becomes occluded, characteristic functional deficits occur in the oxygen-deprived brain areas supplied by the occluded vessel. In many cases the affected artery can be identified based on the associated neurological deficit:

- Bladder weakness (cortical bladder center) and paralysis of the lower limb (hemiplegia with or without hemisensory deficit, predominantly affecting the leg) on the side opposite the occlusion indicate an infarction in the territory of the **anterior cerebral artery**.
- Contralateral hemiplegia affecting the arm and face more than the leg indicates an infarction in the territory of the **middle cerebral artery**. If the dominant hemisphere is affected, aphasia also occurs (the patient cannot name objects, for example).
- Visual disturbances affecting the contralateral visual field (hemianopia) may signify an infarction in the territory of the **posterior cerebral artery**, because the structures supplied by this artery include the visual cortex in the calcarine sulcus of the occipital lobe. If branches to the thalamus are also affected, the patient may also exhibit a contralateral hemisensory deficit because the afferent sensory fibers have already crossed below the thalamus.

The extent of the infarction depends partly on whether the occlusion is proximal or distal. Generally a proximal occlusion will cause a much more extensive infarction than a distal occlusion. MCA infarctions are the most common because the middle cerebral artery is essentially a direct continuation of the internal carotid artery.

Meninges

The brain and spinal cord are covered by membranes called meninges. The meninges are composed of three layers: dura mater (dura), arachnoid (arachnoid membrane), and pia mater.

The subarachnoid space, located between the arachnoid and pia, contains cerebrospinal fluid (CSF, see p. 100). See p. 80 for the coverings of the spinal cord.

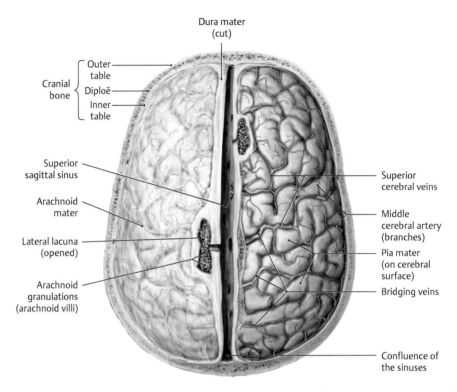

Dura mater
(cut)

Cranial bone
— Outer table
— Diploë
— Inner table

Superior sagittal sinus

Arachnoid mater

Lateral lacuna (opened)

Arachnoid granulations (arachnoid villi)

Superior cerebral veins

Middle cerebral artery (branches)

Pia mater (on cerebral surface)

Bridging veins

Confluence of the sinuses

Fig. 4.56 Layers of the Meninges
Superior view of opened cranium. *Left side:* Dura mater (outer layer) cut to reveal arachnoid (middle layer). *Right side:* Dura mater and arachnoid removed to reveal pia mater (inner layer) lining the surface of the brain. *Note:* Arachnoid granulations, sites for loss of cerebrospinal fluid into the venous blood, are protrusions of the arachnoid layer of the meninges into the venous sinus system.

Migraines are caused by the dilation of blood vessels in the pia mater and dura mater surrounding the brain which triggers the release of neuropeptides, e.g., substance P, from parasympathetic nerve fibers approx-

imating these vessels and excites nociceptive fibers that travel in the trigeminal nerve (CN V) back to the brain. They are characterized by a severe, unilateral throbbing headache, which is often preceded by an aura (usually visual), and may be accompanied by nausea, vomiting, and photophobia (sensitivity to light).

Meningitis is inflammation of the meninges of the brain (pia mater and arachnoid), usually due to a viral infection. Symptoms include headache, stiff neck, photophobia, irritability, drowsiness, vomiting, fever, seizures, and rash (viral or meningococcal meningitis).

Fig. 4.57 Dural septa (folds)
Left anterior oblique view. Two layers of meningeal dura come together, after separating from the periosteal dura during formation of a dural (venous) sinus, to form a dural fold or septa. These include the falx cerebri (separating right and left cerebral hemispheres); the tentorium cerebelli (supporting the cerebrum to keep it from crushing the underlying cerebellum); the falx cerebelli (not shown, that separates right and left cerebellar lobes under the tentorium); and the diaphragma sellae (forms the roof over the pituitary (hypophyseal) fossa and is invaginated by the pituitary gland).

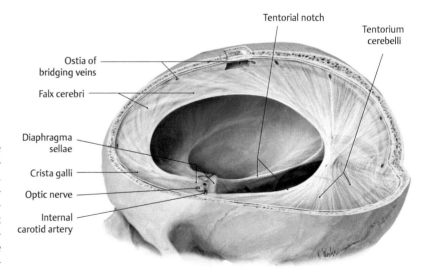

Tentorial notch

Tentorium cerebelli

Ostia of bridging veins

Falx cerebri

Diaphragma sellae

Crista galli

Optic nerve

Internal carotid artery

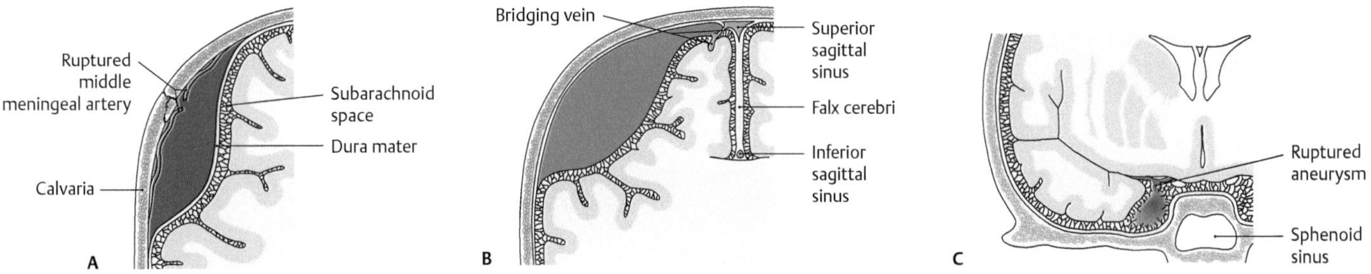

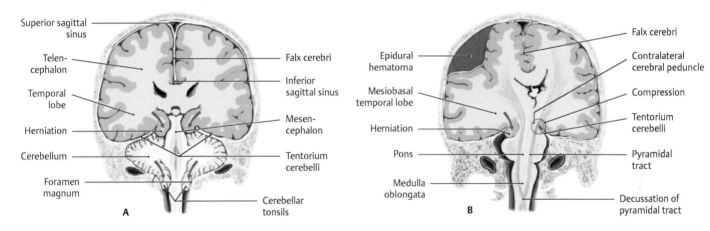

Fig. 4.58 Extracerebral hemorrhages

Bleeding between the bony calvarium and the soft tissues of the brain (extracerebral hemorrhage) exerts pressure on the brain. A rise of intracranial pressure may damage brain tissue both at the bleeding site and in more remote brain areas. Three types of extracerebral hemorrhage are distinguished based on the relationship to the dura mater: (**A**) epidural hematoma, (**B**) subdural hematoma, or (**C**) subarachnoid hemorrhage. **A** Epidural hematomas generally develop after a head injury involving a skull fracture, causing rupture of the middle meningeal artery. The hematoma forms between the calvaria and the periosteal layer of the dura ma-

ter. **B** Subdural hematomas usually form when trauma to the head causes the rupture of bridging veins. Bleeding occurs between the dura mater and the arachnoid mater. Because the source of the bleeding is venous, a subdural hematoma may develop over a period of weeks. **C** Subarachnoid hemorrhage is an arterial bleed caused by the rupture of an aneurysm of an artery at the base of the brain (see **Fig. 4.47**). It is typically caused by a brief, sudden rise in blood pressure, like that produced by a sudden rise in intra-abdominal pressure, e.g. straining at stool. Because the hemorrhage is into the CSF-filled subarachnoid space, blood can be detected in the CSF by means of a lumbar puncture (see **Fig. 4.9**).

Fig. 4.59 Potential sites of brain herniation beneath the free edges of the meninges

Coronal section, anterior view. The tentorium cerebelli divides the cranial cavity into a supratentorial and an infratentorial space. The telencephalon is supratentorial, and the cerebellum is infratentorial (**A**). Because the dura is composed of tough, collagenous connective tissue, it creates a rigid intracranial framework. As a result, a mass lesion within the cranium may displace the cerebral tissue and cause portions of the cerebrum to become entrapped (herniate) beneath the rigid dural septa (= duplication of the meningeal layer of the dura).

A Axial herniation. This type of herniation is usually caused by generalized brain edema. It is a symmetrical herniation in which the middle and lower portions of both temporal lobes of the cerebrum herniate down through the tentorial notch, exerting pressure on the upper portion of

the midbrain (bilateral uncal herniation). If the pressure persists, it will force the cerebellar tonsils through the foramen magnum and also compress the lower part of the brainstem (tonsillar herniation). Because respiratory and circulatory centers are located in the brainstem, this type of herniation is life-threatening. Concomitant vascular compression may cause brainstem infarction.

B Lateral herniation. This type is caused by a unilateral mass effect (e.g., from a brain tumor or intracranial hematoma), as illustrated here on the right side. Compression of the ipsilateral cerebral peduncle usually produces contralateral hemiparesis. Sometimes, the herniating mesiobasal portions of the temporal lobe press the opposite cerebral peduncle against the sharp edge of the tentorium. This damages the pyramidal tract above the level of its decussation, causing hemiparesis to develop on the side opposite the injury.

Sensory Pathways (Excluding the Head)

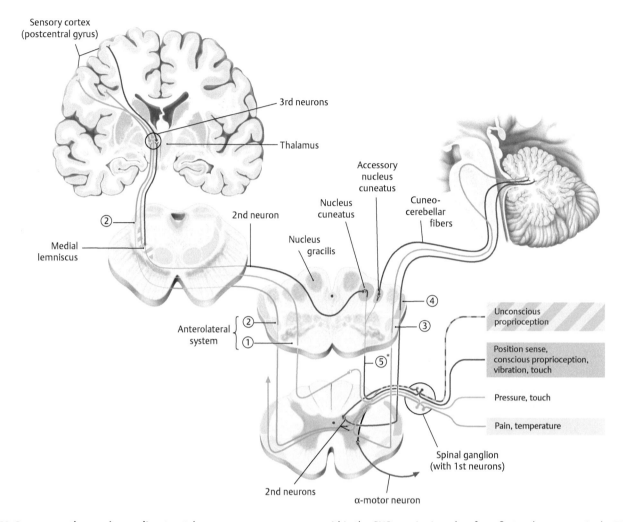

Fig. 4.60 Sensory pathways (ascending tracts)
Spinal nerve sensory pathways involve a three neuron chain: first-order, second-order, and third order. First-order sensory neurons, with cell bodies located outside the CNS, collect sensory data from the sensory organ and convey it to the CNS. The axons of first-order neurons enter the CNS, through the posterior (sensory) root and posteior horn, to synapse on second-order sensory neurons. Second-order sensory neurons, located within the CNS, receive impulses from first-order neurons in the PNS. The axons of second-order neurons ascend as tracts to synapse on third-order sensory neurons located in the thalamus; some second-order neurons project to the cerebellum via the spinocerebellar and cuneocerebellar tracts. Third-order sensory neurons project axons to the sensory cortex. See **Table 4.7** for more details.

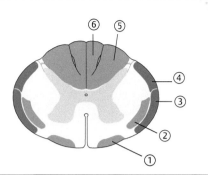

Table 4.7 Ascending tracts of the spinal cord

Tract		Location	Function		Neurons
①	Anterior spinothalamic tract	Anterior funiculus	Pathway for crude touch and pressure sensation		1st order afferent neurons located in spinal ganglia; contain 2nd order neurons and cross in the anterior commissure
②	Lateral spinothalamic tract	Anterior and lateral funiculi	Pathway for pain, temperature, tickle, itch, and sexual sensation		
③	Anterior spinocerebellar tract	Lateral funiculus	Pathway for unconscious coordination of motor activities (unconscious proprioception, automatic processes, e.g., jogging, riding a bike) to the cerebellum		Projection (2nd order) neurons receive proprioceptive signals from 1st order afferent fibers originating at the 1st order neurons of spinal ganglia
④	Posterior spinocerebellar tract				
⑤	Fasciculus cuneatus	Posterior funiculus	Pathway for position sense (conscious proprioception) and fine cutaneous sensation (touch, vibration, fine pressure sense, two-point discrimination)	Conveys information from *upper* limb (not present below T3)	Cell bodies of 1st order neurons located in spinal ganglion; pass uncrossed to the dorsal column nuclei
⑥	Fasciculus gracilis*			Conveys information from *lower* limb	

* The fasciculi cuneatus and gracilis convey information from the upper and lower limbs, respectively. At lower spinal cord levels, only the fasciculus gracilis is present.

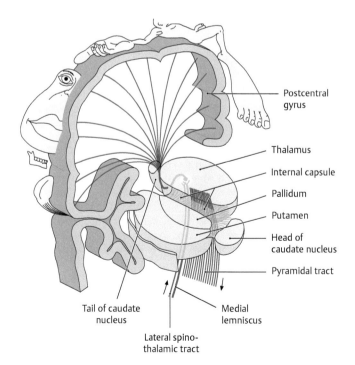

Postcentral gyrus

Thalamus

Internal capsule

Pallidum

Putamen

Head of caudate nucleus

Pyramidal tract

Tail of caudate nucleus

Medial lemniscus

Lateral spino-thalamic tract

Fig. 4.61 Arrangement of sensory pathways in the cerebrum
Anterior view of the right postcentral gyrus. The cell bodies of the third order neurons of the sensory pathways are located in the thalamus. Their axons project to the postcentral gyrus, where the primary somatosensory cortex is located. The postcentral gyrus has a somatotopic organization, meaning that each body region is represented in a particular cortical area. The body regions in the cortex are not represented in proportion to their actual size, but in proportion to the density of their sensory innervation. The fingers and head have abundant sensory receptors, and so their cortical representation is correspondingly large. Conversely, the less dense sensory innervation of the buttocks and legs results in smaller areas of representation. Based on these varying numbers of peripheral receptors, we can construct a "sensory homunculus" whose parts correspond to the cortical areas concerned with their perception.
Note: The head of the homunculus is upright while the trunk is upside down.
The axons of the sensory neurons ascending from the thalamus travel side by side with the axons forming the pyramidal tract (red) in the posterior part of the internal capsule. Because of this arrangement, a large cerebral hemorrhage involving the internal capsule produces sensory as well as motor deficits (see Kell et al.).

111

Sensory Pathways: Pain Pathways in the Head & the Central Analgesic System

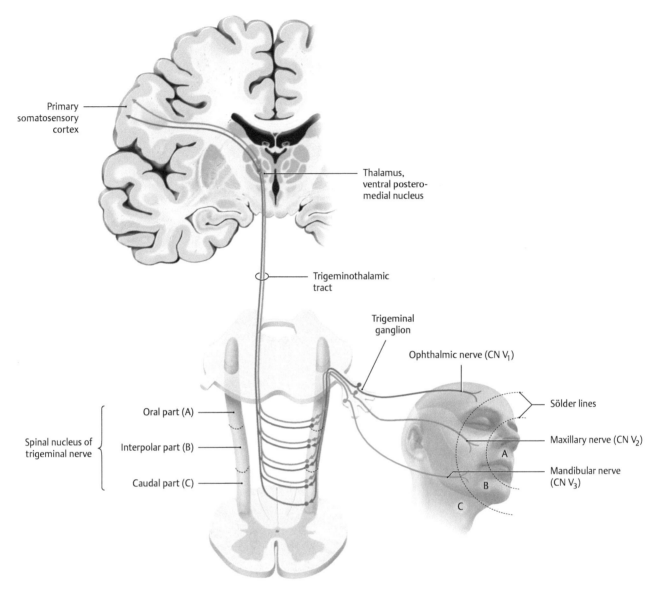

Primary somatosensory cortex

Thalamus, ventral postero-medial nucleus

Trigeminothalamic tract

Trigeminal ganglion

Ophthalmic nerve (CN V₁)

Sölder lines

Maxillary nerve (CN V₂)

Mandibular nerve (CN V₃)

Spinal nucleus of trigeminal nerve
- Oral part (A)
- Interpolar part (B)
- Caudal part (C)

A
B
C

Fig. 4.62 Pain pathways in the head (after Lorke)

The pain fibers in the head accompany the principal divisions of the trigeminal nerve (CN V₁–V₃). The cell bodies of these first order afferent neurons of the pain pathway are located in the trigeminal ganglion. Their axons terminate in the spinal nucleus of the trigeminal nerve.

Note the somatotopic organization of this nuclear region: The perioral region (**A**) is cranial and the occipital regions (**C**) are caudal. Because of this arrangement, central lesions lead to deficits that are distributed along the Sölder lines.

The axons of the second order neurons cross the midline and travel in the trigeminothalamic tract to the ventral posteromedial nucleus and to the intralaminar thalamic nuclei on the opposite side, where they terminate. The third order (thalamic) neuron of the pain pathway ends in the primary somatosensory cortex. Only the pain fibers of the trigeminal nerve

are pictured in the diagram. In the trigeminal nerve itself, the other sensory fibers run parallel to the pain fibers but terminate in various trigeminal nuclei.

Oral dysaesthesia, or *burning mouth syndrome*, is a debilitating, intractable, burning sensation of the oral mucosa that is present without evidence of clinical disease. The precise cause of oral dysaesthesia is unknown but derangements in central and peripheral pain pathways have been implicated and it is also thought to have a strong psycogenic component. It is many times more common in women and tends to affect those in the 40–50 years age range, many of whom are suffering from depression. Diagnosis is made by exclusion of all organic and prosthetic causes. Treatment is usually with antidepressant drugs, which treat both any precipitating or coexisting depression, and affect central pain pathways.

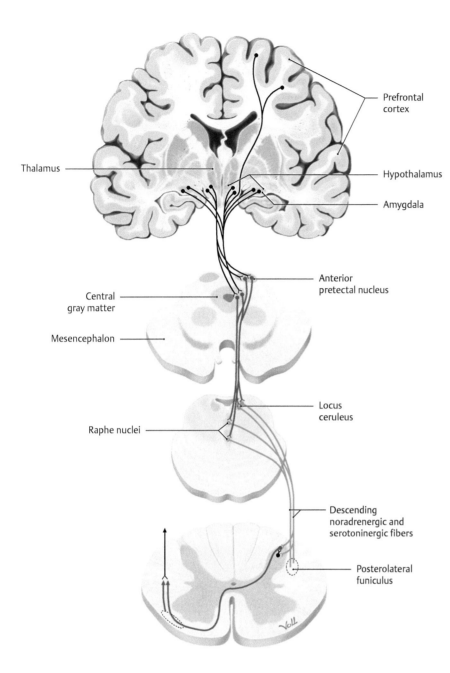

Fig. 4.63 **Pathways of the central descending analgesic system** (after Lorke)

Besides the ascending pathways that carry pain sensation to the primary somatosensory cortex, there are also descending pathways that have the ability to suppress pain impulses. The central relay station for the descending analgesic (pain-relieving) system is the central gray matter of the mesencephalon. It is activated by afferent input from the hypothalamus, the prefrontal cortex, and the amygdaloid bodies (part of the limbic system, not shown). It also receives afferent input from the spinal cord. The axons from the excitatory glutaminergic neurons (red) of the central gray matter terminate on serotoninergic neurons in the raphe nuclei and on noradrenergic neurons in the locus ceruleus (both shown in blue). The axons from both types of neuron descend in the posterolateral funiculus. They terminate directly or indirectly (via inhibitory neurons) on the analgesic projection neurons (second order afferent neuron of the pain pathway), thereby inhibiting the further conduction of pain impulses.

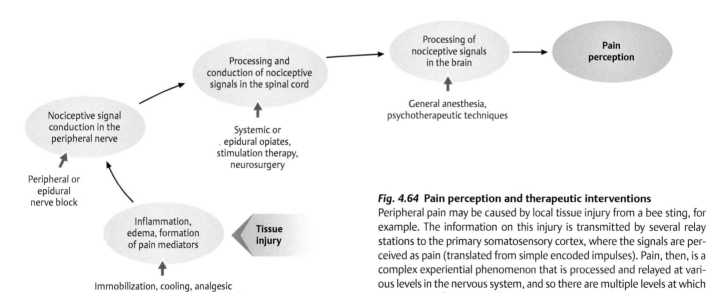

Fig. 4.64 **Pain perception and therapeutic interventions**

Peripheral pain may be caused by local tissue injury from a bee sting, for example. The information on this injury is transmitted by several relay stations to the primary somatosensory cortex, where the signals are perceived as pain (translated from simple encoded impulses). Pain, then, is a complex experiential phenomenon that is processed and relayed at various levels in the nervous system, and so there are multiple levels at which pain may be alleviated by therapeutic measures (red arrows).

113

Motor Pathways

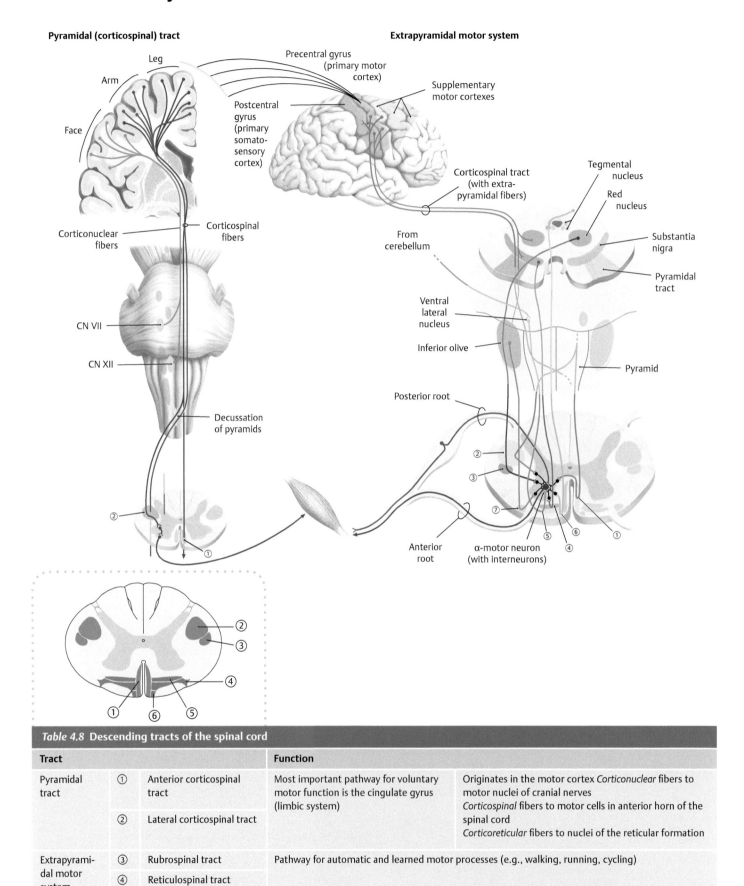

Pyramidal (corticospinal) tract

Leg
Arm
Face

Precentral gyrus (primary motor cortex)

Supplementary motor cortexes

Postcentral gyrus (primary somato-sensory cortex)

Corticonuclear fibers

Corticospinal fibers

CN VII

CN XII

Decussation of pyramids

② ①

Extrapyramidal motor system

Corticospinal tract (with extra-pyramidal fibers)

Tegmental nucleus

Red nucleus

From cerebellum

Substantia nigra

Pyramidal tract

Ventral lateral nucleus

Inferior olive

Pyramid

Posterior root

② ③ ⑦

Anterior root

α-motor neuron (with interneurons)

⑤ ④ ⑥ ①

② ③ ④ ⑤ ⑥ ①

Table 4.8 Descending tracts of the spinal cord

Tract			Function	
Pyramidal tract	①	Anterior corticospinal tract	Most important pathway for voluntary motor function is the cingulate gyrus (limbic system)	Originates in the motor cortex *Corticonuclear* fibers to motor nuclei of cranial nerves
	②	Lateral corticospinal tract		*Corticospinal* fibers to motor cells in anterior horn of the spinal cord *Corticoreticular* fibers to nuclei of the reticular formation
Extrapyramidal motor system	③	Rubrospinal tract	Pathway for automatic and learned motor processes (e.g., walking, running, cycling)	
	④	Reticulospinal tract		
	⑤	Vestibulospinal tract		
	⑥	Tectospinal tract		
	⑦	Olivospinal tract		

Fig. 4.65 Motor pathways (descending tracts)

The motor pathway for the innervation of skeletal muscle involves two neurons, an upper motor neuron and a lower motor neuron. The cell bodies of the upper motor neurons, which are associated with both cranial nerves and spinal nerves, are located in the gray matter of the precentral gyrus of the cerebral cortex. The axons of the upper motor neurons descend via white matter tracts to reach the lower motor neurons, which are located in motor nuclei of in the brainstem and in the anterior horn of the spinal cord. The majority of upper motor neurons descending in the corticospinal tract cross to the contralateral side at the pyramidal decus-

sation at the spinomeduallary junction. The anterior horn is the anterior portion of the gray matter of the spinal cord, containing exclusively motor neurons. The axons of these neurons leave the CNS as the anterior (motor) root of the spinal nerves to synapse on target cells. The anterior (motor) root combines with the posterior (sensory) root, in the intervertebral foramen, to form a mixed spinal nerve. Lower motor neurons in the motor nuclei of the brainstem (cranial nerves) project axons that emerge from the CNS as the motor roots of cranial nerves. See **Table 4.8** for more details.

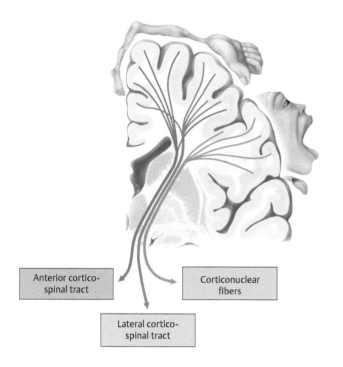

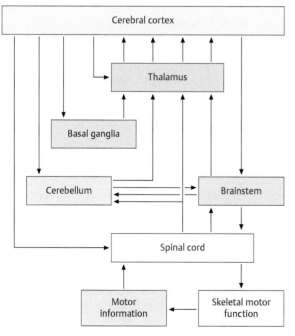

Fig. 4.66 Somatotopic representation of the skeletal muscle in the precentral gyrus (motor homunculus)

Anterior view. Regions in which the muscles are very densely innervated (e.g., the hand) must be supplied by many neurons in the precentral gyrus. As a result, they require a larger representation area in the cortex than regions supplied by fewer neurons (e.g., the trunk). This cortical representation is analogous to that in sensory innervation, where areas of varying size are also represented in the cortex (postcentral gyrus; compare with the sensory homunculus in **Fig. 4.61**). One cortical area is devoted to the trunk and limbs and another to the head. The axons for the head area are the corticonuclear fibers, and the axons for the trunk and limbs are the corticospinal fibers. The latter fibers split into two groups below the telencephalon, forming the lateral and anterior corticospinal tracts.

Fig. 4.67 Simplified diagram of the sensorimotor system role in movement control

Voluntary movements require constant feedback from the periphery (muscle spindles, Golgi tendon organs) in order to remain within the desired limits. Because the motor and sensory systems are so closely interrelated functionally, they are often described jointly as the sensorimotor system. The spinal cord, brainstem, cerebellum, and cerebral cortex are the three control levels of the sensorimotor system. All information from periphery, cerebellum, and the basal ganglia passes through the thalamus on its way to the cerebral cortex. The clinical importance of the sensory system in movement is seen in sensory ataxia (loss of coordination) which may occur when sensory input into the control of movement is lost. The oculomotor component of the sensorimotor system is not shown.

Autonomic Nervous System (I): Overview

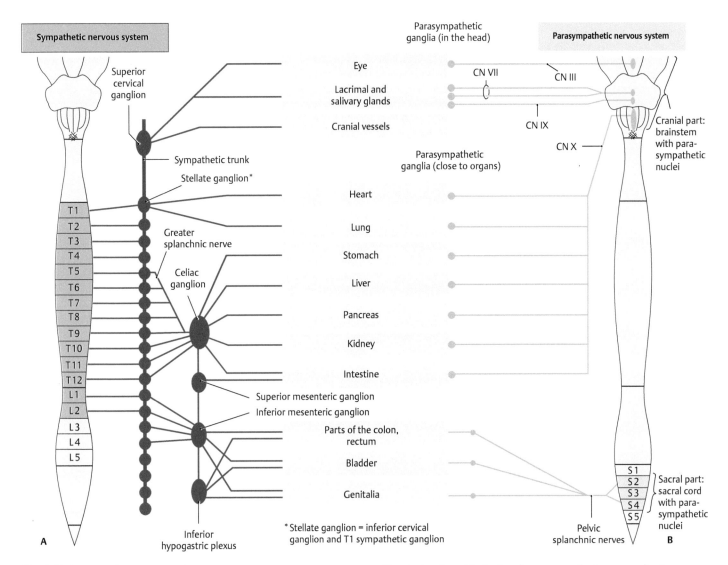

Sympathetic nervous system

- Superior cervical ganglion
- Sympathetic trunk
- Stellate ganglion*
- T1
- T2
- Greater splanchnic nerve
- T3
- T4
- T5
- Celiac ganglion
- T6
- T7
- T8
- T9
- T10
- T11
- T12
- L1
- L2
- Superior mesenteric ganglion
- L3
- Inferior mesenteric ganglion
- L4
- L5

A

Inferior hypogastric plexus

Parasympathetic ganglia (in the head)

- Eye
- Lacrimal and salivary glands
- Cranial vessels
- CN VII
- CN III
- CN IX

Parasympathetic ganglia (close to organs)

- Heart
- Lung
- Stomach
- Liver
- Pancreas
- Kidney
- Intestine
- Parts of the colon, rectum
- Bladder
- Genitalia

CN X

Parasympathetic nervous system

Cranial part: brainstem with para-sympathetic nuclei

- S1
- S2
- S3
- S4
- S5

Sacral part: sacral cord with para-sympathetic nuclei

* Stellate ganglion = inferior cervical ganglion and T1 sympathetic ganglion

Pelvic splanchnic nerves

B

Fig. 4.68 Autonomic nervous system

The autonomic nervous system is the part of the peripheral nervous system that innervates smooth muscle, cardiac muscle, and glands. It is subdivided into the sympathetic (red) and the parasympathetic (blue) nervous systems, which often act in antagonistic fashion to regulate blood flow, secretions, and organ function.

Both the sympathetic and parasympathetic nervous systems have a two-neuron pathway, which is under central nervous system control via an upper motor neuron with its cell body in the hypothalamus.

In the sympathetic system, the preganglionic neuron synapses within the ganglia of the sympathetic trunk (paired, one on each side of vertebral column) or on one of the unpaired prevertebral ganglia located at the base of the artery for which the ganglion was named (celiac, superior and inferior mesenteric). Sympathetic postganglionic neurons then either re-enter spinal nerves via grey rami communicantes and are distributed to their target structure or they reach their target structure by travelling

with arteries. Except in the head, parasympathetic preganglionic neurons synapse in ganglia in the wall of the target organ. Short postganglioinc parasympathetic neurons then innervate the organ. In the head there are four parasympathetic ganglia: ciliary ganglion, pterygopalatine ganglion, submandibular ganglion, otic ganglion, which are associated with cranial nerves III, VII, and IX, respectively. These four ganglia are responsible to distributing fibers to smooth muscle within the eye and to the salivary glands and glands of the nasal cavity, paranasal sinuses, hard and soft palate, and pharynx.

Both sympathetic and parasympathetic preganglionic neurons secrete acetylcholine, which acts upon nicotinic receptors in the ganglia. Sympathetic postganglionic neurons secrete norepinephrine, which acts upon adrenoceptors (α or β) in target tissues. Parasympathetic postganglionic neurons secrete acetylcholine, which acts upon muscarinic receptors in target tissues.

Table 4.9 Parasympathetic pathways

Neuron	Location of cell body (soma)	
Upper motor neuron	**Hypothalamus:** The cell bodies of parasympathetic upper motor neurons are located in the hypothalamus. Their axons descend via white matter tracts to synapse with the lower motor neuron in the brainstem and sacral spinal cord (S2–S4).	
Preganglionic neuron (lower motor neuron)	The parasympathetic nervous system is divided into two parts (cranial and sacral), based on the location of the preganglionic parasympathetic neurons.	
	Brainstem cranial nerve nuclei: The axons of these secondary neurons leave the CNS as the motor root of cranial nerves III, VII, IX, and X.	**Spinal cord (S2–S4):** The axons of these secondary neurons leave the CNS (S2–S4) as the pelvic splanchnic nerves. These nerves travel in the posterior rami of the S2–S4 spinal nerves and are distributed via the sympathetic plexuses to the pelvic viscera.
Postganglionic neuron	**Cranial nerve parasympathetic ganglia:** The parasympathetic cranial nerves of the head each have at least one ganglion: • CN III: Ciliary ganglion • CN VII: Pterygopalatine ganglion and submandibular ganglion • CN IX: Otic ganglion • CN X: Small unnamed ganglia close to target structures	
Distribution of postganglionic fibers	Parasympathetic fibers course with other fiber types to their targets. In the head, the postganglionic fibers from the pterygopalatine ganglion (CN VII) and otic ganglion (CN IX) are distributed via branches of the trigeminal nerve (CN V). Postganglionic fibers from the ciliary ganglion (CN III) course with sympathetic and sensory fibers in the short ciliary nerves (preganglionic fibers travel with the somatomotor fibers of CN III). In the thorax, abdomen, and pelvis, preganglionic parasympathetic fibers from CN X and the pelvic splanchnic nerves combine with postganglionic sympathetic fibers to form plexuses (e.g., cardiac, pulmonary, esophageal).	

Table 4.10 Sympathetic pathways

Neuron	Location of cell body (soma)	
Upper motor neuron	**Hypothalamus:** The cell bodies of sympathetic upper motor neurons are located in the hypothalamus. Their axons descend via white matter tracts to synapse with the lower motor neuron in the lateral horn of the spinal cord (T1–L2).	
Preganglionic neuron (lower motor neuron)	**Lateral horn of spinal cord (T1–L2):** The lateral horn is the middle portion of the gray matter of the spinal cord, situated between the anterior and posterior horns. It contains exclusively autonomic (sympathetic) neurons. The axons of these neurons leave the CNS as the motor root of the spinal nerves and enter the paravertebral ganglia via the white rami communicantes (myelinated).	
Preganglionic neurons in paravertebral ganglia	All preganglionic sympathetic neurons enter the sympathetic chain. There they may synapse in a chain ganglion or ascend or descend to synapse. Preganglionic sympathetic neurons synapse in one of two places, yielding two types of sympathetic ganglia.	
	Synapse *in* the paravertebral ganglia	Pass without synapsing *through* the parasympathetic ganglia. These fibers travel in the thoracic, lumbar, and sacral splanchnic nerves to synapse in the prevertebral ganglia.
Postganglionic neuron	**Paravertebral ganglia:** These ganglia form the sympathetic nerve trunks that flank the spinal cord. Postganglionic axons leave the sympathetic trunk via the gray rami communicantes (unmyelinated).	**Prevertebral ganglia:** Associated with peripheral plexuses, which spread along the abdominal aorta. There are three primary prevertebral ganglia: • Celiac ganglion • Superior mesenteric ganglion • Inferior mesenteric ganglion
Distribution of postganglionic fibers	Postganglionic fibers are distributed in two ways: 1. Spinal nerves: Postganglionic neurons may re-enter the spinal nerves via the gray rami communicantes. These sympathetic neurons induce constriction of blood vessels, sweat glands, and arrector pili (muscle fibers attached to hair follicles, "goose bumps"). 2. Arteries and ducts: Nerve plexuses may form along existing structures. Postganglionic sympathetic fibers may travel with arteries to target structures. Viscera are innervated by this method (e.g., sympathetic innervation concerning vasoconstriction, bronchial dilatation, glandular secretions, pupillary dilatation, smooth muscle contraction).	

Autonomic Nervous System (II): Connections

Fig. 4.69 Parasympathetic nervous system (cranial part): Overview

There are four parasympathetic nuclei in the brainstem. The visceral efferent fibers of these nuclei travel along particular cranial nerves, listed below.

- Visceral oculomotor (Edinger–Westphal) nucleus: oculomotor nerve (CN III)
- Superior salivatory nucleus: facial nerve (CN VII)
- Inferior salivatory nucleus: glossopharyngeal nerve (CN IX)
- Dorsal motor nucleus: vagus nerve (CN X)

The presynaptic parasympathetic fibers often travel with multiple cranial nerves to reach their target organs. The vagus nerve supplies all of the thoracic and abdominal organs as far as a point near the left colic flexure.
Note: The sympathetic fibers to the head travel along the arteries to their target organs.

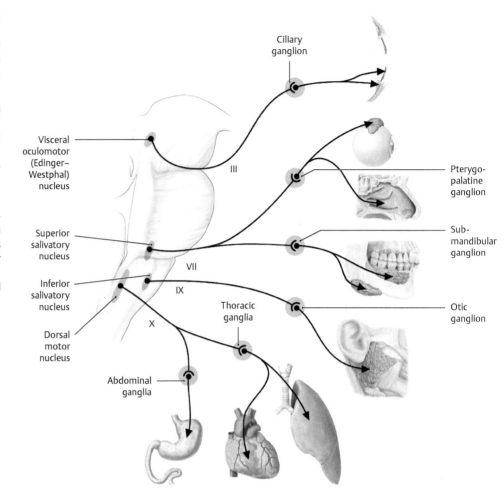

Table 4.11 Parasympathetic ganglia in the head

Nucleus	Path of presynaptic fibers	Ganglion	Postsynaptic fibers	Target organs
Edinger-Westphal nucleus	Oculomotor nerve (CN III)	Ciliary ganglion	Short ciliary nerves (CN V$_1$)	Ciliary muscle (accommodation) Pupillary sphincter (miosis)

Superior salivary nucleus	Nervus intermedius (CN VII root) → greater petrosal nerve → nerve of pterygoid canal	Pterygopalatine ganglion	• Maxillary nerve (CN V$_2$)
			  → zygomatic nerve →
			  anostomosis → lacrimal nerve
			  (CN V$_1$)
			• Orbital branches
			• Posterior superior nasal branches
			• Nasopalatine nerves
			• Greater and lesser palatine nerves
				• Lacrimal gland
				• Glands of nasal cavity and paranasal sinuses
				• Glands of gingiva
				• Glands of hard and soft palate
				• Glands of pharynx

	Nervus intermedius (CN VII root) → chorda tympani → lingual nerve (CN V$_3$)	Submandibular ganglion	Glandular branches	Submandibular gland Sublingual gland
Inferior salivatory nucleus	Glossopharyngeal nerve (CN IX) → tympanic nerve → lesser petrosal nerve	Otic ganglion	Auriculotemporal nerve (CN V$_3$)	Parotid gland
Dorsal motor (vagal) nucleus	Vagus nerve (X)	Ganglia near organs	Fine fibers in organs, not individually named	Thoracic and abdominal viscera

→ = is continuous with

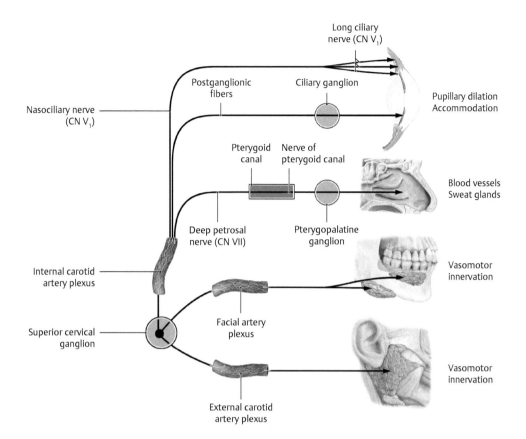

Fig. 4.70 Sympathetic innervation of the head

Sympathetic preganglionic neurons of the head originate in the lateral horn of the spinal cord (TI–L2). They exit into the sympathetic chain ganglia and ascend to synapse in the superior cervical ganglion. Postganglionic neurons then travel with arterial plexuses. Postganglionic fibers that travel with the carotid plexus (on the internal carotid artery) join with the nasociliary nerves (of CN V_1) and then the long ciliary nerves to reach the dilator pupillae muscle (pupillary dilation); other postganglionic fibers travel through the ciliary ganglion (without synapsing) to reach the ciliary muscle (accommodation). Still other postganglionic fibers from the carotid plexus leave with the deep petrosal nerve, which joins with the greater petrosal nerve (CN VII), to form the nerve of the pterygoid canal (vidian nerve). This nerve travels to the pterygopalatine ganglion where it distributes fibers via branches of the maxillary nerve to the glands of the nasal cavity, maxillary sinus, hard and soft palate, gingiva, and pharynx, and to sweat glands and blood vessels in the head.

Postganglionic fibers from the superior cervical ganglion that travel with the facial artery plexus pass through the submandibular ganglion (without synapsing) to the submandibular and sublingual glands. Other postganglionic fibers travel with the middle meningeal plexus, through the otic ganglion (without synapsing), to the parotid gland.

Table 4.12 Sympathetic fibers in the head				
Nucleus	**Path of presynaptic fibers**	**Ganglion**	**Postsynaptic fibers**	**Target organs**
Lateral horn of spinal cord (TI–L2)	Enter sympathetic chain ganglia and ascend to superior cervical ganglion	Superior cervical ganglion	ICA plexus → nasociliary nn. (CN V_1) → long ciliary nn. (CN V_1)	Dilator pupillae muscle (mydriasis)
			Postganglionic fibers→ciliary ganglion* → short ciliary nerves	Ciliary muscle (accommodation)
			ICA plexus → deep petrosal n. → n. of pterygoid canal → pterygopalatine ganglion* → branches of maxillary n. (CN V_2)	Glands of nasal cavity Sweat glands Blood vessels
			Facial artery plexus → submandibular ganglion*	Submandibular gland Sublingual gland
			External carotid artery plexus	Parotid gland

*passes through without synpasing; → = is continuous with
ICA, internal carotid artery

Cranial Nerves: Overview

Table 4.13 Cranial nerves

Cranial nerve	Attachment to brain	Fiber type (Table 4.11) Afferent				Efferent		
CN I: Olfactory n.	Telencephalon			●				
CN II: Optic n.	Diencephalon	●						
CN III: Oculomotor n.	Mesencephalon					●	●	
CN IV: Trochlear n.						●		
CN V: Trigeminal n.	Pons							●
CN VI: Abducent n.	Pontomedullary junction					●		
CN VII: Facial n.				●			●	●
CN VIII: Vestibulocochlear n.		●						
CN IX: Glossopharyngeal n.	Medulla oblongata			●		●	●	●
CN X: Vagus n.				●		●	●	●
CN XI: Accessory n.						●		●
CN XII: Hypoglossal n.						●		

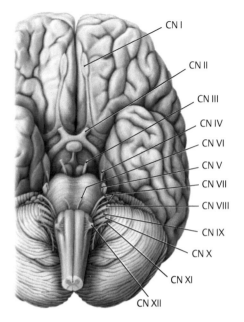

Fig. 4.71 Cranial nerves
Whereas the 31 spinal nerve pairs emerge from the spinal cord, the 12 pairs of cranial nerves emerge from the brain at various levels (**Table 4.13**). They are numbered according to the order of their emergence. (*Note:* Cranial nerves I and II are not true peripheral nerves but are instead extensions of the telencephalon [CN I] and diencephalon [CN II].) Unlike the spinal nerves, which each have a posterior sensory and an anterior motor root, the cranial nerves may contain afferent (sensory) and/or efferent (motor) fibers. The types of fibers (**Table 4.14**) correspond to the function of the nerve (**Table 4.15**).

Table 4.14 Cranial nerve fiber types

The seven types of cranial nerve fibers are classified according to three criteria (reflected in the three-letter codes): 1. General (G) vs. Special (S), 2. Somatic (S) vs. Visceral (V), 3. Afferent (A) vs. Efferent (E). Each fiber type has an associated color used throughout this chapter.

	Afferent (sensory) fibers			Efferent (motor) fibers		
General fibers	GSA	General somatosensory	General sensation (touch, pain, and temperature) from somite derivatives (skin, skeletal muscle, and mucosa)	GSE	Somatomotor	Motor innervation to striated (skeletal) muscle derived from somites
	GVA	General viscerosensory	General sensation from viscera (smooth muscle, cardiac muscle, and glands)	GVE	Parasympathetic	Motor innervation to viscera (smooth muscle, cardiac muscle, glands, etc.)
Special fibers	SSA	Special somato-sensory	Sight, hearing, and balance			
	SVA	Special viscerosensory	Taste and smell	SVE	Branchiomotor	Fibers to striated (skeletal) muscle derived from the branchial arches

Table 4.15 Cranial nerve function

Cranial nerve		Passage through skull	Fiber A	Fiber E	Sensory territory (afferent) / Target organ (efferent)
CN I: Olfactory n. (p. 124)		Ethmoid bone (cribriform plate)	○		Smell: special viscerosensory fibers from olfactory mucosa of nasal cavity
CN II: Optic n. (p. 125)		Optic canal	●		Sight: special somatosensory fibers from retina
CN III: Oculomotor n. (pp. 126–127)		Superior orbital fissure		●	Somatomotor innervation: to levator palpebrae superioris and four extraocular mm. (superior, medial, and inferior rectus, and inferior oblique)
				○	Parasympathetic innervation: preganglionic fibers to ciliary ganglion; postganglionic fibers to intraocular mm. (ciliary mm. and pupillary sphincter)
CN IV: Trochlear n. (pp. 126–127)		Superior orbital fissure		●	Somatomotor innervation: to one extraocular m. (superior oblique)
CN V: Trigeminal n. (pp. 128–135)	CN V₁ (pp. 130–131)	Superior orbital fissure	○		General somatic sensation: from orbit, nasal cavity, paranasal sinuses, and face
	CN V₂ (pp. 132–133)	Foramen rotundum	○		General somatic sensation: from nasal cavity, paranasal sinuses, superior nasopharynx, upper oral cavity, internal skull, and face
	CN V₃ (pp. 134–135)	Foramen ovale	○		General somatic sensation: from lower oral cavity, ear, internal skull, and face
				●	Branchiomotor innervation: to the eight mm. derived from the 1st pharyngeal (branchial) arch (including mm. of mastication)
CN VI: Abducent n. (pp. 126–127)		Superior orbital fissure		●	Somatomotor innervation: to one extraocular m. (lateral rectus)
CN VII: Facial n. (pp. 136–139)		Internal acoustic meatus	○		General somatic sensation: from external ear
			○		Taste: special viscerosensory fibers from tongue (anterior ⅔) and soft palate
				○	Parasympathetic innervation: preganglionic fibers to submandibular and pterygopalatine ganglia; postganglionic fibers to glands (e.g., lacrimal, submandibular, sublingual, palatine) and mucosa of nasal cavity, palate, and paranasal sinuses
				●	Branchiomotor innervation: to mm. derived from the 2nd pharyngeal arch (including mm. of facial expression, stylohyoid, and stapedius)
CN VIII: Vestibulocochlear n. (pp. 140–141)		Internal acoustic meatus	○		Hearing and balance: special somatosensory fibers from cochlea (hearing) and vestibular apparatus (balance)
CN IX: Glossopharyngeal n. (pp. 142–143)		Jugular foramen	○		General somatic sensation: from oral cavity, pharynx, tongue (posterior ⅓), and middle ear
			○		Taste: special visceral sensation from tongue (posterior ⅓)
			●		General visceral sensation: from carotid body and sinus
				○	Parasympathetic innervation: preganglionic fibers to otic ganglion; postganglionic fibers to parotid gland and inferior labial glands
				●	Branchiomotor innervation: to the one m. derived from the 3rd pharyngeal arch (stylopharyngeus)
CN X: Vagus n. (pp. 144–145)		Jugular foramen	○		General somatic sensation: from ear and internal skull
			○		Taste: special visceral sensation from epiglottis and root of tongue
			●		General visceral sensation: from aortic body, laryngopharynx and larynx, respiratory tract, and thoracoabdominal viscera
				○	Parasympathetic innervation: preganglionic fibers to small, unnamed ganglia near target organs or embedded in smooth muscle walls; postganglionic fibers to glands, mucosa, and smooth muscle of pharynx, larynx, and thoracic and abdominal viscera
				●	Branchiomotor innervation: to pharyngeal and laryngeal mm. derived from the 4th and 6th pharyngeal arches; also distributes branchiomotor fibers from CN XI
CN XI: Accessory n. (p. 146)		Jugular foramen		●	Somatomotor innervation: to trapezius and sternocleidomastoid
				●	Branchiomotor innervation: to laryngeal mm. (except cricothyroid) via pharyngeal plexus and CN X (*Note:* The branchiomotor fibers from the cranial root of CN XI are distributed by CN X [vagus n.].)
CN XII: Hypoglossal n. (p. 147)		Hypoglossal canal		●	Somatomotor innervation: to all intrinsic and extrinsic lingual mm. (except palatoglossus)

Cranial Nerve Nuclei

Fig. 4.72 Cranial nerve nuclei: topographic arrangement

Cross sections through the spinal cord and brainstem, superior view. Yellow = Somatic sensation. Green = Visceral sensation. Blue = Visceromotor function. Red = Somatomotor function.

The nuclei of the spinal and cranial nerves have a topographic arrangement based on embryonic migration of neuron populations.

A Embryonic spinal cord: Initially, the developing spinal cord demonstrates a posteroanterior arrangement in which the sensory (afferent) neurons are posterior and the motor (efferent) neurons are anterior. This pattern is continued into the adult spinal cord: the cell bodies of afferent neurons (generally secondary neurons) are located in the posterior horn, and the cell bodies of efferent neurons (lower motor neurons and preganglionic autonomic neurons) are located in the anterior and lateral horns, respectively.

B Early embryonic brainstem: Sensory neurons (in the alar plate) migrate laterally, whereas motor nuclei (in the basal plate) migrate medially. This produces a mediolateral arrangement of nuclear columns (functionally similar nuclei stacked longitudinally).

C Adult brainstem: The four longitudinal nuclear columns have a mediolateral arrangement (from medial to lateral): somatic efferent, visceral efferent, visceral afferent, and somatic afferent.

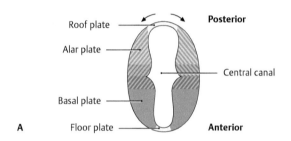

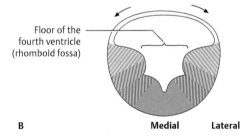

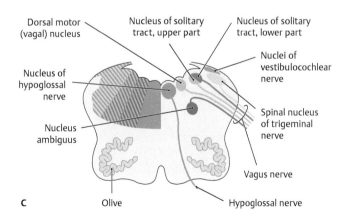

Table 4.16 Cranial nerve nuclei	
There is not a 1-to-1 relationship between cranial nerve fiber types and cranial nerve nuclei. Some nerves derive similar fibers from multiple nuclei (e.g., CN V and CN VIII). Other nuclei are associated with multiple nerves. *Note:* The five sensory cranial nerves have eight associated sensory ganglia (cell bodies of first-order sensory neurons). The three parasympathetic cranial nerves have four associated autonomic ganglia (cell bodies of postganglionic neurons).	
Nuclei	**Cranial nerve**
Somatic afferent nuclear column (yellow)	
General somatosensory: Three nuclei that are primarily associated with CN V but receive fibers from other nerves.	
• Mesencephalic nucleus	CN V (via trigeminal ganglion)
• Principal (pontine) sensory nucleus	CN IX (via superior ganglion)
• Spinal nucleus	CN X (via superior ganglion)
	Possibly CN VII (via geniculate ganglion)
Special somatosensory: Six nuclei that are associated with CN VIII.* The nerve and nuclei are divided into a vestibular part (balance) and a cochlear part (hearing).	
• Medial, lateral, superior, and inferior vestibular nuclei	CN VIII, vestibular root (via vestibular ganglion)
• Anterior and posterior cochlear nuclei	CN VIII, cochlear root (via spiral ganglia)
Visceral afferent nuclear column (green)	
General and special viscerosensory: One nuclear complex in the brainstem that consists of a superior (taste) and inferior (general visceral sensation) part and is associated with three cranial nerves.**	
• Nucleus of the solitary tract, inferior part	CN IX (via inferior ganglion)
	CN X (via inferior ganglion)
• Nucleus of the solitary tract, superior part	CN VII (via geniculate ganglion)
	CN IX (via inferior ganglion)
	CN X (via inferior ganglion)
Visceral motor nuclear column (blue)	
Parasympathetic (general visceromotor): Four nuclei that each have an associated cranial nerve and one or more ganglia.	
• Edinger-Westphal nucleus	CN III (via ciliary ganglion)
• Superior salivatory nucleus	CN VII (via submandibular and pterygopalatine ganglia)
• Inferior salivatory nucleus	CN IX (via otic ganglion)
• Dorsal motor (vagal) nucleus	CN X (via myriad unnamed ganglia near target organs)
Branchiomotor (special visceromotor): Three nuclei that innervate the muscles of the pharyngeal arches via four cranial nerves.	
• Trigeminal motor nucleus	CN V
• Facial nucleus	CN VII
• Nucleus ambiguus	CN IX
	CN X (with fibers from CN XI)
Somatomotor nuclear column (red)	
Five nuclei, each associated with a separate nerve.	
• Nucleus of the oculomotor n.	CN III
• Nucleus of the trochlear n.	CN IV
• Nucleus of the abducent n.	CN VI
• Nucleus of the accessory n.	CN XI
• Nucleus of the hypoglossal n.	CN XII

*There are no brainstem nuclei associated with CN II because it emerges from the diencephalon.

**The special visceral afferent fibers in the olfactory nerve (CN I) project to the telencephalon.

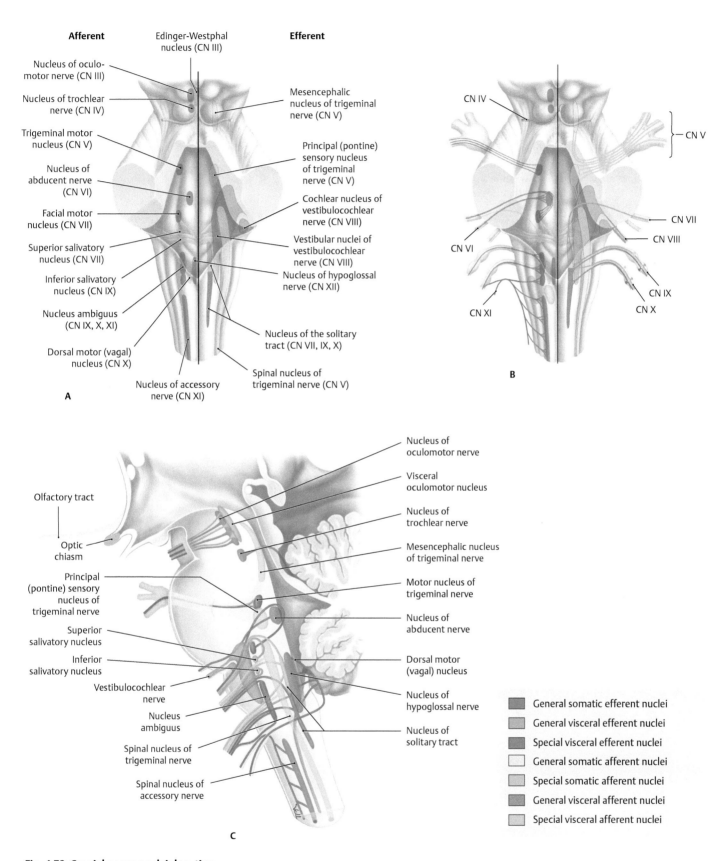

Afferent   Edinger-Westphal nucleus (CN III)   **Efferent**

Nucleus of oculomotor nerve (CN III)

Nucleus of trochlear nerve (CN IV)

Trigeminal motor nucleus (CN V)

Nucleus of abducent nerve (CN VI)

Facial motor nucleus (CN VII)

Superior salivatory nucleus (CN VII)

Inferior salivatory nucleus (CN IX)

Nucleus ambiguus (CN IX, X, XI)

Dorsal motor (vagal) nucleus (CN X)

Mesencephalic nucleus of trigeminal nerve (CN V)

Principal (pontine) sensory nucleus of trigeminal nerve (CN V)

Cochlear nucleus of vestibulocochlear nerve (CN VIII)

Vestibular nuclei of vestibulocochlear nerve (CN VIII)

Nucleus of hypoglossal nerve (CN XII)

Nucleus of the solitary tract (CN VII, IX, X)

Spinal nucleus of trigeminal nerve (CN V)

Nucleus of accessory nerve (CN XI)

A

CN IV

CN V

CN VI

CN VII

CN VIII

CN IX

CN X

CN XI

B

Olfactory tract

Optic chiasm

Principal (pontine) sensory nucleus of trigeminal nerve

Superior salivatory nucleus

Inferior salivatory nucleus

Vestibulocochlear nerve

Nucleus ambiguus

Spinal nucleus of trigeminal nerve

Spinal nucleus of accessory nerve

Nucleus of oculomotor nerve

Visceral oculomotor nucleus

Nucleus of trochlear nerve

Mesencephalic nucleus of trigeminal nerve

Motor nucleus of trigeminal nerve

Nucleus of abducent nerve

Dorsal motor (vagal) nucleus

Nucleus of hypoglossal nerve

Nucleus of solitary tract

C

- General somatic efferent nuclei
- General visceral efferent nuclei
- Special visceral efferent nuclei
- General somatic afferent nuclei
- Special somatic afferent nuclei
- General visceral afferent nuclei
- Special visceral afferent nuclei

Fig. 4.73 Cranial nerve nuclei: location
A, B Posterior view of brainstem (cerebellum removed). **C** Left lateral view of midsagittal section. *Note:* The cranial nerves are numbered and described according to the level of their *emergence* from the brainstem. This does not necessarily correspond to the level of the cranial nerve nuclei associated with the nerve.

CN I & II: Olfactory & Optic Nerves

Neither the olfactory nerve nor the optic nerve is a true peripheral nerve. They are extensions of the brain (telencephalon and diencephalon, respectively). They are therefore both sheathed in meninges (removed here) and contain CNS-specific cells (oligodendrocytes and microglia).

Fig. 4.74 **Olfactory nerve (CN I)**

A Left lateral view of left nasal septum and right lateral nasal wall (the posterior part of the nasal septum is cut). **B** Inferior view of brain. (*Shaded structures are deep to the basal surface.)

The olfactory nerve relays smell information (special visceral afferent) to the cortex via a classical three-neuron pathway.

1. First-order sensory neurons are located in the mucosa of the upper nasal septum and superior nasal concha (**A**). These bipolar neurons form 20 or so fiber bundles collectively called the olfactory nerves (CN I). As the "olfactory region" is limited by the extent of these fibers (2–4 cm²), the nasal conchae create turbulence, which ensures that air (and olfactory stimuli) passes over this area. The thin, unmyelinated olfactory fibers enter the anterior cranial fossa via the cribriform plate of the ethmoid bone.
2. Second-order sensory neurons are located in the olfactory bulb (**B**). Their axons course in the olfactory tract to the medial or lateral olfactory striae. These axons synapse in the amygdala, the prepiriform area, or neighboring areas.
3. Third-order neurons relay the information to the cerebral cortex.

The first-order neurons have a limited lifespan (several months) and are continuously replenished from a pool of precursor cells in the olfactory mucosa. The regenerative capacity of the olfactory mucosa diminishes with age. Injuries to the cribriform plate may damage the meningeal covering of the olfactory fibers, causing olfactory disturbances and cerebrospinal fluid leakage ("runny nose" after head trauma). See pp. 194–195 for the mechanisms of smell.

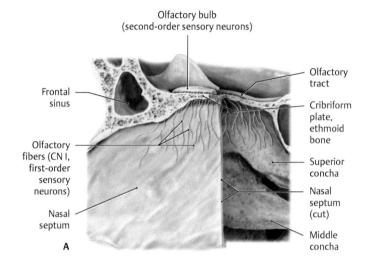

A

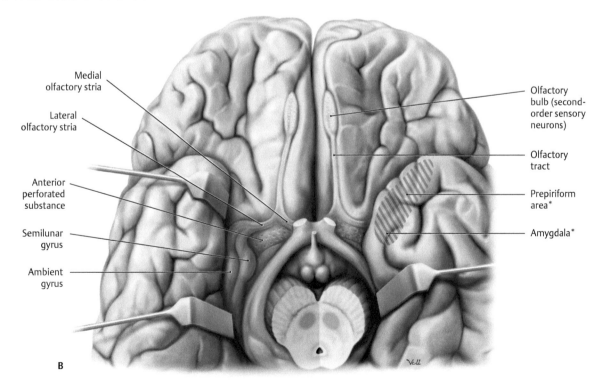

B

Fig. 4.75 Optic nerve (CN II)

A Inferior view of brain. **B** Left lateral view of opened orbit. **C** Left posterolateral view of brainstem. The optic nerve (special somatic afferent) relays sight information from the retina to the visual cortex (striate area) via a four-neuron pathway (see p. 268). First-order neurons (rods and cones) in the retina translate incoming photons into impulses, which are relayed to second-order bipolar neurons and third-order ganglion cells. These retinal ganglion cells combine to form the optic nerve (CN II). The optic nerve passes from the orbit into the middle cranial fossa via the optic canal (the optic canal is medial to the superior orbital fissure by which the other cranial nerves enter the orbit, **B**). Ninety percent of the third-order neurons in the optic nerve synapse in the lateral geniculate body (**C**), which then projects to the striate area. Ten percent of the third-order neurons synapse in the mesencephalon. This nongeniculate part of the visual pathway functions in unconscious and reflex action. See p. 270 for the mechanisms of sight. Lesion of the optic nerve may cause partial or complete loss of vision, depending on the point at which the nerve is disrupted (see p. 270).

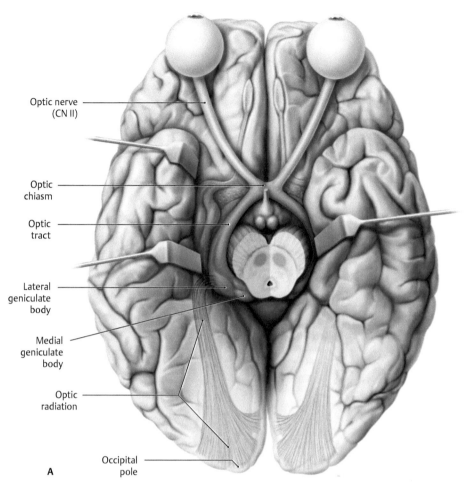

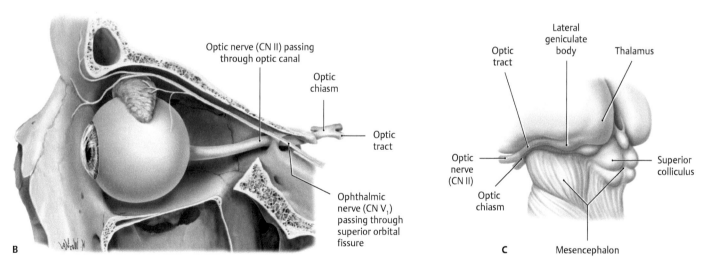

125

CN III, IV, & VI: Oculomotor, Trochlear, & Abducent Nerves

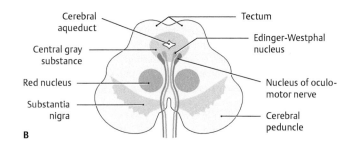

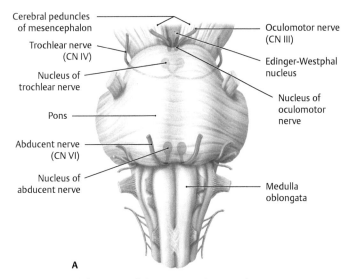

Fig. 4.76 Cranial nerves of the extraocular muscles
A Anterior view of brainstem. **B** Superior view of cross section through the mesencephalon.

CN III, IV, and VI are the three cranial nerves that collectively innervate the six extraocular muscles. (*Note:* CN III is also involved with the parasympathetic supply to the intraocular muscles.) CN III and IV arise from nuclei in the mesencephalon (midbrain, the highest level of the brainstem) and emerge at roughly the same level. CN VI arises from nuclei in the pons and emerges from the brainstem at the pontomedullary junction.

Table 4.17 Oculomotor nerve (CN III)

Nuclei, ganglion, and fiber distribution

Somatomotor (red)

Nucleus of the oculomotor nerve (mesencephalon)	Lower motor neurons innervate: • Levator palpebrae superioris • Superior, medial, and inferior rectus muscles • Inferior oblique

Parasympathetic (blue)

Edinger-Westphal nucleus (mesencephalon)	Preganglionic neurons travel in the inferior division of CN III
	Postganglionic neurons in the **ciliary ganglion** innervate: Intraocular muscles (pupillary sphincter and ciliary muscle)

Course

CN III emerges from the mesencephalon, the highest level of the brainstem. It runs anteriorly through the lateral wall of the cavernous sinus to enter the orbit through the **superior orbital fissure**. After passing *through* the common tendinous ring, CN III divides into a superior and an inferior division.

Lesions

Lesions cause oculomotor palsy of various extents. Complete oculomotor palsy is marked by paralysis of all the innervated muscles, causing:
• Ptosis (drooping of eyelid) = disabled levator palpebrae superioris
• Inferolateral deviation of affected eye, causing diplopia (double vision) = disabled extraocular muscles
• Mydriasis (pupil dilation) = disabled pupillary sphincter
• Accommodation difficulties (difficulty focusing) = disabled ciliary muscle

Table 4.18 Trochlear nerve (CN IV)

Nucleus and fiber distribution

Somatomotor (red)

Nucleus of the trochlear nerve (mesencephalon)	Lower motor neurons innervate: • Superior oblique

Course

CN IV is the only cranial nerve to emerge from the posterior surface of the brainstem. After emerging from the mesencephalon, it courses anteriorly around the cerebral peduncle. CN IV then enters the orbit through the **superior orbital fissure**, passing *lateral* to the common tendinous ring. It has the longest *intra*dural course of the three extraocular motor nerves.

Lesions

Lesions cause trochlear nerve palsy:
• Superomedial deviation of the affected eye, causing diplopia (double vision) = disabled superior oblique
Note: Because CN IV crosses to the opposite side, lesions close to the nucleus result in trochlear nerve palsy on the opposite side (contralateral palsy). Lesions past the site where the nerve crosses the midline cause palsy on the same side (ipsilateral palsy).

Table 4.19 Abducent nerve (CN VI)

Nucleus and fiber distribution

Somatomotor (red)

Nucleus of the abducent nerve (pons)	Lower motor neurons innervate: • Lateral rectus

Course

CN VI follows a long *extra*dural path. It emerges from the pontomedullary junction (inferior border of pons) and runs through the cavernous sinus in close proximity to the internal carotid artery. CN VI enters the orbit through the **superior orbital fissure** and courses *through* the common tendinous ring.

Lesions

Lesions cause abducent nerve palsy:
• Medial deviation of the affected eye, causing diplopia = disabled lateral rectus
Note: The path of CN VI through the cavernous sinus exposes it to injury. Cavernous sinus thrombosis, aneurysms of the internal carotid artery, meningitis, and subdural hemorrhage may all compress the nerve, resulting in nerve palsy. Excessive fall in CSF pressure (e.g., due to lumbar puncture) may cause the brainstem to descend, exerting traction on the nerve.

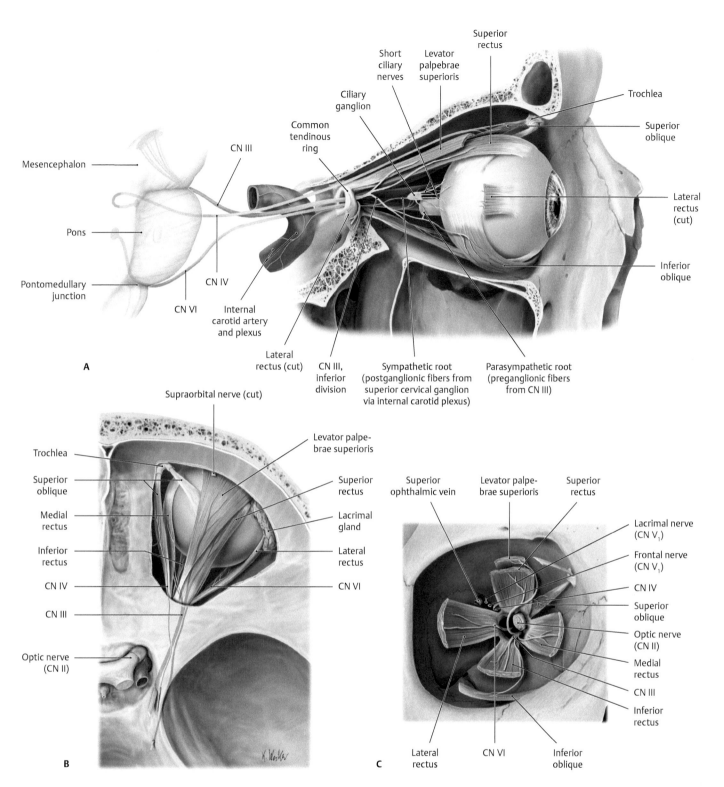

Fig. 4.77 Nerves supplying the ocular muscles

Right orbit. **A** Lateral view with temporal wall removed. **B** Superior view of opened orbit. **C** Anterior view. Cranial nerves III, IV, and VI enter the orbit through the superior orbital fissure, lateral to the optic canal (CN IV then passes lateral to the common tendinous ring, and CN III and VI pass through it). All three nerves supply somatomotor innervation to the extraocular muscles. The ciliary ganglion communicates three types of fibers (parasympathetic, sympathetic, and sensory) to and from the intraocular muscles via the short ciliary nerves. (Only parasympathetics synapse in the ciliary ganglion. All other fibers pass through without synapsing.) The ciliary ganglion therefore has three roots:

• Parasympathetic (motor) root: Preganglionic parasympathetic fibers travel with the inferior division of CN III to the ciliary ganglion. Only

the parasympathetic fibers synapse in the ciliary ganglion (the other two fiber types pass through the ganglion without synapsing).
• Sympathetic root: Postganglionic sympathetic fibers from the superior cervical ganglion travel on the internal carotid artery to enter the superior orbital fissure, where they may course along the ophthalmic artery to enter the short ciliary nerves via the ciliary ganglion.
• Sensory root: Sensory fibers (from the eyeball) travel to the nasociliary nerve (CN V₁) via the ciliary ganglion.

The short ciliary nerves therefore contain sensory fibers from the eyeball and postganglionic sympathetic and parasympathetic fibers from the superior cervical and ciliary ganglion, respectively. *Note:* Sympathetic fibers from the superior cervical ganglion may also travel with the nasociliary nerve (CN V₁) and reach the intraocular muscles via the long ciliary nerves.

127

CN V: Trigeminal Nerve, Nuclei, & Divisions

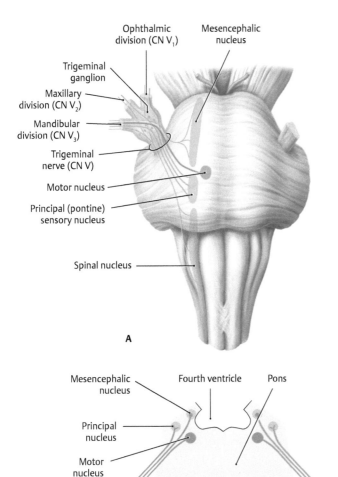

A

B

Fig. 4.78 Trigeminal nerve nuclei
A Anterior view of brainstem. **B** Superior view of cross section through the pons.

Afferent neurons in the trigeminal nerve divisions convey general somatic sensation (touch, pain, and temperature) to the CNS. The neurons from all three divisions synapse in three brainstem nuclei named for their locations (see **Table 4.20**):

- **Mesencephalic nucleus**
- **Principal (pontine) sensory nucleus**
- **Spinal nucleus**

Efferent fibers arise from lower motor neurons in the **motor nucleus**. These fibers exit at the motor root of the trigeminal nerve and unite with the mandibular division (CN V₃) in the foramen ovale. The branchiomotor fibers innervate the muscles of the first pharyngeal (brachial) arch.

Fig. 4.79 Trigeminal nerve lesions
Lesions of the trigeminal nerve divisions (peripheral nerves) will produce sensory loss following the pattern in **Fig. 4.80B** and potentially motor paralysis. Lesions of the spinal nucleus of the trigeminal cord will produce sensory loss (pain and temperature) in the pattern shown here (Sölder lines). These concentric circles correspond to the somatotopic organization of the spinal cord nucleus: more cranial portions receive axons from the center of the face, and more caudal portions receive axons from the periphery.

Table 4.20 Trigeminal nerve nuclei and lesions

Nuclei

Somatosensory (yellow)

Afferent neurons from the sensory territories of all three trigeminal divisions synapse in three brainstem nuclei named for their location.

Nucleus	Location	Sensation
Mesencephalic nucleus	Mesencephalon	Proprioception (*Note:* The first-order sensory cell bodies of proprioceptive fibers associated with CN V have their cell bodies located in the mesencephalic nucleus.)
Principal (pontine) sensory nucleus	Pons	Touch
Spinal nucleus	Medulla oblongata	Pain and temperature

Note: These sensory nuclei contain the cell bodies of second-order neurons. The mesencephalic nucleus is an exception — it contains the cell bodies of first-order pseudounipolar neurons, which have migrated into the brain.

Branchiomotor (purple)

Lower motor neurons are located in the motor nucleus of the trigeminal nerve. They innervate the eight muscles derived from the 1st branchial arch:

- Masseter
- Temporalis
- Lateral pterygoid
- Medial pterygoid
- Tensor veli palatini
- Tensor tympani
- Mylohyoid
- Digastric, anterior belly

Lesions

Traumatic lesions of the trigeminal nerve may cause sensory loss in corresponding territories or paralysis to the target muscles. *Note:* The afferent fibers of the trigeminal nerve compose the afferent limb of the corneal reflex (reflex eyelid closure).

- Trigeminal neuralgia is a disorder of CN V causing intense, crippling pain in the sensory territories.

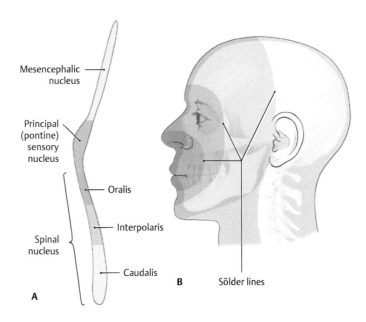

A   **B**   Sölder lines

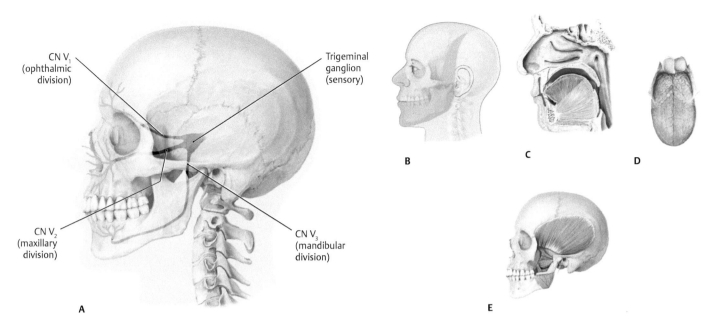

Fig. 4.80 Trigeminal nerve divisions and distribution
A Left lateral view of trigeminal divisions. **B–D** Somatosensory nerve territories. **E** Branchiomotor nerve territories.
The trigeminal nerve is the major sensory nerve of the face. It has three major divisions (**A**) that convey general somatic sensation (touch, pain, and proprioception) from the face (**B**) and select mucosa (**C** and **D**). The trigeminal nerve also contains branchiomotor fibers that innervate the eight muscles derived from the first branchial arch (**E**).

Table 4.21 Trigeminal nerve (CN V) divisions and distribution		
CN V consists of a large sensory root and a small motor root, which emerge from the brainstem separately in the middle cranial fossa at the level of the pons.		
Sensory root		
Fibers	**General somatosensory** (yellow): Convey general sensation (touch, pain, and temperature) from the sensory territories of CN V (see **Fig. 4.80**). The cell bodies of these first-order pseudounipolar neurons are primarily located in the trigeminal ganglion.	
Course	The sensory root is formed by three divisions that unite as the **trigeminal ganglion** in the middle cranial fossa.	**Division** / **Distribution**

Division	Distribution
CN V₁ (ophthalmic division)	From orbit via superior orbital fissure (see pp. 130, 252)
CN V₂ (maxillary division)	From pterygopalatine fossa via foramen rotundum (see pp. 132, 181)
CN V₃ (mandibular division)	From inferior skull base via foramen ovale (see pp. 134, 169)

| **Nuclei** | Afferent axons from all three divisions synapse on three brainstem nuclei located in the mesencephalon, pons, and medulla oblongata of the spinal cord. | |

Nuclei	Sensation
Mesencephalic nucleus	Proprioception (see **Table 4.20**)
Principal (pontine) sensory nucleus	Touch
Spinal nucleus	Pain and temperature

Motor root		
Fibers	**Branchiomotor** (purple): Conveys motor fibers to the eight muscles derived from the 1st branchial (pharyngeal) arch:	• Masseter • Temporalis • Lateral pterygoid • Medial pterygoid • Tensor veli palatini • Tensor tympani • Mylohyoid • Digastric, anterior belly
Course	The motor root emerges separately from the pons and unites with CN V₃ in the foramen ovale.	
Nucleus	Motor nucleus (located in pons)	
"Scaffolding": CN V is used as scaffolding for the distribution of autonomic (sympathetic and parasympathetic) and taste fibers from other cranial nerves.		
Parasympathetic	All three branches of CN V are used to convey postganglionic parasympathetic fibers from parasympathetic ganglia. • CN VII: Preganglionic fibers from CN VII synapse in the pterygopalatine or the submandibular ganglion, associated with CN V₂ and CN V₃, respectively. Postganglionic parasympathetic fibers then travel with the sensory branches of CN V to reach their targets. • CN IX: Preganglionic fibers synapse in the otic ganglion; postganglionic fibers are distributed along branches of CN V₃.	
Sympathetic	Postganglionic sympathetic fibers from the superior cervical ganglion may also be distributed by the sensory branches of CN V.	
Taste	Taste fibers from the presulcal tongue (anterior two thirds) travel via the lingual nerve (CN V₃) to the chorda tympani (CN VII) and nuclei of CN VII.	

CN V₁: Trigeminal Nerve, Ophthalmic Division

***Fig. 4.81* Ophthalmic division (CN V₁) of the trigeminal nerve**

Lateral view of the partially opened right orbit. The ophthalmic nerve divides into three major branches *before* reaching the superior orbital fissure: the lacrimal (L), frontal (F), and nasociliary (N) nerves. These nerves run roughly in the lateral, middle, and medial portions of the upper orbit, respectively. The lacrimal and frontal nerves enter the orbit superior to the common tendinous ring, and the nasociliary nerve enters through it. See **Table 4.22** for labels.

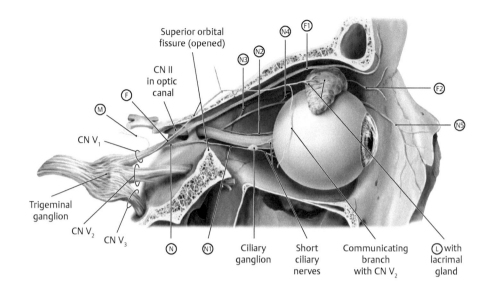

***Fig. 4.82* Ophthalmic nerve divisions in the orbit**

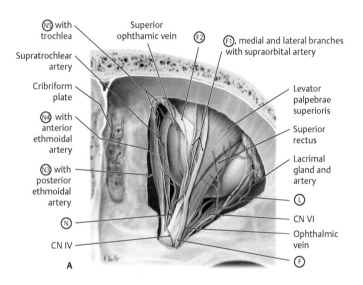

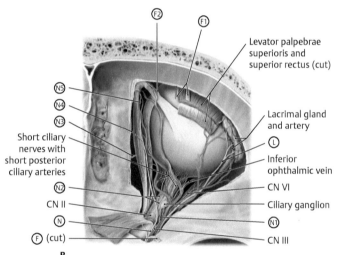

Superior view of orbit. (*Removed:* Bony roof, periorbita, and periorbital fat.) See **Table 4.22** for labels. **A** Lacrimal, frontal, and nasociliary divisions. **B** Nasociliary nerve and ciliary ganglion. (*Cut:* Superior rectus and levator palpebrae superioris.)

The *extra*ocular muscles receive somatomotor innervation from the oculomotor (CN III), trochlear (CN IV), and abducent (CN VI) nerves. The *intra*ocular muscles receive autonomic (sympathetic and parasympathetic) innervation via the short and long ciliary nerves. Sympa-

thetic fibers from the superior cervical ganglion ascend on the internal carotid artery and travel in two manners: they may join the nasociliary nerve (CN V₁), which distributes them as the long ciliary nerves, or they may course along the ophthalmic artery to enter the ciliary ganglion as the *sympathetic root*. The ciliary ganglion also receives parasympathetic fibers from CN III (via the *parasympathetic root*). The ganglion distributes these sympathetic and parasympathetic fibers via the short ciliary nerves. The short ciliary nerves contain sensory fibers, which enter the nasociliary nerve via the *sensory root* of the ciliary ganglion.

Table 4.22 Ophthalmic nerve (CN V₁)

The ophthalmic nerve (CN V₁) is a sensory nerve* that conveys fibers from structures of the superior facial skeleton to the trigeminal ganglion. CN V₁ gives off one branch in the middle cranial fossa before dividing into three major branches, which pass through the superior orbital fissure into the orbit. The lacrimal, frontal, and nasociliary nerves travel in the lateral, middle, and medial portions of the upper orbit, respectively.

Ⓜ **Meningeal n.**	Sensory: Dura mater of the middle cranial fossa.
Ⓛ **Lacrimal n.**	The smallest of the three major branches, the lacrimal nerve runs in the superolateral orbit.
Opening	Superior orbital fissure (above the common tendinous ring).
Course	Runs (with the lacrimal artery) along the superior surface of the lateral rectus, through the lacrimal gland and orbital septum to the skin of the upper eyelid.
Innervation	Sensory: Upper eyelid (skin and conjunctiva) and lacrimal gland.
	Sensory and parasympathetic: Lacrimal gland. Postganglionic parasympathetic secretomotor fibers from the pterygopalatine ganglion of the facial nerve (CN VII) travel with the zygomatic and zygomaticotemporal nerves (CN V₂). They enter the sensory lacrimal nerve (CN V₁) via a communicating branch and are distributed to the gland. Postganglionic sympathetic fibers follow a similar path.
Ⓕ **Frontal n.**	The largest of the three major branches, the frontal nerve runs in the middle of the upper orbit.
Opening	Superior orbital fissure (above the common tendinous ring).
Course and branches	Runs along the superior surface of the levator palpebrae superioris, below the periosteum. At roughly the level of the posterior eyeball, the frontal nerve divides into two terminal branches:

	Ⓕ₁ **Supraorbital n.**	Continues on the superior surface of the levator palpebrae superioris and passes through the supraorbital foramen (notch).
	Ⓕ₂ **Supratrochlear n.**	Courses anteromedially with the supratrochlear artery toward the trochlea (tendon of superior oblique) and passes through the frontal notch.

Innervation	Sensory: Upper eyelid (skin and conjunctiva) and the skin of the forehead (both branches). The supraorbital n. also receives fibers from frontal sinus mucosa; the supratrochlear n. communicates with the infratrochlear nerve.
Ⓝ **Nasociliary n.**	The nasociliary nerve runs in the middle and medial parts of the upper orbit.
Opening	Superior orbital fissure (via the common tendinous ring).
Course and branches	Runs medially (across the optic nerve [CN II]) and then anteriorly between the superior oblique and medial rectus. Gives off three branches (two sensory and one sympathetic) before dividing into two terminal branches (anterior ethmoid and infratrochlear nerves).

	Ⓝ₁ **Sensory root of the ciliary ganglion**	Sensory: Fibers from the **short ciliary nerves** pass without synapsing through the ciliary ganglion and enter the nasociliary nerve via the sensory root.
	Ⓝ₂ **Long ciliary nn.**	Sensory: Eye (e.g., cornea and sclera).
	Ⓝ₃ **Posterior ethmoid n.**	Sensory: Ethmoid air cells and sphenoid sinus. Fibers run in the ethmoid bone (posterior ethmoid canal) to the nasociliary nerve.
	Ⓝ₄ **Anterior ethmoid n.**	Sensory: Superficial nose and anterior nasal cavity. • **Internal nasal n.:** Mucosa of the anterior portions of the nasal septum (medial internal nasal n.) and lateral nasal wall (lateral internal nasal n.). • **External nasal n.:** Skin of the nose (courses under the nasalis muscle). Fibers from these two terminal branches ascend via the nasal bone, course posteriorly in the cranial cavity over the cribriform plate, and enter the orbit via the anterior ethmoid canal.
	Ⓝ₅ **Infratrochlear n.**	Sensory: Medial aspect of the upper eyelid (skin and conjunctiva) and the lacrimal sac. Fibers enter the orbit near the trochlea (tendon of superior oblique) and course posteriorly to the nasociliary nerve.

Innervation	Sensory: Ethmoid air cells, sphenoid sinus, anterior nasal cavity, superficial nose, upper eyelid, lacrimal sac, and eye.

*Note: Nerve courses are traditionally described proximal to distal (CNS to periphery). However, for sensory nerves, the sensory relay is in the opposite direction. It is more appropriate to talk of sensory nerves collecting fibers than to talk of them branching to supply a region.

CN V₂: Trigeminal Nerve, Maxillary Division

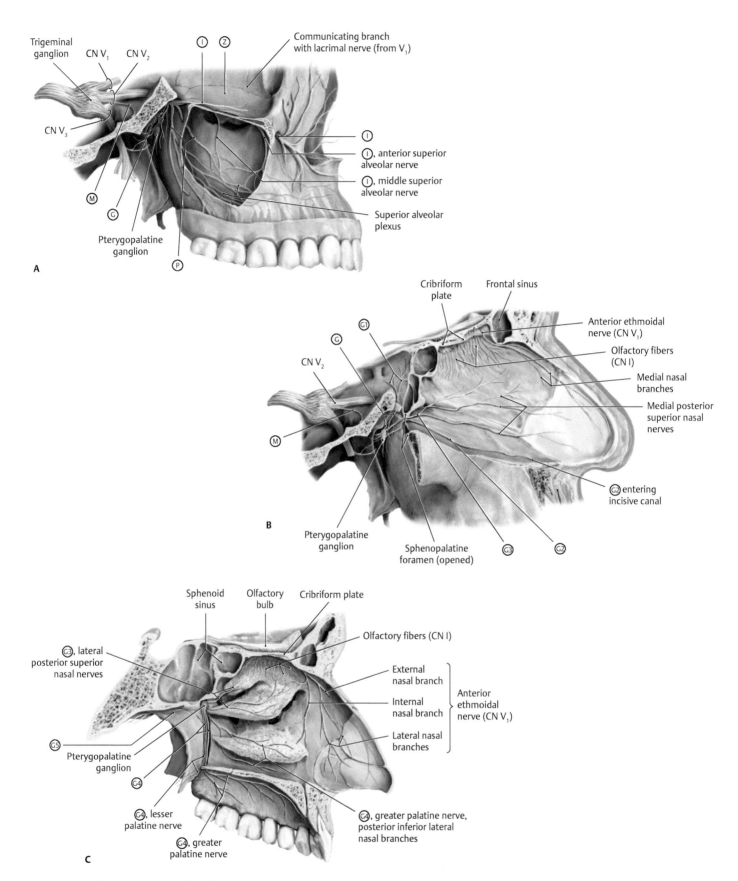

Fig. 4.83 Maxillary division (CN V₂) of the trigeminal nerve
Right lateral view. See **Table 4.23** for labels. **A** Opened right maxillary sinus. **B** Nasal septum in right nasal cavity. **C** Left lateral nasal wall.

Table 4.23 Maxillary nerve (CN V₂)

Like the ophthalmic nerve (CN V₁), the maxillary nerve (CN V₂) is a sensory nerve* that conveys fibers from structures of the facial skeleton to the trigeminal ganglion. CN V₂ gives off one branch in the middle cranial fossa before entering the foramen rotundum to the pterygopalatine fossa. In the pterygopalatine fossa, the maxillary nerve divides into branches (e.g., zygomatic, posterior superior alveolar, and infraorbital nerves) and receives ganglionic branches from the pterygopalatine ganglion. This ganglion has five major branches, which distribute CN V₂ fibers. These sensory CN V₂ fibers convey autonomic fibers from the pterygopalatine ganglion.

Direct branches of the maxillary n. (CN V₂)

Ⓜ **Middle meningeal n.**	Sensory: Meninges of the middle cranial fossa.
Ⓖ **Ganglionic branches**	Generally, two ganglionic branches suspend (pass through) the **pterygopalatine ganglion** from CN V₂ (see below).
Ⓩ **Zygomatic n.**	Sensory: Skin of the temple (**zygomaticotemporal nerve**) and cheek (**zygomaticofacial nerve**). Fibers enter the orbit via canals in the zygomatic bone and course in the lateral orbit wall to CN V₂ via the inferior orbital fissure.
Ⓟ **Posterior superior alveolar n.**	Sensory: Maxillary molars (with associated gingivae and buccal mucosa) and maxillary sinus. Fibers course on the infratemporal surface of the maxilla. The posterior superior alveolar nerve contributes to the **superior alveolar plexus** (anterior, middle, and superior alveolar nn.).
Ⓘ **Infraorbital n.**	Sensory: Lower eyelid (skin and conjunctiva), maxillary sinus, and maxillary teeth (via anterior and middle superior alveolar branches). • **Middle superior alveolar nerve:** Sensory fibers from the maxillary premolars (with associated gingivae, buccal mucosa, and maxillary sinus). (The occurance is variable). • **Anterior superior alveolar nerve:** Sensory fibers from the maxillary incisors and canines (with associated gingivae, lingual mucosa, and maxillary sinus). Nasal branch: Sensory fibers from anterior portions of the nasal wall, floor, and septum. These fibers enter the infraorbital canal and emerge from the infraorbital groove.

Branches passing through the pterygopalatine ganglion: The pterygopalatine ganglion is a parasympathetic ganglion of the facial nerve (CN VII). It conveys first-order sensory fibers to CN V₂ from five major branches supplying the orbit, nasal cavity, hard and soft palates, and nasopharynx.

Ⓖ₁ **Orbital branches**	Sensory: Orbital periosteum (via inferior orbital fissure) and paranasal sinuses (ethmoid air cells and sphenoid sinus, via the posterior ethmoid canal).
Ⓖ₂ **Nasopalatine n.**	Sensory: Anterior hard palate and the inferior nasal septum. The left and right nasopalatine nerves ascend (in the anterior and posterior incisive foramina, respectively) and converge in the incisive fossa. They travel posterosuperiorly on the nasal septum (vomer) through the sphenopalatine foramen.
Ⓖ₃ **Posterior superior nasal nn.**	Sensory: Posterosuperior nasal cavity. (*Note:* The anterior ethmoid nerve [CN V₁] conveys fibers from the anterosuperior portion.) • **Lateral posterior superior nasal nn.:** Posterior ethmoid air cells and mucosa in the posterior of the superior and middle nasal conchae. • **Medial posterior superior nasal nn.:** Mucosa of the posterior nasal roof and septum.
Ⓖ₄ **Palatine nn.**	Sensory: Hard and soft palates. • **Greater palatine n.:** Hard palate (gingivae, mucosa, and glands) and soft palate via greater palatine canal. Receives fibers from the inferior nasal concha and walls of the middle and inferior nasal meatuses through the perpendicular plate of the ethmoid bone (posterior inferior nasal branches). • **Lesser palatine n.:** Soft palate, palatine tonsils, and uvula via lesser palatine canal. The greater and lesser palatine nerves converge in the greater palatine canal.
Ⓖ₅ **Pharyngeal n.**	Sensory: Mucosa of the superior nasopharynx via palatovaginal (pharyngeal) canal.

Autonomic scaffolding: The pterygopalatine ganglion is affiliated with the sensory CN V₂. Postganglionic autonomic fibers are distributed by sensory fibers of CN V₂.

Pterygopalatine ganglion (CN VII)	**Motor root:** Preganglionic parasympathetic fibers from the facial nerve (CN VII) travel in the **greater petrosal nerve** (joins with deep petrosal nerve to form nerve of pterygoid canal).
	Sympathetic root: Postganglionic sympathetic fibers from the superior cervical ganglion ascend (via the internal carotid plexus) and travel in the **deep petrosal nerve** (joins with greater petrosal nerve to form nerve of pterygoid canal).
	Sensory root: Sensory fibers pass through the ganglion from five sensory branches (see above).

• **Lacrimal gland:** Postganglionic parasympathetic secretomotor fibers to the lacrimal gland leave the pterygopalatine ganglion on the zygomatic nerve (CN V₂). They travel with the zygomaticotemporal nerve to the lacrimal nerve (CN V₁) via a communicating branch.
• **Glands of the oral cavity:** Postganglionic parasympathetic fibers to the glands of the palatine, pharyngeal, and nasal mucosa reach their targets via corresponding sensory branches of CN V₂.
• **Blood vessels:** Postganglionic sympathetic fibers are distributed by CN V₂.
• **Taste (CN VII):** Taste fibers (special visceral afferent) associated with CN VII ascend from the palate to the greater petrosal nerve and geniculate ganglion of CN VII via the palatine nerves.

*Note: Nerve courses are traditionally described proximal to distal (CNS to periphery). However, for sensory nerves, the sensory relay is in the opposite direction. It is more appropriate to talk of sensory nerves collecting fibers than to talk of them branching to supply a region.

CN V₃: Trigeminal Nerve, Mandibular Division

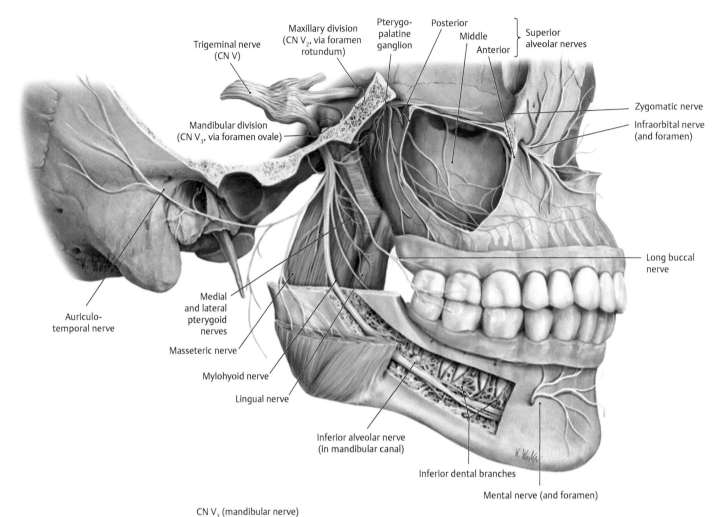

Trigeminal nerve (CN V)

Maxillary division (CN V₂, via foramen rotundum)

Pterygopalatine ganglion

Posterior
Middle
Anterior

Superior alveolar nerves

Mandibular division (CN V₃, via foramen ovale)

Zygomatic nerve

Infraorbital nerve (and foramen)

Long buccal nerve

Auriculotemporal nerve

Medial and lateral pterygoid nerves

Masseteric nerve

Mylohyoid nerve

Lingual nerve

Inferior alveolar nerve (in mandibular canal)

Inferior dental branches

Mental nerve (and foramen)

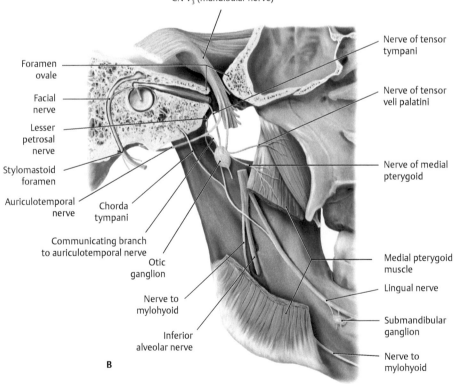

CN V₃ (mandibular nerve)

Foramen ovale

Facial nerve

Lesser petrosal nerve

Stylomastoid foramen

Auriculotemporal nerve

Chorda tympani

Communicating branch to auriculotemporal nerve

Otic ganglion

Nerve to mylohyoid

Inferior alveolar nerve

Nerve of tensor tympani

Nerve of tensor veli palatini

Nerve of medial pterygoid

Medial pterygoid muscle

Lingual nerve

Submandibular ganglion

Nerve to mylohyoid

B

Fig. 4.84 Mandibular division (CN V₃) of the trigeminal nerve

Right lateral view. **A** Partially opened mandible with middle cranial fossa windowed. **B** Opened oral cavity (right half of mandible removed).

The trunk of CN V₃ gives off two branches (recurrent meningeal and medial pterygoid nerves) before splitting into an anterior and a posterior division (see **Table 4.24**). The nerve to the medial pterygoid conveys branchiomotor fibers to the otic ganglion; these fibers pass without synapsing to innervate the tensors tympani and veli palatini. The otic ganglion is the parasympathetic ganglion of the glossopharyngeal nerve (CN IX). Preganglionic fibers enter via the lesser petrosal nerve (reconstituted from the tympanic plexus; see p. 143). Postganglionic fibers leave with the auriculotemporal nerve (CN V₃) to innervate the buccal and parotid glands. Taste fibers of CN VII travel in the lingual nerve (CN V₃) to the chorda tympani (which they enter either directly or indirectly via the otic ganglion). These fibers ascend in the chorda tympani via the tympanic cavity to the facial nerve (CN VII; see p. 137).

Table 4.24 Mandibular nerve (CN V₃)

The mandibular nerve (CN V_3) is the mixed afferent-efferent branch of CN V, containing general sensory fibers and branchiomotor fibers to the eight muscles derived from the 1st pharyngeal arch. The large sensory and small motor roots of CN V leave the middle cranial fossa via the foramen ovale. In the infratemporal fossa, they unite to form the CN V_3 trunk. The trunk gives off two branches before splitting into an anterior and a posterior division. Of the eight branchial arch muscles, three are supplied by the trunk, three by the anterior division, and two by the posterior division.

Trunk: The trunk of CN V_3 gives off one sensory and one motor branch. The motor branch conveys branchiomotor fibers to three of the eight muscles of the 1st pharyngeal arch.

Ⓡ **Recurrent meningeal branch** (nervus spinosum)	Sensory: Dura of the middle cranial fossa (also anterior cranial fossa and calvarium). The nervus spinosum arises in the infratemporal fossa and re-enters the middle cranial fossa via the foramen spinosum.
Ⓜ **Medial pterygoid n.**	Branchiomotor: Directly to the **medial pterygoid**. Certain fibers enter the otic ganglion via the motor root and pass without synapsing to: • N. to tensor veli palatini: **Tensor veli palatini**. • N. to tensor tympani: **Tensor tympani**.

Anterior division: The anterior division of CN V_3 contains predominantly efferent fibers (with one sensory branch, the buccal nerve.) The branchiomotor fibers innervate three of the eight muscles of the 1st pharyngeal arch.

Ⓜ **Masseter n.**	Branchiomotor: **Masseter**. Sensory: Temporomandibular joint (articular branches).
Ⓣ **Deep temporal nn.**	Branchiomotor: **Temporalis** via two branches: • Anterior deep temporal n. • Posterior deep temporal n.
Ⓛ **Lateral pterygoid n.**	Branchiomotor: **Lateral pterygoid**.
Ⓑ **Long buccal n.**	Sensory: Cheek (skin and mucosa) and buccal gingivae of the molars.

Posterior division: The larger posterior division of CN V_3 contains predominantly afferent fibers (with one motor branch, the mylohyoid nerve). The mylohyoid nerve arises from the inferior alveolar nerve and supplies the remaining two muscles of the 1st pharyngeal arch.

Ⓐ **Auriculotemporal n.**	Sensory: Skin of the ear and temple. Fibers pass through the parotid gland, behind the temporomandibular joint, and into the infratemporal fossa. The nerve typically splits around the middle meningeal artery (a branch of the maxillary artery) before joining the posterior division. Distributes postganglionic parasympathetic fibers from the otic ganglion.
Ⓛ **Lingual n.**	Sensory: Mucosa of the oral cavity (presulcal tongue, oral floor, and gingival covering of lingual surface of mandibular teeth). In the infratemporal fossa, the lingual nerve combines with the chorda tympani (CN VII).
Ⓘ **Inferior alveolar n.**	Sensory: Mandibular teeth and chin: • **Incisive branch:** Incisors, canines, and 1st premolars (with associated labial gingivae). • **Mental n.:** Labial gingivae of the incisors and the skin of the lower lip and chin. The mental nerve enters the mental foramen and combines with the incisive branch in the mandibular canal. The inferior alveolar nerve exits the mandible via the mandibular foramen and combines to form the posterior division of CN V_3. *Note:* 2nd premolars and mandibular molars are supplied by the inferior alveolar nerve before it splits into its terminal branches. Branchiomotor: Fibers branch just proximal to the mandibular foramen: • **Mylohyoid n.: Mylohyoid** and anterior belly of the **digastric**.

Autonomic scaffolding: The parasympathetic ganglia of CN VII (submandibular ganglion) and CN IX (otic ganglion) are functionally associated with CN V_3.

Submandibular ganglion (CN VII)	Parasympathetic root	Preganglionic parasympathetic fibers from the facial nerve (CN VII) travel to the ganglion in the **chorda tympani**, facial nerve, and lingual nerve (CN V_3).
	Sympathetic root	Sympathetic fibers from the **superior cervical ganglion** ascend (via the internal carotid plexus) and travel in a plexus on the facial artery.
Otic ganglion (CN IX)	Parasympathetic root	Preganglionic parasympathetic fibers enter from CN IX via the **lesser petrosal nerve**.
	Sympathetic root	Postganglionic sympathetic fibers from the **superior cervical ganglion** enter via a plexus on the middle meningeal artery.

• **Parotid gland:** Postganglionic parasympathetic fibers from the otic ganglion travel to the parotid gland via the auriculotemporal n. (CN V_3).
• **Submandibular and sublingual glands:** Postganglionic autonomic fibers to the submandibular and sublingual glands travel from the submandibular ganglion via glandular branches.

• **Taste** (CN VII): Taste fibers (special viscerosensory fibers) to CN VII may travel via the lingual nerve (CN V_3) to the chorda tympani (CN VII).

Note: Nerve courses are traditionally described proximal to distal (CNS to periphery). However, for sensory nerves, the sensory relay is in the opposite direction. It is more appropriate to talk of sensory nerves collecting fibers than to talk of them branching to supply a region.

CN VII: Facial Nerve, Nuclei & Internal Branches

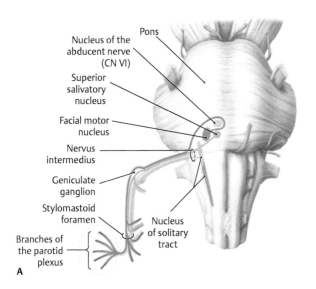

Pons
Nucleus of the abducent nerve (CN VI)
Superior salivatory nucleus
Facial motor nucleus
Nervus intermedius
Geniculate ganglion
Stylomastoid foramen
Branches of the parotid plexus
Nucleus of solitary tract

A

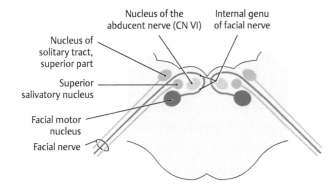

Nucleus of the abducent nerve (CN VI)
Internal genu of facial nerve
Nucleus of solitary tract, superior part
Superior salivatory nucleus
Facial motor nucleus
Facial nerve

B

Fig. 4.85 Facial nerve (CN VII)
A Anterior view of brainstem. **B** Superior view of cross section through pons.
Fibers: The facial nerve provides branchiomotor innervation to the muscles of the second pharyngeal arch and parasympathetic motor innervation to most salivary glands (via the pterygopalatine and submandibular ganglia). Taste fibers are conveyed via pseudounipolar sensory neurons with cell bodies in the geniculate ganglion. The facial nerve also receives general sensation from the external ear.
Branches: The superficial branches of CN VII are primarily branchiomotor (only the posterior auricular nerve may contain sensory fibers as well as motor). Taste and preganglionic parasympathetic fibers travel in both the chorda tympani and greater petrosal nerves. These fibers converge in the external genu and enter the brainstem together as the nervus intermedius.

Table 4.25 Facial nerve (CN VII)	
Nuclei, ganglia, and fiber distribution	
Branchiomotor (purple)	
Facial motor nucleus	Lower motor neurons innervate all muscles of the 2nd pharyngeal (branchial) arch: • Muscles of facial expression • Stylohyoid • Digastric, posterior belly • Stapedius
Parasympathetic (blue)	
Superior salivatory nucleus	Preganglionic neurons synapse in the **pterygo-palatine** or **submandibular ganglion**. Postganglionic neurons innervate: • Lacrimal gland • Submandibular and sublingual glands • Small glands of the oral and nasal cavities
Special visceral afferent (light green)	
Nucleus of the solitary tract, superior part	First-order pseudounipolar cells in the **geniculate ganglion** relay taste sensation from the presulcal tongue (anterior two thirds) and soft palate (via the chorda tympani and greater petrosal nerve).
General somatic afferent (yellow)	
First-order pseudounipolar cells in the **geniculate ganglion** relay general sensation from the external ear (auricle and skin of the auditory canal) and lateral tympanic membrane.	

Course

Emergence: Axons from the superior salivatory nucleus and the nucleus of the solitary tract form the **nervus intermedius**. These combine with the branchiomotor and somatosensory fibers to emerge from the brainstem as CN VII.
Internal branches: CN VII enters the petrous bone via the internal acoustic meatus. Within the facial canal, it gives off one branchiomotor branch (nerve to the stapedius) and two nerves (greater petrosal nerve and chorda tympani) containing both parasympathetic and taste fibers.
External branches: The remaining fibers emerge via the stylomastoid foramen. Three direct branches arise before the fibers enter the parotid gland (nerve to posterior belly of digastric, nerve to stylohyoid, and posterior auricular nerve). In the gland, the branchiomotor fibers branch to form the parotid plexus, which innervates the muscles of the 2nd pharyngeal arch.

Lesions

CN VII is most easily injured in its distal portions (after emerging from the parotid gland). Nerve lesions of the parotid plexus cause muscle paralysis. Temporal bone fractures may injure the nerve within the facial canal, causing disturbances of taste, lacrimation, salivation, etc. (see **Fig. 4.86**).

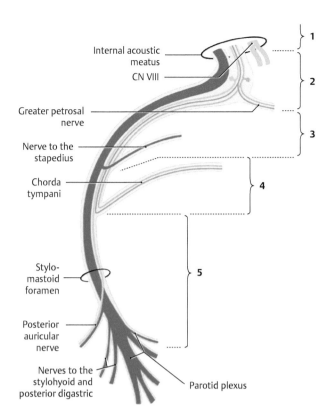

Fig. 4.87 Course of the facial nerve
Right lateral view of right temporal bone (petrous part). Both the facial nerve and vestibulocochlear nerve (CN VIII, not shown) pass through the internal acoustic meatus on the posterior surface of the petrous bone. The facial nerve courses laterally in the bone to the external genu, which contains the **geniculate ganglion** (cell bodies of first-order pseudounipolar sensory neurons). At the genu (L. *genu* = knee), CN VII bends and descends in the facial canal. It gives off three branches between the geniculate ganglion and the stylomastoid foramen:

- **Greater petrosal nerve:** Parasympathetic and taste (special visceral afferent) fibers branch from the geniculate ganglion in the greater petrosal canal. They emerge on the anterior surface of the petrous pyramid and continue across the surface of the foramen lacerum. The greater petrosal nerve combines with the deep petrosal nerve in the pterygoid canal (nerve of the pterygoid canal, vidian nerve). The greater petrosal nerve contains the fibers that form the motor root of the pterygopalatine ganglion (the parasympathetic ganglion of CN VII). The pterygopalatine ganglion distributes autonomic fibers via the trigeminal nerve (primarily the maxillary division, CN V$_2$).
- **Stapedial nerve:** Branchiomotor fibers innervate the stapedius muscle.
- **Chorda tympani:** The remaining parasympathetic and taste fibers leave the facial nerve as the chorda tympani. This nerve runs through the tympanic cavity and petrotympanic fissure to the infratemporal fossa, where it unites with the lingual nerve (CN V$_3$).

The remaining fibers (branchiomotor with some general sensory) exit via the stylomastoid foramen.

Fig. 4.86 Branches of the facial nerve
The facial nerve enters the facial canal of the petrous bone via the internal acoustic meatus. Most branchiomotor fibers and all somatosensory fibers emerge via the stylomastoid foramen. Within the facial canal, CN VII gives off one branchiomotor branch and two nerves containing both parasympathetic and taste fibers (greater petrosal nerve and chorda tympani). Temporal bone fractures may injure the facial nerve at various levels:

1 Internal acoustic meatus: Lesions affect CN VII and the vestibulocochlear nerve (CN VIII). Peripheral motor facial paralysis is accompanied by hearing loss and dizziness.
2 External genu of facial nerve: Peripheral motor facial paralysis is accompanied by disturbances of taste sensation, lacrimation, and salivation (greater petrosal nerve).
3 Motor paralysis is accompanied by disturbances of salivation and taste (chorda tympani). Paralysis of the stapedius causes hyperacusis (hypersensitivity to normal sounds).
4 Facial paralysis is accompanied by disturbances of taste and salivation (chorda tympani).
5 Facial paralysis is the only manifestation of a lesion at this level.

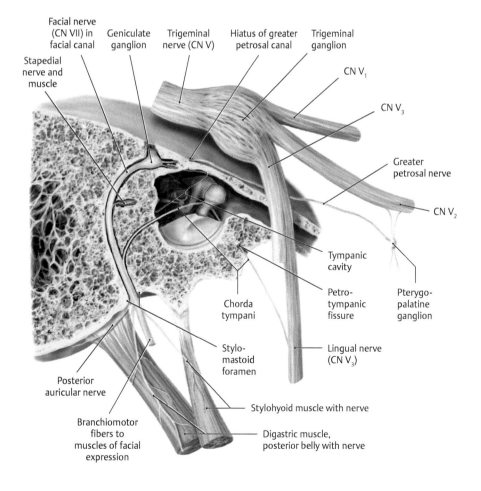

CN VII: Facial Nerve, External Branches & Ganglia

Fig. 4.88 **Innervation of the second branchial arch muscles**

Left lateral view. The branchiomotor fibers of CN VII innervate all the muscles derived from the second pharyngeal arch. With the exception of the stapedial nerve (to the stapedius), all branchiomotor fibers in the facial nerve emerge from the facial canal via the stylomastoid foramen. Three branches arise *before* the parotid plexus:

- Posterior auricular nerve (*Note:* This may also contain general somatosensory fibers.)
- Nerve to the digastric (posterior belly)
- Nerve to the stylohyoid

The remaining branchiomotor fibers then enter the parotid gland where they divide into two trunks (temporofacial and cervicofacial) and five major branches, which innervate the muscles of facial expression:

- Temporal
- Zygomatic
- Buccal
- Mandibular (marginal mandibular)
- Cervical

The branching of the plexus is variable.

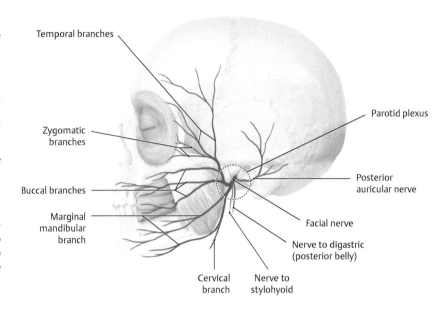

Fig. 4.89 **Facial paralysis**

A Upper motor neurons in the primary somatomotor cortex (precentral gyrus) descend to the cell bodies of lower motor neurons in the facial motor nucleus. The axons of these lower motor neurons innervate the muscles derived from the second branchial arch. The facial motor nucleus has a "bipartite" structure: its cranial (upper) part supplies the muscles of the calvaria and palpebral fissure, and its caudal (lower) part supplies the muscles of the lower face. The cranial part of the nucleus receives bilateral innervation (from upper motor neurons in both hemispheres). The caudal part receives contralateral innervation (from cortical neurons on the other side).

B Central (supranuclear) paralysis: Loss of upper motor neurons (shown here for the left hemisphere) causes contralateral paralysis in the lower half of the face but no paralysis in the upper half. For example, the patient's mouth will sag on the right (contralateral paralysis of lower muscles), but the ability to wrinkle the forehead and close the eyes is intact.

C Peripheral (infranuclear) paralysis: Loss of lower motor neurons (shown here for right brainstem) causes complete ipsilateral paralysis. For example, the whole right side of the face is paralyzed. Depending on the site of the lesion, additional deficits may be present (decreased lacrimation or salivation, loss of taste sensation in the presulcal (anterior two thirds) tongue).

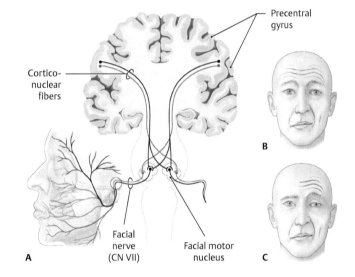

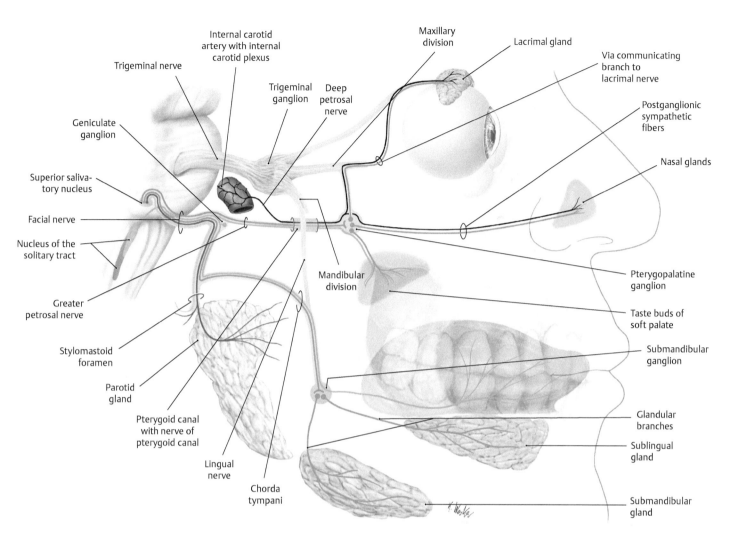

Fig. 4.90 Facial nerve ganglia
Autonomic and taste fibers often travel with sensory fibers from other nerves to reach their targets. Parasympathetic and taste fibers leave the facial nerve via two branches: the greater petrosal nerve and the chorda tympani.

- **Greater petrosal nerve:** Preganglionic parasympathetic and taste fibers from the geniculate ganglion course in the greater petrosal canal. They are joined by the deep petrosal nerve, which conveys postganglionic sympathetic fibers from the superior cervical ganglion (via the internal carotid plexus). The greater and deep petrosal nerves combine to form the nerve of the pterygoid canal (vidian nerve), which conveys sympathetic, parasympathetic, and taste fibers to the pterygopalatine ganglion (only parasympathetics will synapse at the ganglion; all other fiber types pass through without synapsing). Branches of CN V_2 then distribute the fibers to their targets:
  - **Lacrimal gland:** Autonomic fibers (sympathetic and parasympathetic) run with branches of CN V_2 (zygomatic and zygomaticotemporal nerves) to a communicating branch, which conveys them to the lacrimal nerve (CN V_1) and thus to the lacrimal gland.
  - **Small glands of the nasal and oral cavities:** Autonomic fibers run with branches of CN V_2 to the small glands in the mucosa of the nasal cavity, maxillary sinuses, and palatine tonsils.
  - **Taste:** Taste fibers run with branches of CN V_2 to the soft palate.

- **Chorda tympani:** Preganglionic parasympathetic and taste fibers course through the chorda tympani. They emerge from the petrotympanic fissure and combine with the lingual nerve (CN V_3) in the infratemporal fossa. They are conveyed to the submandibular ganglion by the lingual nerve, and from there, postganglionic branches travel to their targets via branches of CN V_3.
  - **Submandibular and sublingual glands:** Postganglionic parasympathetic fibers run with branches of CN V_3 to the glands.
  - **Taste buds of tongue:** The taste buds on the presulcal portion (anterior two thirds) of the tongue receive taste fibers from the chorda tympani via the lingual nerve (CN V_3). *Note:* The postsulcal portion (posterior one third) of the tongue and the oropharynx receive taste fibers from CN IX. The root of the tongue and epiglottis receive taste fibers from CN X.

Note: The **lesser petrosal nerve** runs in the lesser petrosal canal roughly parallel to the greater petrosal nerve. The lesser petrosal nerve conveys preganglionic parasympathetic fibers from the tympanic plexus (CN IX) to the otic ganglion. These fibers innervate the parotid, buccal, and inferior labial glands, with postganglionic fibers distributed via branches of CN V_3.

139

CN VIII: Vestibulocochlear Nerve

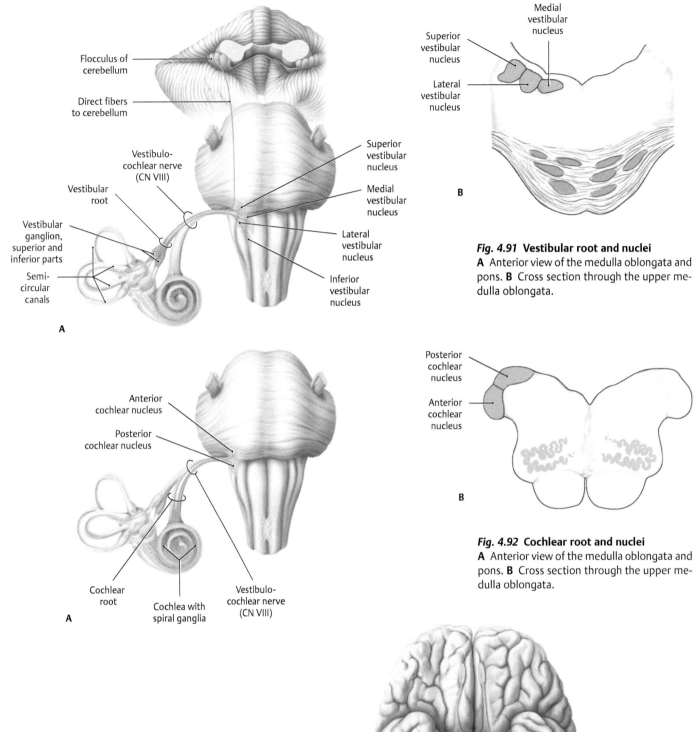

Fig. 4.91 Vestibular root and nuclei
A Anterior view of the medulla oblongata and pons. **B** Cross section through the upper medulla oblongata.

Fig. 4.92 Cochlear root and nuclei
A Anterior view of the medulla oblongata and pons. **B** Cross section through the upper medulla oblongata.

Fig. 4.93 Acoustic neuroma in the cerebellopontine angle
Acoustic neuromas (more accurately, vestibular schwannomas) are benign tumors of the cerebellopontine angle arising from the Schwann cells of the vestibular root of CN VIII. As they grow, they compress and displace the adjacent structures and cause slowly progressive hearing loss and gait ataxia. Large tumors can impair the egress of CSF from the 4th ventricle, causing hydrocephalus and symptomatic intracranial hypertension (vomiting, impairment of consciousness).

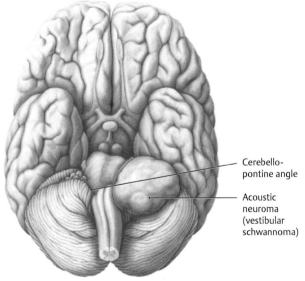

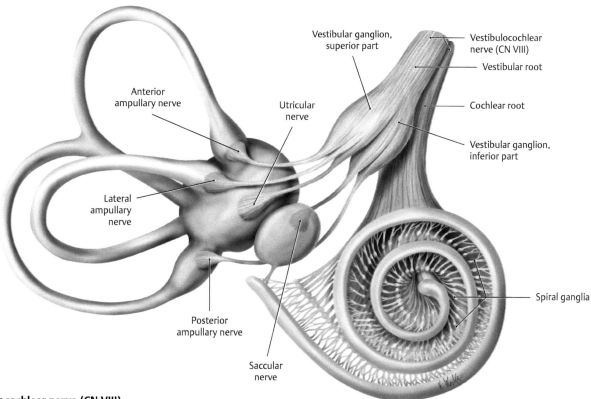

Fig. 4.94 Vestibulocochlear nerve (CN VIII)
The vestibulocochlear nerve consists of two parts. The vestibular root conveys afferent impulses from the vestibular apparatus (balance). The cochlear root conveys afferent impulses from the auditory apparatus (hearing).

Table 4.26 Vestibulocochlear nerve (CN VIII)

Nuclei, ganglia, and fiber distribution

Special somatic afferent (orange): Special somatic sensory neurons convey sensory fibers from the vestibular apparatus (balance) and auditory apparatus (hearing). Both parts of the nerve contain first-order bipolar sensory neurons.

Neurons	Vestibular root	Cochlear root
Peripheral processes	In the sensory cells of the semicircular canals, the saccule, and the utricle.	In the hair cells of the organ of Corti.
Cell bodies	**Vestibular ganglion** • Inferior part: Peripheral processes from saccule and posterior semicircular canal. • Superior part: Peripheral processes from anterior and lateral semicircular canals and utricle.	**Spiral ganglia.** The peripheral processes from the neurons in these myriad ganglia radiate outward to receive sensory input from the spiral modiolus.
Central processes (axons)	To four **vestibular nuclei** in the medulla oblongata (floor of the rhomboid fossa). A few pass directly to the cerebellum via the inferior cerebellar peduncle.	To two **cochlear nuclei** lateral to the vestibular nuclei.
Nuclei	Superior, lateral, medial, and inferior vestibular nuclei.	Anterior and posterior cochlear nuclei.
Lesions	Dizziness and vertigo.	Hearing loss (ranging to deafness).

Course

The vestibular and cochlear roots unite in the internal acoustic meatus to form the vestibulocochlear nerve, which is covered by a common connective tissue sheath. The nerve emerges from the internal acoustic meatus on the medial surface of the petrous temporal bone and enters the brainstem at the level of the pontomedullary junction, in particular at the cerebellopontine angle.

CN IX: Glossopharyngeal Nerve

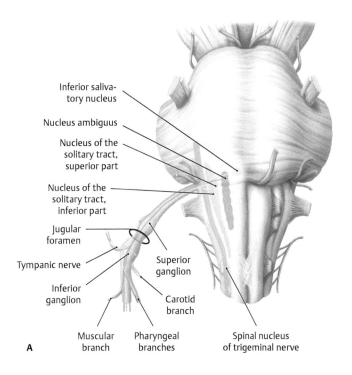

A

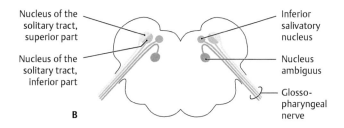

B

Fig. 4.95 Glossopharyngeal nerve nuclei
A Anterior view of brainstem. **B** Cross section through the medulla oblongata.

Table 4.27 Glossopharyngeal nerve (CN IX)	
Nuclei, ganglia, and fiber distribution	
Branchiomotor (purple)	
Nucleus ambiguus	Lower motor neurons innervate the muscles derived from the 3rd, 4th, and 6th pharyngeal (branchial) arches via CN IX, X, and XI. • CN IX innervates the derivative of the 3rd branchial arch (stylopharyngeus)
Parasympathetic (blue)	
Inferior salivatory nucleus	Preganglionic neurons synapse in the **otic ganglion**.
	Postganglionic neurons innervate: • Parotid gland (**Fig. 4.96A**) • Buccal glands • Inferior labial glands
General somatic afferent (yellow)	
Spinal nucleus of CN V	First-order pseudounipolar cells in the **superior ganglion** of CN IX innervate: • Nasopharynx (inferior torus tubarius), oropharynx, postsulcal tongue, palatine tonsils, and uvula (**Fig. 4.96C**). These fibers include the afferent limb of the gag reflex. • Tympanic cavity and pharyngotympanic tube (**Fig. 4.96D**).
Viscerosensory (green)	
First-order pseudounipolar cells in the **inferior ganglion** relay taste and visceral sensation to the **nucleus of the solitary tract**. This nuclear complex consists of a superior part (taste) and inferior part (general visceral sensation).	
Nucleus of the solitary tract	Taste (**Fig. 4.96E**): Special viscerosensory fibers from the postsulcal tongue synapse in the **superior part**.
	Visceral sensation (**Fig. 4.96F**): General viscerosensory fibers from the carotid body (chemoreceptors) and carotid sinus (pressure receptors) synapse in the **inferior part**.
Course	
The glossopharyngeal nerve arises from the medulla oblongata and exits the skull by passing through the jugular foramen. It has two sensory ganglia with first-order pseudounipolar sensory cells: the superior ganglion (somatosensory) is within the cranial cavity, and the inferior ganglion (viscerosensory) is distal to the jugular foramen.	
Lesions	
Isolated CN IX lesions are rare. Lesions tend to occur during basal skull fractures, which disrupt the jugular foramen. Such injuries would affect CN IX, X, and XI.	

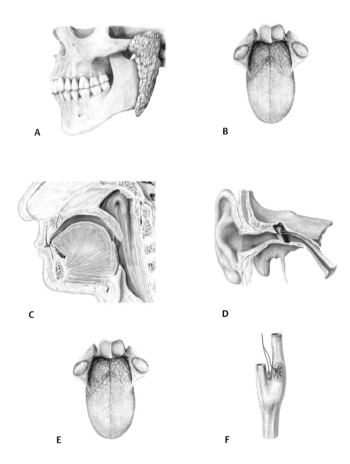

Fig. 4.96 Distribution of CN IX fibers

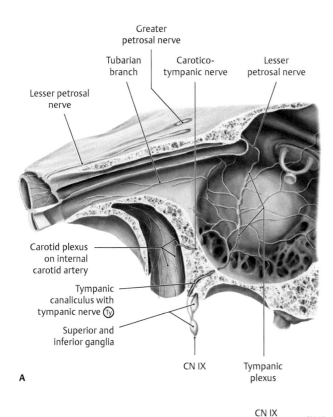

A

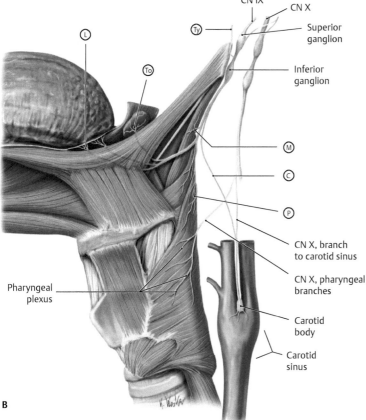

B

Fig. 4.97 Glossopharyngeal nerve branches
A Left anterolateral view of opened tympanic cavity. **B** Left lateral view.

Table 4.28 Glossopharyngeal nerve branches

Ⓣⱽ **Tympanic n.**

Somatosensory and preganglionic parasympathetic fibers branch at the inferior ganglion and travel through the tympanic canaliculus as the tympanic nerve.

- **Tympanic plexus:** The tympanic nerve combines with postganglionic sympathetic fibers from the superior cervical ganglion (via carotid plexus and caroticotympanic nerve) and branches to form the tympanic plexus. This plexus provides general somatosensory innervation to the tympanic cavity, pharyngotympanic tube, and mastoid air cells.
- **Lesser petrosal n.:** The preganglionic parasympathetic fibers in the tympanic plexus are reconstituted as the lesser petrosal nerve, which runs in the lesser petrosal canal to synapse in the otic ganglion.
- **Otic ganglion:** The postganglionic parasympathetic fibers innervate the parotid, buccal, and inferior labial glands by traveling with branches of CN V_3.

Ⓒ **Carotid branch**

General viscerosensory fibers from the carotid sinus (pressure receptors) and carotid body (chemoreceptors) ascend on the internal carotid artery to join CN IX or X on their way to the inferior part of the nucleus of the solitary tract.

Ⓟ **Pharyngeal branches**

The **pharyngeal plexus** consists of general somatosensory fibers (from CN IX), sympathetic fibers (from the sympathetic trunk), and motor fibers (from CN X).

- CN IX receives sensory fibers from the mucosa of the naso- and oropharynx via the pharyngeal plexus.

Ⓜ **Muscular branch**

The branchiomotor fibers in CN IX innervate the derivative of the 3rd pharyngeal (branchial) arch, the **stylopharyngeus**.

Ⓣ° **Tonsillar branches**

General somatosensory fibers from the palatine tonsils and mucosa of the oropharynx.

Ⓛ **Lingual branches**

General somatosensory and special viscerosensory (taste) fibers from the postsulcal tongue (posterior one third).

143

CN X: Vagus Nerve

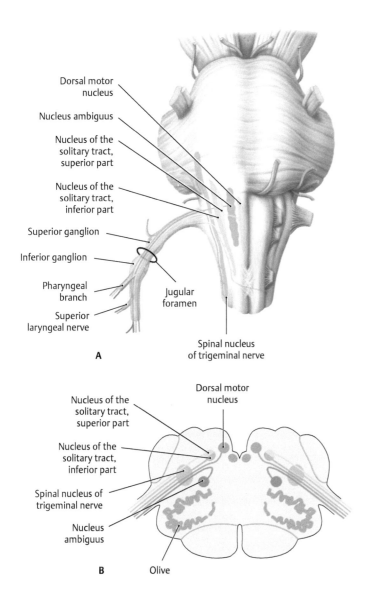

A

B   Olive

Fig. 4.98 Vagus nerve nuclei
A Anterior view of medulla oblongata. **B** Cross section through the medulla oblongata.
The vagus nerve has the most extensive distribution of all the cranial nerves (L. *vagus* = vagabond). Parasympathetic fibers descend into the thorax and abdomen. These fibers form autonomic plexuses with post-ganglionic sympathetic fibers (from the sympathetic trunk and abdominal ganglia). The plexuses extend along organs and blood vessels and provide motor innervation to the thoracic and abdominal viscera. General viscerosensory fibers ascend via CN X to the inferior part of the nucleus of the solitary tract.

Table 4.29 Vagus nerve (CN X)

Nuclei, ganglia, and fiber distribution

Branchiomotor (purple)

Nucleus ambiguus	Lower motor neurons innervate the muscles derived from the 3rd, 4th, and 6th pharyngeal (branchial) arches via CN IX, X, and XI. CN X innervates the derivatives of the 4th and 6th branchial arches: • Pharyngeal muscles (pharyngeal constrictors) • Muscles of the soft palate (levator veli palatini, musculus uvulae, palatoglossus, palatopharyngeus) • Intrinsic laryngeal muscles

Parasympathetic (blue)

Dorsal motor nucleus	Preganglionic neurons synapse in small, unnamed ganglia close to target structures.
	Postganglionic neurons innervate: • Smooth muscles and glands of thoracic and abdominal viscera (**Fig. 4.100G**)

General somatic afferent (yellow)

Spinal nucleus of CN X	First-order pseudounipolar cells in the **superior (jugular) ganglion** innervate: • Dura of the posterior cranial fossa (**Fig. 4.100F**) • External auditory canal, and lateral tympanic membrane (**Fig. 4.100C**) • Mucosa of the oropharynx and laryngopharynx

Viscerosensory (green)

First-order pseudounipolar cells in the **inferior (nodose) ganglion** relay taste and visceral sensation to the **nucleus of the solitary tract**. This nuclear complex consists of a superior part (taste) and inferior part (general visceral sensation).

Nucleus of the solitary tract	Taste (**Fig. 4.100D**): Fibers from the epiglottis and the root of the tongue are conveyed to the **superior part** of the nucleus of the solitary tract.
	Visceral sensation (**Fig. 4.100G**): Fibers are relayed to the **inferior part** of the nucleus of the solitary tract from: • Mucosa of the laryngopharynx and larynx (**Fig. 4.100A**) • Aortic arch (pressure receptors) and para-aortic body (chemoreceptors) (**Fig. 4.100E**) • Thoracic and abdominal viscera (**Fig. 4.100G**)

Course

The vagus nerve arises from the medulla oblongata and emerges from the skull via the jugular foramen. It has two sensory ganglia with first-order pseudounipolar cells: the superior (jugular) ganglion (somatosensory) is within the cranial cavity, and the inferior (nodose) ganglion (viscerosensory) is distal to the jugular foramen.

Lesions

The recurrent laryngeal nerve supplies parasympathetic innervation to the intrinsic laryngeal muscles (except the cricothyroid). This includes the posterior cricoarytenoid, the only muscle that abducts the vocal cords. Unilateral lesions of this nerve cause hoarseness; bilateral destruction leads to respiratory distress (dyspnea).

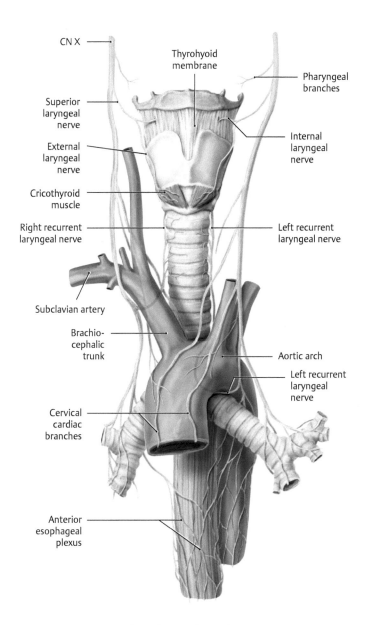

Fig. 4.99 Vagus nerve branches in the neck
Anterior view.

Table 4.30 Vagus nerve branches
Meningeal branches
General somatosensory fibers from the dura of the posterior cranial fossa.
Auricular branch
General somatosensory fibers from external ear (auricle, external acoustic canal, and part of lateral side of tympanic membrane).
Pharyngeal branches
The **pharyngeal plexus** consists of general somatosensory fibers (from CN IX), sympathetic fibers (from the sympathetic trunk), and motor fibers (from CN X). • CN X conveys branchiomotor fibers to the pharyngeal muscles.
Carotid branch
General viscerosensory fibers from the carotid body (chemoreceptors) ascend on the internal carotid artery to join CN IX or X on their way to the inferior part of the nucleus of the solitary tract.
Superior laryngeal n.
Combines with a sympathetic branch from the superior cervical ganglion and divides into: • **Internal laryngeal n.:** Sensory fibers from the mucosa of the laryngopharynx, larynx, and root of the tongue • **External laryngeal n.:** Parasympathetic motor innervation to the cricothyroid.
Recurrent laryngeal n.
The recurrent laryngeal nerve is asymmetrical: • Right recurrent laryngeal n.: Recurs behind the right subclavian artery. • Left recurrent laryngeal n.: Recurs behind the aortic arch. Ascends between the trachea and esophagus. The recurrent laryngeal nerves supply: • Motor innervation to the laryngeal muscles (except the cricothyroid). • Viscerosensory innervation to the laryngeal mucosa.
Branches to the thorax and abdomen
The vagus nerve also conveys parasympathetic and general viscerosensory fibers from the cardiac, pulmonary, esophageal, celiac, renal, hepatic, and gastric plexuses (**Fig. 4.100G**)

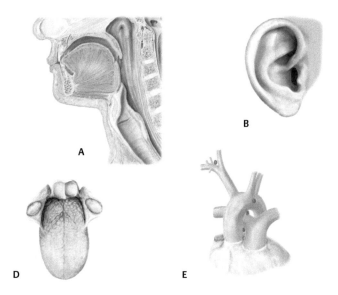

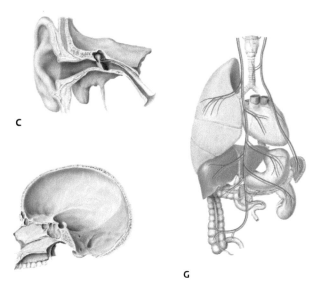

Fig. 4.100 Distribution of the vagus nerve (CN X)

CN XI & XII: Accessory Spinal & Hypoglossal Nerves

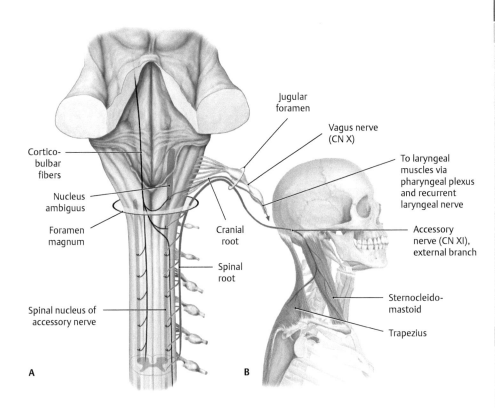

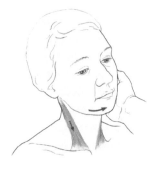

Fig. 4.101 Accessory nerve
A Posterior view of brainstem. **B** Right lateral view of sternocleidomastoid and trapezius.

(*Note:* For didactic reasons, the right muscles are displayed though they are innervated by the right cranial nerve nuclei.)

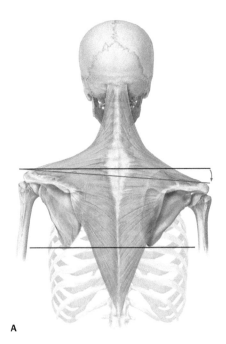

Fig. 4.102 Accessory nerve lesions
Accessory nerve lesions cause partial paralysis of the trapezius and complete (flaccid) paralysis of the sternocleidomastoid (see **Table 4.28**). Both lesions shown here are unilateral (right side). **A** Posterior view. Partial paralysis of the trapezius causes drooping of the shoulder on the affected side. **B** Right anterolateral view. Flaccid paralysis of the sternocleidomastoid causes torticollis (wry neck).

Table 4.31 Accessory nerve (CN XI)

Nuclei, ganglia, and fiber distribution

Branchiomotor (purple)

Nucleus ambiguus	Lower motor neurons innervate the muscles derived from the 3rd, 4th, and 6th branchial arches via CN IX, X, and XI. • CN XI innervates the laryngeal muscles (except cricoarytenoid) with motor fibers being distributed by branches of CN X.

General somatomotor (red)

Spinal nucleus of CN XI	Lower motor neurons in the lateral part of the anterior horn of C2–C6 spinal cord segments innervate: • Trapezius (upper part). • Sternocleidomastoid.

Course

CN XI arises and courses in two parts that unite briefly distal to the jugular foramen:

Cranial root: Branchiomotor fibers emerge from the medulla oblongata and pass through the jugular foramen. They briefly unite with the spinal root before joining CN X at the inferior ganglion. CN X distributes the branchiomotor fibers via the pharyngeal plexus and the external and recurrent laryngeal nerves.

Spinal root: General somatomotor fibers emerge as rootlets from the spinal medulla. They unite and ascend through the foramen magnum. The spinal root then passes through the jugular foramen, courses briefly with the cranial root, and then descends to innervate the sternocleidomastoid and trapezius.

Lesions

The sternocleidomastoid is exclusively innervated by CN XI, and the lower portions of the trapezius may be innervated by C3–C5. Accessory nerve lesions therefore cause complete (flaccid) sternocleidomastoid paralysis but only partial trapezius paralysis.

Trapezius paralysis: Unilateral lesions may occur during operations in the neck (e.g., lymph node biopsies), causing:
• Drooping of the shoulder on the affected side.
• Difficulty raising the arm above the horizontal.

Sternocleidomastoid paralysis:
• Unilateral lesions: Flaccid paralysis causes torticollis (wry neck, i.e., difficulty turning the head to the opposite side).
• Bilateral lesions: Difficulty holding the head upright.

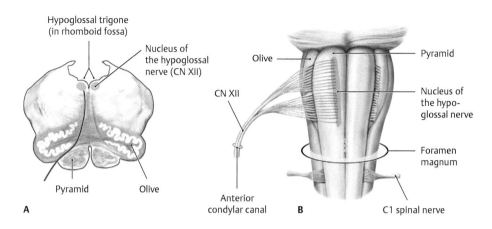

A

B

Fig. 4.103 Hypoglossal nerve nuclei
The nucleus of the hypoglossal nerve is located in the floor of the rhomboid fossa. Rootlets emerge between the pyramid and the olive.

A Cross section through the medulla oblongata. The proximity of the nuclei to the midline causes extensive lesions to involve both nuclei. **B** Anterior view of medulla oblongata.

Table 4.32 Hypoglossal nerve (CN XII)

Nuclei, ganglia, and fiber distribution

General somatomotor (red)

Nucleus of CN XII	Lower motor neurons innervate: • Extrinsic lingual muscles (except palatoglossus). • Intrinsic lingual muscles.

Course

The hypoglossal nerve emerges from the medulla oblongata as rootlets between the olive and pyramid. These rootlets combine into CN XII, which courses through the hypoglossal (anterior condylar) canal. CN XII enters the root of the tongue superior to the hyoid bone and lateral to the hyoglossus.
• C1 motor fibers from the cervical plexus travel with the hypoglossal nerve: some branch to form the superior root of the ansa cervicalis (not shown), whereas others continue with CN XII to supply the geniohyoid and thyrohyoid muscles.

Lesions

Upper motor neurons innervate the lower motor neurons in the contralateral nucleus of the hypoglossal nerve. Supranuclear lesions (central hypoglossal paralysis) will therefore cause the tongue to deviate away from the affected side. Nuclear or peripheral lesions will cause the tongue to deviate toward the affected side (**Fig. 4.104C**).

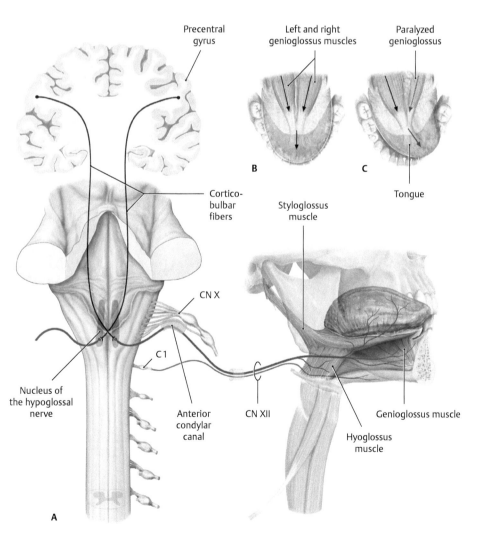

A

B

C

Fig. 4.104 Hypoglossal nerve
A Course of the hypoglossal nerve. Upper motor neurons synapse on lower motor neurons on the contralateral nucleus of the hypoglossal nerve. Supranuclear lesions will therefore cause contralateral paralysis; peripheral lesions will cause ipsilateral paralysis (same side). **B** The functional genioglossus extends the tongue anteriorly. **C** Unilateral paralysis due to a peripheral lesion causes the tongue to deviate *toward* the affected side (dominance of the intact genioglossus).

147

Radiographs of the Cranial Nerves Exiting the Brain (I)

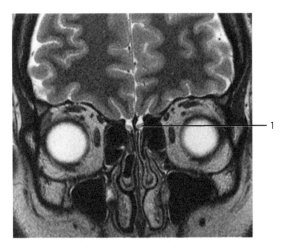

Fig. 4.105 Cranial nerve I
Coronal plane. Compare the structures here and in **Fig. 4.106** to those in **Fig. 4.74**. **Figures 4.105** to **4.108** form a series from anterior to posterior. 1 = olfactory bulb

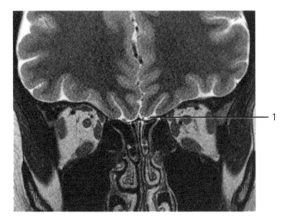

Fig. 4.106 Cranial nerve I
Coronal plane. 1 = olfactory tract

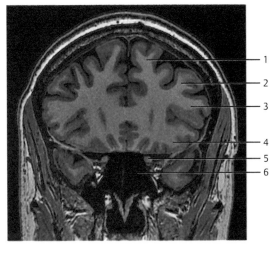

Fig. 4.107 Cranial nerve II
Coronal plane. Compare the structures here and in **Figs. 4.108** and **4.109** to those in **Fig. 4.75**. 1 = Superior frontal gyrus, 2 = middle frontal gyrus, 3 = inferior frontal gyrus, 4 = orbital gyri, 5 = optic nerve, 6 = sphenoid sinus

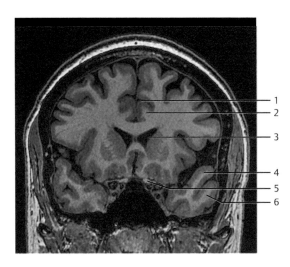

Fig. 4.108 Cranial nerve II
Coronal plane. 1 = Cingulate sulcus, 2 = cingulate gyrus, 3 = anterior horn of lateral ventricle, 4 = superior temporal gyrus, 5 = optic nerve, 6 = middle temporal gyrus

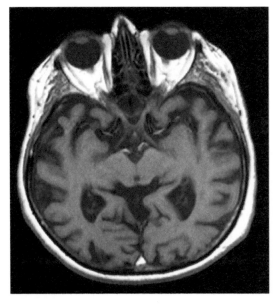

Fig. 4.109 Cranial nerve II
Axial plane. Note the optic nerve, chiasm, and optic tract.

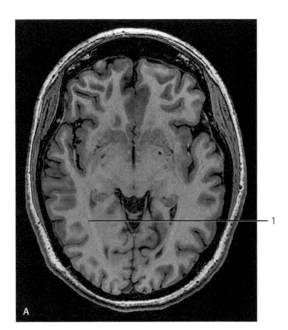

Fig. 4.110 Cranial nerve II
Axial plane. The two images show the same structures but with different weightings. **A** T1w sequence. **B** T2w sequence. 1 = Optic radiation

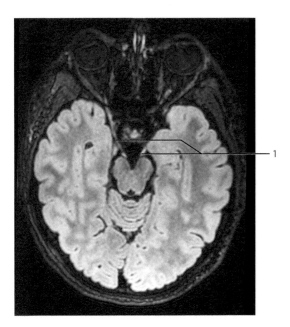

Fig. 4.111 Cranial nerve III
Axial plane. Compare the structures here and in Fig. 4.112 to those in **Fig. 4.76**. 1 = Oculomotor nerve

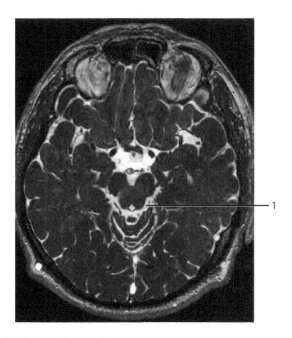

Fig. 4.112 Cranial nerve IV
Axial plane. 1 = Trochlear nerve

Radiographs of the Cranial Nerves Exiting the Brain (II)

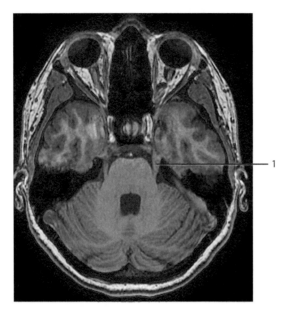

Fig. 4.113 Cranial nerve V
Axial plane. Compare the structures here to those in **Fig. 4.78**. 1 = Trigeminal nerve

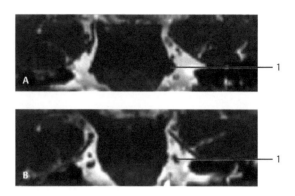

Fig. 4.114 Cranial nerve V
Axial plane. **A** Trigeminal nerve in the reentry zone of the pons. **B** Trigeminal nerve in its course through the CSF space toward the trigeminal cave (Meckel's cave). 1 = Trigeminal nerve

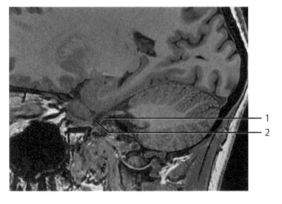

Fig. 4.115 Cranial nerve V
Parasagittal plane. 1 = Trigeminal nerve, 2 = trigeminal cave (Meckel's cave)

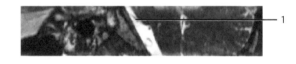

Fig. 4.116 Cranial nerve VI
Parasagittal plane through the pons. Compare the structures here and in **Fig. 4.116** to those in **Fig. 4.76**. 1 = Abducent nerve

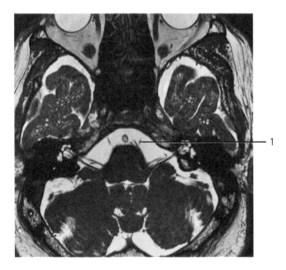

Fig. 4.117 Cranial nerve VI
Axial plane. 1 = Abducent nerve

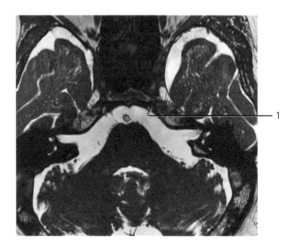

Fig. 4.118 Cranial nerve VI
Axial plane. The abducent nerve is passing through the periosteum of the clivus. 1 = Abducent nerve

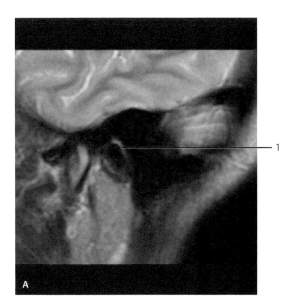
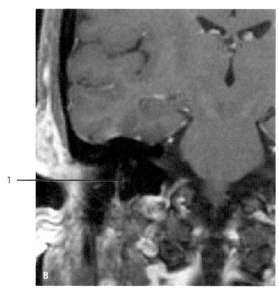

Fig. 4.119 Cranial nerve VII
A Parasagittal plane. **B** Coronal plane. Compare the structures here to those in **Fig. 4.87**. 1 = Facial canal

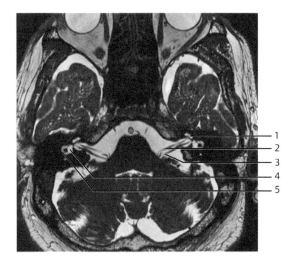
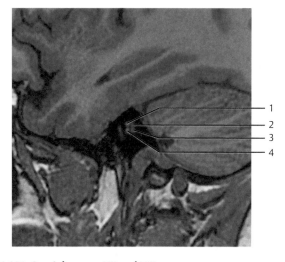

Fig. 4.120 Cranial nerves VII and VIII
Axial plane. 1 = cochlea, 2 = facial nerve, 3 = vestibulocochlear nerve, 4 = vestibule, 5 = lateral semicircular canal

Fig. 4.121 Cranial nerves VII and VIII
Parasagittal plane. 1 = Facial nerve and nervus intermedius, 2 = superior vestibular nerve, 3 = inferior vestibular nerve, 4 = cochlear nerve

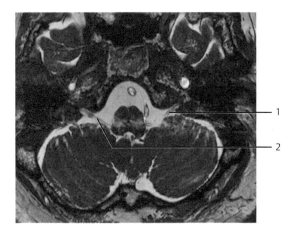
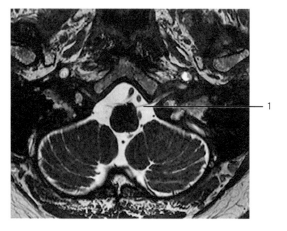

Fig. 4.122 Cranial nerve IX
Axial plane. Compare the structures here to those in **Figs. 4.95** and **4.98**. 1 = Glossopharyngeal nerve and vagus nerve (accessory nerve is also exiting the jugular foramen here, but is not easily seen), 2 = glossopharyngeal nerve

Fig. 4.123 Cranial nerve XII
Axial plane. Compare the structures here to those in **Fig. 4.103**. 1 = Hypoglossal nerve

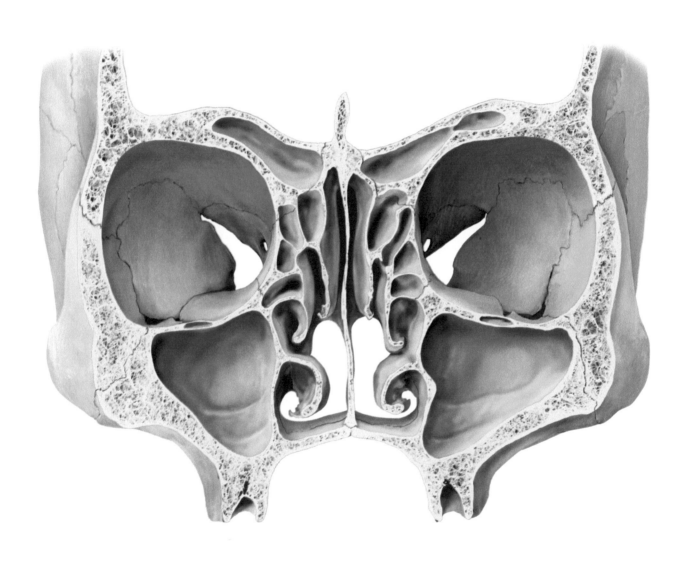

Regions of the Head

Muscles of the Face

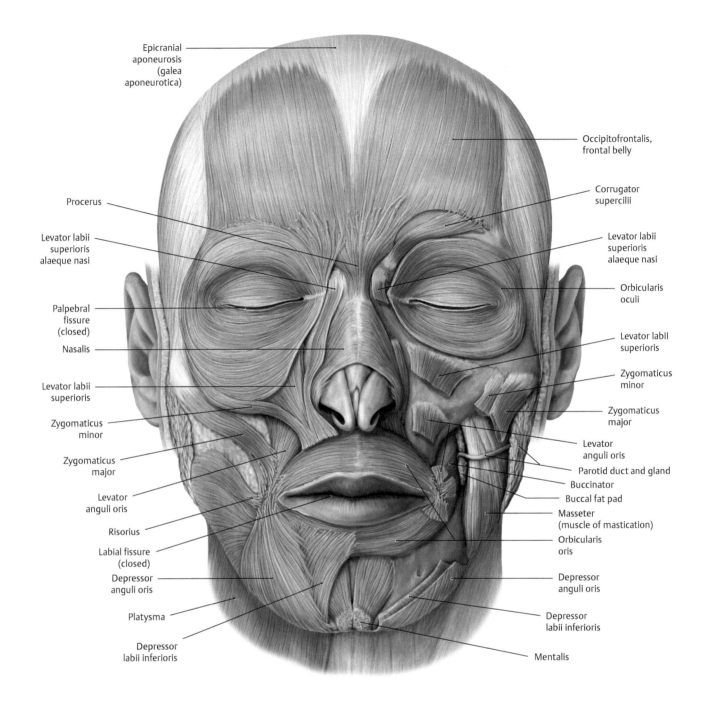

Epicranial
aponeurosis
(galea
aponeurotica)

Occipitofrontalis,
frontal belly

Corrugator
supercilii

Procerus

Levator labii
superioris
alaeque nasi

Levator labii
superioris
alaeque nasi

Orbicularis
oculi

Palpebral
fissure
(closed)

Nasalis

Levator labii
superioris

Levator labii
superioris

Zygomaticus
minor

Zygomaticus
minor

Zygomaticus
major

Zygomaticus
major

Levator
anguli oris

Levator
anguli oris

Parotid duct and gland

Risorius

Buccinator

Buccal fat pad

Labial fissure
(closed)

Masseter
(muscle of mastication)

Orbicularis
oris

Depressor
anguli oris

Depressor
anguli oris

Platysma

Depressor
labii inferioris

Depressor
labii inferioris

Mentalis

Fig. 5.1 Superficial facial muscles

Anterior view. The superficial layer of muscles is shown on the right side of the face. Certain muscles have been cut on the left to expose deeper muscles. The muscles of facial expression are the superficial layer of muscles that arise either directly from the periosteum or from adjacent muscles and insert onto other facial muscles or directly into the connective tissue of the skin. Because of their cutaneous attachments, the muscles of facial expression are able to move the facial skin (an action that may be temporarily abolished by botulinum toxin injection). They also serve a protective function (especially for the eyes) and are active during food ingestion (closing the labial fissure). The muscles of facial expression are innervated by branches of the facial nerve (CN VII). As these muscles are located in the subcutaneous fat, and because

the superficial body fascia is absent in the face, surgeons must be particularly careful when dissecting this region. The lack of fascia on the face and the loose connective tissue between the cutaneous attachments of the facial muscles also means that facial lacerations, following a blow to the face for example, tend to gape widely. This necessitates careful suturing of these lacerations to approximate the edges of the wound and to prevent scarring. The loose nature of the connective tissue also provides a place for blood and fluid to accumulate, leading to swelling and bruising of the face. Such swelling may also be apparent following an inflammatory insult, such as a bee sting. The muscles of mastication lie deep to the muscles of facial expression. They control the movement of the mandible and are innervated by branches of the trigeminal nerve (CN V).

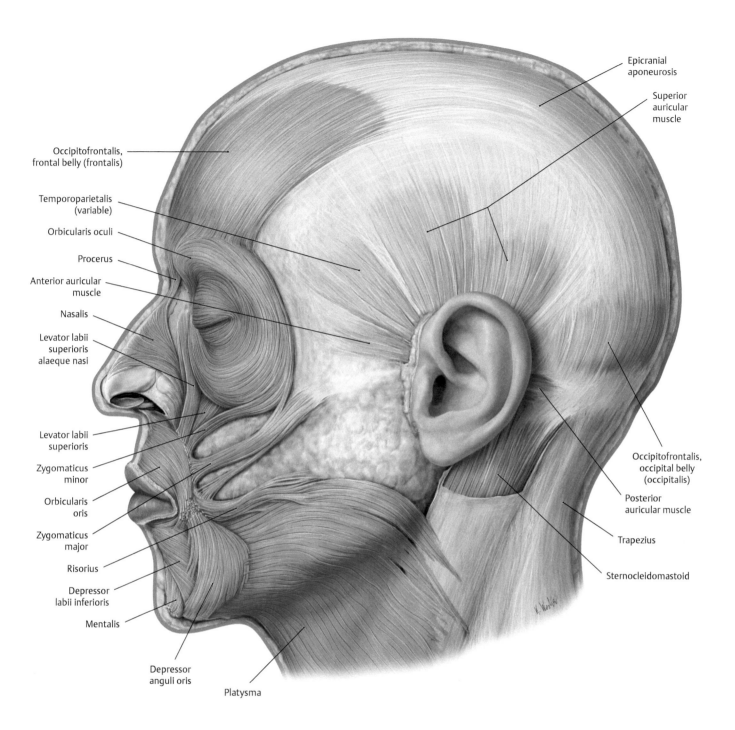

Epicranial aponeurosis

Superior auricular muscle

Occipitofrontalis, frontal belly (frontalis)

Temporoparietalis (variable)

Orbicularis oculi

Procerus

Anterior auricular muscle

Nasalis

Levator labii superioris alaeque nasi

Levator labii superioris

Zygomaticus minor

Orbicularis oris

Zygomaticus major

Risorius

Depressor labii inferioris

Mentalis

Depressor anguli oris

Platysma

Occipitofrontalis, occipital belly (occipitalis)

Posterior auricular muscle

Trapezius

Sternocleidomastoid

Fig. 5.2 **Superficial facial muscles**
Lateral view. The epicranial aponeurosis (galea aponeurotica) is a tough tendinous sheet stretching over the calvaria; it is loosely attached to the periosteum. The muscles of the calvaria that arise from the epicranial aponeurosis (temporoparietalis and occipitofrontalis) are collectively known as the "epicranial muscles." The occipitofrontalis has two bellies: frontal (frontalis) and occipital (occipitalis). The trapezius and sternocleidomastoid muscles are superficial neck muscles.

155

Muscles of Facial Expression: Calvaria, Ear, & Eye

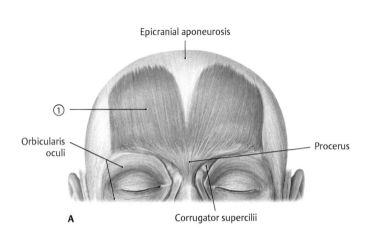

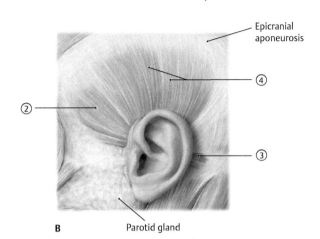

Epicranial aponeurosis

Epicranial aponeurosis

④

②

③

Orbicularis oculi

Procerus

A

Corrugator supercilii

B

Parotid gland

Fig. 5.3 Muscles of facial expression: calvaria and ear
A Anterior view of calvaria. **B** Left lateral view of auricular muscles.

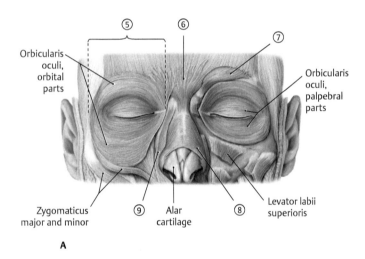

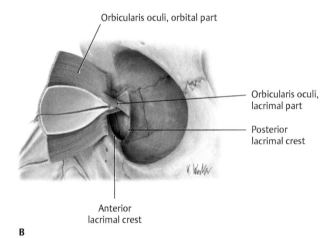

⑤ ⑥ ⑦

Orbicularis oculi, orbital parts

Orbicularis oculi, palpebral parts

Orbicularis oculi, orbital part

Orbicularis oculi, lacrimal part

Posterior lacrimal crest

Zygomaticus major and minor

⑨ Alar cartilage

⑧ Levator labii superioris

Anterior lacrimal crest

A

B

Fig. 5.4 Muscles of facial expression: palpebral fissure and nose

A Anterior view. The most functionally important muscle of this region is the orbicularis oculi, which closes the palpebral fissure (a protective reflex against foreign matter). As the orbicularis oculi closes the palpebral fissure, it does so by closing from lateral to medial, thus spreading lacrimal secretions across the cornea (p. 257). If the action of the orbicularis oculi is lost because of facial nerve paralysis, the loss of this protective reflex will be accompanied by drying of the cornea from prolonged exposure to the air. The function of the orbicularis oculi is tested by asking the patient to squeeze the eyelids tightly shut. Other symptoms of facial nerve paralysis (Bell's palsy)

include ipsilateral drooping of the corner of the mouth, eyebrow, and lower eyelid, and the inability to smile, whistle, blow out cheeks, or wrinkle the forehead (due to paralysis of the other muscles of facial expression).

B The orbicularis oculi has been dissected from the left orbit to the medial canthus of the eye and reflected anteriorly to demonstrate its lacrimal part (called the Horner muscle). This part of the orbicularis oculi arises mainly from the posterior lacrimal crest, and its action is a subject of debate (it may have a functional role in drainage of the lacrimal sac).

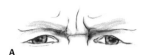
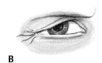

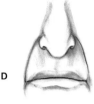

A   B   C   D

***Fig. 5.5* Changes of facial expression: palpebral fissure and nose**
Anterior view.
A Corrugator supercilii. **B** Orbicularis oculi. **C** Nasalis. **D** Levator labii superioris alaeque nasi.

Table 5.1 Muscles of facial expression: calvaria and ear, palbebral fissure, and nose

Muscle and parts	Origin	Insertion	I*	Main action(s)
Calvaria and ear				
① Occipitofrontalis, frontal belly	Epicranial aponeurosis near coronal suture	Skin and subcutaneous tissue of eyebrows and forehead	T	Elevates eyebrows; wrinkles skin of forehead
Auricular muscles			T	Elevate ear
② Anterior	Temporal fascia (anterior portion)	Helix of the ear		• Pull ear superiorly and anteriorly
③ Posterior	Epicranial aponeurosis on side of head	Upper portion of auricle		• Elevate ear
④ Superior	Temporal fascia	Helix of the ear	PA	• Pull ear superiorly and posteriorly
Occipitofrontalis, occipital belly	Occipital bone (highest nuchal line) and temporal bone (mastoid part)	Epicranial aponeurosis near coronal suture		Pulls scalp backward
Palpebral fissure and nose				
⑤ Orbicularis oculi				Whole muscle acts as orbital sphincter (closes eyelids)
• Orbital part	Medial orbital margin (frontal bone and maxilla) and medial palpebral ligament	Adjacent muscles (occipitofrontalis, corrugator supercilii, levator labii, etc.)	T/Z	• Voluntary closure of eyelids, furrowing of nose and eyebrows during squinting
• Palpebral part	Medial palpebral ligament	Eyelids (as lateral palpebral raphe)		• Voluntary (sleeping) and involuntary closure (blinking) of eyelids
• Lacrimal part	Lacrimal crest	Tarsi of eyelids, lateral palpebral raphe		• Pulls eyelids medially
⑥ Procerus	Fascial aponeurosis of lower nasal bone	Skin between eyebrows	T/Z	Pulls eyebrows medially and inferiorly (frowning)
⑦ Corrugator supercilii	Bone of superciliary arch (medial end)	Skin above supraorbital margin	T	Acts with orbicularis oculi to pull eyebrows medially and inferiorly (during squinting)
⑧ Nasalis				
• Transverse part	Maxilla	Aponeurosis at bridge of nose	B/Z	• Compresses nasal aperture (compressor naris)
• Alar part		Ala nasi		• Widens nasal aperture (flares nostril) by drawing ala toward nasal septum
⑨ Levator labii superioris alaeque nasi	Frontal process of maxilla	Greater alar cartilage and orbital muscles (levator labii superioris and orbicularis oris)	B/Z	Elevates upper lip, increases the curvature of the nasolabial furrow, dilates nostril

* Innervation: The muscles of facial expression are innervated by six branches of the facial nerve (CN VII). The posterior muscles are innervated by the posterior auricular (PA) nerve, which arises before the facial nerve enters the parotid gland (see p. 137). The anterior muscles are innervated by five branches off the parotid plexus of the facial nerve: temporal (T), zygomatic (Z), buccal (B), marginal mandibular (M), and cervical (C).

Muscles of Facial Expression: Mouth

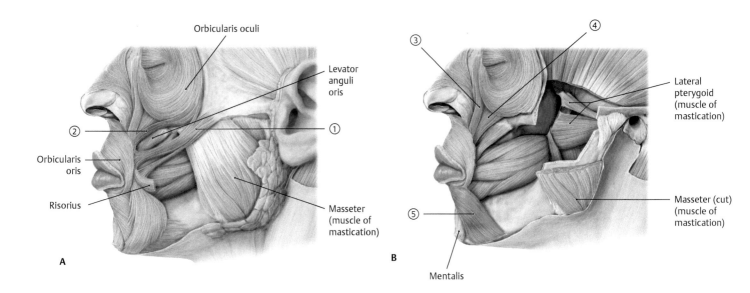

A

Orbicularis oculi

Levator anguli oris

② Orbicularis oris

①

Risorius

Masseter (muscle of mastication)

B

③ ④

Lateral pterygoid (muscle of mastication)

⑤

Masseter (cut) (muscle of mastication)

Mentalis

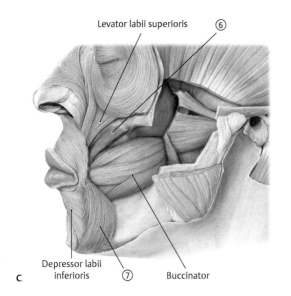

C

Levator labii superioris

⑥

Depressor labii inferioris ⑦ Buccinator

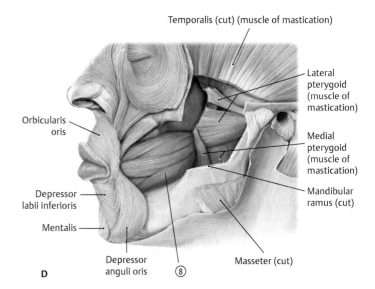

D

Temporalis (cut) (muscle of mastication)

Lateral pterygoid (muscle of mastication)

Orbicularis oris

Medial pterygoid (muscle of mastication)

Mandibular ramus (cut)

Depressor labii inferioris

Mentalis

Depressor anguli oris ⑧ Masseter (cut)

Fig. 5.6 Muscles of facial expression: mouth
A–D Left lateral view. **E** Anterior view.
A Zygomaticus major and minor. **B** Levator labii superioris and depressor labii inferioris (exposed by removal of the depressor anguli oris). **C** Levator anguli oris and depressor anguli oris. **D** Buccinator. **E** Muscles of facial expression of the mouth.

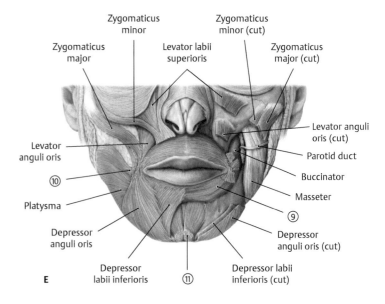

E

Zygomaticus minor

Zygomaticus minor (cut)

Zygomaticus major

Levator labii superioris

Zygomaticus major (cut)

Levator anguli oris (cut)

Parotid duct

Buccinator

Masseter

⑨

Depressor anguli oris (cut)

Levator anguli oris

⑩

Platysma

Depressor anguli oris

Depressor labii inferioris ⑪ Depressor labii inferioris (cut)

158

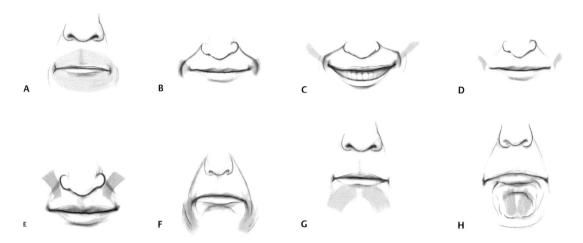

Fig. 5.7 Changes of facial expression: mouth
Anterior view.
A Orbicularis oris. **B** Buccinator. **C** Zygomaticus major. **D** Risorius. **E** Levator anguli oris. **F** Depressor anguli oris. **G** Depressor labii inferioris. **H** Mentalis.

Table 5.2 Muscles of facial expression: mouth

Muscle	Origin	Insertion	I*	Main action(s)
① Zygomaticus major	Zygomatic bone (lateral surface, posterior part)	Muscles at the angle of the mouth	Z	Pulls corner of mouth superiorly and laterally
② Zygomaticus minor		Upper lip just medial to corner of the mouth		Pulls upper lip superiorly
③ Levator labii superioris alaeque nasi	Maxilla (frontal process)	Upper lip and alar cartilage of nose	B/Z	Elevates upper lip; flares nostril
④ Levator labii superioris	Maxilla (frontal process) and infraorbital margin	Skin of upper lip		Elevates upper lip
⑤ Depressor labii inferioris	Mandible (anterior portion of oblique line)	Lower lip at midline; blends with muscle from opposite side	M	Pulls lower lip inferiorly and laterally, also contributes to eversion (pouting)
⑥ Levator anguli oris	Maxilla (canine fossa, below infraorbital foramen)	Muscles at the angle of mouth	B/Z	Raises angle of mouth; helps form nasolabial furrow
⑦ Depressor anguli oris	Mandible (oblique line below canine, premolar, and 1st molar teeth)	Skin at corner of mouth; blends with orbicularis oris	B/M	Pulls angle of mouth inferiorly and laterally
⑧ Buccinator	Alveolar processes of maxilla and mandible (by molars); pterygomandibular raphe	Lips, orbicularis oris, submucosa of lips and cheek	B	• Suckling in nursing infant • Presses cheek against molar teeth, working with tongue to keep food between occlusal surfaces and out of oral vestibule; expels air from oral cavity/resists distention when blowing *Unilateral:* draws mouth to one side
⑨ Orbicularis oris	Deep surface of skin Superiorly: Maxilla (median plane) Inferiorly: Mandible	Mucous membrane of lips	B/M	Acts as oral sphincter • Compresses and protrudes lip (e.g., whistling, sucking, kissing) • Resists distention (when blowing)
⑩ Risorius	Fascia and superficial muscles over masseter	Skin of corner of mouth	B	Retracts corner of mouth as in smiling, laughing, grimacing
⑪ Mentalis	Anterior surface of body of mandible	Skin of chin	M	Elevates and protrudes lower lip (drinking)
Platysma	Mandible (inferior border); skin over lower face; angle of mouth	Skin over lower neck and upper lateral thorax	C	Depresses and wrinkles skin of lower face and mouth; tenses skin of neck; aids in forced depression of the mandible

* Innervation: The muscles of facial expression are innervated by six branches of the facial nerve (CN VII). The posterior muscles are innervated by the posterior auricular (PA) nerve, which arises before the facial nerve enters the parotid gland. The anterior muscles are innervated by five branches off the parotid plexus of the facial nerve: temporal (T), zygomatic (Z), buccal (B), marginal mandibular (M), and cervical (C).

Neurovascular Topography of the Anterior Face & Scalp: Superficial Layer

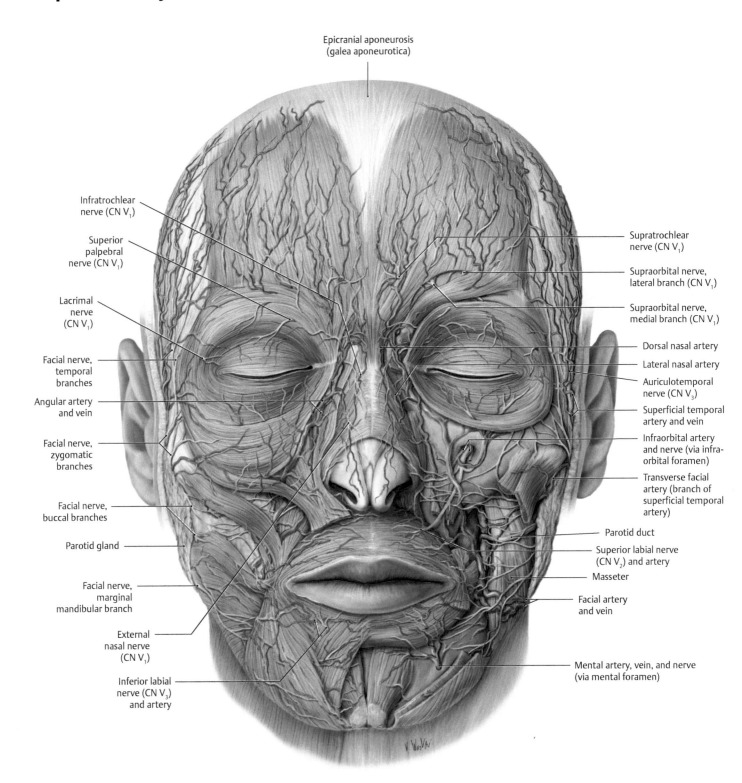

Epicranial aponeurosis (galea aponeurotica)

Infratrochlear nerve (CN V₁)

Superior palpebral nerve (CN V₁)

Lacrimal nerve (CN V₁)

Facial nerve, temporal branches

Angular artery and vein

Facial nerve, zygomatic branches

Facial nerve, buccal branches

Parotid gland

Facial nerve, marginal mandibular branch

External nasal nerve (CN V₁)

Inferior labial nerve (CN V₃) and artery

Supratrochlear nerve (CN V₁)

Supraorbital nerve, lateral branch (CN V₁)

Supraorbital nerve, medial branch (CN V₁)

Dorsal nasal artery

Lateral nasal artery

Auriculotemporal nerve (CN V₃)

Superficial temporal artery and vein

Infraorbital artery and nerve (via infra-orbital foramen)

Transverse facial artery (branch of superficial temporal artery)

Parotid duct

Superior labial nerve (CN V₂) and artery

Masseter

Facial artery and vein

Mental artery, vein, and nerve (via mental foramen)

Fig. 5.8 Neurovasculature of the superficial layer of the anterior face

Anterior view. *Removed:* Skin and fatty tissue. The muscles of facial expression have been partially removed on the left side to display underlying musculature and neurovascular structures. The muscles of facial expression receive motor innervation from the facial nerve (CN VII), which emerges laterally from the parotid gland. The muscles of mastication receive motor innervation from the mandibular division of the trigeminal nerve (CN V₃). The face receives sensory innervation primarily from the terminal branches of the three divisions of the trigeminal nerve (CN V), but also from the great auricular nerve, which arises from the cervical plexus (see pp. 336 and 337). The face receives blood supply primarily from branches of the external carotid artery, though these do anastomose on the face with facial branches of the internal carotid artery (see **Fig. 3.12**).

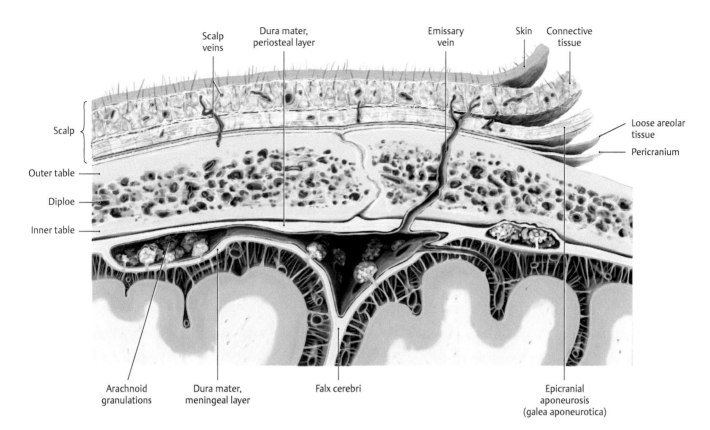

Scalp veins — Dura mater, periosteal layer — Emissary vein — Skin — Connective tissue

Scalp

Outer table

Diploe

Inner table

Loose areolar tissue

Pericranium

Arachnoid granulations — Dura mater, meningeal layer — Falx cerebri — Epicranial aponeurosis (galea aponeurotica)

Fig. 5.9 Scalp
The scalp consists of five layers. From superficial to deep, these are **S**kin, **C**onnective tissue, epicranical **A**poneurosis (galea aponeurotica), **L**oose areolar tissue, and **P**ericranium.
Scalp infections are able to spread easily through the loose connective tissue layer. They may spread intracranially to the dural venous sinuses through emissary veins, causing meningitis, or to the eyelids or nose because the frontalis muscle inserts into the skin and subcutaneous tissue but does not attach to bone. Infections that spread to the eyelid cause rapid swelling because the skin of the eyelid is very thin and it covers a loose connective tissue layer. Scalp infections are unable to spread into the neck because the occipital bellies of the occipitofrontalis muscles attach to the occipital bone and the mastoid process of

the temporal bone. Likewise they are prevented from spreading laterally beyond the zygomatic arches because the epicranial aponeurosis is continuous with the temporal fascia, which attaches to the zygomatic arches.
Scalp lacerations bleed profusely because the arteries entering the periphery of the scalp bleed from both ends owing to extensive anastomoses. Furthermore, the arteries do not contract to arrest bleeding because they are held open by the dense connective tissue layer of the scalp. The occipitofrontalis may go into spasm following scalp laceration causing the wound to gape. Scalp lacerations should be sutured or otherwise controlled as soon as possible after injury to prevent serious, sometimes fatal, loss of blood.

Fig. 5.10 Venous "danger zone" in the face
The superficial veins of the face have extensive connections with the deep veins of the head (e.g., the pterygoid plexus) and dural sinuses (e.g., the cavernous sinus) (see p. 70). Veins in the triangular danger zone are, in general, valveless. There is therefore a particularly high risk of bacterial dissemination into the cranial cavity. For example, bacteria from a boil on the lip may enter the facial vein and cause meningitis by passing through venous communications with the cavernous sinus.

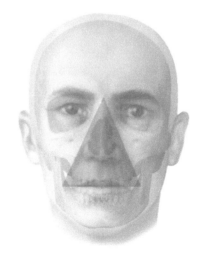

Neurovascular Topography of the Lateral Head: Superficial Layer

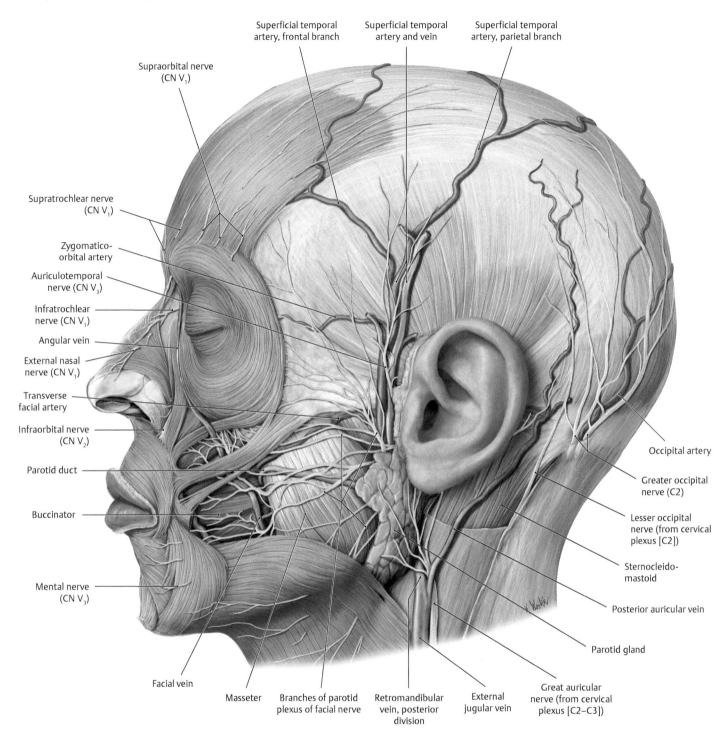

Fig. 5.11 Neurovasculature of the superficial layer of the lateral head

Left lateral view. The arteries supplying the lateral head arise from branches of the external carotid artery (see **Fig. 5.12**). Blood drains primarily into the internal, external, and anterior jugular veins (see p. 62). The muscles of facial expression receive motor innervation from the facial nerve (CN VII), which emerges laterally from the parotid gland (see p. 139). The muscles of mastication receive motor innervation from the mandibular division of the trigeminal nerve (CN V$_3$, see p. 134). The sensory innervation of the face is shown in **Fig. 5.13**.

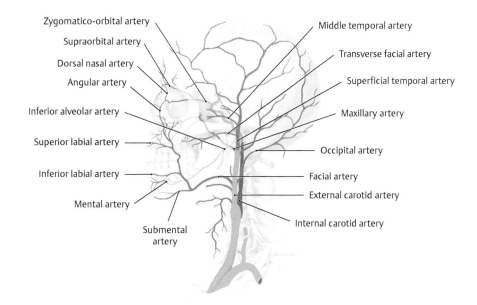

Fig. 5.12 Superficial arteries of the head
Left lateral view. The superficial face is supplied primarily by branches of the external carotid artery (e.g., facial, superficial temporal, and maxillary arteries). However, there is a limited contribution from branches derived from the internal carotid artery in the region of the orbital rim. *Note:* The internal carotid artery is colored purple and the anterior, medial, posterior, and terminal branches of the external carotid artery are colored red, blue, green, and yellow, respectively.

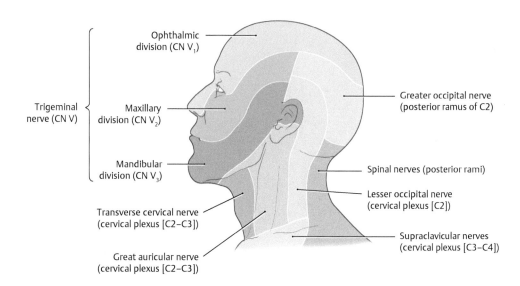

Fig. 5.13 Sensory innervation of the lateral head and neck
Left lateral view. The head receives sensory innervation primarily from the trigeminal nerve (orange), the cervical plexus (green and gray), and the posterior rami of the spinal nerves (blue). Sensory supply to the face is primarily from the terminal branches of the three trigeminal nerve divisions. The occiput and nuchal region are supplied primarily by posterior rami of the spinal nerves. The anterior rami of the first four spinal nerves combine to form the cervical plexus. The cervical plexus gives off four cutaneous branches that supply the lateral head and neck (nerves listed with their associated spinal nerve fibers): lesser occipital (C2, occasionally C3), great auricular (C2–C3), transverse cervical (C2–C3), and supraclavicular (C3–C4) nerves (see **Fig. 12.3**).

Neurovascular Topography of the Lateral Head: Intermediate & Deep Layers

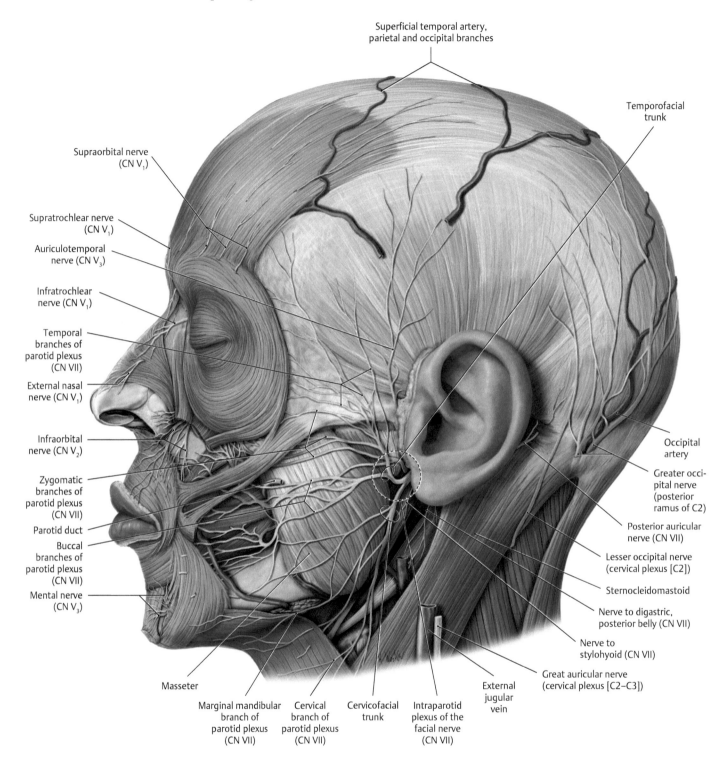

Superficial temporal artery, parietal and occipital branches

Temporofacial trunk

Supraorbital nerve (CN V$_1$)

Supratrochlear nerve (CN V$_1$)

Auriculotemporal nerve (CN V$_3$)

Infratrochlear nerve (CN V$_1$)

Temporal branches of parotid plexus (CN VII)

External nasal nerve (CN V$_1$)

Infraorbital nerve (CN V$_2$)

Zygomatic branches of parotid plexus (CN VII)

Parotid duct

Buccal branches of parotid plexus (CN VII)

Mental nerve (CN V$_3$)

Occipital artery

Greater occipital nerve (posterior ramus of C2)

Posterior auricular nerve (CN VII)

Lesser occipital nerve (cervical plexus [C2])

Sternocleidomastoid

Nerve to digastric, posterior belly (CN VII)

Nerve to stylohyoid (CN VII)

Great auricular nerve (cervical plexus [C2–C3])

External jugular vein

Masseter

Marginal mandibular branch of parotid plexus (CN VII)

Cervical branch of parotid plexus (CN VII)

Cervicofacial trunk

Intraparotid plexus of the facial nerve (CN VII)

Fig. 5.14 Nerves of the intermediate layer of the lateral head
Left lateral view. The parotid gland has been removed to demonstrate the structure of the parotid plexus of the facial nerve (see **Fig. 4.88**). The occiput receives sensory innervation from the greater occipital nerve, which arises from the posterior primary ramus of C2, and the lesser occipital nerve, which arises from the cervical plexus (anterior rami of C2).

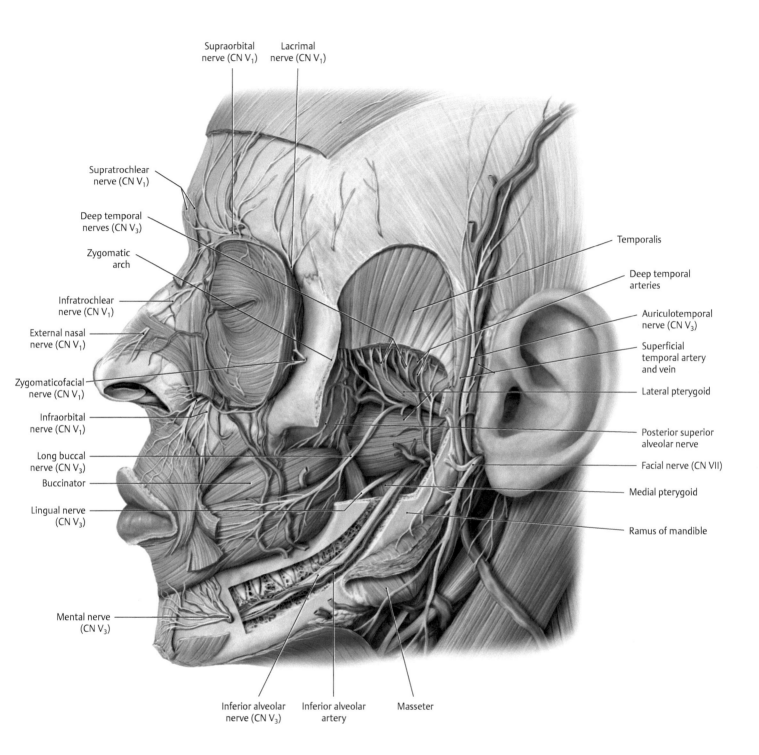

Supraorbital nerve (CN V$_1$)

Lacrimal nerve (CN V$_1$)

Supratrochlear nerve (CN V$_1$)

Deep temporal nerves (CN V$_3$)

Zygomatic arch

Infratrochlear nerve (CN V$_1$)

External nasal nerve (CN V$_1$)

Zygomaticofacial nerve (CN V$_1$)

Infraorbital nerve (CN V$_1$)

Long buccal nerve (CN V$_3$)

Buccinator

Lingual nerve (CN V$_3$)

Mental nerve (CN V$_3$)

Temporalis

Deep temporal arteries

Auriculotemporal nerve (CN V$_3$)

Superficial temporal artery and vein

Lateral pterygoid

Posterior superior alveolar nerve

Facial nerve (CN VII)

Medial pterygoid

Ramus of mandible

Inferior alveolar nerve (CN V$_3$)

Inferior alveolar artery

Masseter

Fig. 5.15 Neurovasculature of the lateral face
Left lateral view. The masseter and zygomatic arch have been windowed to reveal the deep structures. Also, the ramus and body of the mandible have been opened to demonstrate neurovascular structures that traverse it.

165

Temporal & Infratemporal Fossae: Contents

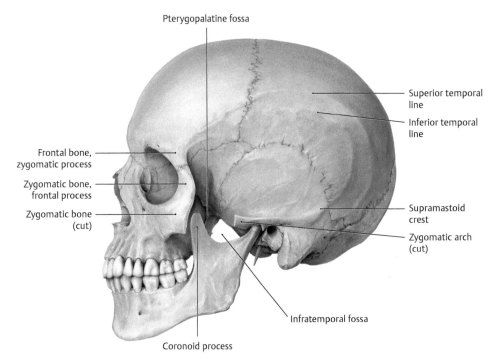

Pterygopalatine fossa

Superior temporal line

Inferior temporal line

Frontal bone, zygomatic process

Zygomatic bone, frontal process

Zygomatic bone (cut)

Supramastoid crest

Zygomatic arch (cut)

Infratemporal fossa

Coronoid process

Fig. 6.1 Temporal fossa
Left lateral view. The temporal fossa is located on the lateral aspect of the skull. Its boundaries are listed in **Table 6.1**. The temporal fossa communicates with the infratemporal fossa inferiorly (medial to the zygomatic arch). The pterygopalatine fossa can also be seen here medial to the infratemporal fossa due to the removal of the zygomatic arch and some of the zygomatic bone.

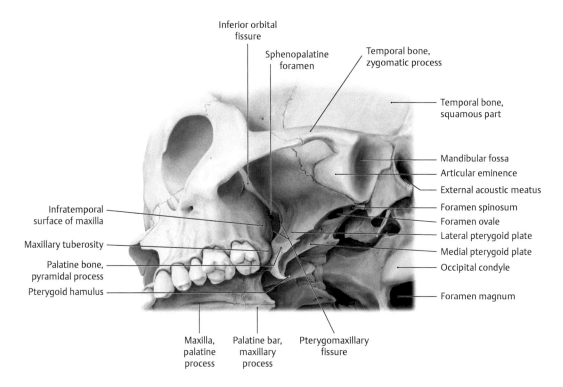

Inferior orbital fissure

Sphenopalatine foramen

Temporal bone, zygomatic process

Temporal bone, squamous part

Mandibular fossa

Articular eminence

External acoustic meatus

Foramen spinosum

Foramen ovale

Lateral pterygoid plate

Medial pterygoid plate

Occipital condyle

Foramen magnum

Infratemporal surface of maxilla

Maxillary tuberosity

Palatine bone, pyramidal process

Pterygoid hamulus

Maxilla, palatine process

Palatine bar, maxillary process

Pterygomaxillary fissure

Fig. 6.2 Infratemporal fossa
Oblique external view of the base of the skull. The infratemporal fossa's bony boundaries are listed in **Table 6.3**. The infratemporal fossa communicates *medially* with the pterygopalatine fossa via the pterygomaxillary fissure; *anteriorly* with the orbit via the inferior orbital fissure; *superiorly* with the middle cranial fossa via foramen ovale and foramen spinosum, and with the temporal fossa passing medial to the zygomatic arch.

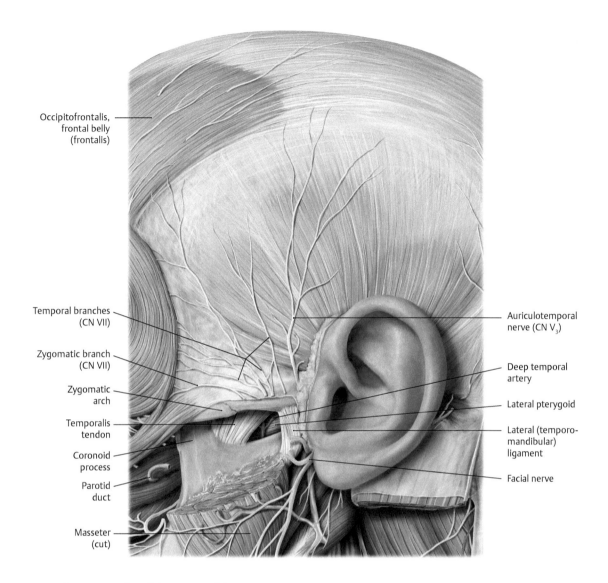

Occipitofrontalis,
frontal belly
(frontalis)

Temporal branches
(CN VII)

Zygomatic branch
(CN VII)

Zygomatic
arch

Temporalis
tendon

Coronoid
process

Parotid
duct

Masseter
(cut)

Auriculotemporal
nerve (CN V₃)

Deep temporal
artery

Lateral pterygoid

Lateral (temporo-
mandibular)
ligament

Facial nerve

Fig. 6.3 Neurovascular topography of the temporal fossa
Left lateral view. *Cut:* Masseter. *Revealed:* Temporal fossa and temporomandibular joint.
The muscles and neurovasculature of the temporal fossa are listed in **Table 6.2**.

Table 6.1 Borders of the temporal fossa	
Superior	Superior and inferior temporal lines
Inferior	Zygomatic arch (laterally); infratemporal crest of the greater wing of sphenoid bone (medially)
Anterior	Frontal process of zygomatic bone; zygomatic process of frontal bone
Posterior	Supramastoid crest
Medial	Sphenoid, temporal, parietal, and frontal bones
Lateral	Temporal fascia

Table 6.2 Muscles and neurovasculature of the temporal fossa		
Muscle	**Vasculature**	**Nerves**
Temporalis	Superficial temporal a. and v.	Auriculotemporal n. (CN V₃)
	Deep temporal aa. and vv.	Deep temporal nn. (CN V₃)
		Temporal branches (CN VII)

167

Infratemporal Fossa: Contents

The infratemporal fossa is located lateral to the lateral pterygoid plate of the sphenoid, medial to the ramus of the mandible, posterior to the maxilla, anterior to the styloid process (and the carotid sheath and its contents), and inferior to the greater wing of the sphenoid and a small part of the temporal bone. It is continuous with the pterygopalatine fossa (through the pterygomaxillary fissure). The maxillary artery gives rise to its mandibular (bony, first part) and pterygoid (muscular, second part) branches in the infratemporal fossa. The mandibular division of the trigeminal nerve (CN V$_3$) divides into its terminal branches in the infratemporal fossa.

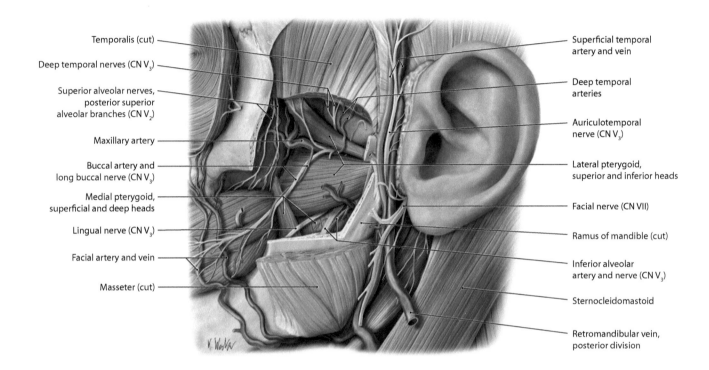

Fig. 6.4 Infratemporal fossa, superficial dissection
Left lateral view. *Removed:* Masseter, anterior portion of the mandibular ramus, and zygomatic arch. The pterygoid plexus normally is embedded between the medial and lateral pterygoids. It drains to the maxillary vein, a tributary of the retromandibular vein. The inferior alveolar artery and nerve can be seen entering the mandibular canal (the accompanying vein has been removed).

Table 6.3 Borders of the infratemporal fossa

Superior*	Inferior surface of the greater wing of the sphenoid bone Squamous part of the temporal bone (small contribution)
Inferior	Demarked by an imaginary line that is an inward extension of the mandibular plane
Anterior	Infratemporal surface of the maxilla
Posterior	Styloid process and contents of carotid sheath
Medial	Lateral surface of the lateral pterygoid plate and pyramidal process of the palatine bone
Lateral	Medial surface of the ramus of the mandible

* The infratemporal crest separates the roof from the temporal fossa above.

Table 6.4 Muscles and vessels of the infratemporal fossa

Muscles	Arteries	Veins
Lateral and medial pterygoids	Maxillary a. • Mandibular branches	Pterygoid plexus and its tributaries
Temporalis tendon	• Pterygoid branches	Maxillary v.
		Deep facial v. (deep portion)
		Emissary vv.

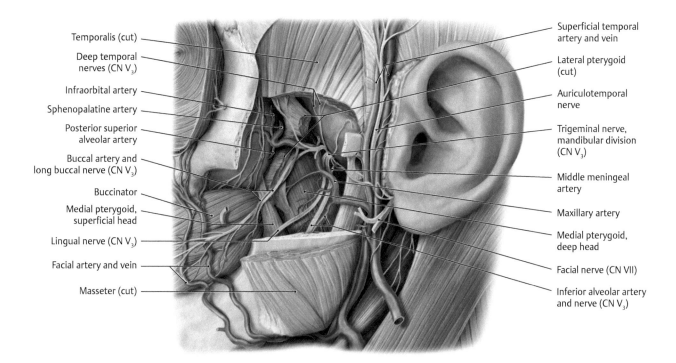

Temporalis (cut)

Deep temporal nerves (CN V₃)

Infraorbital artery

Sphenopalatine artery

Posterior superior alveolar artery

Buccal artery and long buccal nerve (CN V₃)

Buccinator

Medial pterygoid, superficial head

Lingual nerve (CN V₃)

Facial artery and vein

Masseter (cut)

Superficial temporal artery and vein

Lateral pterygoid (cut)

Auriculotemporal nerve

Trigeminal nerve, mandibular division (CN V₃)

Middle meningeal artery

Maxillary artery

Medial pterygoid, deep head

Facial nerve (CN VII)

Inferior alveolar artery and nerve (CN V₃)

Fig. 6.5 **Infratemporal fossa, deep dissection**
Left lateral view. *Removed:* Both heads of the lateral pterygoid muscle. The branches of the maxillary artery and mandibular division of the trigeminal nerve (CN V₃) can be identified. *Note:* By careful observation, it is possible to define the site where the auriculotemporal nerve (branch of the mandibular division) splits around the middle meningeal artery before the artery enters the middle cranial fossa through the foramen spinosum. Branches of the third part of the maxillary artery can be observed in the pterygopalatine fossa, which is medial to the infratemporal fossa.

Table 6.5 Nerves in the infratemporal fossa

CN V₃	Trunk of CN V₃ and direct branches:
	 • Recurrent meningeal branch (nervus spinosus)
	 • Medial pterygoid n.
	   • Tensor veli palatini
	   • Tensor tympani
		Anterior division:
		 • Masseteric n.
		 • Deep temporal nn.
		 • Long buccal n.
		 • Lateral pterygoid n.
			Posterior division:
			 • Auriculotemporal n.
			 • Lingual n.
			 • Inferior alveolar n.
			   • Mylohyoid n.

CN V₂	Posterior superior alveolar n.		
Other	Otic ganglion	Lesser petrosal n. (CN IX)	Chorda tympani (CN VII)

The anterior aspect of the infratemporal fossa is the site of needle placement for a posterior superior alveolar nerve block.

Muscles of Mastication: Overview

The muscles of mastication are located at various depths in the parotid and infratemporal regions of the face. They attach to the mandible and receive their motor innervation from the mandibular division of the trigeminal nerve (CN V$_3$).

Table 6.6 Masseter and temporalis muscles

Muscle		Origin	Insertion	Innervation*	Action
Masseter	① Superficial head	Zygomatic bone (maxillary process) and zygomatic arch (lateral aspect of anterior ⅔)	Mandibular angle and ramus (inferior lateral surface)	Masseteric n. (anterior division of CN V$_3$)	*Bilateral:* Elevates mandible, also assists in protraction *Unilateral:* Lateral movement of mandible (chewing)
	Middle head	Zygomatic arch (medial aspect of anterior ⅔)	Mandibular ramus (central part of lateral surface)		
	② Deep head	Zygomatic arch (deep surface of posterior ⅓)	Mandibular ramus (superior lateral surface) and inferior coronoid process		
Temporalis	③ Superficial head	Temporal fascia	Coronoid process of mandible (apex, medial surface, and anterior surface of mandibular ramus)	Deep temporal nn. (anterior division of CN V$_3$)	*Vertical (anterior) fibers:* Elevate mandible *Horizontal (posterior) fibers:* Retract (retrude) mandible *Unilateral:* Lateral movement of mandible (chewing)
	④ Deep head	Temporal fossa (inferior temporal line)			

* The muscles of mastication are innervated by motor branches of the mandibular nerve (CN V$_3$), the 3rd division of the trigeminal nerve (CN V).

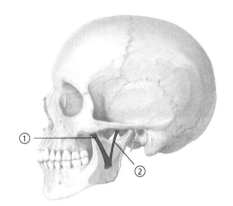

Fig. 6.6 Masseter

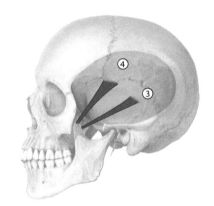

Fig. 6.7 Temporalis

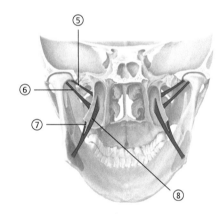

Fig. 6.8 Pterygoids

Table 6.7 Lateral and medial pterygoid muscles

Muscle		Origin	Insertion	Innervation	Action
Lateral pterygoid	⑤ Superior (upper) head	Greater wing of sphenoid bone (infratemporal crest)	Mandible (pterygoid fovea) and temporomandibular joint (articular disk)	Lateral pterygoid nerve (anterior division of CN V$_3$)	*Bilateral:* Protrudes mandible (pulls articular disk forward) and opens mouth. *Unilateral:* Alternating actions, along with ipsilateral medial pterygoid, result in side-to-side movements necessary for grinding.
	⑥ Inferior (lower) head	Lateral pterygoid plate (lateral surface)	Mandible (pterygoid fovea and condylar process) and neck of mandible		
Medial pterygoid	⑦ Superficial (external) head	Maxilla (maxillary tuberosity) and palatine bone (pyramidal process)	Pterygoid rugosity on medial surface of the mandibular angle	Medial pterygoid nerve (trunk of CN V$_3$)	*Bilateral:* Elevation of mandible; also acts with lateral pterygoid to assist in protrusion of mandible. *Unilateral:* Acts with ipsilateral lateral pterygoid to protrude mandible and produce medial movement toward the opposite side. Alternating actions between right and left sides results in side-to-side chewing movements.
	⑧ Deep (internal) head	Medial surface of lateral pterygoid plate and pterygoid fossa			

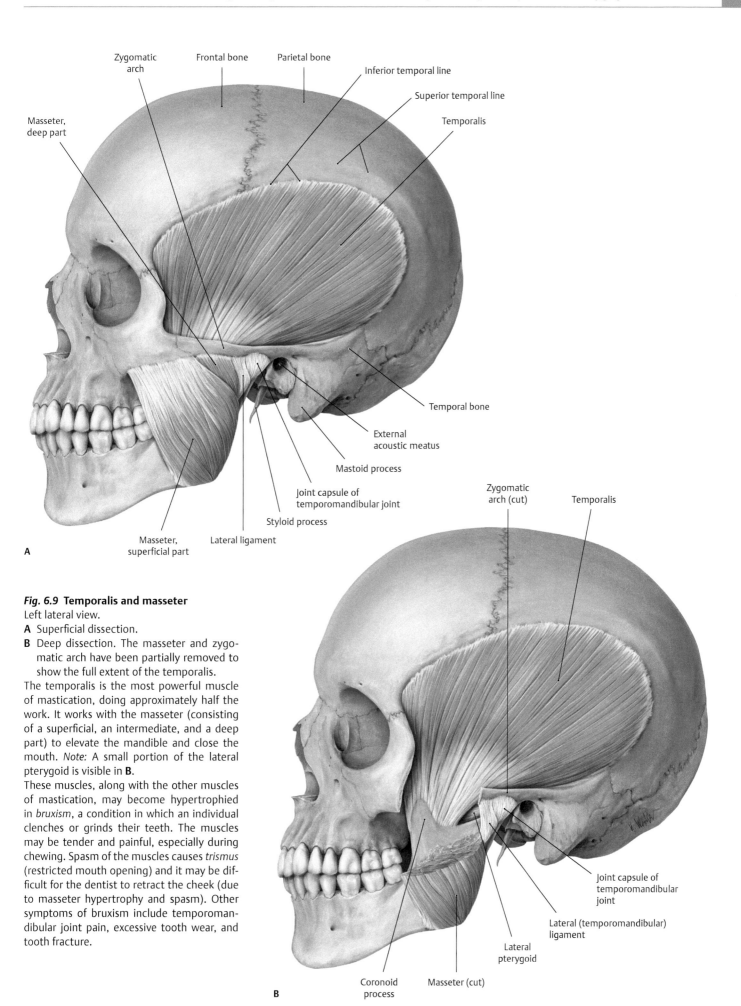

A

Zygomatic arch

Masseter, deep part

Frontal bone

Parietal bone

Inferior temporal line

Superior temporal line

Temporalis

Temporal bone

External acoustic meatus

Mastoid process

Joint capsule of temporomandibular joint

Styloid process

Lateral ligament

Masseter, superficial part

Zygomatic arch (cut)

Temporalis

Joint capsule of temporomandibular joint

Lateral (temporomandibular) ligament

Lateral pterygoid

Masseter (cut)

Coronoid process

B

***Fig. 6.9* Temporalis and masseter**
Left lateral view.
A Superficial dissection.
B Deep dissection. The masseter and zygomatic arch have been partially removed to show the full extent of the temporalis.

The temporalis is the most powerful muscle of mastication, doing approximately half the work. It works with the masseter (consisting of a superficial, an intermediate, and a deep part) to elevate the mandible and close the mouth. *Note:* A small portion of the lateral pterygoid is visible in **B**.

These muscles, along with the other muscles of mastication, may become hypertrophied in *bruxism*, a condition in which an individual clenches or grinds their teeth. The muscles may be tender and painful, especially during chewing. Spasm of the muscles causes *trismus* (restricted mouth opening) and it may be difficult for the dentist to retract the cheek (due to masseter hypertrophy and spasm). Other symptoms of bruxism include temporomandibular joint pain, excessive tooth wear, and tooth fracture.

171

Muscles of Mastication: Deep Muscles

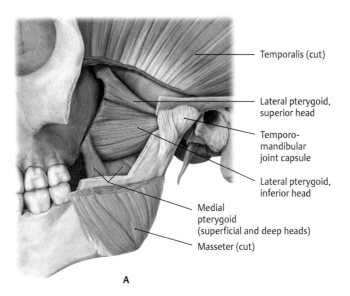

Temporalis (cut)

Lateral pterygoid, superior head

Temporo-mandibular joint capsule

Lateral pterygoid, inferior head

Medial pterygoid (superficial and deep heads)

Masseter (cut)

A

Lateral pterygoid, superior head (cut)

Articular disk

Lateral pterygoid, inferior head (cut)

Medial pterygoid, deep (internal) head

Pterygoid process, lateral plate

Medial pterygoid, superficial (external) head

B

Fig. 6.10 Lateral and medial pterygoid muscles
Left lateral views.
A The coronoid process of the mandible has been removed here along with the lower part of the temporalis so that both pterygoid muscles are observed (see **Fig. 6.9B**).
B Here the temporalis has been completely removed, and the inferior head of the lateral pterygoid has been windowed. The *lateral* pterygoid initiates depression of the mandible, which is then continued by the suprahyoid and infrahyoid muscles and gravity. With the temporomandibular joint opened, we can see that fibers from the superior head of the lateral pterygoid blend with the articular disk. The lateral pterygoid functions as the guide muscle of the temporomandibular joint. The *medial* pterygoid runs almost perpendicular to the lateral pterygoid and contributes to the formation of a muscular sling that partially encompasses the mandible (see **Fig. 6.11**). Note how the inferior head of the lateral pterygoid originates between the two heads of the medial pterygoid.

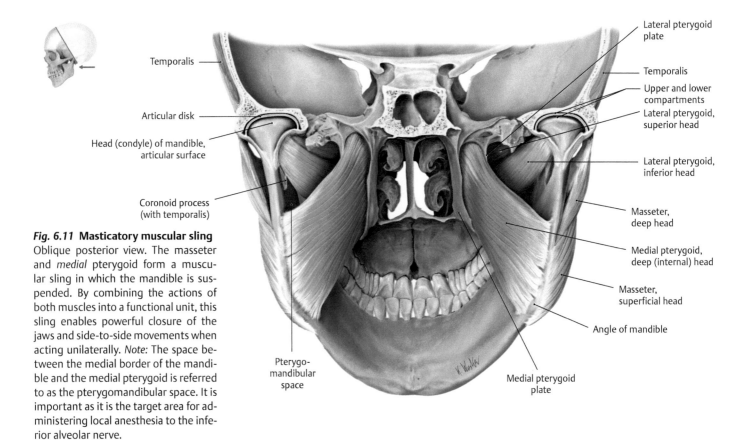

Temporalis

Articular disk

Head (condyle) of mandible, articular surface

Coronoid process (with temporalis)

Pterygo-mandibular space

Lateral pterygoid plate

Temporalis

Upper and lower compartments

Lateral pterygoid, superior head

Lateral pterygoid, inferior head

Masseter, deep head

Medial pterygoid, deep (internal) head

Masseter, superficial head

Angle of mandible

Medial pterygoid plate

Fig. 6.11 Masticatory muscular sling
Oblique posterior view. The masseter and *medial* pterygoid form a muscular sling in which the mandible is suspended. By combining the actions of both muscles into a functional unit, this sling enables powerful closure of the jaws and side-to-side movements when acting unilaterally. *Note:* The space between the medial border of the mandible and the medial pterygoid is referred to as the pterygomandibular space. It is important as it is the target area for administering local anesthesia to the inferior alveolar nerve.

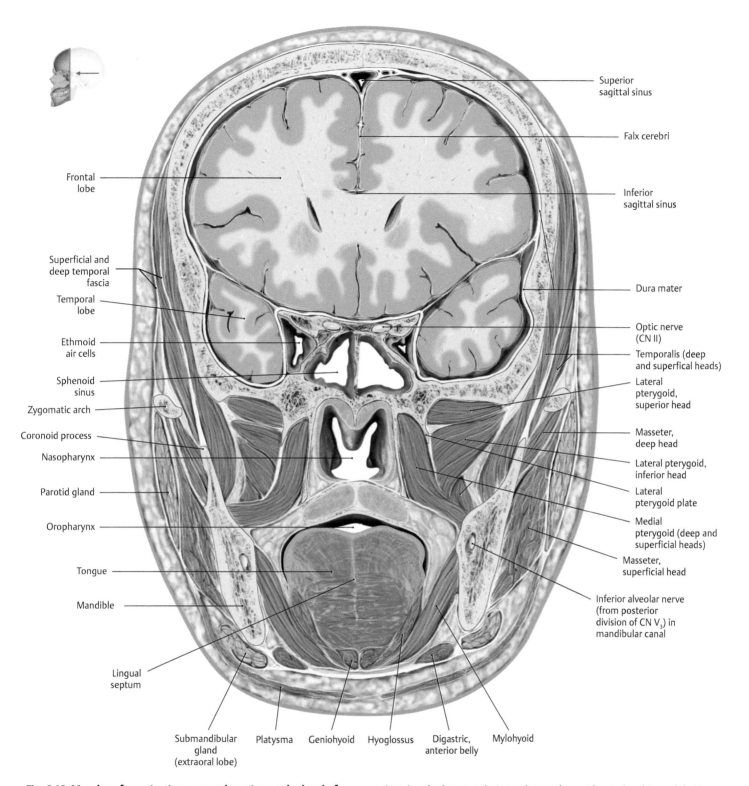

Superior
sagittal sinus

Falx cerebri

Frontal
lobe

Inferior
sagittal sinus

Superficial and
deep temporal
fascia

Dura mater

Temporal
lobe

Optic nerve
(CN II)

Ethmoid
air cells

Temporalis (deep
and superfical heads)

Sphenoid
sinus

Lateral
pterygoid,
superior head

Zygomatic arch

Masseter,
deep head

Coronoid process

Lateral pterygoid,
inferior head

Nasopharynx

Lateral
pterygoid plate

Parotid gland

Medial
pterygoid (deep and
superficial heads)

Oropharynx

Masseter,
superficial head

Tongue

Inferior alveolar nerve
(from posterior
division of CN V₃) in
mandibular canal

Mandible

Lingual
septum

Submandibular   Platysma   Geniohyoid   Hyoglossus   Digastric,   Mylohyoid
gland   anterior belly
(extraoral lobe)

***Fig. 6.12 Muscles of mastication, coronal section at the level of
the sphenoid sinus***

Posterior view. The topography of the muscles of mastication and
neighboring structures is particularly well displayed in this section.
The muscles of mastication can be bimanually palpated to assess for hypertrophy or tenderness. To palpate the temporalis, the clinician places
his fingers over the temporal region and works his way down the length
of this muscle from superior to inferior; to palpate the masseter the patient is asked to put their teeth together without clenching while the
clinician palpates over the lateral cheek from superior to inferior; the
lateral pterygoid is palpated by the clinician placing his index or little
finger in the buccal sulcus as far posteriorly as possible and palpating in
a posterior, superior, and medial direction (it is a source of some debate
whether this actually allows for palpation of the lateral pterygoid); the
medial pterygoid is palpated along the medial border of the body and
angle of the mandible.

Temporomandibular Joint (TMJ)

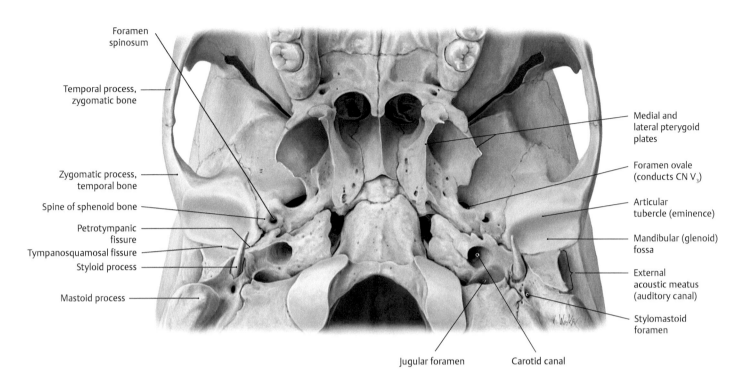

Foramen spinosum

Temporal process, zygomatic bone

Zygomatic process, temporal bone

Spine of sphenoid bone

Petrotympanic fissure

Tympanosquamosal fissure

Styloid process

Mastoid process

Medial and lateral pterygoid plates

Foramen ovale (conducts CN V₃)

Articular tubercle (eminence)

Mandibular (glenoid) fossa

External acoustic meatus (auditory canal)

Stylomastoid foramen

Jugular foramen

Carotid canal

Fig. 6.13 Mandibular (glenoid) fossa of the TMJ
Inferior view. The head of the mandible articulates with the articular disk in the mandibular (glenoid) fossa of the temporal bone. The mandibular fossa is a depression in the squamous part of the temporal bone. The articular tubercle is located on the anterior side of the mandibular fossa. The head of the mandible is markedly smaller than the mandibular fossa, allowing it to have an adequate range of movement. Unlike other articular surfaces, the mandibular fossa is covered by fibrocartilage rather than hyaline cartilage. As a result, it is not as

clearly delineated on the skull as other articular surfaces. The external auditory canal lies just posterior to the mandibular fossa. Trauma to the mandible may damage the auditory canal. *Note:* The mandibular fossa is divided into two compartments (anterior and posterior), separated by the tympanosquamosal and petrotympanic fissures. The posterior compartment is nonarticulatory, and the chorda tympani nerve and anterior tympanic artery are able to pass through this space without being compressed. The glenoid lobe of the parotid gland may also project into the posterior compartment.

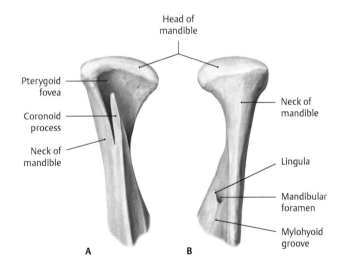

Head of mandible

Pterygoid fovea

Coronoid process

Neck of mandible

Neck of mandible

Lingula

Mandibular foramen

Mylohyoid groove

A   B

Fig. 6.14 Processes of the mandible
A Anterior view. **B** Posterior view. The head of the mandible not only is markedly smaller than the articular fossa but also has a cylindrical shape. This shape increases the mobility of the mandibular head, as it allows rotational movements about a vertical axis (condular–hinge axis).

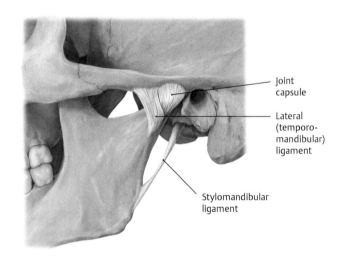

Joint capsule

Lateral (temporomandibular) ligament

Stylomandibular ligament

Fig. 6.15 Ligaments of the left TMJ
Lateral view. The TMJ is surrounded by a relatively lax capsule, which permits physiological dislocation during jaw opening. The joint is stabilized by three ligaments: lateral (temporomandibular), stylomandibular, and sphenomandibular (see **Fig. 6.16**). This lateral view demonstrates the strongest of these ligaments, the lateral ligament, which stretches over the capsule and is blended with it.

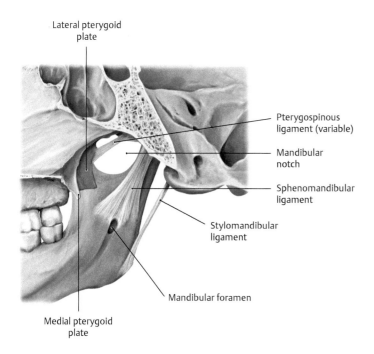

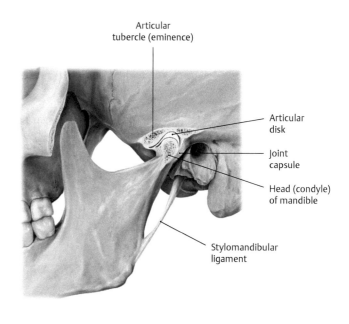

Fig. 6.16 Ligaments of the right TMJ
Medial view. The sphenomandibular ligament can be identified in this view.

Fig. 6.17 Opened left TMJ
Lateral view. The capsule extends posteriorly to the petrotympanic fissure (not shown here). Interposed between the mandibular head and fossa is the articular disk, which is attached to the joint capsule on all sides. *Note:* The articular disk (meniscus) divides the TMJ into upper and lower compartments. Gliding (translational) movement occcurs in the upper compartment, hinge (rotational) movement in the lower compartment.

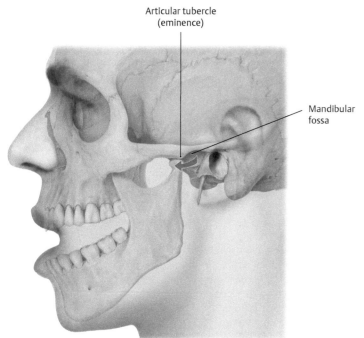

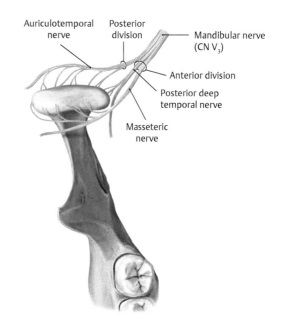

Fig. 6.18 Dislocation of the TMJ
The head of the mandible may slide past the articular tubercle when the mouth is opened, dislocating the TMJ. This may result from heavy yawning or a blow to the opened mandible. When the joint dislocates, the mandible becomes locked in a protruded position and can no longer be closed. This condition is easily diagnosed clinically and is reduced by pressing on the mandibular row of teeth.

Fig. 6.19 Sensory innervation of the TMJ capsule (after Schmidt)
Superior view. The TMJ capsule is supplied by articular branches arising from three branches of the mandibular division of the trigeminal nerve (CN V$_3$):

- Auriculotemporal nerve (posterior division of CN V$_3$)
- Posterior deep temporal nerve (anterior division of CN V$_3$)
- Masseteric nerve (anterior division of CN V$_3$)

Note: While the masseteric and posterior deep temporal nerves are generally considered to be motor nerves, they also innervate the TMJ.

175

Temporomandibular Joint (TMJ): Biomechanics

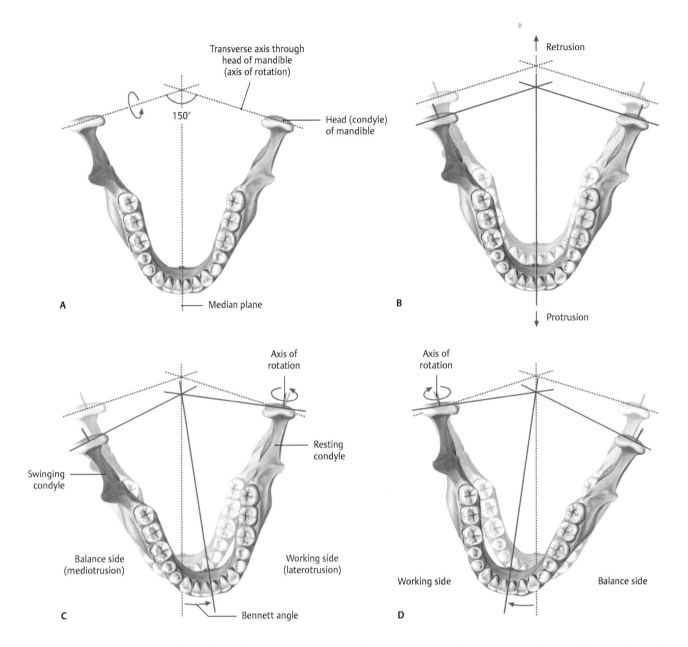

Fig. 6.20 Movements of the mandible in the TMJ
Superior view. Most of the movements in the TMJ are complex motions that have three main components:

- Rotation (opening and closing the mouth)
- Translation (protrusion and retrusion of the mandible)
- Grinding movements during mastication

A Rotation. The axis for joint rotation runs transversely through both heads of the mandible. The two axes intersect at an angle of approximately 150 degrees (range of 110–180 degrees between individuals). During this movement the TMJ acts as a hinge joint (abduction/depression and adduction/elevation of the mandible). In humans, pure rotation in the TMJ usually occurs only during sleep with the mouth slightly open (aperture angle up to approximately 15 degrees, see **Fig. 6.21B**). When the mouth is opened past 15 degrees, rotation is combined with translation (gliding) of the mandibular head.

B Translation. In this movement the mandible is advanced (protruded) and retracted (retruded). The axes (condylar–hinge axes) for this movement are parallel to the median axes through the center of the mandibular heads.

C Grinding movements in the left TMJ. In describing these lateral movements, a distinction is made between the "resting condyle" and the "swinging condyle." The resting condyle on the left working side rotates about an almost vertical axis through the head of the mandible (also a rotational axis), whereas the swinging condyle on the right balance side swings forward and inward in a translational movement. The lateral excursion of the mandible is measured in degrees and is called the Bennett angle. During this movement the mandible moves in laterotrusion on the working side and in mediotrusion on the balance side.

D Grinding movements in the right TMJ. Here, the right TMJ is the working side. The right resting condyle rotates about an almost vertical axis, and the left condyle on the balance side swings forward and inward.

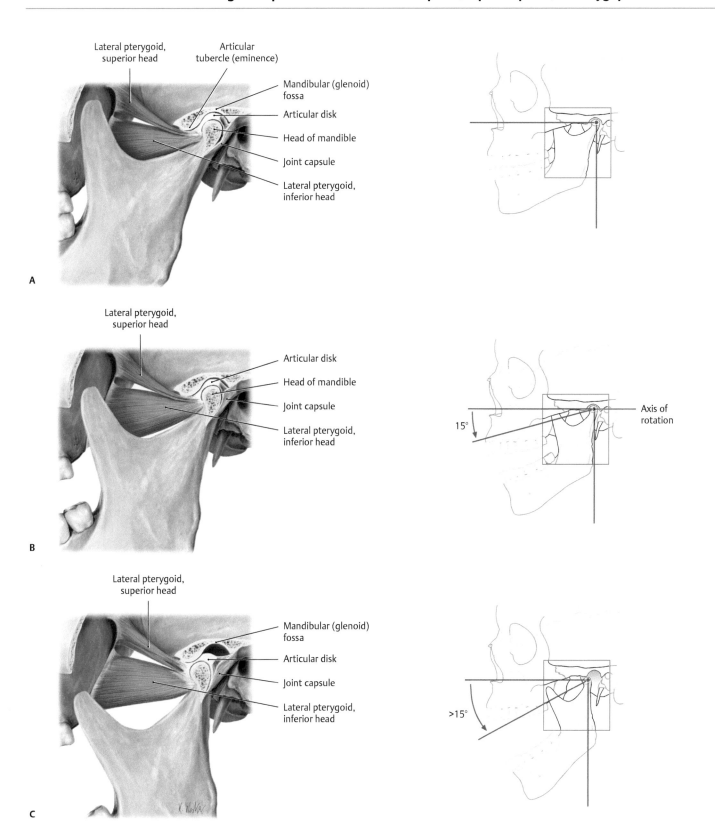

Fig. 6.21 Movements of the TMJ
Left lateral view. Each drawing shows the left TMJ (including the articular disk and capsule) and the lateral pterygoid muscle. *Note:* The gap between the heads of the lateral pterygoid is exaggerated. Each schematic diagram at right shows the corresponding axis of joint movement. The muscle, capsule, and disk form a functionally coordinated musculo-disco-capsular system and work closely together when the mouth is opened and closed.

A **Mouth closed, teeth in occlusion.** When the mouth is in the closed position with teeth in occlusion, the head (condyle) of the mandible maintains its contact with the articular disk, and the space of the upper compartment is maintained between the articular disk and the mandibular (glenoid) fossa of the temporal bone.

B **Mouth opened to 15 degrees.** Up to 15 degrees of abduction, the head of the mandible remains in the mandibular fossa.

C **Mouth opened past 15 degrees.** At this point the head of the mandible glides (translates) forward onto the articular tubercle (eminence). The joint axis that runs transversely through the mandibular head is shifted forward. The articular disk is pulled forward by the superior part of the lateral pterygoid muscle, and the head (condyle) of the mandible is drawn forward by the inferior part of that muscle.

Pterygopalatine Fossa: Overview

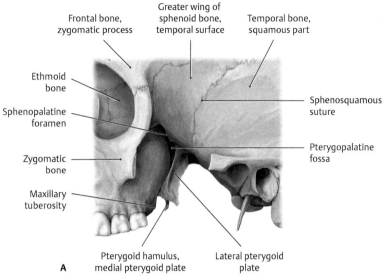

Frontal bone, zygomatic process
Greater wing of sphenoid bone, temporal surface
Temporal bone, squamous part
Ethmoid bone
Sphenopalatine foramen
Zygomatic bone
Maxillary tuberosity
Sphenosquamous suture
Pterygopalatine fossa
Pterygoid hamulus, medial pterygoid plate
Lateral pterygoid plate

A

Fig. 6.22 Pterygopalatine fossa

A Left lateral view of left infratemporal fossa and pterygopalatine fossa. **B** Inferior view of right infratemporal fossa and lateral approach to pterygopalatine fossa. The sphenoid bone is shaded green. The pterygopalatine fossa is a crossroads between the orbit, nasal cavity, oral cavity, nasopharynx, and middle cranial fossa. It is traversed by many nerves and vessels supplying these structures. The pterygopalatine fossa is continuous laterally with the infratemporal fossa through the pterygopalatine fissure. The lateral approach through the infratemporal fossa is used in surgical operations on tumors of the pterygopalatine fossa (e.g., nasopharyngeal fibroma).

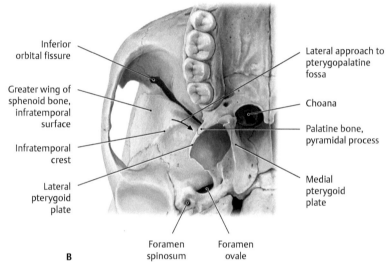

Inferior orbital fissure
Greater wing of sphenoid bone, infratemporal surface
Infratemporal crest
Lateral pterygoid plate
Lateral approach to pterygopalatine fossa
Choana
Palatine bone, pyramidal process
Medial pterygoid plate
Foramen spinosum
Foramen ovale

B

Table 6.8 Borders and openings of the pterygopalatine fossa		
Border	**Structure**	**Foramen/fissures/canals**
Superior	Sphenoid bone (greater wing)	Inferior orbital fissure (runs beside sphenoid bone in roof of pterygopalatine fossa)
Inferior	Greater palatine canal	Greater and lesser palatine foramina
Anterior	Maxilla (infratemporal [posterior] surface)	
Posterior	Sphenoid, root of the pterygoid process	Foramen rotundum
		Pterygoid (vidian) canal
		Palatovaginal (pharyngeal) canal
Medial	Palatine bone (perpendicular plate)	Sphenopalatine foramen
Lateral	Pterygomaxillary fissure	Pterygomaxillary fissure

Fig. 6.23 Communications of the pterygopalatine fossa

Left lateral view of left fossa (detail from **Fig. 6.22A**). The pterygopalatine fossa contains the pterygopalatine ganglion, the parasympathetic ganglion of CN VII that is affiliated with the maxillary nerve (CN V_2, sensory). Sensory fibers from the face, maxillary dentition, nasal cavity, oral cavity, nasopharynx, and paranasal sinuses pass through the ganglion without synapsing and enter the middle cranial fossa as the maxillary nerve (CN V_2). These sensory fibers also serve as "scaffolding" for the peripheral distribution of postganglionic autonomic parasympathetic fibers from the pterygopalatine ganglion and postganglionic sympathetic fibers derived from the internal carotid plexus. See **Table 4.23** for a complete treatment of the maxillary nerve and pterygopalatine ganglion.

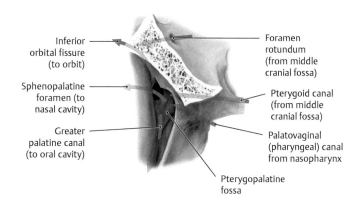

Inferior orbital fissure (to orbit)

Sphenopalatine foramen (to nasal cavity)

Greater palatine canal (to oral cavity)

Foramen rotundum (from middle cranial fossa)

Pterygoid canal (from middle cranial fossa)

Palatovaginal (pharyngeal) canal from nasopharynx

Pterygopalatine fossa

Table 6.9 Communications of the pterygopalatine fossa

Communication	Direction	Via	Transmitted structures
Middle cranial fossa	Posterosuperiorly	Foramen rotundum	• Maxillary n. (CN V_2)
Middle cranial fossa	Posteriorly in anterior wall of foramen lacerum	Pterygoid canal	• N. of pterygoid canal (Vidian n.), formed from: 　○ Greater petrosal n. (preganglionic parasympathetic fibers from CN VII) 　○ Deep petrosal n. (postganglionic sympathetic fibers from internal carotid plexus) • A. of pterygoid canal • Vv. of pterygoid canal
Orbit	Anterosuperiorly	Inferior orbital fissure	• Branches of maxillary n. (CN V_2): 　○ Infraorbital n. 　○ Zygomatic n. • Infraorbital a. and vv. • Communicating vv. between inferior ophthalmic v. and pterygoid plexus of vv.
Nasal cavity	Medially	Sphenopalatine foramen	• Nasopalatine n. (CN V_2), lateral and medial superior posterior nasal branches • Sphenopalatine a. and vv.
Oral cavity	Inferiorly	Greater palatine canal (foramen)	• Greater (descending) palatine n. (CN V_2) and a. • Branches that emerge through lesser palatine canals: 　○ Lesser palatine nn. (CN V_2) and aa.
Nasopharynx	Inferoposteriorly	Palatovaginal (pharyngeal) canal	• CN V_2, pharyngeal branches, and pharyngeal a.
Infratemporal fossa	Laterally	Pterygomaxillary fissure	• Maxillary a., pterygopalatine (third) part • Posterior superior alveolar n., a., and v.

Topography of the Pterygopalatine Fossa

The pterygopalatine fossa is a small inverted pyramidal space just inferior to the apex of the orbit. It is continuous with the infratemporal fossa through the pterygopmaxillary fissure. The pterygopalatine fossa is a crossroads for neurovascular structures traveling between the middle cranial fossa, orbit, nasal cavity, and oral cavity.

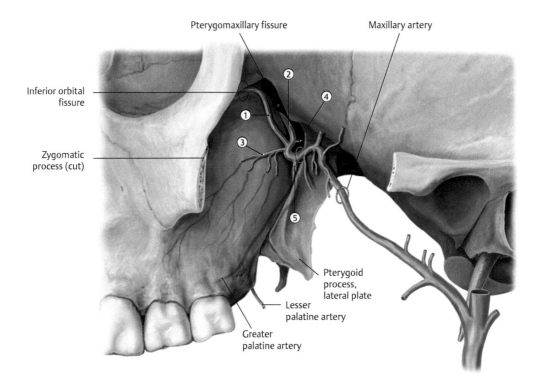

Fig. 6.24 Arteries in the pterygopalatine fossa
Left lateral view into area. The maxillary artery passes either superficial or deep to the lateral pterygoid in the infratemporal fossa and enters the pterygopalatine fossa through the pterygomaxillary fissure.

Table 6.10 Branches of the maxillary artery within the pterygopalatine fossa			
Part of maxillary artery	**Artery**		**Distribution**
Pterygopalatine part	① Infraorbital a.		Cheek, upper lip, nose, lower eyelid
		Anterior and middle superior alveolar aa.	Maxillary anterior teeth (to premolars), maxillary sinus
	② Sphenopalatine a.	Lateral posterior nasal aa.	Lateral wall of nasal cavity, choanae, paranasal sinuses (frontal, maxillary, ethmoidal, and sphenoidal)
		Posterior septal branches	Nasal septum and conchae
	③ Posterior superior alveolar a.		Maxillary premolars, molars, gingiva, maxillary sinus
	④ A. of pterygoid canal		Pharyngotympanic (auditory) tube, tympanic cavity, upper pharynx
	⑤ Descending palatine a.	Greater palatine a.	Hard palate, nasal cavity (inferior meatus), maxillary gingiva
		Lesser palatine a.	Soft palate, palatine tonsil, pharyngeal wall

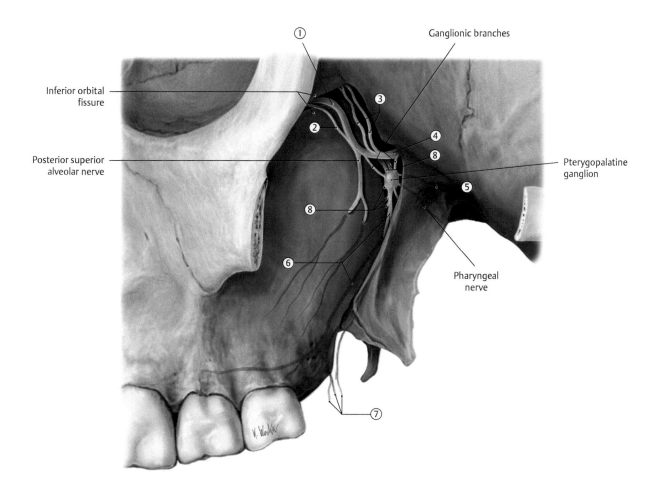

Fig. 6.25 Nerves in the pterygopalatine fossa
Left lateral view.
The maxillary division of the trigeminal nerve (CN V₂) passes from the middle cranial fossa through the foramen rotundum into the pterygopalatine fossa (see **Table 6.11**). The parasympathetic pterygopalatine ganglion receives presynaptic fibers from the greater petrosal nerve (the fibers ultimately derive from the parasympathetic root of the nervus intermedius branch of the facial nerve). The preganglionic fibers of the pterygopalatine ganglion synapse with ganglion cells that innervate the lacrimal, small palatal, and small nasal glands. The sympathetic fibers of the deep petrosal nerve (sensory root) pass through the pterygoapaltine ganglion without synapsing.

Transmitted nerves	Distribution
① Infraorbital n.	Sensory to lower eyelid, maxillary sinus, and upper incisors, canines, and premolars.
② Zygomatic n.	Sensory to skin of the temple (zygomaticotemporal n.) and cheek (zygomaticofacial n.)
③ Orbital branches (from CN V₂)	Sensory to orbital periosteum, sphenoid sinus, and ethmoidal air cells
④ Maxillary n. (CN V₂)	Gives off only sensory branches within pterygopalatine fossa
⑤ N. of pterygoid canal (Vidian n.)	• Greater petrosal n. carries preganglionic parasympathetic fibers to the pterygopalatine ganglion (from CN VII); • Deep petrosal n. carries postganglionic sympathetic fibers to the pterygopalatine ganglion
⑥ Greater palatine n.	Sensory to gingiva, mucosa, and glands of the posterior two thirds of the hard palate
⑦ Lesser palatine nn.	Sensory to soft palate, palatine tonsils, and uvula
⑧ Medial and lateral posterior superior and posterior inferior nasal branches (from nasopalatine n., CN V₂)	Sensory to the posterosuperior nasal cavity; medial branches also sensory to posterior nasal roof and septum; lateral branches also sensory to posterior ethmoid air cells and mucosa overlying the superior and middle nasal conchae

Table 6.11 Nerves that emerge from pterygopalatine fossa*

*Because the pterygopalatine fossa contains all branches of CN V₂, it is the site of needle placement for a maxillary division block.

Radiographs of the Infratemporal Fossa

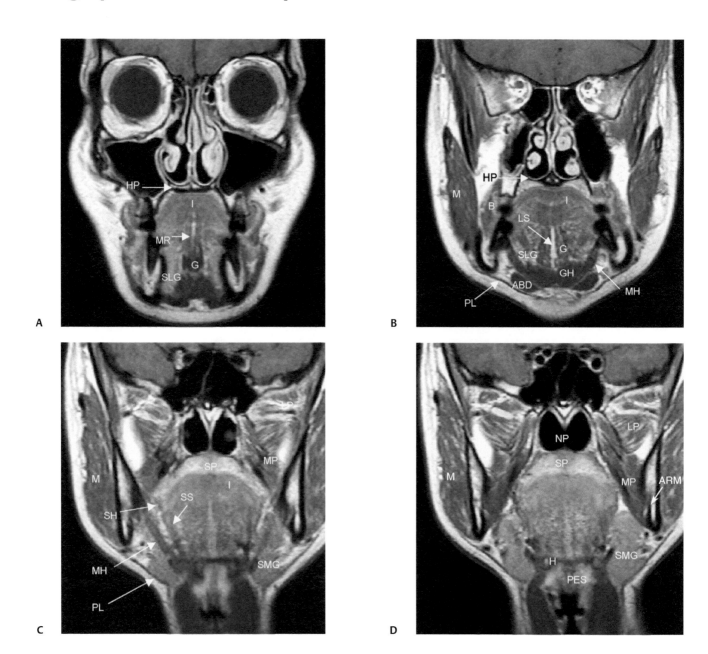

Fig. 6.26 Radiographs of the infratemporal fossa
A–D Normal anatomy as seen on coronal contrast-enhanced T1W MR images. ABD = anterior belly of the digastric muscle; ARM = ascending ramus of the mandible; ATP = anterior tonsillar pillar; B = buccinator muscle; G = genioglossus muscle; GH = geniohyoid muscle; H = hyoid bone; HP = hard palate; I = intrinsic muscles of the tongue; LP = lateral pterygoid muscle; LS = lingual septum; M = masseter muscle; MH = mylohyoid muscle; MP = medial pterygoid muscle; MR = median raphe; NP = nasopharynx; PES = preepiglottic space; PL = platysma; SLG = sublingual gland; SMG = submandibular gland; SH = stylohyoid muscle; SP = soft palate; SS = styloglossus muscle; (Reproduced from Becker M. Normal Anatomy. In: Valvassori G, Mafee M, Becker M, Hrsg. Imaging of the Head and Neck. 2nd edition. Thieme; 2004.)

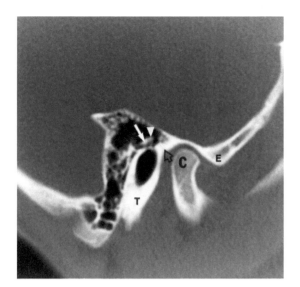

A

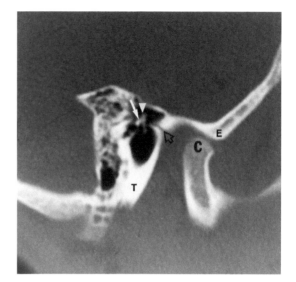

B

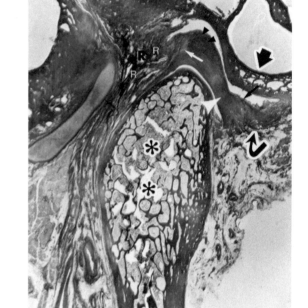

C

***Fig. 6.27* Normal TMJ anatomy.**
A, B Sagittal CT scans show a central section of the TMJ, in the closed-mouth (a) and open-mouth (b) positions. The relationship between the normal condyle (C), glenoid fossa, and anterior articular eminence (E) is clearly seen. Note the tympanic bone (T), incus (long arrow), malleus (arrowhead), and squamotympanic fissure (open arrow).
C Sagittal microscopic section of the right TMJ, demonstrating the posterior band (black arrowheads), intermediate zone (arrowhead), anterior band (small black arrow), anterior eminence (large black arrow), and condyle (stars). Note the anterior attachment (curved arrow), which blends with the anterior joint capsule and is composed of a looser fibrous connective tissue than the anterior band (small black arrow). The posterior attachment (white solid arrow) blends with the posterior band (black arrowheads). The disk can clearly be demarcated from the retrodiskal tissue (R).

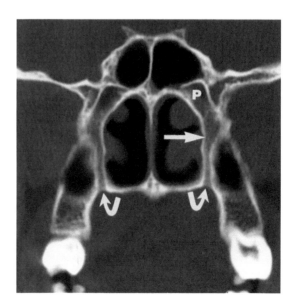

***Fig. 6.28* Radiograph of pterygopalatine fossa**
Coronal CT scan showing the pterygopalatine fossa (P), greater palatine canal (straight arrow), and greater palatine foramina (curved arrows).

183

Nose: Nasal Skeleton

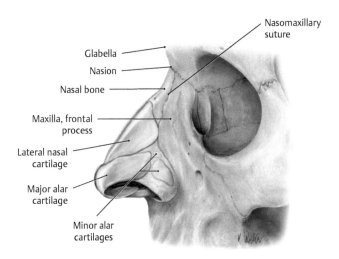

Fig. 7.1 Skeleton of the external nose
Left lateral view. The skeleton of the nose is composed of bone, cartilage, and connective tissue. Its upper portion is bony and frequently involved in midfacial fractures, whereas its lower, distal portion is cartilaginous and therefore more elastic and less susceptible to injury. The proximal lower portion of the nostrils (alae) is composed of connective tissue with small embedded pieces of cartilage. The lateral nasal cartilage is a winglike lateral expansion of the cartilaginous part of the nasal septum rather than a separate piece of cartilage.

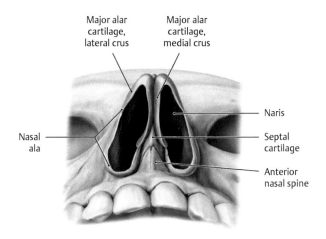

Fig. 7.2 Nasal cartilage
Inferior view. Viewed from below, each of the major alar cartilages is seen to consist of a medial and lateral crus. This view also displays the two nares, which open into the nasal cavities. The right and left nasal cavities are separated by the nasal septum, whose inferior cartilaginous portion is just visible in the diagram.

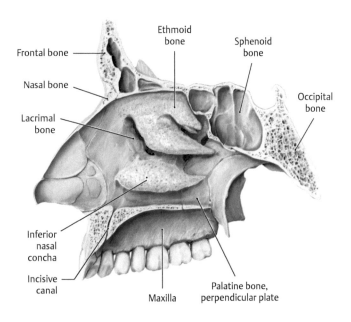

Fig. 7.3 Bones of the lateral wall of the right nasal cavity
Left lateral view. The lateral wall of the right nasal cavity is formed by seven bones: the maxilla, nasal bone, ethmoid bone, inferior nasal concha, palatine bone, lacrimal bone, and sphenoid bone. Of the nasal concha, only the inferior is a separate bone; the middle and superior conchae are parts of the ethmoid bone.

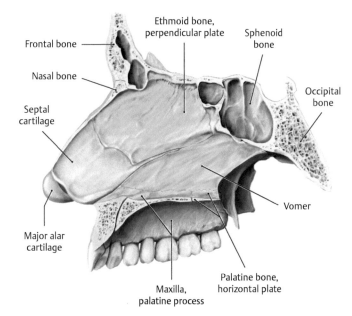

Fig. 7.4 Bones of the nasal septum
Parasagittal section. The nasal septum is formed by six bones. The ethmoid and vomer bones are the major components of the septum. The sphenoid bone, palatine bone, maxilla, and nasal bone (roof of the septum) contribute only small bony projections to the nasal septum.

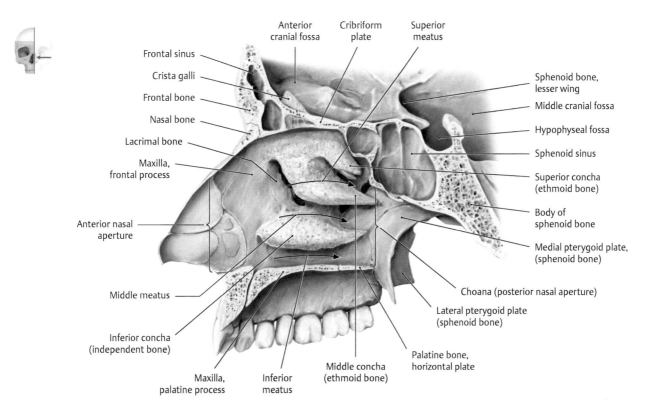

Fig. 7.5 Lateral wall of the right nasal cavity
Medial view. Air enters the bony nasal cavity through the anterior nasal aperture and travels through the three nasal passages: the superior meatus, middle meatus, and inferior meatus, which are the spaces inferolateral to the superior, middle, and inferior conchae, respectively. Air leaves the nose through the choanae (posterior nasal apertures), entering the nasopharynx.

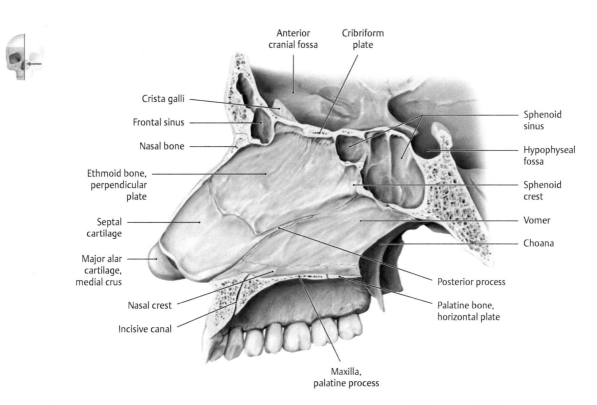

Fig. 7.6 Nasal septum
Parasagittal section viewed from the left. The left lateral wall of the nasal cavity has been removed with the adjacent bones. The nasal septum consists of an anterior septal cartilage and a posterior bony part composed of several bones. The posterior process of the cartilaginous septum extends deep into the bony septum. Deviations of the nasal septum are common and may involve the cartilaginous part of the septum, the bony part, or both. Cases in which the septal deviation is sufficient to cause obstruction of nasal breathing can be surgically corrected.

Overview of the Nasal Cavity & Paranasal Sinuses

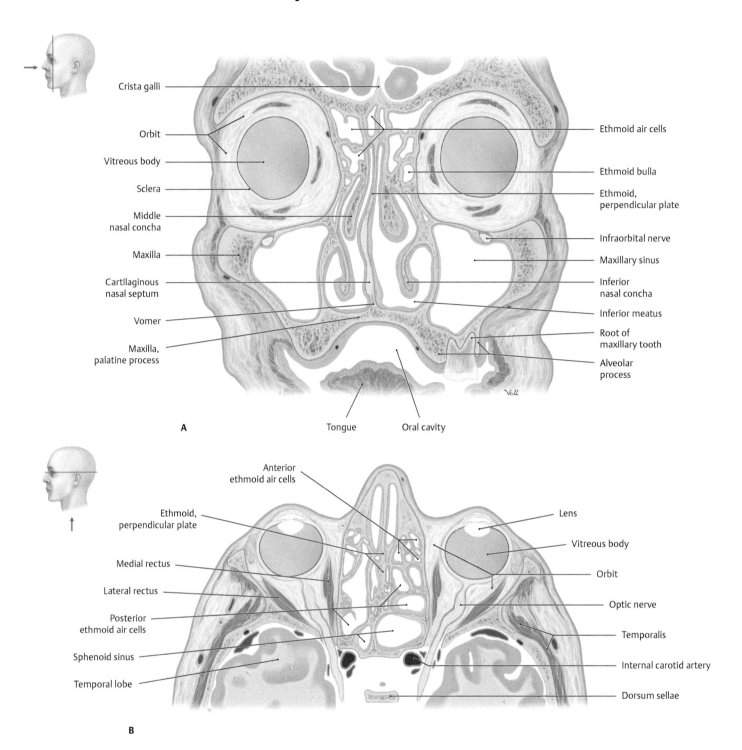

A

Crista galli
Orbit
Vitreous body
Sclera
Middle nasal concha
Maxilla
Cartilaginous nasal septum
Vomer
Maxilla, palatine process

Ethmoid air cells
Ethmoid bulla
Ethmoid, perpendicular plate
Infraorbital nerve
Maxillary sinus
Inferior nasal concha
Inferior meatus
Root of maxillary tooth
Alveolar process

Tongue   Oral cavity

B

Anterior ethmoid air cells
Ethmoid, perpendicular plate
Medial rectus
Lateral rectus
Posterior ethmoid air cells
Sphenoid sinus
Temporal lobe

Lens
Vitreous body
Orbit
Optic nerve
Temporalis
Internal carotid artery
Dorsum sellae

Fig. 7.7 Overview of the nose and paranasal sinuses
A Coronal section through nasal cavity, anterior view. **B** Transverse section, inferior view.

The nasal cavities and paranasal sinuses are arranged in pairs. The left and right nasal cavities are separated by the nasal septum and have an approximately triangular shape. Below the base of the triangle is the oral cavity. Note the relations of the infraorbital nerve and maxillary dentition to the maxillary sinus.

The close proximity of the roots of the maxillary teeth (canine to second molar) to the maxillary sinus (antrum) is very significant in clinical dentistry. Sinus pathology, for example, acute maxillary sinusitis due to an upper respiratory infection (URTI), can often be confused as dental pain originating from these teeth. Diagnosis is made by exclusion of dental pathology and observation of URTI symptoms, such as nasal dis-

charge and stuffiness. Furthermore, the pain of acute maxillary sinusitis is often worsened by bending the head forward. There would also be tenderness on palpation of the cheeks.

The close proximity is also significant because the roots or the entire tooth can be displaced into the maxillary sinus during extractions, requiring surgical removal (see **Fig. 7.17**).

Extracted upper molars may also cause an oro-antral fistula, an abnormal communication between the oral cavity and the maxillary sinus. Post-extraction reflux of fluids into the nose or minor nosebleeds should raise the dentist's index of suspicion of this condition. Diagnosis is confirmed by getting the patient to hold their nose and blow: air bubbles will be seen at the tooth socket. Small oro-antral fistulas close spontaneously; others require suturing of the mucosal flap.

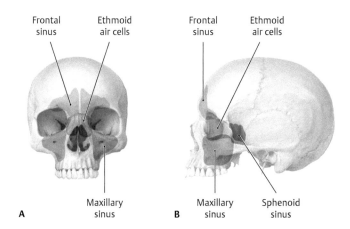

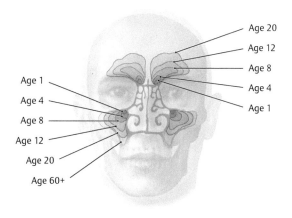

Fig. 7.8 Projection of the paranasal sinuses onto the skull
A Anterior view. **B** Left lateral view.
The paranasal sinuses are air-filled cavities that reduce the weight of the skull. They are subject to inflammation that may cause pain over the affected sinus (e.g., frontal headache due to frontal sinusitis). Knowing the location and sensory supply of the sinuses is helpful in making the correct diagnosis.

Fig. 7.9 Pneumatization of the maxillary and frontal sinuses
Anterior view. The frontal and maxillary sinuses develop gradually during the course of cranial growth (pneumatization), unlike the ethmoid air cells, which are already pneumatized at birth. As a result, sinusitis in children is most likely to involve the ethmoid air cells (with risk of orbital penetration: red, swollen eye).

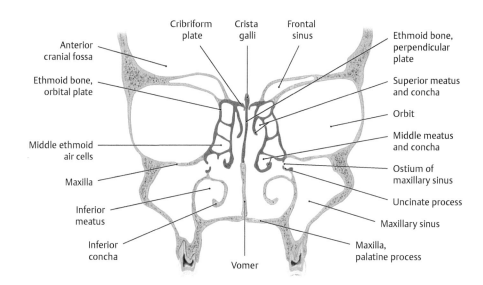

Fig. 7.10 Bony structure of the paranasal sinuses
Anterior view. The central structure of the *paranasal sinuses* is the ethmoid bone (red). Its cribriform plate forms a portion of the anterior skull base. The frontal and maxillary sinuses are grouped around the ethmoid bone. The inferior, middle, and superior meatuses of the nasal cavity are bounded by the accordingly named conchae. The bony ostium of the maxillary sinus opens into the middle meatus, lateral to the middle concha. Below the middle concha and above the maxillary sinus ostium is the ethmoid bulla, which con-tains the middle ethmoid air cells. At its anterior margin is a bony hook, the uncinate process, which bounds the maxillary sinus ostium anteriorly. The middle concha is a useful landmark in surgical procedures on the maxillary sinus and anterior ethmoid. The lateral wall separating the ethmoid bone from the orbit is the paper-thin orbital plate (= lamina papyracea). Inflammatory processes and tumors may penetrate this thin plate in either direction. *Note:* The maxilla forms the floor of the orbit and roof of the maxillary sinus. In addition, roots of the maxillary dentition may project into the maxillary sinus.

Fig. 7.11 Nasal cavity and paranasal sinuses
Transverse section viewed from above. The mucosal surface anatomy has been left intact to show how narrow the nasal passages are. Even relatively mild swelling of the mucosa may obstruct the nasal cavity, impeding aeration of the paranasal sinuses.
The pituitary gland, located behind the sphenoid sinus in the hypophyseal fossa, is accessible via transnasal surgical procedures.

187

Nasal Cavity

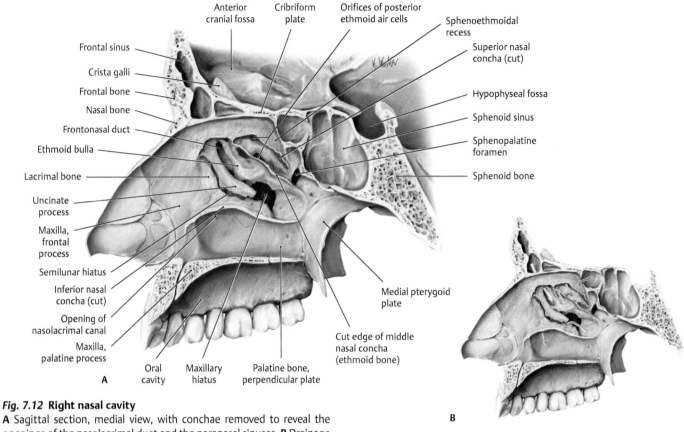

Fig. 7.12 Right nasal cavity
A Sagittal section, medial view, with conchae removed to reveal the openings of the nasolacrimal duct and the paranasal sinuses. **B** Drainage of the nasolacrimal duct and the paranasal sinuses (see Table 7.1); arrows indicate flow of mucosal secretions into the nasal cavity.

Table 7.1 Drainage of the nasolacrimal duct and the paranasal sinuses		
Duct/Sinuses	**Via**	**Drains to**
Nasolacrimal duct (red)	Nasolacrimal canal	Inferior meatus
Frontal sinus (yellow)	Frontonasal duct	Middle meatus
Maxillary sinus (orange)	Direct	Middle meatus
Anterior and middle ethmoid air cells (green)		
Posterior ethmoid air cells (green)	Direct	Superior meatus
Sphenoid sinus (blue)	Direct	Sphenoethmoid recess

Fig. 7.13 Osteomeatal unit (complex)
Coronal section. Arrows indicate flow of mucosal secretions. The osteomeatal unit (complex) is that part of the middle meatus into which the frontal and maxillary sinuses drain along with the anterior and middle ethmoid air cells. When the mucosa (ciliated respiratory epithelium) in the ethmoid air cells (green) becomes swollen due to inflammation (sinusitis), it blocks the flow of secretions from the frontal sinus (yellow) and maxillary sinus (orange) in the osteomeatal unit (red). Because of this blockage, microorganisms also become trapped in the other sinuses, where they may incite an inflammation. Thus, whereas the anatomical focus of the disease lies in the ethmoid air cells, inflammatory symptoms are also manifested in the frontal and maxillary sinuses. In patients with *chronic sinusitis*, the narrow sites can be surgically widened to establish an effective drainage route.

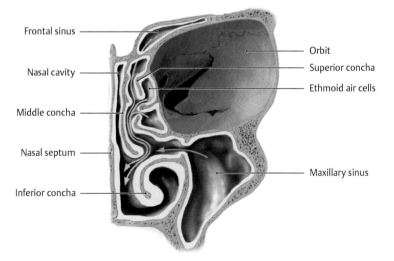

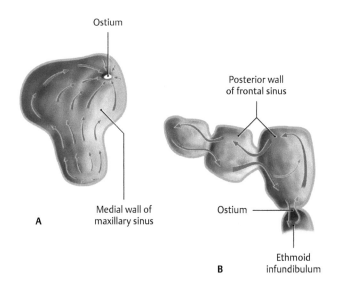

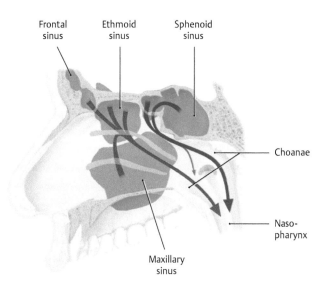

Fig. 7.14 Ciliary beating and fluid flow in the right maxillary and frontal sinuses
Schematic coronal sections of the right maxillary sinus (**A**) and frontal sinus (**B**), anterior view.
Beating of the cilia produces a flow of fluid in the paranasal sinuses that is always directed toward the sinus ostium. This clears the sinus of particles and microorganisms that are trapped in the mucous layer. If the ostium is obstructed due to swelling of the mucosa, inflammation may develop in the affected sinus (*sinusitis*). This occurs most commonly in the osteomeatal complex of the middle meatus.

Fig. 7.15 Normal drainage of secretions from the paranasal sinus
Left lateral view. The beating cilia propel the mucous blanket over the cilia and through the choana into the nasopharynx, where it is swallowed.

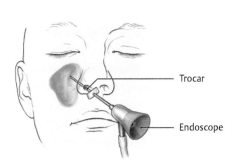

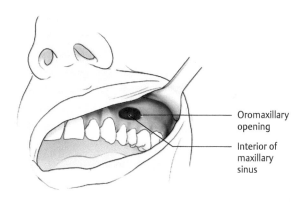

Fig. 7.16 Endoscopy of the maxillary sinus
Anterior view. The maxillary sinus is not accessible to direct inspection and must therefore be examined with an endoscope. To enter the maxillary sinus, the examiner pierces the thin bony wall below the inferior concha with a trocar and advances the endoscope through the opening. The scope can then be angled and rotated to inspect all of the mucosal surfaces. Attachment of a suction device also facilitates the drainage of secretions. Drainage of the maxillary sinus can also be achieved via the Caldwell-Luc procedure (see **Fig. 7.17**).

Fig. 7.17 Caldwell-Luc Procedure
In the Caldwell-Luc procedure, a window (fenestration) is created in the anterior wall of the maxillary sinus. It is used to remove teeth or tooth roots that have been displaced during extractions (see **Fig. 7.7**); to remove cysts, polyps, tumors, and other foreign bodies; to close oroantral fistulas; to reduce facial fractures; and to drain the sinus (rare now due to endoscopy). It can also be used to gain access to the ethmoid air cells, the sphenoid sinus, and the pterygomaxillary fissure (which lies behind maxillary sinus).

Mucosa of the Nasal Cavity

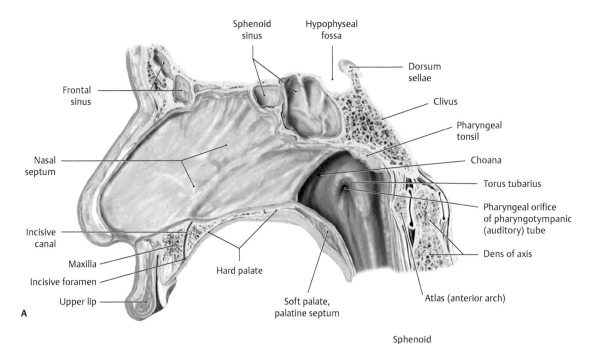

A

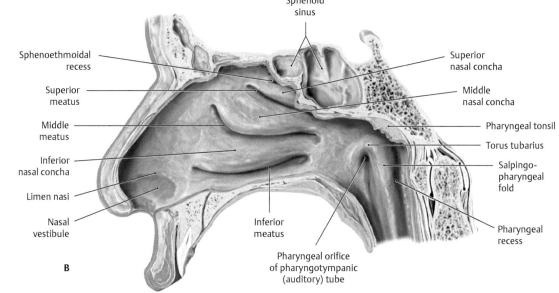

B

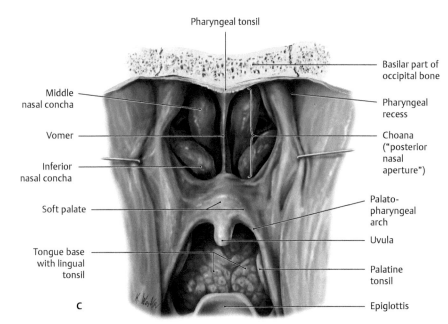

C

Fig. 7.18 Mucosa of the nasal cavity
A Mucosa of the nasal septum, parasagittal section viewed from the left side. **B** Mucosa of the right lateral nasal wall, viewed from the left side. **C** Posterior view through the choanae into the nasal cavity.

Although the medial wall of the nasal cavity is smooth, its lateral wall is raised into folds by the three conchae (superior, middle, and inferior concha), which increase the surface area of the nasal cavity, enabling it to warm and humidify the inspired air more efficiently. They also create turbulence, mixing olfactory stimulants (see p. 124 for olfactory nerve). The choanae (posterior nasal apertures) (**C**) are the posterior openings by which the nasal cavity communicates with the nasopharynx. Note the close proximity of the choanae to the pharyngotympanic (auditory) tube and pharyngeal tonsil in **A**.

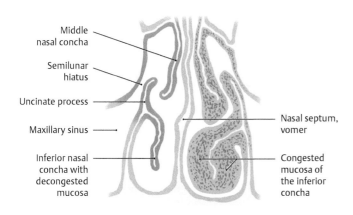

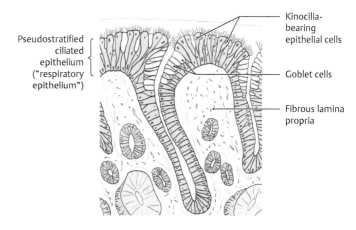

Fig. 7.19 Functional states of the nasal mucosa
Coronal section, anterior view. The function of the nasal mucosa is to warm and humidify the inspired air and mix olfactory stimulants. This is accomplished by an increase of blood flow through the mucosa, placing it in a congested (swollen) state. The mucous membranes are not simultaneously congested on both sides, but undergo a normal cycle of congestion and decongestion that lasts approximately six hours (the right side is decongested in the drawing). Examination of the nasal cavity can be facilitated by first administering a decongestant to shrink the mucosa.

Fig. 7.20 Histology of the nasal mucosa
The surface of the pseudostratified respiratory epithelium of the nasal mucosa consists of kinocilia-bearing cells and goblet cells, which secrete their mucus into a watery film on the epithelial surface. Serous and seromucous glands are embedded in the connective tissue and also release secretions into the superficial fluid film. The directional fluid flow produced by the cilia is an important component of the non-specific immune response. If coordinated beating of the cilia is impaired, the patient will suffer chronic recurring infections of the respiratory tract.

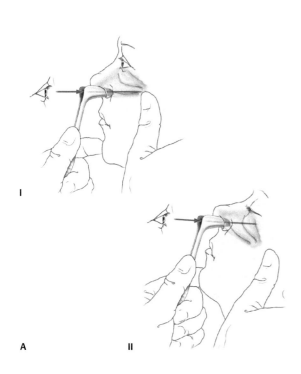

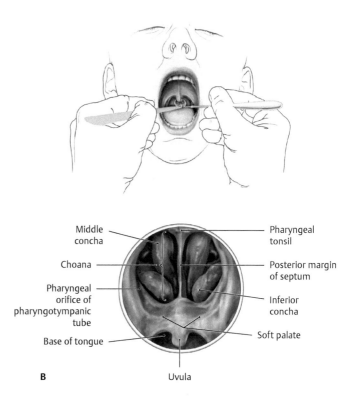

Fig. 7.21 Anterior and posterior rhinoscopy
A **Anterior rhinoscopy** is a procedure for inspection of the nasal cavity. Two different positions (I, II) are used to ensure that all of the anterior nasal cavity is examined.
B In **posterior rhinoscopy**, the choanae and pharyngeal tonsil are accessible to clinical examination. The rhinoscope can be angled and rotated to demonstrate the structures shown in the composite image. Today the rhinoscope is frequently replaced by an endoscope.

Nose & Paranasal Sinuses: Histology & Clinical Anatomy

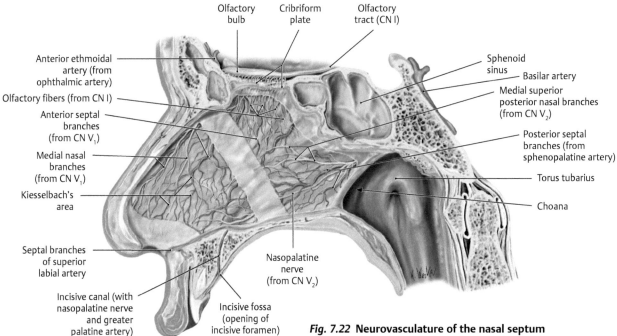

Fig. 7.22 Neurovasculature of the nasal septum
Parasagittal section, left lateral view. The nasal septum is supplied anterosuperiorly by CN V$_1$ and posteroinferiorly by CN V$_2$. It receives blood primarily from branches of the ophthalmic and maxillary arteries, with contribution from the facial artery (septal branches of the superior labial artery).

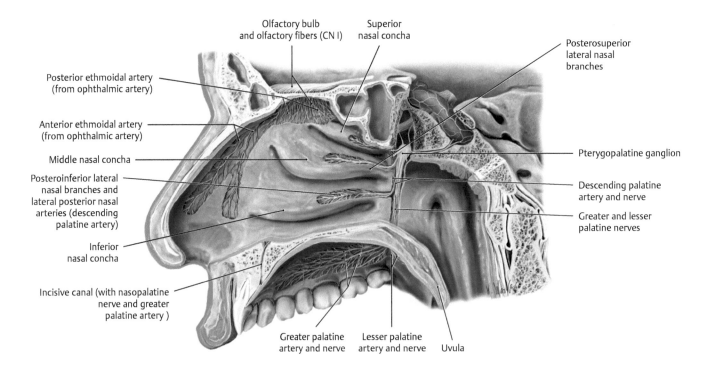

Fig. 7.23 Neurovasculature of the lateral nasal wall
Left medial view of right lateral nasal wall. The pterygopalatine ganglion (located in the pterygopalatine fossa but exposed here) is an important relay in the parasympathetic nervous system. The CN V$_2$ nerve fibers pass through it to the small nasal glands of the nasal conchae, along with palatine glands. The anterosuperior portion of the lateral nasal wall is supplied by branches of the ophthalmic artery and CN V$_1$. *Note:* Olfactory fibers (CN I) pass through the cribriform plate to the olfactory mucosa at the level of the superior concha.

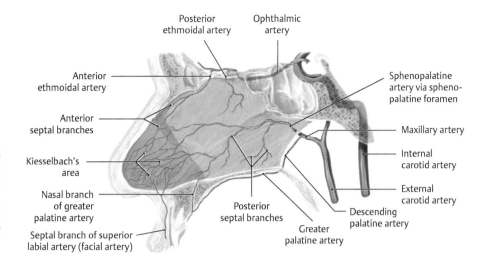

Fig. 7.24 Arteries of the nasal septum
Left lateral view of left side of septum. The vessels of the nasal septum arise from branches of the external and internal carotid arteries. The anterior part of the septum contains a highly vascularized area called Kiesselbach's area, which is supplied by vessels from both major arteries. This area is the most common site of significant nosebleed due to anastomoses.

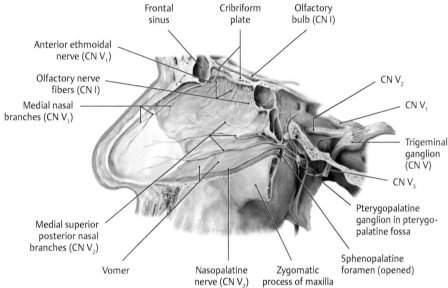

Fig. 7.25 Nerves of the nasal septum
Left lateral view of right lateral nasal wall. The nasal septum receives its general sensory innervation from branches of the trigeminal nerve (CN V). The anterosuperior part of the septum is supplied by branches of the ophthalmic division (CN V₁) and the rest by branches of the maxillary division (CN V₂). Bundles of olfactory nerve fibers (CN I) arise from receptors in the olfactory mucosa on the superior part of the septum, pass through the cribriform plate, and enter the olfactory bulb. (see p. 124 for discussion of olfactory nerve [CN I]).

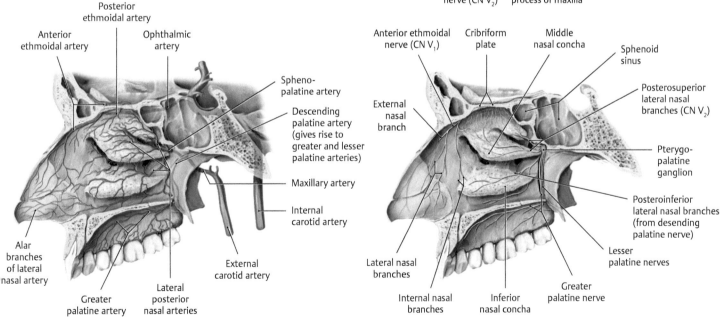

Fig. 7.26 Arteries of the right lateral nasal wall
Left lateral view of right lateral nasal wall. The nasal wall is supplied primarily by branches of the ophthalmic artery (anterosuperiorly) and maxillary artery (posteroinferiorly), with contributions from the facial artery (alar branches of the lateral nasal artery).

Fig. 7.27 Nerves of the right lateral nasal wall
Left lateral view of the right lateral nasal wall. The nasal wall derives its sensory innervation from branches of the ophthalmic division (CN V₁) and the maxillary division (CN V₂). Receptor neurons in the olfactory mucosa send their axons in the olfactory nerve (CN I) to the olfactory bulb.

Olfactory System (Smell)

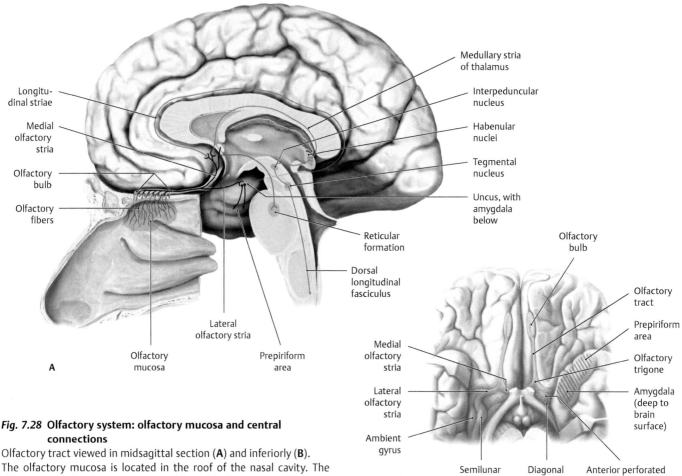

Fig. 7.28 Olfactory system: olfactory mucosa and central connections

Olfactory tract viewed in midsagittal section (**A**) and inferiorly (**B**). The olfactory mucosa is located in the roof of the nasal cavity. The olfactory cells (= primary sensory cells) are bipolar neurons. Their peripheral receptor-bearing processes terminate in the epithelium of the nasal mucosa, and their central processes pass to the olfactory bulb. The olfactory bulb, where the second neurons of the olfactory pathway (mitral and tufted cells) are located, is considered an extension of the telencephalon. The axons of these second neurons pass centrally as the *olfactory tract*. In front of the anterior perforated substance, the olfactory tract widens to form the olfactory trigone and splits into the lateral and medial olfactory striae.

- Some of the axons of the olfactory tract run in the **lateral olfactory stria** to the olfactory centers: the amygdala, semilunar gyrus, and ambient gyrus. The prepiriform area (Brodmann area 28) is considered to be the primary olfactory cortex in the strict sense. It contains the third neurons of the olfactory pathway. *Note:* The prepiriform area is shaded in **B**, lying at the junction of the basal side of the frontal lobe and the medial side of the temporal lobe.
- Other axons of the olfactory tract run in the **medial olfactory stria** to nuclei in the septal (subcallosal) area, which is part of the limbic system, and to the olfactory tubercle, a small elevation in the anterior perforated substance.
- Yet other axons of the olfactory tract terminate in the **anterior olfactory nucleus**, where the fibers that cross to the opposite side branch off and are relayed. This nucleus is located in the olfactory trigone, which lies between the two olfactory striae and in front of the anterior perforated substance.

Note: None of these three tracts are routed through the thalamus. Thus, the olfactory system is the only sensory system that is not relayed in the thalamus before reaching the cortex. There is, however, an indirect route from the primary olfactory cortex to the neocortex passing through the thalamus and terminating in the basal forebrain. The olfactory signals are further analyzed in these basal portions of the forebrain (not shown).

The olfactory system is linked to other brain areas well beyond the primary olfactory cortical areas, with the result that olfactory stimuli can evoke complex emotional and behavioral responses. Noxious smells induce nausea, and appetizing smells evoke watering of the mouth. Presumably these sensations are processed by the hypothalamus, thalamus, and limbic system via connections established mainly by the medial forebrain bundle and the medullary striae of the thalamus. The medial forebrain bundle distributes axons to the following structures:

- Hypothalamic nuclei
- Reticular formation
- Salivatory nuclei
- Dorsal motor nucleus

The axons that run in the medullary striae of the thalamus terminate in the habenular nuclei. This tract also continues to the brainstem, where it stimulates salivation in response to smell.

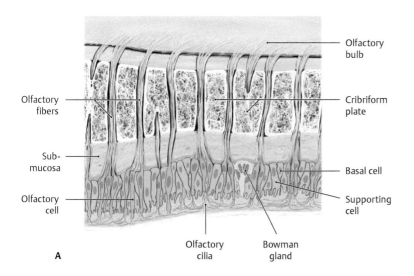

Olfactory bulb

Cribriform plate

Basal cell

Supporting cell

Olfactory fibers

Sub-mucosa

Olfactory cell

Olfactory cilia

Bowman gland

A

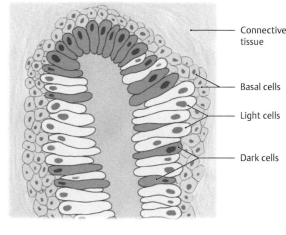

Connective tissue

Basal cells

Light cells

Dark cells

C

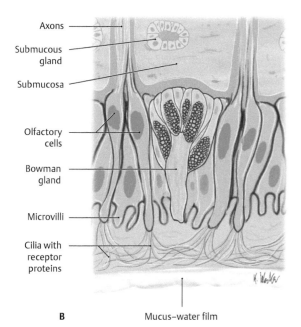

Axons

Submucous gland

Submucosa

Olfactory cells

Bowman gland

Microvilli

Cilia with receptor proteins

B

Mucus–water film

Fig. 7.29 Olfactory mucosa and vomeronasal (Jacobson's) organ (VNO)

The **olfactory mucosa** occupies an area of approximately 2 cm^2 on the roof of each nasal cavity, and 10^7 primary sensory cells are concentrated in each of these areas (**A**). At the molecular level, the olfactory receptor proteins are located in the cilia of the sensory cells (**B**). Each sensory cell has only one specialized receptor protein that mediates signal transduction when an odorant molecule binds to it. Although humans are microsmatic, having a sense of smell that is feeble compared with other mammals, the olfactory receptor proteins still make up 2% of the human genome. This underscores the importance of olfaction in humans. The primary olfactory sensory cells have a life span of approximately 60 days and regenerate from the basal cells (lifelong division of neurons). The bundled central processes (axons) from hundreds of olfactory cells form olfactory fibers (**A**) that pass through the cribriform plate of the ethmoid bone and terminate in the *olfactory bulb*, which lies above the cribriform plate. The VNO (**C**) is located on both sides of the anterior nasal septum. It is an accessory olfactory organ and is generally considered vestigial in adult humans. However, it responds to steroids and evokes subconscious reactions in subjects (possibly influences the choice of a mate). Mate selection in many animal species is known to be mediated by olfactory impulses that are perceived in the VNO.

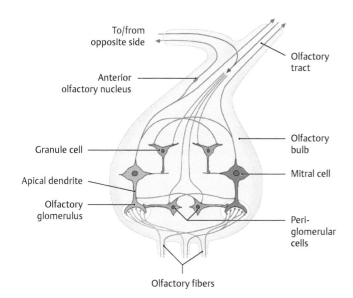

To/from opposite side

Anterior olfactory nucleus

Granule cell

Apical dendrite

Olfactory glomerulus

Olfactory tract

Olfactory bulb

Mitral cell

Peri-glomerular cells

Olfactory fibers

Fig. 7.30 Synaptic patterns in an olfactory bulb

Specialized neurons in the olfactory bulb, called mitral cells, form apical dendrites that receive synaptic contact from the axons of thousands of primary sensory cells. The dendrite plus the synapses make up the *olfactory glomeruli*. Axons from sensory cells with the same receptor protein form glomeruli with only one or a small number of mitral cells. The basal axons of the mitral cells form the olfactory tract. The axons that run in the olfactory tract project primarily to the olfactory cortex but are also distributed to other nuclei in the central nervous system. The axon collaterals of the mitral cells pass to granule cells: both granule cells and periglomerular cells inhibit the activity of the mitral cells, causing less sensory information to reach higher centers. These inhibitory processes are believed to heighten olfactory contrast, which aids in the more accurate perception of smells. The tufted cells, which also project to the primary olfactory cortex, are not shown.

Radiographs of the Nasal Cavity

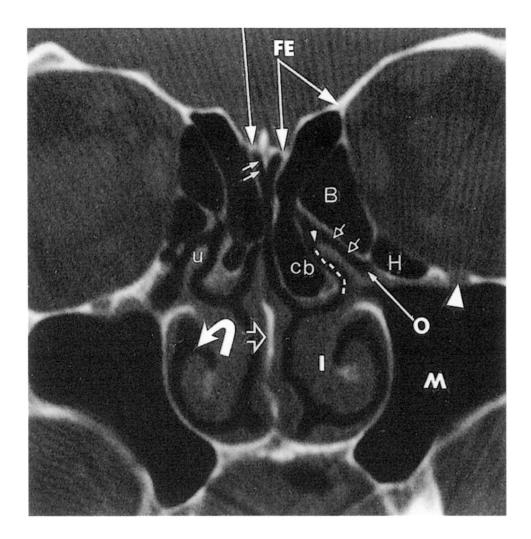

Fig. 7.31
Coronal CT scan showing the inferior turbinate (I), nasal septum (hollow arrow), inferior meatus (curved arrow), uncinate process (u), superior nasal cavity (small double arrows), cribriform plate (long arrow), fovea ethmoidalis (FE), bulla ethmoidalis (B), infundibulum (double hollow arrows), pneumatized middle turbinate, so-called concha bullosa (cb), maxillary sinus ostium (O), infraorbital canal (large arrowhead), and maxillary sinuses (M). The small arrowhead points to the region of the hiatus semilunaris, which allows communication of the middle meatus (dashed line) with the infundibulum.

Radiographs of the Paranasal Sinuses

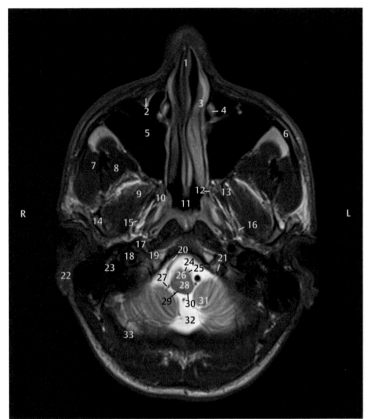

A

1 Nasal septum	18 Internal jugular vein
2 Infraorbital canal with infraorbital nerve	19 Hypoglossal canal
	20 Vertebral artery
3 Inferior nasal concha	21 Hypoglossal nerve
4 Lacrimal duct	22 External ear
5 Maxillary sinus	23 Mastoid process
6 Zygomatic bone	24 Anterior median fissure
7 Masseter	25 Pyramid
8 Temporalis	26 Inferior olivary nucleus
9 Lateral pterygoid	27 Posterior inferior cerebellar artery (PICA)
10 Medial pterygoid	
11 Pharynx, nasopharynx	28 Medulla oblongata
12 Medial part of pterygoid process	29 Gracile tubercle
	30 Cuneate tubercle
13 Lateral part of pterygoid process	31 Tonsils of cerebellum (H IX)
14 Mandible	32 Posterior cerebellomedullary cistern (magna)
15 Mandibular nerve	
16 Pterygoid venous plexus	
17 Internal carotid artery	33 Occipital bone

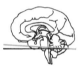

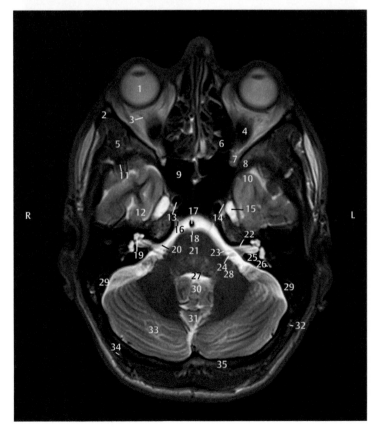

B

1 Eyeball (with lens)	20 Anterior inferior cerebellar artery (AICA)
2 Zygomatic bone	
3 Ophthalmic vein	21 Pons
4 Inferior rectus	22 Internal acoustic canal
5 Temporalis	23 Facial nerve with intermediate nerve
6 Ethmoidal air cells	
7 Pterygopalatine fossa	24 Vestibulocochlear nerve
8 Sphenoid bone	25 Temporal bone, petrous part
9 Sphenoid sinus	
10 Temporal lobe	26 Posterior semicircular canal
11 Middle meningeal artery, frontal branch	
	27 Fourth ventricle
12 Inferior temporal gyrus	28 Middle cerebellar peduncle
13 Internal carotid artery	
14 Cavernous sinus	29 Sigmoid sinus
15 Trigeminal nerve, Gasserian ganglion	30 Uvula of vermis (IX)
	31 Vermis of cerebellum
16 Abducens nerve at the dural aperture	32 Emissary vein
	33 Posterior lobe of cerebellum, hemisphere
17 Basilar artery	
18 Basilar sulcus	34 Occipital artery
19 Cochlea	35 Occipital bone

Fig. 7.32

A Axial T2w MRI showing the maxillary sinuses (5) and the nasal cavity communicating with the nasopharynx.

B Axial T2w MRI, superior to the plane of the previous image, showing the ethmoid air cells (6) and the sphenoid sinus (9).

Oral Cavity: Overview

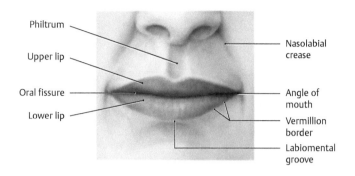

- Philtrum
- Upper lip
- Oral fissure
- Lower lip
- Nasolabial crease
- Angle of mouth
- Vermillion border
- Labiomental groove

Fig. 8.1 Lips and labial creases

Anterior view. The upper and lower lips (labia) meet at the angle of the mouth. The oral fissure opens into the oral cavity. Changes in the lips noted on visual inspection may yield important diagnostic clues: Blue lips (cyanosis) suggest a disease of the heart, lung, or both, and deep nasolabial creases may reflect chronic diseases of the digestive tract.

Fig. 8.2 Oral cavity

A Anterior view. **B** Anterior view showing ventral surface of tongue. **C** Left lateral view.

The dental arches (with the alveolar processes of the maxilla and mandible) subdivide the oral cavity into two parts:

- **Oral vestibule:** portion outside the dental arches, bounded on one side by the lips and cheeks and on the other side by the dental arches.
- **Oral cavity proper:** region within the dental arches.

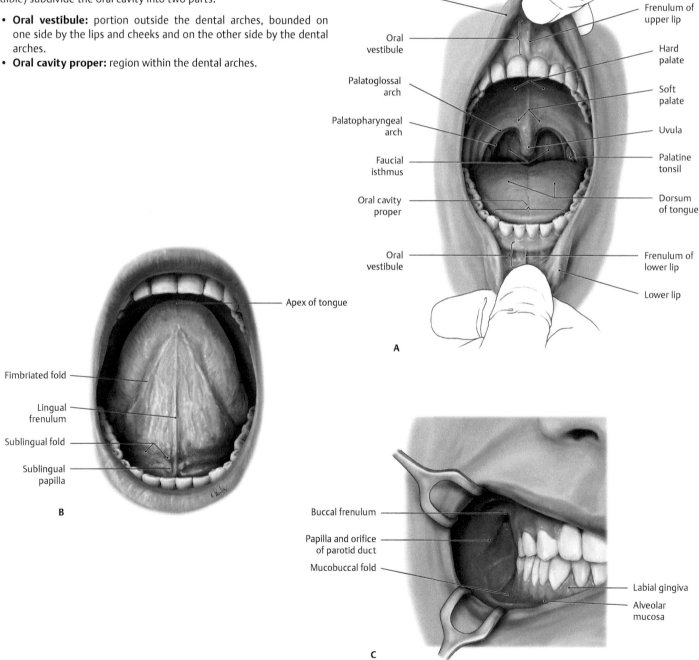

- Upper lip
- Oral vestibule
- Palatoglossal arch
- Palatopharyngeal arch
- Faucial isthmus
- Oral cavity proper
- Oral vestibule
- Frenulum of upper lip
- Hard palate
- Soft palate
- Uvula
- Palatine tonsil
- Dorsum of tongue
- Frenulum of lower lip
- Lower lip

A

- Apex of tongue
- Fimbriated fold
- Lingual frenulum
- Sublingual fold
- Sublingual papilla

B

- Buccal frenulum
- Papilla and orifice of parotid duct
- Mucobuccal fold
- Labial gingiva
- Alveolar mucosa

C

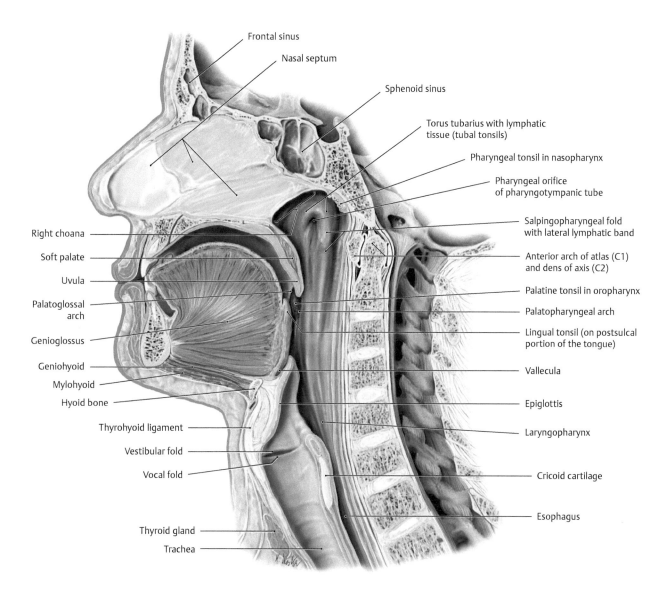

Frontal sinus

Nasal septum

Sphenoid sinus

Torus tubarius with lymphatic tissue (tubal tonsils)

Pharyngeal tonsil in nasopharynx

Pharyngeal orifice of pharyngotympanic tube

Right choana

Salpingopharyngeal fold with lateral lymphatic band

Soft palate

Anterior arch of atlas (C1) and dens of axis (C2)

Uvula

Palatine tonsil in oropharynx

Palatoglossal arch

Palatopharyngeal arch

Genioglossus

Lingual tonsil (on postsulcal portion of the tongue)

Geniohyoid

Vallecula

Mylohyoid

Hyoid bone

Epiglottis

Thyrohyoid ligament

Laryngopharynx

Vestibular fold

Vocal fold

Cricoid cartilage

Esophagus

Thyroid gland

Trachea

Fig. 8.3 Topography of the oral cavity and pharynx
Midsagittal section, left lateral view. The oral cavity is located inferior to the nasal cavity and anterior to the pharynx. The roof of the oral cavity is formed by the hard palate in its anterior two thirds and by the soft palate (velum) in its posterior one third. Its inferior boundary is formed by the mylohyoid muscle. Laterally, the oral cavity is bounded by the cheeks; posteriorly, it is continuous with the oropharynx.

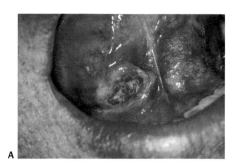

A

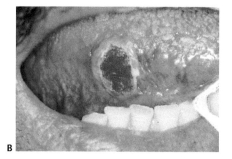

B

Fig. 8.4 Oral cancer
A Cancerous lesion of the oral floor. **B** Cancerous lesion of the tongue. Most oral cancers are squamous cell carcinomas and can be attributed to the use of alcohol and tobacco (synergistic effect). They typically occur on the oral floor or the ventral (inferior) or lateral surface of the tongue and present as a painless ulcer which is firm with raised edges and an indurated, inflamed base. Other presentations include an area of leukoplakia (a white patch), erythroplakia (red patch), or a combination of the two. Lesions that occur on the oral floor tend to undergo malignant transformation more readily than those in other locations in the oral cavity. Pain from oral cancer occurs later in the pathogenesis and is usually due to superinfection.

199

Vasculature of the Oral Cavity

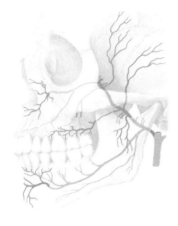

A

Fig. 8.5 Maxillary artery

Left lateral view. **A** Schematic. **B** Course of the maxillary artery.

A The maxillary artery can be divided into three parts: mandibular (blue); pterygoid (green), and pterygopalatine (yellow).

B The maxillary artery is the principle artery supplying the oral cavity. The mandibular part supplies the mandibular teeth, gingiva, and mucosa, and contributes to the supply of certain muscles of mastication and of the soft palate. The pterygoid part supplies the muscles of mastication and the buccal mucosa. The pterygopalatine part supplies the maxillary teeth, gingiva, mucosa, hard palate, and soft palate, and contributes to the supply of the upper lip. Note. This only represents those parts of the maxillary artery that contribute to the blood supply of the structures of the oral cavity only. For full details of the structures that the maxillary artery supplies, see **Table 3.6,** p. 61.

Other arteries that contribute to the blood supply of the oral cavity include the lingual artery (p. 56), which supplies the tongue and oral floor, and the facial artery (p. 57), which supplies the lower lip (inferior labial branch) and upper lip (superior labial branch).

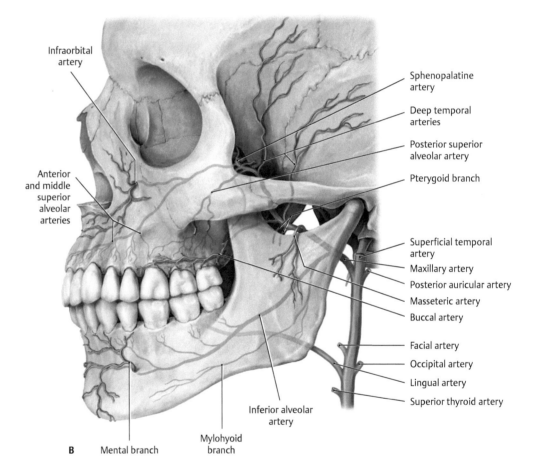

B   Mental branch   Mylohyoid branch   Inferior alveolar artery

Infraorbital artery

Anterior and middle superior alveolar arteries

Sphenopalatine artery

Deep temporal arteries

Posterior superior alveolar artery

Pterygoid branch

Superficial temporal artery

Maxillary artery

Posterior auricular artery

Masseteric artery

Buccal artery

Facial artery

Occipital artery

Lingual artery

Superior thyroid artery

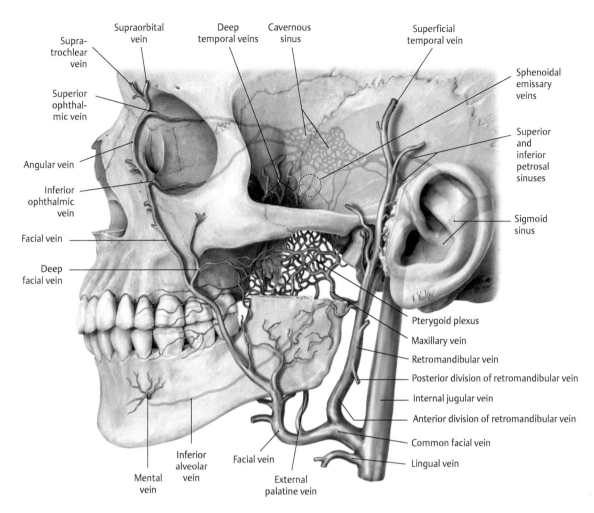

Fig. 8.6 Venous drainage of the oral cavity

Left lateral view. Veins within the mandibular teeth, gingiva, and mucosa combine to form inferior alveolar veins, which drain to the pterygoid plexus. Likewise, veins within the maxillary teeth, gingiva, and mucosa form the superior alveolar veins, which drain to the pterygoid plexus. Veins from the hard and soft palate also drain to the pterygoid plexus. Middle and anterior superior alveolar veins drain into the infraorbital vein which drains into the pterygoid plexus of veins. The lingual vein drains the tongue and oral floor. The facial vein contributes to the venous drainage of the mandibular teeth.

Innervation of the Oral Cavity

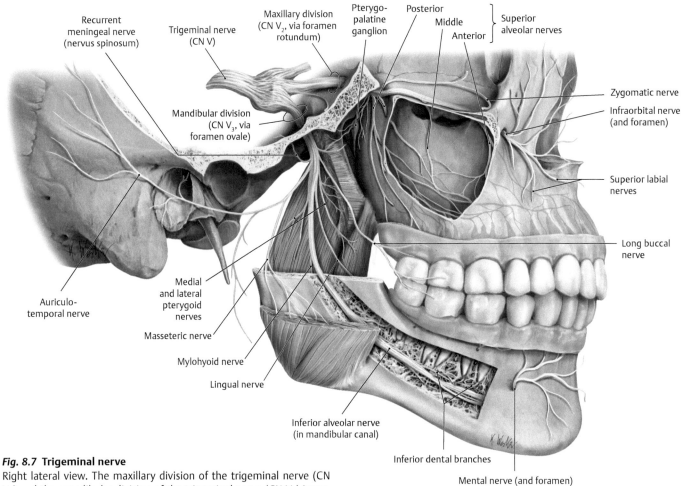

Fig. 8.7 Trigeminal nerve

Right lateral view. The maxillary division of the trigeminal nerve (CN V$_2$) and the mandibular division of the trigeminal nerve (CN V$_3$) innervate the structures of the oral cavity via their many branches. For full details see pp. 132–135.

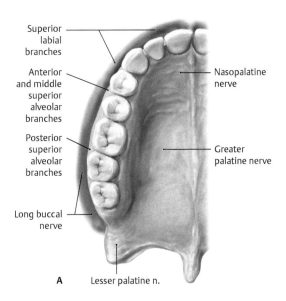

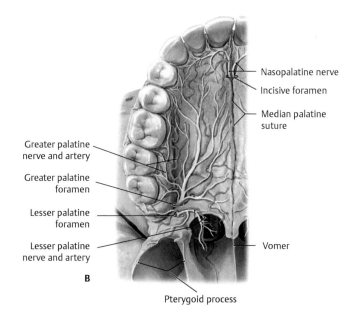

Fig. 8.8 Neurovasculature of the hard palate

Inferior view. **A** The hard palate receives sensory innervation primarily from the terminal branches of the maxillary division of the trigeminal nerve (CN V$_2$). *Note:* The long buccal nerve is a branch of the mandibular division of the trigeminal nerve (CN V$_3$).

B The arteries of the hard palate arise from the maxillary artery (a branch of the external carotid artery)

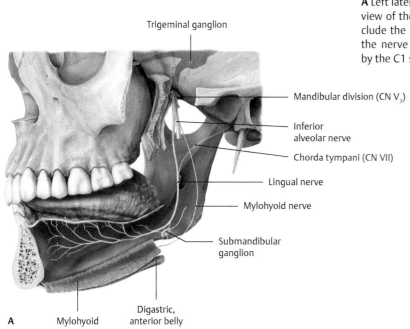

Trigeminal ganglion

Mandibular division (CN V₃)

Inferior alveolar nerve

Chorda tympani (CN VII)

Lingual nerve

Mylohyoid nerve

Submandibular ganglion

Digastric, anterior belly

A Mylohyoid

Fig. 8.9 Innervation of the muscles of the oral floor
A Left lateral view with left half of the mandible removed. **B** Left lateral view of the muscles of the oral floor. The muscles of the oral floor include the mylohyoid and geniohyoid. The mylohyoid is innervated by the nerve to mylohyoid (from CN V₃); the geniohyoid is innervated by the C1 spinal nerve via the hypoglossal nerve (CN XII).

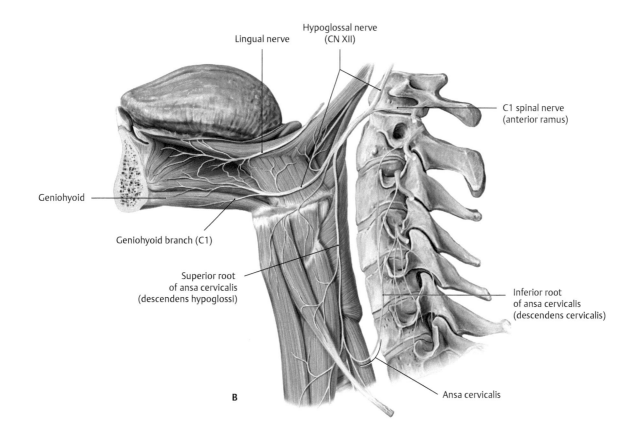

Lingual nerve

Hypoglossal nerve (CN XII)

C1 spinal nerve (anterior ramus)

Geniohyoid

Geniohyoid branch (C1)

Superior root of ansa cervicalis (descendens hypoglossi)

Inferior root of ansa cervicalis (descendens cervicalis)

Ansa cervicalis

B

Teeth in situ & Terminology

Humans have two successive sets of teeth: deciduous teeth and their permanent replacements. There are four different forms of teeth: incisor, canine, premolar (not present in the deciduous dentition), and molar. Teeth are set in sockets composed of alveolar bone and held in place by the elastic connective tissue.

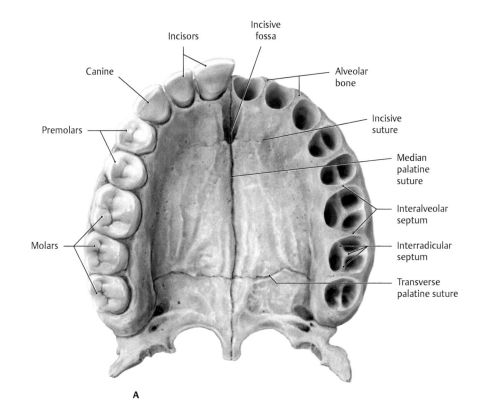

A

Fig. 8.10 Permanent teeth in adults
A Inferior view of the maxilla (with teeth removed on left side).
B Superior view of the mandible (with teeth removed on left side).
The 16 teeth in both the maxilla and the mandible in humans are aligned in a bilateral, symmetrical fashion to suit their different chewing functions. The teeth in each half of the maxilla and mandible consist of: two incisors, one canine, two premolars, and three molars. The incisors and canine are responsible for ripping the food while the molars are responsible for grinding it.

The teeth have been removed on right side of each image to reveal the alveoli, which hold the teeth. In the anterior area (where the incisors and canines are located), the labial plate of compact bone is extremely thin (approximately 0.1 mm) and the roots of these teeth are palpable. The interalveolar septa separate the alveoli of two adjacent teeth. The interradicular septa separate the roots of teeth with multiple roots.

Alveolar ostitis (dry socket), an inflammation of the alveolar bone, may occur following tooth extraction when the blood clot that would normally occupy the socket does not form properly (e.g., due to smoking) or is displaced (e.g., by mouth rinsing), exposing the underlying bone and nerves and allowing an infection to flourish.

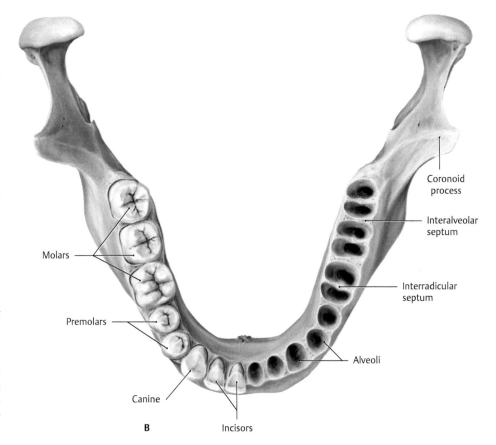

B

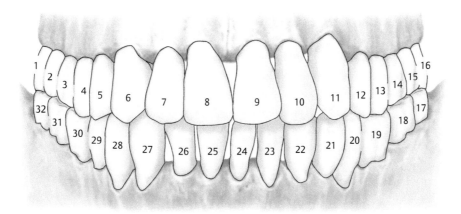

Fig. 8.11 Coding the permanent teeth

In the United States, the permanent teeth are numbered sequentially, not assigned to quadrants. Progressing in a clockwise fashion (from the perspective of the dentist), the teeth of the upper arc are numbered 1 to 16, and those of the lower are considered 17 to 32. *Note:* The third upper molar (wisdom tooth) on the patient's right is considered 1.

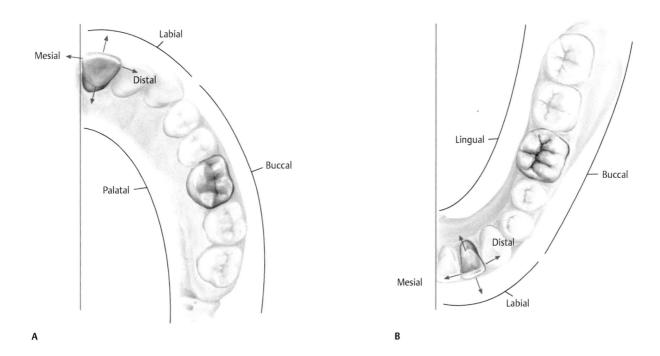

A

B

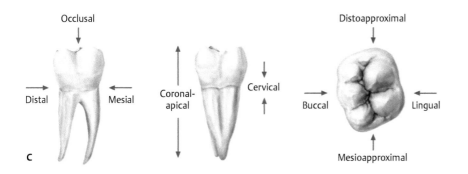

C

Fig. 8.12 Designation of tooth surfaces

A Inferior view of the maxillary dental arch.
B Superior view of the mandibular dental arch.
C Buccal, distal, and occlusal views of the right mandibular first molar (tooth 30).
The *mesial* and *distal* tooth surfaces are those closest to and farthest from the midline, respectively. The term *labial* is used for incisors and canine teeth, and *buccal* is used for premolar and molar teeth. *Palatal* denotes the inside surface of maxillary teeth, and *lingual* denotes the inside surface of mandibular teeth. **C** shows the coronal, apical, and cervical directions of a tooth and the approximal surfaces, which *contact*, or *face*, the adjacent teeth. These designations are used to describe the precise location of small carious lesions.

Structure of the Teeth & Periodontium

The periodontium includes all the structures that bind the tooth to its bony socket:

- gingiva,
- cementum,
- periodontal ligament, and
- alveolar bone.

Its essential functions include:

- anchoring the teeth in alveolar bone and transforming chewing pressure into tensile stress,
- mediating the sensation of pain and regulating chewing pressure through nerve fibers and sensitive nerve endings,
- defending against infection through efficient separation of the oral cavity and the dental root region and by having a large number of defense cells, and
- rapid metabolism and high regenerative capacity, via its rich blood supply

Fig. 8.13 Parts of the tooth
Cross section of a tooth (mandibular incisor). The teeth consist of an enamel-covered crown that meets the cementum-covered roots at the neck (cementoenamel junction). The body of the tooth is primarily dentine.

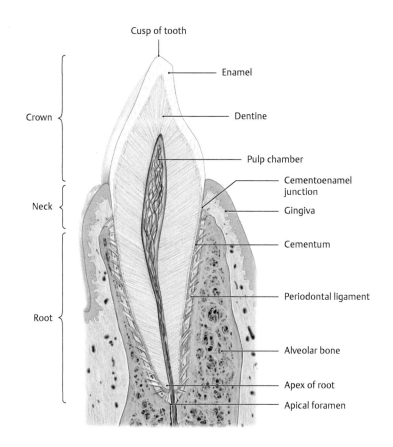

Cusp of tooth
Enamel
Dentine
Crown
Pulp chamber
Cementoenamel junction
Gingiva
Neck
Cementum
Periodontal ligament
Root
Alveolar bone
Apex of root
Apical foramen

Table 8.1 Structures of the tooth

Protective coverings: These hard, avascular layers of tissue protect the underlying body of the tooth. They meet at the cervical margin (neck, cementoenamel junction). Failure to do so exposes the underlying dentine, which has extremely sensitive pain responses.	**Enamel:** Hard, translucent covering of the crown of the tooth. Maximum thickness (2.5 mm) occurs over the cusps. Enamel prisms lie parallel to each other and are composed of hydroxyapatite [$Ca_5 (PO_4)_3(OH)$]. The enamel covering meets the cementum at the neck (cervical margin, cementoenamel junction). **Cementum:** Bonelike covering of the dental roots, lacking neurovascular structures.
Body of the tooth: The tooth is primarily composed of dentine, which is supported by the vascularized dental pulp.	**Dentine:** Tough tissue composing the majority of the body of the tooth. It consists of extensive networks of S-shaped tubules (intratubular dentine) surrounded by peritubular dentine. The tubules connect the underlying dental pulp to the overlying tissue. Exposed dentine is extremely sensitive due to extensive innervation via the dental pulp. **Dental pulp:** Located in the pulp chamber and root canals, the dental pulp is a well-vascularized layer of loose connective tissue. Neurovascular structures enter the apical foramen at the apex of the root. The dental pulp receives sympathetic innervation from the superior cervical ganglion and sensory innervation from the trigeminal ganglion (CN V).
Periodontium: The tooth is anchored and supported by the periodontium, which consists of several tissue types. *Note:* The cementum is also considered part of the periodontium.	**Periodontal ligament:** Dense connective tissue fibers that connect the cementum of the roots in the osseous socket to the alveolar bone. **Alveolar bone** (alveolar processes of maxilla and mandible)**:** The portion of the maxilla or mandible in which the dental roots are embedded are considered the alveolar processes (the more proximal portion of the bones are considered the body). **Gingiva:** The attached gingivae bind the alveolar periosteum to the teeth; the free gingiva composes the 1 mm tissue radius surrounding the neck of the tooth. A mucogingival line marks the boundary between the keratinized gingivae of the mandibular arch and the nonkeratinized lingual mucosa. The palatal mucosa is masticatory (orthokeratinized), so no visual distinction can be made with the gingiva of the maxillary arch. Third molars (wisdom teeth) often erupt through the mucosogingival line. The oral mucosa cannot support the tooth, and food can become trapped in the regions lacking attached gingiva.

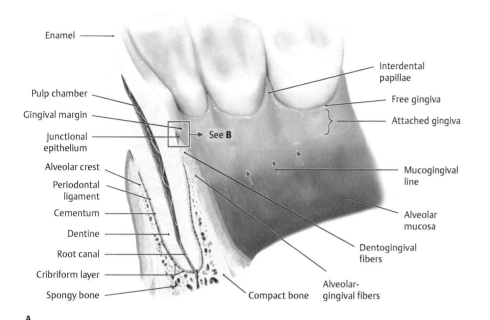

Labels for Fig. A:
- Enamel
- Pulp chamber
- Gingival margin
- Junctional epithelium
- Alveolar crest
- Periodontal ligament
- Cementum
- Dentine
- Root canal
- Cribriform layer
- Spongy bone
- See B
- Compact bone
- Interdental papillae
- Free gingiva
- Attached gingiva
- Mucogingival line
- Alveolar mucosa
- Dentogingival fibers
- Alveolar-gingival fibers

A

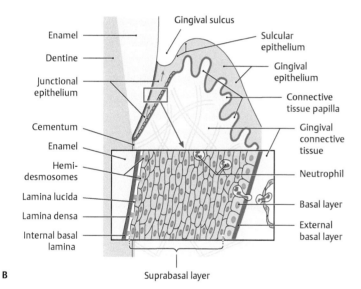

Labels for Fig. B:
- Enamel
- Dentine
- Junctional epithelium
- Cementum
- Enamel
- Hemi-desmosomes
- Lamina lucida
- Lamina densa
- Internal basal lamina
- Gingival sulcus
- Sulcular epithelium
- Gingival epithelium
- Connective tissue papilla
- Gingival connective tissue
- Neutrophil
- Basal layer
- External basal layer
- Suprabasal layer

B

Fig. 8.14 Gingiva
A Gingiva. **B** Junctional epithelium.

A The gingiva extends from the gingival margin to the mucogingival border. There, the gingival epithelium blends into the considerably more reddish alveolar epithelium.

There is a clinical distinction between two types of gingiva:

- **Free gingiva** surrounds the neck of the tooth like a cuff and is attached only to the cervical enamel. The gingiva sulcus is a channel that runs around the tooth between the free gingival and the junctional epithelium.
- **Attached gingiva** extends from the gingival sulcus to the mucogingival border. It is tightly bound to both the cementum at the neck of the tooth and the alveolar crest by dentogingival fibers.

B The junctional epithelium attaches to the surface of the cementum by hemidesmosomes and basal lamina, thereby ensuring a complete attachment of the oral mucosa to the tooth surface. The junctional epithelium becomes broader in the apical-coronal direction.

Note: The integrity of the junctional epithelium is a precondition for the health of the entire periodontium. If bacterial colonization from dental plaque leads to inflammation of the neck of tooth, the junctional epithelium detaches from the tooth and so-called "gingival pockets" form in the area around the gingival sulcus. This is called *periodontitis*.

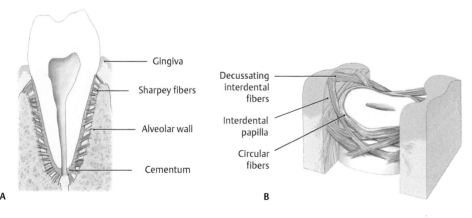

Labels for Fig. A:
- Gingiva
- Sharpey fibers
- Alveolar wall
- Cementum

Labels for Fig. B:
- Decussating interdental fibers
- Interdental papilla
- Circular fibers

A   **B**

Fig. 8.15 Peridontal ligament
A The Sharpey fibers of the periodontal ligament pass obliquely downward from the alveolar bone and insert into the cementum of the tooth. This arrangement transforms masticatory pressures on the dental arch into tensile stresses acting on the fibers and anchored bone (pressure would otherwise lead to alveolar bone atrophy).

B Many of the tough collagenous fiber bundles in the connective tissue core of the gingiva above the alveolar bone are arranged in a screwlike pattern around the tooth further strengthening its attachment.

Maxillary Permanent Teeth

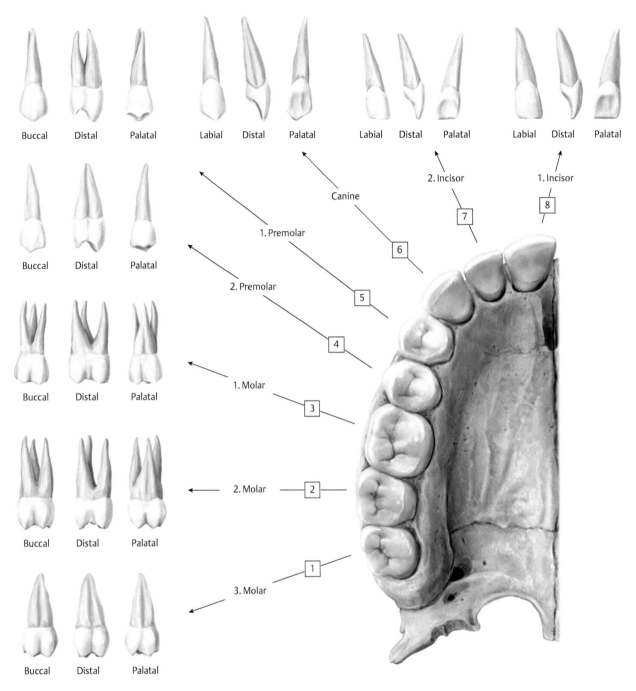

Buccal Distal Palatal   Labial Distal Palatal   Labial Distal Palatal   Labial Distal Palatal

2. Incisor

1. Incisor

Canine

7

8

1. Premolar

6

Buccal Distal Palatal

2. Premolar

5

Buccal Distal Palatal

4

1. Molar

3

Buccal Distal Palatal

2. Molar   2

Buccal Distal Palatal

1

3. Molar

Buccal Distal Palatal

Fig. 8.16 Morphology of the maxillary permanent teeth
Right maxilla, occlusal view and isolated teeth shown in various views.
Incisors: Incisors are used for cutting off chunks of food. Accordingly, they are sharp-edged (scoop-shaped). In addition, they largely determine the esthetic appearance of the oral region. In general, all incisors are single-rooted and have one root canal. The upper central incisor is the largest, the lower central incisor the smallest. The palatal surfaces of the two upper incisors often bear a blind pit, the foramen cecum, which is a site of predilection for dental caries. The maxillary incisors are considerably larger than the mandibular incisors, resulting in a cusp-and-fissure occlusion (see **Fig. 8.18**).
Canines: Canines consist of a single cusp. Typically they have one long root (the longest root of all teeth) containing one root canal, and they support the incisors. Eruption of the maxillary canine tends to correct the splayed orientation of the maxillary lateral incisor and any median diastema (space between the two maxillary central incisors) and so often orthodontic treatment is delayed until this tooth erupts to

monitor how much the teeth will "self-correct". The canine teeth (both maxillary and mandibular) also play an important role in occlusion.
Premolars: Premolars represent a transitional form between the incisors and the molars. They have cusps and fissures. They are more important in grinding than biting off food. Maxillary premolars have two cusps, one buccal and one palatal, separated by a central fissure. The first maxillary premolar has two roots, each containing a root canal. The second maxillary premolar typically has one root, but this may contain one or two root canals.
Molars: Molars are the largest of the permanent teeth and have an occlusal suface with multiple cusps. In order to absorb the powerful chewing pressure, the maxillary molars have three roots, each of which contains a root canal (although the mesial root may contain two canals). Third molars (wisdom teeth) are the exception. The roots of third molars are often fused and therefore their root canal system is complex (root canal therapy is rarely attempted in these teeth).

Table 8.2 Morphology of the maxillary permanent teeth

Tooth	Crown	Surfaces	Root(s)	Root canal(s)
Central incisors (8, 9) Lateral incisors (7, 10)	Roughly trapezoidal in the labial view; contains an incisal edge with 3 tubercles (mamelons)	Labial: convex Palatal: concavoconvex	1 rounded root	Usually 1
Canines (6, 11)	Roughly trapezoidal with 1 labial cusp	Labial: convex Palatal: concavoconvex	1 root; the longest of the teeth	Usually 1
1st premolar (5, 12)	2 cusps (1 buccal, 1 palatal), separated by a central fissure	Buccal, distal, palatal, and mesial: all convex, slightly flattened. The mesial surface often bears a small pit that is difficult to clean and vulnerable to caries Occlusal: more oval than the mandibular premolars	2 roots (1 buccal, 1 palatal)	Usually 2, one per root
2nd premolar (4, 13)			1 root divided by a longitudinal groove and containing 2 root canals	1 or 2
1st molar (3, 14)	4 cusps (1 at each corner of its occlusal surface); a ridge connects the mesiopalatal and distobuccal cusps	Buccal, distal, palatal, and mesial: all convex, slightly flattened Occlusal: rhomboid	3 roots (2 buccal, 1 palatal)	3 or 4 (mesial root may have 2 canals)
2nd molar (2, 15)	4 cusps (though the distopalatal is often small or absent		3 roots (2 buccal, 1 palatal), occasionally fused	3 or 4 (mesial root may have 2 canals)
3rd molar (1, 16)	3 cusps (no distopalatal)		3 roots (2 buccal, 1 palatal), often fused	Complex canal system

The maxillary teeth are supplied by the posterior superior alveolar a. (molars), middle superior alveolar a. (premolars), and the anterior superior alveolar a. (incisors and canines); venous drainage is via the alveolar vv. that drain to the pterygoid plexus. Innervation is via the posterior, middle, and anterior superior alveolar nn. (same distribution as the arteries). Lymph from the maxillary teeth drain to the submandibular nodes.

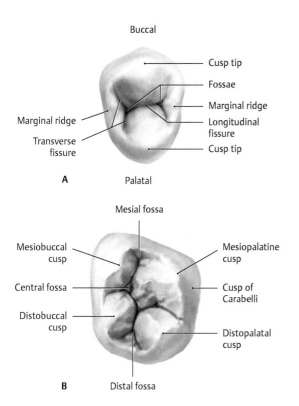

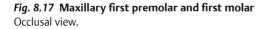

Fig. 8.17 Maxillary first premolar and first molar
Occlusal view.

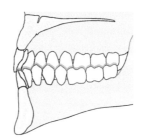

Fig. 8.18 Cusp-and-fissure occlusion
With the mouth closed (occlusal position), the maxillary teeth are opposed to their mandibular counterparts. They are offset relative to one another such that the cusps of one tooth fit into the fissures of the two opposing teeth (cusp-and-fissure occulsion). Because of this arrangement, every tooth comes into contact with two opposing teeth. This offset results from the slightly greater width of the maxillary incisors.
A class I occlusion is a "normal" occlusion where the lower anterior teeth occlude with the cingulum of the upper anterior teeth. A class II occlusion is when the lower teeth occlude behind the cingulum of the upper anterior teeth. A class III occlusion is when the lower anterior teeth occlude in front of the cingulum of the upper anterior teeth. Crossbites are when the teeth are not in the usual buccal-lingual relationship.

209

Mandibular Permanent Teeth

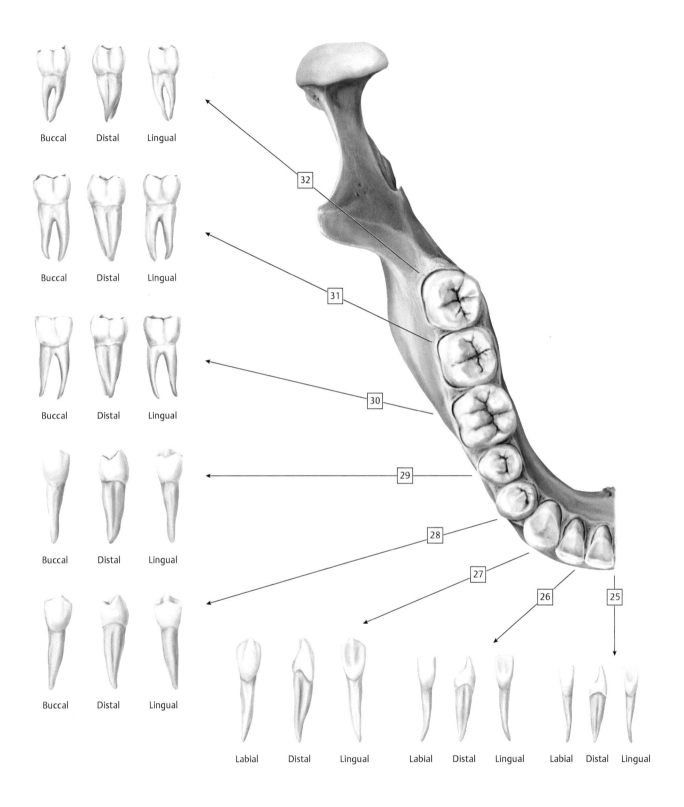

Fig. 8.19 Morphology of the mandibular permanent teeth
The general morphology of the mandibular teeth is similar to that of the maxillary teeth.

Incisors: Mandibular incisors are smaller than their maxillary counterparts but have one root containing one root canal.

Canines: The mandibular canine is similar to the maxillary canine.

Premolars: The mandibular first premolar has a less well defined lingual cusp. It typically has one root with one canal.

Molars: Mandibular first molars have five cusps, two roots, and between two and four root canals. Mandibular second molars have four cusps but are otherwise similar to the first molars. Mandibular third molars are often impacted (do not erupt into the arch) and have two fused roots with a complex canal system.

Table 8.3 Morphology of the mandibular permanent teeth

Tooth	Crown	Surfaces	Root(s)	Root canal(s)
Central incisors (24, 25) Lateral incisors (23, 26)	Roughly trapezoidal in the labial view; contains an incisal edge with 3 tubercles (mamelons)	Labial: convex Palatal: concavoconvex	1 root, slightly flattened	1
Canines (22, 27)	Roughly trapezoidal with 1 labial cusp	Labial: convex Palatal: concavoconvex	1 root; the longest of the teeth (*Note:* mandibular canines are occassionally bifid)	1
1st premolar (21, 28)	2 cusps (1 tall buccal cusp connected to 1 smaller lingual cusp; the groove between the cusps creates a mesial and distal occlusal pit.	Buccal, distal, lingual, and mesial: all convex, slightly flattened. The mesial surface often bears a small pit that is difficult to clean and vulnerable to caries Occlusal: more oval than the mandibular premolars	1 root (occasaionally bifid)	1
2nd premolar (20, 29)	3 cusps (1 tall buccal cusp separated from 2 smaller lingual cusps by a mesiodistal fissure)	mandibular premolars	1 root	1
1st molar (19, 30)	5 cusps (3 buccal and 2 lingual), all of which are separated by fissures	Buccal, distal, lingual, and mesial: all convex, slightly flattened Occlusal: rectangular	2 roots (1 mesial and 1 distal); widely spaced	2–4
2nd molar (18, 31)	4 cusps (2 buccal; 2 lingual)		2 roots (1 mesial and 1 distal)	2–4
3rd molar (17, 32)	May resemble either the 1st or 2nd molar		2 roots, often fused	Complex canal system

The mandibular teeth are supplied by the inferior alveolar a. (molars and premolars) or its incisive branch (incisors and canines); venous drainage is via the inferior alveolar v., which drains to the pterygoid plexus. Innervation is via the inferior alveolar n. (molars and second premolar) or its incisive branch (incisors, canines, and first premolars). Lymph from these teeth drain to the submandibular nodes.

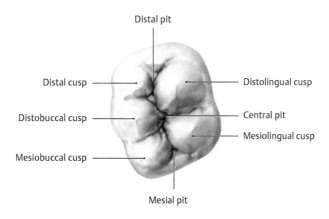

Fig. 8.20 Mandibular first molar
Occlusal view.

Deciduous Teeth

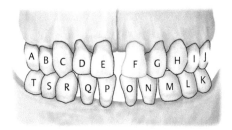

Fig. 8.21 Coding the deciduous teeth
The upper right molar is considered A. The lettering then proceeds clockwise along the upper arc and back across the lower.

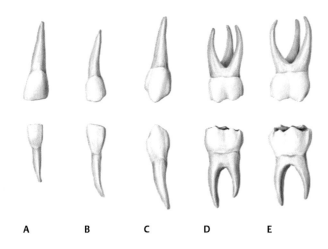

A   B   C   D   E

Fig. 8.22 Deciduous teeth
Left side. The deciduous dentition consists of only 20 teeth. Each of the four quadrants contains the following teeth: **A** Central incisor. **B** Lateral incisor. **C** Canine. **D** First molar. **E** Second molar. To distinguish the deciduous teeth from the permanent teeth, they are coded with letters. The upper arch is labeled A to J, the lower is labeled K to T.

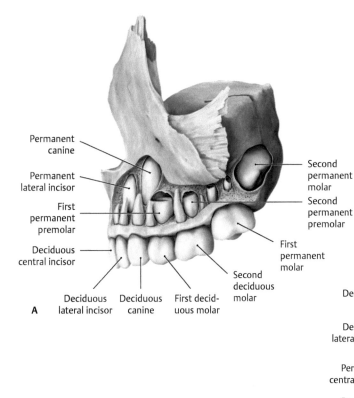

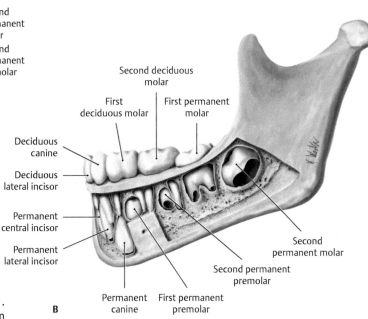

Fig. 8.23 Teeth of a 6-year-old child
A Maxillary teeth, left lateral view. **B** Mandibular teeth, left lateral view . The anterior bony plate over the roots of the deciduous teeth has been removed to display the underlying permanent tooth buds (blue). At six years of age, all the deciduous teeth have erupted and are still present along with the first permanent tooth, the first molar.
Note: The roots of deciduous molars are more divergent than those of permanent molars. This is because the permanent premolars form in between these roots and they are guided by them into the dental arch as they erupt. In addition to this difference between deciduous teeth and permanent teeth, deciduous teeth have thinner enamel, larger pulp horns, their pulpal outline follows the cementoenamel junction (CEJ) more closely, they have narrower occlusal surfaces, broader contact points, thin pulpal floors, and the pulp within the root canals is more tortuous and branching. Furthermore, alveolar bone is more permeable in young children often allowing the clinician to achieve adequate anesthesia via infiltration injections (see p. 498).

Table 8.4 Eruption of the teeth

The eruptions of the deciduous and permanent teeth are called the first and second dentitions, respectively. Types of teeth are ordered by the time of eruption; individual teeth are listed from left to right (viewer's perspective).

Type of tooth	Tooth		Time of eruption
First dentition (deciduous teeth)			
Central incisor	E, F	P, O	6–8 months
Lateral incisor	D, G	Q, N	8–12 months
First molar	B, I	S, L	12–16 months
Canine	C, H	R, M	15–20 months
Second molar	A, J	T, K	20–40 months
Second dentition (permanent teeth)			
First molar	3, 14	30, 19	6–8 years ("6-yr molar")
Central incisor	8, 9	25, 24	6–9 years
Lateral incisor	7, 10	26, 23	7–10 years
First premolar	5, 12	28, 21	9–13 years
Canine	6, 11	27, 22	9–14 years
Second premolar	4, 13	29, 20	11–14 years
Second molar	2, 15	31, 18	10–14 years ("12-yr molar")
Third molar	1, 16	32, 17	16–30 years ("wisdom tooth")

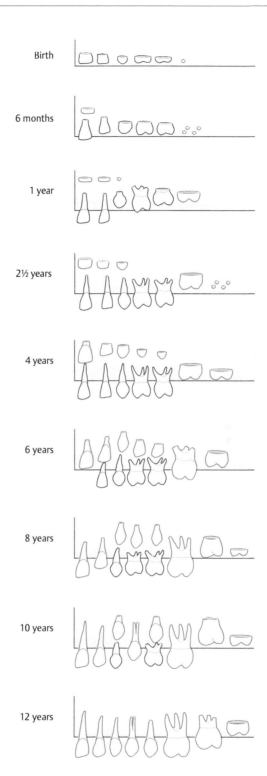

Fig. 8.24 Eruption pattern of the deciduous and permanent teeth
Left maxillary teeth. Deciduous teeth (black), permanent teeth (red). Eruption times can be used to diagnose growth delays in children.

213

Radiographs of Teeth

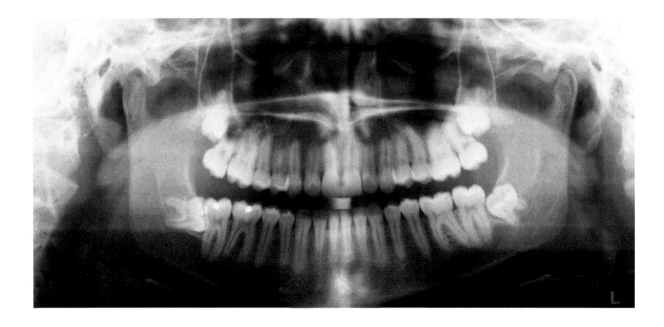

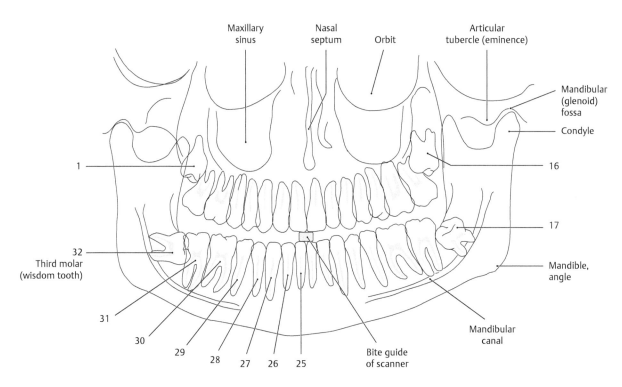

Fig. 8.25 Dental panoramic tomogram

The dental panoramic tomogram (DPT) is a survey radiograph that allows a preliminary assessment of the temporomandibular joints, maxillary sinuses, maxilla, mandible, and dental status (carious lesions, location of the wisdom teeth). It is based on the principle of conventional tomography in which the x-ray tube and film are moved about the plane of interest to blur out the shadows of structures outside the sectional plane. The plane of interest in the DPT is shaped like a parabola, conforming to the shape of the jaws. If the DPT raises suspicion of caries or root disease, it should be followed with spot radiographs so that specific regions of interest can be evaluated at higher resolution. (Tomogram courtesy of Prof. Dr. U. J. Rother, director of the Department of Diagnostic Radiology, Center for Dentistry and Oromaxillofacial Surgery, Eppendorf University Medical Center, Hamburg, Germany.)

Generally, radiographic images of the teeth and gums are taken by directing the X-ray beam perpendicular to a tangent to the dental arch, or, to put it more simply, perpendicular to the outer surface of the tooth or teeth. Thus, the radiograph shows all consecutive structures in the beam path and so they overlap. In teeth with multiple roots, the individual root canals cannot be clearly evaluated. This is only possible with the help of so-called eccentric images, in which the X-ray beam is directed to the tangent at a particular angle, so that the consecutive structures are clearly distinguishable. Bitewing radiographs (see **Fig. 8.31**) only show the crown of the tooth, and not the entire tooth. The patient bites down on a mount that holds a small piece of film perpendicular to it. The resulting radiograph shows the crown of both maxillary and mandibular teeth in the same radiograph, which helps in detection of caries (tooth decay) underneath fillings or on the contact surfaces. (Radiographs courtesy of Christian Friedrichs, DDM.)

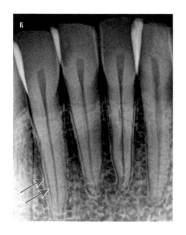

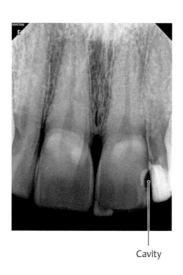

Cavity

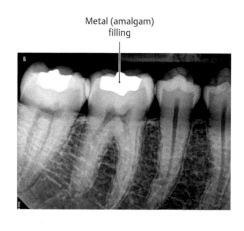

Metal (amalgam) filling

Fig. 8.26 Mandibular incisors
Single-rooted teeth have two root canals in one third of all cases. This radiograph shows a cross section of the dental root and a double periodontal space (see arrows).

Fig. 8.27 Maxillary incisors
The radiolucent spots shown here distally on tooth 9 could indicate caries, open cavities, or non-radioopaque filling material (as in the case here).

Fig. 8.28 Mandibular teeth 28–31
Radiopacities, such as those seen here near the crowns of teeth 30 and 31, can be the result of metal inlays, crowns, amalgam fillings, or modern zinc oxide ceramics.

Zygomatic arch

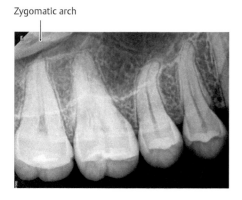

Root filling

Periapical area

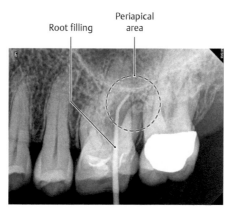

Pulp stone   Dentine caries

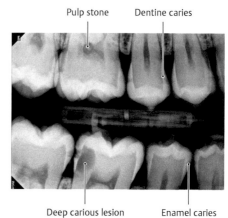

Deep carious lesion   Enamel caries

Fig. 8.29 Maxillary teeth 2–5
In this area of the maxilla, superimposition of teeth and the zygomatic arch frequently occurs (see the upper left margin). The roots of the molars are less clearly visible.

Fig. 8.30 Maxillary teeth 12–15
An infection of the root canal system, which has spread to the periapical bone can lead to the formation of a fistula. In order to be able to exactly locate the infection, a gutta-percha root-filling point is inserted into the fistula from outside. Around the distobuccal root of tooth 14, a periapical radioopaque area indicating the infection is visible. Tooth 15 has been capped with a crown.

Fig. 8.31 Bitewings for the diagnosis of caries
There is massive carious damage on the distal surface of tooth 30 and there are also enamel caries and the beginning of dentine caries at the contact points of almost all teeth. In addition to the occlusal surfaces, the contact points represent sites of predilection for caries. Note the pulp stones visible in the lumen of the pulp chambers.

215

Lingual Mucosa

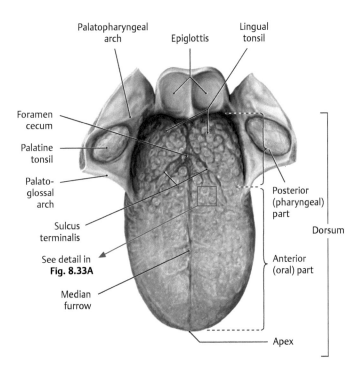

Fig. 8.32 Surface anatomy of the lingual mucosa
Superior view. The parts of the tongue are the root, the ventral (inferior) surface, the apex, and the dorsal (superior) surface. The V-shaped furrow on the dorsum (sulcus terminalis) divides the dorsal surface into an oral portion (comprising the anterior two thirds) and a pharyngeal portion (comprising the posterior one third).
The tongue's very powerful muscular body make possible its motor functions in mastication, swallowing, and speaking. Its specialized mucosal coat covering the dorsum of the tongue make possible its equally important sensory functions (including taste and fine tactile discrimination). The human tongue contains approximately 4600 taste buds, in which the secondary sensory cells for taste perception are collected. The taste buds are embedded in the epithelium of the lingual mucosa and its surface expansions, the papillae (see **Fig. 8.33**). Additionally, isolated taste buds are located in the mucous membranes of the soft palate and pharynx. Humans can perceive five basic taste qualities: sweet, sour, salty, bitter, and umami.

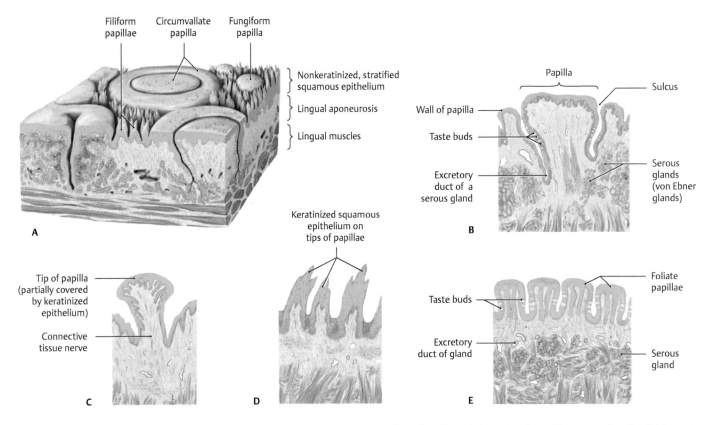

Fig. 8.33 Papillae of the tongue
The mucosa of the anterior dorsum is composed of numerous papillae (A) and the connective tissue between the mucosal surface and musculature, which contains many small salivary glands. The papillae are divided into four morphologically distinct types (see **Table 8.5**):

- Circumvallate (B): Encircled and containing taste buds.
- Fungiform (C): Mushroom-shaped and containing mechanical and thermal receptors and taste buds.

- Filiform (D): Thread-shaped and sensitive to tactile stimuli (the only lingual papillae without taste buds).
- Foliate (E): Containing taste buds.

The surrounding serous glands of the tongue (Von Ebner glands), which are most closely associated with circumvallate papilla, constantly wash the taste buds clean to allow for new tasting.

Table 8.5 Regions and structures of the tongue

Region	Structures
Anterior (oral, presulcal) portion of the tongue	

The anterior ⅔ of the tongue contains the apex and the majority of the dorsum. It is tethered to the oral floor by the lingual frenulum.
• **Mucosa:**
  ◦ Dorsal lingual mucosa: This portion (with no underlying submucosa) contains numerous papillae.
  ◦ Ventral mucosa: Covered with the same smooth (nonkeratinized, stratified squamous epithelial) mucosa that lines the oral floor and gingiva.
• **Innervation:** The anterior portion is derived from the first (pharyngeal) arch and is therefore innervated by the lingual nerve, a branch of the mandibular nerve (CN V$_3$).
	Median furrow (midline septum): The furrow running anteriorly down the midline of the tongue; this corresponds to the position of the lingual septum. *Note:* Muscle fibers do not cross the lingual septum.
	
	Papillae (Fig. 8.33A): The dorsal mucosa, which has no submucosa, is covered with nipplelike projections (papillae) that increase the surface area of the tongue. There are four types, all of which occur in the presulcal but not postsulcal portion of the tongue.
	• Circumvallate (**Fig. 8.33B**): Encircled by a wall and containing abundant taste buds.
	• Fungiform (**Fig. 8.33C**): Mushroom-shaped papillae located on the lateral margin of the posterior oral portion near the palatoglossal arches. These have mechanical receptors, thermal receptors, and taste buds.
	• Filiform (**Fig. 8.33D**): Thread-shaped papillae that are sensitive to tactile stimuli. These are the only papillae that do not contain taste buds.
	• Foliate (**Fig. 8.33E**): Located near the sulcus terminalis, these contain numerous taste buds.

Sulcus terminalis	
The sulcus terminalis is the V-shaped furrow that divides the tongue functionally and anatomically into an anterior and a posterior portion.	**Foramen cecum:** The embryonic remnant of the passage of the thyroid gland that migrates from the dorsum of the tongue during development. The foramen cecum is located at the convergence of the sulci terminalis.
Posterior (pharyngeal, postsulcal) portion of the tongue	
The base (root) of the tongue is located posterior to the palatoglossal arches and sulcus terminalis. • **Mucosa:** The same mucosa that lines the palatine tonsils, pharyngeal walls, and epiglottis. The pharyngeal portion of the tongue does not contain papillae. • **Innervation:** The posterior portion is innervated by the glossopharyngeal nerve (CN IX). A small midline area at the root of the tongue is innervated by the vagus nerve (CN X).	**Lingual tonsils:** The submucosa of the posterior portion contains embedded lymph nodes known as the lingual tonsils, which create the uneven surface of the posterior portion. **Oropharynx:** The region posterior to the palatoglossal arch. The oropharynx, which contains the palatine tonsils, communicates with the oral cavity via the oropharyngeal isthmus (defined by the palatoglossal arches).

Glossoepiglottic folds and epiglottic valleculae: The (nonkeratinized, stratified squamous) mucosal covering of the posterior tongue and pharyngeal walls is reflected onto the anterior aspect of the epiglottis, forming one median and two lateral glossoepiglottic folds. The median glossoepiglottic fold is flanked by two depressions, the epiglottic valleculae.

Glossal Muscles

There are two sets of lingual muscles: extrinsic and intrinsic. The extrinsic muscles, which are attached to specific bony sites outside the tongue, move the tongue as a whole. The intrinsic muscles, which have no attachments to skeletal structures, alter the shape of the tongue. With the exception of the palatoglossus, the glossal muscles are innervated by the hypoglossal nerve (CN XII).

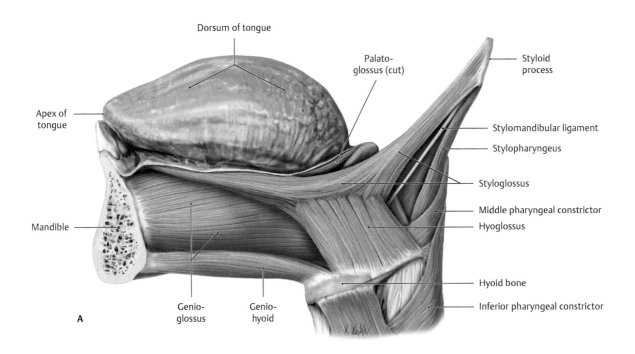

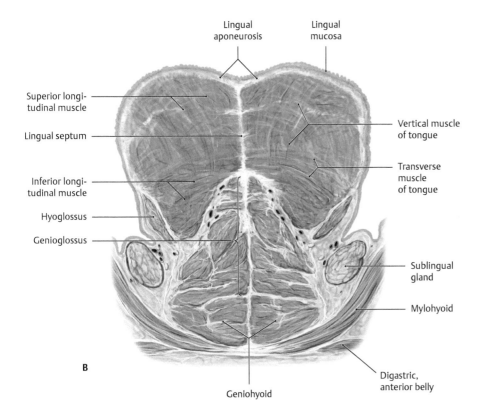

Fig. 8.34 Extrinsic and intrinsic lingual muscles
A Left lateral view. **B** Anterior view of coronal section.

Table 8.6 Muscles of the tongue

Muscle	Origin	Insertion	Innervation	Action
Extrinsic lingual muscles				
Genioglossus	Mandible (superior genial [mental] spine via an intermediate tendon); more posteriorly the two genioglossi are separated by the lingual septum	Inferior fibers: Hyoid body (anterosuperior surface) Intermediate fibers: Posterior tongue Superior fibers: Ventral surface of tongue (mix with intrinsic muscles)	Hypoglossal n. (CN XII)	Protrusion of the tongue *Bilaterally:* Makes dorsum concave *Unilaterally:* Deviation to opposite side
Hyoglossus	Hyoid bone (greater horn and anterior body)	Lateral tongue, between styloglossus and inferior longitudinal muscle		Depresses the tongue
Styloglossus	Styloid process of temporal bone (anterolateral aspect of apex) and stylomandibular ligament	Longitudinal part: Dorsolateral tongue (mix with inferior longitudinal muscle) Oblique part: Mix with fibers of the hyoglossus		Elevates and retracts the tongue
Palatoglossus	Palatine aponeurosis (oral surface)	Lateral tongue to dorsum and fibers of the transverse muscle	Vagus n. (CN X) via the pharyngeal plexus	Elevates the root of the tongue; closes the oropharyngeal isthmus by contracting the palatoglossal arch
Intrinsic lingual muscles				
Superior longitudinal muscle	Thin layer of muscle inferior to the dorsal mucosa; fibers run anterolaterally from the epiglottis and median lingual septum		Hypoglossal n. (CN XII)	Shortens tongue; makes dorsum concave (pulls apex and lateral margin upward)
Inferior longitudinal muscle	Thin layer of muscle superior to the genioglossus and hyoglossus; fibers run anteriorly from the root to the apex of the tongue			Shortens tongue; makes dorsum convex (pulls apex down)
Transverse muscle	Fibers run laterally from the lingual septum to the lateral tongue			Narrows tongue; elongates tongue
Vertical muscle	In the anterior tongue, fibers run inferiorly from the dorsum of the tongue to its ventral surface			Widens and flattens tongue

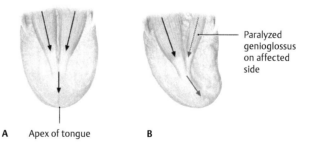

A Apex of tongue **B** Paralyzed genioglossus on affected side

Fig. 8.35 **Unilateral hypoglossal nerve palsy**
Active protrusion of the tongue with an intact hypoglossal nerve (**A**) and with a unilateral hypoglossal nerve lesion (**B**).
When the hypoglossal nerve is damaged on one side, the genioglossus muscle is paralyzed on the affected side. As a result, the healthy (innervated) genioglossus on the opposite side dominates the tongue across the midline toward the affected side. When the tongue is protruded, therefore, it deviates *toward* the paralyzed side.

Neurovasculature of the Tongue

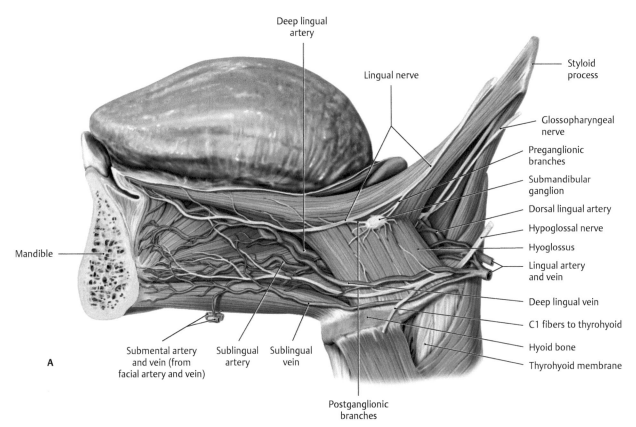

Deep lingual artery

Lingual nerve

Styloid process

Glossopharyngeal nerve

Preganglionic branches

Submandibular ganglion

Dorsal lingual artery

Hypoglossal nerve

Hyoglossus

Lingual artery and vein

Deep lingual vein

C1 fibers to thyrohyoid

Hyoid bone

Thyrohyoid membrane

Mandible

Submental artery and vein (from facial artery and vein)

Sublingual artery

Sublingual vein

A

Postganglionic branches

Fig. 8.36 Nerves and vessels of the tongue
A Left lateral view. **B** View of the inferior surface of the tongue.
The tongue is supplied by the *lingual artery* (from the external carotid artery), which divides into its terminal branches, the deep lingual artery and the sublingual artery. The dorsal lingual artery supplies the root of the tongue in the oropharynx. The lingual vein usually runs parallel to the artery but on the medial surface of the hyoglossus muscle and drains into the *internal jugular vein*. The anterior two thirds of the lingual mucosa receives its *somatosensory* innervation (sensitivity to thermal and tactile stimuli) from the *lingual nerve*, which is a branch of the trigeminal nerve's mandibular division (CN V$_3$). The lingual nerve transmits fibers from the chorda tympani of the facial nerve (CN VII), among them the afferent taste fibers for the anterior two thirds of the tongue. The chorda tympani also contains presynaptic, parasympathetic visceromotor axons that synapse in the submandibular ganglion, whose neurons in turn innervate the submandibular and sublingual glands. The palatoglossus receives its *somatomotor* innervation from the vagus nerve (CN X) via the pharyngeal plexus, the other glossal muscles from the hypoglossal nerve (CN XII). The hyoglossus muscle serves as a useful landmark for some of the tongue's neurovasculature: the glossopharyngeal nerve and the lingual artery travel deep to the hyoglossus, while the lingual nerve and the hypoglossal nerve travel superficial to it.

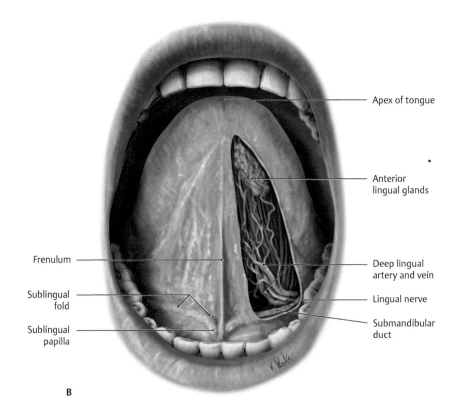

Apex of tongue

Anterior lingual glands

Frenulum

Sublingual fold

Sublingual papilla

Deep lingual artery and vein

Lingual nerve

Submandibular duct

B

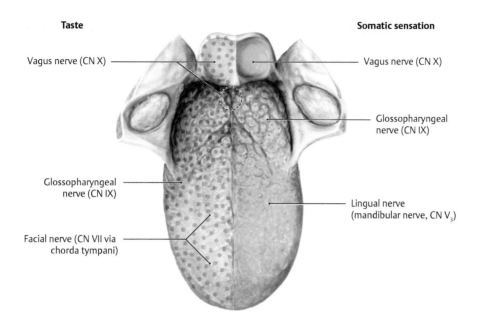

Fig. 8.37 Innervation of the tongue

Anterior view. Left side: Somatosensory innervation. Right side: Taste innervation.

The posterior one third of the tongue (postsulcal part) primarily receives somatosensory and taste innervation from the glossopharyngeal nerve (CN IX), with additional taste sensation conveyed by the vagus nerve (CN X) via the internal laryngeal nerve. The anterior two thirds of the tongue (presulcal part) receives its somatosensory innervation (e.g., touch, pain, and temperature) from the lingual nerve (branch of CN V$_3$) and its taste sensation from the chorda tympani branch of the facial nerve (CN VII) distributed by the lingual nerve (CN V$_3$). Disturbances of sensation in the presulcal tongue can therefore be used to determine facial or trigeminal nerve lesions.

Table 8.7 Blood supply to the tongue

Blood supply	Source	Branches	Distribution
Lingual a.	External carotid a.	Dorsal lingual aa.	Dorsal surface of posterior one third of tongue, palatoglossal arch, palatine tonsil, epiglottis, soft palate
		Sublingual a.	Floor of oral cavity, sublingual gland and surrounding mucosa and muscles
		Deep lingual a.	Ventral surface of tongue
		Terminal branches	Dorsal surface of anterior two thirds of tongue
Submental a.	Facial a. (from external carotid a.)		Anatomoses with sublingual a. to supply sublingual gland and surrounding floor of mouth
Tonsillar a.	Facial a. (from external carotid a.)		Root of tongue
Ascending pharyngeal a.	External carotid a.		Root of tongue

Table 8.8 Venous drainage of the tongue

Vein	Tributaries	Region drained	Drains to
Lingual v.	Deep lingual vv.	Ventral surface of tongue	Internal jugular v.
	Dorsal lingual vv.	Dorsum of tongue	
Submental v.		Anastomoses with branches of lingual vv. to help drain tongue	Facial v.

221

Gustatory Pathway

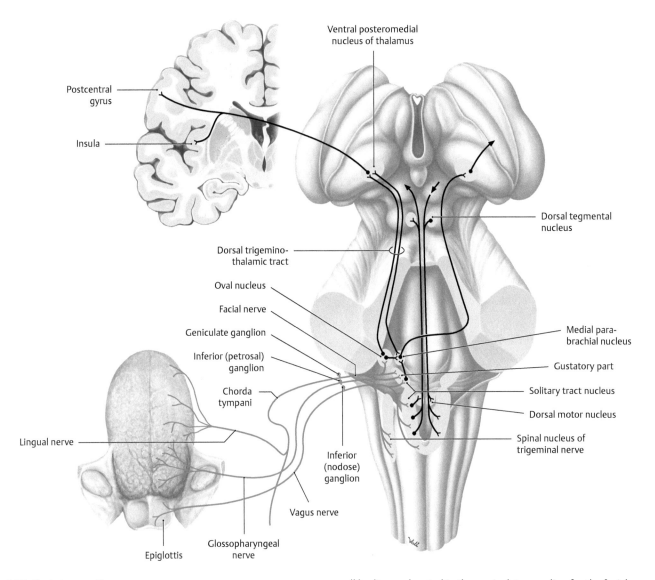

Fig. 8.38 Gustatory pathway

The receptors for the sense of taste are the taste buds of the tongue (see **Fig. 8.39**). Unlike other receptor cells, the receptor cells of the taste buds are specialized epithelial cells (secondary sensory cells, as they do not have an axon). When these epithelial cells are chemically stimulated, the base of the cells releases glutamate, which stimulates the peripheral processes of afferent cranial nerves. These different cranial nerves serve different areas of the tongue. It is rare, therefore, for a complete loss of taste (ageusia) to occur.

- The *anterior two thirds* of the tongue is supplied by the facial nerve (CN VII), the afferent fibers first passing in the lingual nerve (branch of the trigeminal nerve) and then in the chorda tympani to the geniculate ganglion of the facial nerve.
- The *posterior third of the tongue* and the *vallate papillae* are supplied by the glossopharyngeal nerve (CN IX). A small area on the posterior third of the tongue is also supplied by the vagus nerve (CN X).
- The *epiglottis* and *valleculae* are supplied by the vagus nerve (CN X).

Peripheral processes from pseudounipolar ganglion cells (which correspond to pseudounipolar spinal ganglion cells) terminate on the taste buds. The central portions of these processes convey taste information to the gustatory part of the nucleus of the solitary tract. Thus, they function as the first afferent neuron of the gustatory pathway. Their

cell bodies are located in the geniculate ganglion for the facial nerve, in the inferior (petrosal) ganglion for the glossopharyngeal nerve, and in the inferior (nodose) ganglion for the vagus nerve. After synapsing in the gustatory part of the nucleus of the solitary tract, the axons from the second neuron are believed to terminate in the medial parabrachial nucleus, where they are relayed to the third neuron. Most of the axons from the third neuron cross to the opposite side and pass in the dorsal trigeminothalamic tract to the contralateral ventral posteromedial nucleus of the thalamus. Some of the axons travel uncrossed in the same structures. The fourth neurons of the gustatory pathway, located in the thalamus, project to the postcentral gyrus and insular cortex, where the fifth neuron is located. Collaterals from the first and second neurons of the gustatory afferent pathway are distributed to the superior and inferior salivatory nuclei. Afferent impulses in these fibers induce the secretion of saliva during eating ("salivary reflex"). The parasympathetic preganglionic fibers exit the brainstem via cranial nerves VII and IX (see the descriptions of these cranial nerves for details). Besides this purely gustatory pathway, spicy foods may also stimulate trigeminal fibers (not shown), which contribute to the sensation of taste. Finally, olfaction (the sense of smell), too, is a major component of the sense of taste as it is subjectively perceived: patients who cannot smell (anosmia) report that their food tastes abnormally bland.

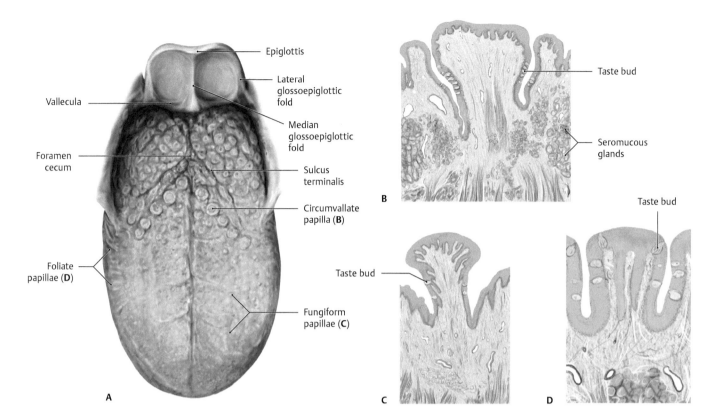

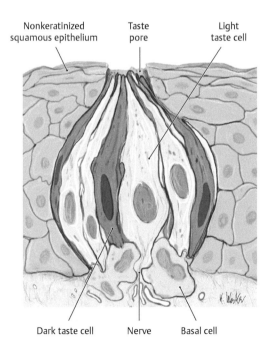

Fig. 8.39 Organization of the taste receptors in the tongue

The human tongue contains approximately 4600 taste buds in which the secondary sensory cells for taste perception are collected. The taste buds are embedded in the epithelium of the lingual mucosa and are located on the surface expansions of the lingual mucosa—the circumvallate papillae (principal site, **B**), the fungiform papillae (**C**), and the foliate papillae (**D**). Additionally, isolated taste buds are located in the mucous membranes of the soft palate and pharynx. The surrounding serous glands of the tongue (Ebner glands), which are most closely associated with the circumvallate papillae, constantly wash the taste buds clean to allow for new tasting. Humans can perceive five basic taste qualities: sweet, sour, salty, bitter, and a fifth "savory" quality, called umami, which is activated by glutamate (a taste enhancer).

Fig. 8.40 Microscopic structure of a taste bud

Nerves induce the formation of taste buds in the oral mucosa. Axons of cranial nerves VII, IX, and X grow into the oral mucosa from the basal side and induce the epithelium to differentiate into the light and dark taste cells (= modified epithelial cells). Both types of taste cell have microvilli that extend to the gustatory pore. For sour and salty, the taste cell is stimulated by hydrogen ions and other cations. The other taste qualities are mediated by receptor proteins to which the low-molecular-weight flavored substances bind (details may be found in textbooks of physiology). When the low-molecular-weight flavored substances bind to the receptor proteins, they induce signal transduction that causes the release of glutamate, which excites the peripheral processes of the pseudounipolar neurons of the three cranial nerve ganglia. The taste cells have a life span of approximately 12 days and regenerate from cells at the base of the taste buds, which differentiate into new taste cells.

Note: The old notion that particular areas of the tongue are sensitive to specific taste qualities has been found to be false.

Floor of the Oral Cavity

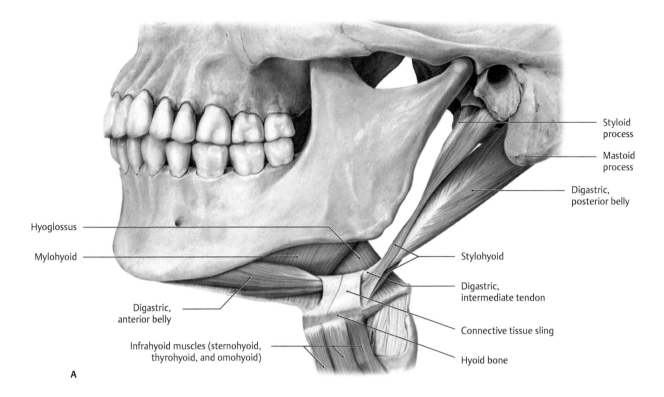

Styloid process

Mastoid process

Digastric, posterior belly

Hyoglossus

Mylohyoid

Stylohyoid

Digastric, intermediate tendon

Digastric, anterior belly

Connective tissue sling

Infrahyoid muscles (sternohyoid, thyrohyoid, and omohyoid)

Hyoid bone

A

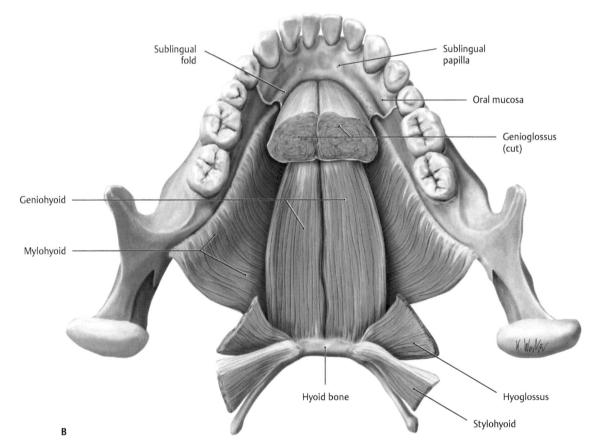

Sublingual fold

Sublingual papilla

Oral mucosa

Genioglossus (cut)

Geniohyoid

Mylohyoid

Hyoid bone

Hyoglossus

Stylohyoid

B

Fig. 8.41 **Muscles of the oral floor**
A Left lateral view. **B** Superior view. Strictly speaking the floor of the oral cavity is composed only of the mylohyoid and geniohyoid muscles. However, other suprahyoid muscles contribute to this region. The suprahyoid muscles also play an important role in swallowing (see **Table 8.6**). The suprahyoid and infrahyoid muscles attach to the hyoid bone inferiorly and superiorly, respectively. The infrahyoid muscles depress the hyoid muscles during phonation and swallowing. These muscles are discussed in detail on pages 330–331.

Table 8.9 Muscles contributing to the oral floor and surrounding regions

Muscle		Origin	Insertion		Innervation	Action
Mylohyoid		Mandible (mylohyoid line)	Hyoid bone (body)	Via median tendon of insertion (mylohyoid raphe)	Mylohyoid n. (CN V₃)	Tightens and elevates oral floor; draws hyoid bone forward (during swallowing); assists in opening mandible and moving it side to side (mastication)
Geniohyoid		Mandible (inferior genial [mental] spines)		Directly inserts into hyoid	Anterior ramus of C1	Draws hyoid bone forward (during swallowing); assists in opening mandible
Digastric*	Anterior belly	Mandible (digastric fossa)		Via an intermediate tendon with a fibrous loop	Mylohyoid n. (CN V₃)	Elevates hyoid bone (during swallowing); assists in depressing mandible
	Posterior belly	Temporal bone (mastoid notch, medial to mastoid process)			Facial n. (CN VII)	
Stylohyoid*		Temporal bone (styloid process)		Via a split tendon	Facial n. (CN VII)	

* Not true muscles of the floor of the oral cavity.

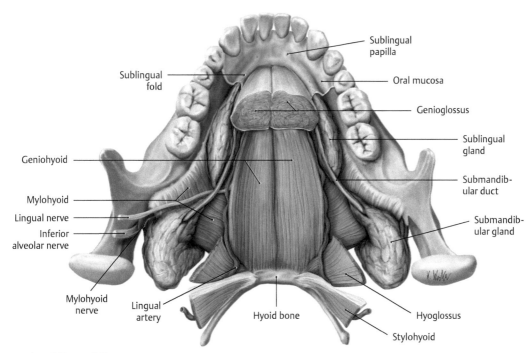

Fig. 8.42 Topography of the oral floor
The geniohyoid muscle is supplied by the sublingual artery, a branch of the lingual artery, and the submental artery, a branch of the facial artery. The sublingual artery also supplies the ventral surface of the tongue and mucosa of the oral floor. The mylohyoid muscle is supplied by the mylohyoid branch of the inferior alveolar artery. Venous drainage is via the sublingual vein, which drains into the internal jugular vein. Sensory innervation is via the lingual nerve (CN V₃). Lymphatic drainage is via the submental and submandibular nodes.

Salivary Glands

***Fig. 8.43* Major salivary glands**
A Left lateral view. **B** Superior view. There are three major (large, paired) salivary glands: parotid, submandibular, and sublingual. They collectively produce 0.5 to 2.0 liters of saliva per day, excreted into the oral cavity via excretory ducts. The saliva keeps the oral mucosa moist. It also has digestive and protective functions: saliva contains the starch-splitting enzyme amylase and the bactericidal enzyme lysozyme.

1. **Parotid glands:** Largest of the salivary glands; wedge-shaped but variable; the facial nerve splits the parotid gland into superficial and deep lobes, which are connected by an isthmus; the parotid duct (Stensen's duct) arises from the deep lobe and crosses the face superficial to the masseter, pierces the buccinators, and opens into the oral vestibule opposite the second upper molar (see **Fig. 8.1C**); it is a purely serous gland (watery secretions). Malignant tumors of the parotid gland may invade surrounding structures directly or indirectly via regional lymph nodes (see **Fig. 3.27**). They may also spread systematically through the vascular system.

2. **Submandibular glands:** Second largest of the salivary glands is located in the floor of the oral cavity, where it wraps around the posterior border of mylohyoid; the submandibular duct (Wharton's duct) opens on to the sublingual papilla behind the lower incisors; it is a mixed seromucous gland (watery and mucus secretions).

3. **Sublingual glands:** The smallest of the three major salivary glands; it is located anterior in the floor of the oral cavity between the oral mucosa and the mylohyoid; the sublingual gland has many smaller excretory ducts that open on the sublingual fold or into the submandibular gland; it is predominantly a mucus-secreting gland (mucoserous).

The salivary glands are a potential site of tumor formation. The majority of such tumors are benign and occur in the superficial lobe of the parotid gland. These are pleomorphic adenomas. The tumors cells can lie outside the capsule and so treatment involves surgical excision of the superficial lobe with a margin. Malignant tumors of the parotid gland, for example, adenolymphoma, are suspected if there is pain, rapid growth, fixation to surrounding tissues, and involvement of the facial nerve. Tumors of the submandibular, sublingual, and minor salivary glands are more likely to be malignant.

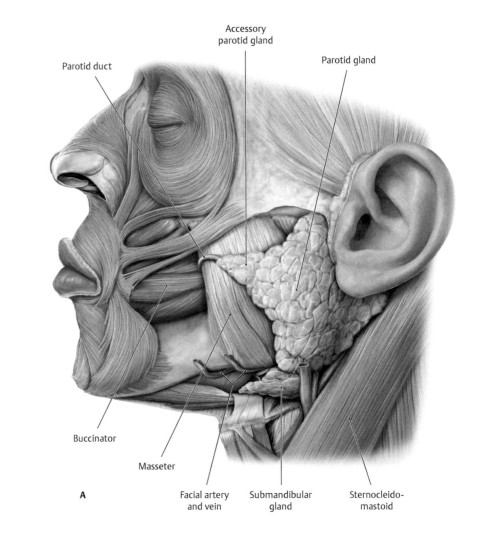

A

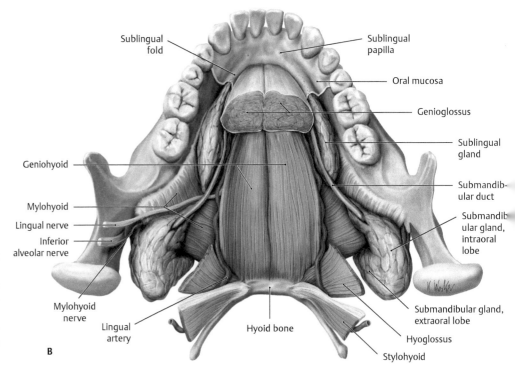

B

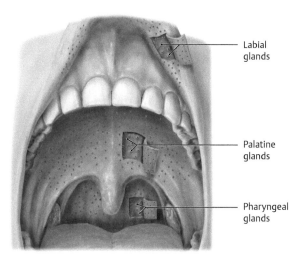

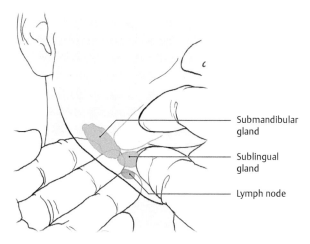

Fig. 8.44 Minor salivary glands
In addition to the three major paired glands, 700 to 1000 minor glands secrete saliva into the oral cavity. They produce only 5 to 8 percent of the total output, but this amount suffices to keep the mouth moist when the major salivary glands are not functioning.

Fig. 8.45 Bimanual examination of the salivary glands
The two salivary glands of the mandible, the submandibular gland and sublingual gland, and the adjacent lymph nodes are grouped around the mobile oral floor and therefore must be palpated against resistance. This is done with bimanual examination.

Table 8.10 Summary of salivary glands

Gland and duct	Autonomic innervation	Blood supply
Parotid - Parotid duct (Stensen's duct)	Glossopharyngeal n. (CN IX) — Preganglionic parasympathetic fibers arise from the inferior salivatory nucleus in the medulla and travel with the inferior petrosal n. (from CN IX) to the otic ganglion — Postganglionic parasympathetic fibers arise in the otic ganglion and travel with the auriculotemporal nerve (of CN V_3) to the parotid gland	Glandular branches from the external carotid a. and superficial temporal a.

Submandibular
- Submandibular duct (Wharton's duct)
 	
Sublingual
- Multiple small ducts that open on the sublingual fold or into the submandibular duct
 	
Minor salivary glands
- Small ducts open directly on the mucosa of the oral cavity and oropharynx
	Facial n. (CN VII)
	— Preganglionic parasympathetic fibers arise from the superior salivary nucleus in the pons. In the facial canal it gives rise to two parasympathetic branches: the greater petrosal n. and the chorda tympani n.
	  o The greater petrosal n. joins the deep petrosal n. (sympathetic) to form the nerve of the pterygoid canal (Vidian n.). It then travels to the pterygopalatine ganglion.
	  o The chorda tympani joins the lingual n. and travels to the submandibular ganglion.
	— Postganglionic parasympathetic fibers from the pterygopalatine ganglion travel with CN V_2 to the nasal, palatine, pharyngeal and superior labial glands. Other postganglionic parasympathetic fibers travel via CN V_2 to the lacrimal n. (of CN V_1) to the lacrimal gland.
	— Postganglionic parasympathetic fibers from the submandibular ganglion travel to the submandibular and sublingual glands.
		Glandular branches of facial a.
		
		Glandular branches of sublingual a.

Lymph from the parotid gland drains to the superficial and deep cervical nodes; lymph from the submandibular gland drains to the deep cervical nodes; lymph from the submandibular gland drains to the submandibular nodes.

Hard & Soft Palates

The palate forms the roof or the oral cavity and the floor of the nasal cavity. It is divided into a bony hard palate and a muscular soft palate.

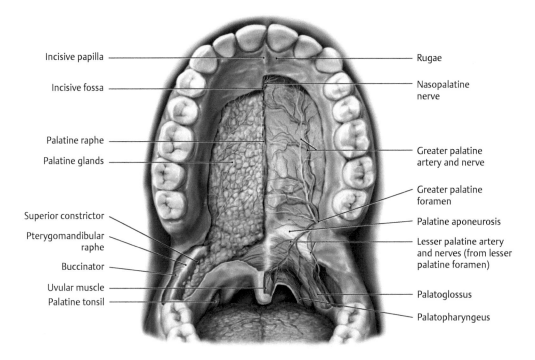

Incisive papilla — Rugae

Incisive fossa — Nasopalatine nerve

Palatine raphe — Greater palatine artery and nerve

Palatine glands — Greater palatine foramen

Superior constrictor — Palatine aponeurosis

Pterygomandibular raphe — Lesser palatine artery and nerves (from lesser palatine foramen)

Buccinator —

Uvular muscle — Palatoglossus

Palatine tonsil — Palatopharyngeus

Fig. 8.46 Hard palate

Anterior view. The hard palate is formed by the palatine process of the maxilla and the horizontal plate of the palatine bone. It is covered with tough masticatory mucosa, which forms irregular folds anteriorly, known as ruggae, which aid in guiding food toward the pharynx. The mucosa is tightly bound to the periosteum of the bones of the hard palate. The mucosa may become stripped off of the periosteum when local anesthetic solution is introduced into the palate, which is very painful.

The hard palate receives it blood supply from the greater palatine artery which arises from the maxillary artery. Veins drain to the pterygoid plexus. Lymph from the hard palate most commonly drains to the submandibular nodes or directly to the superior deep cervical nodes. The hard palate is innervated by branches of the maxillary division of

the trigeminal nerve (CN V$_2$). The anterior one third of the palate is innervated by the nasopalatine nerve, which emerges from the incisive foramen. The posterior two thirds is innervated by the greater palatine nerve, which emerges from the greater palatine foramen along with the greater palatine artery (and the lesser palatine nerves and artery, which innervates and supplies the soft palate).

This view also shows the pterygomandibular raphe, which is a ligament formed from the buccopharyngeal fascia. It attaches superiorly to the pterygoid hamulus and inferiorly to the mylohyoid line of the mandible. The buccinator muscle is attached to the pterygomandibular raphe anteriorly and the superior constrictor of the pharynx posteriorly. The raphe forms an important landmark for the administration of an inferior alveolar nerve block (see p. 511).

Table 8.11 Neurovasculature of the hard palate			
Blood supply	**Venous drainage**	**Innervation**	**Lymphatic drainage**
Greater palatine a., sphenopalatine a.*	Pterygoid plexus	- Anterior one third: nasopalatine n. (from CN V$_2$) - Posterior two thirds: greater palatine n. (from CN V$_2$)	- Submandibular nodes - Superior deep cervical nodes - Retropharyngeal nodes (rarely)

*Supplies the aspect of the hard palate that forms the floor of the nasal cavity.

Table 8.12 Muscles of the soft palate

Muscle	Origin	Insertion	Innervation	Action
Tensor veli palatini	Sphenoid bone (scaphoid fossa of pterygoid process and medial aspect of the spine; it is connected to the anterolateral membranous wall of the pharyngotympanic (auditory tube)	Palatine aponeurosis and palatine bone (horizontal plate) via a tendon that is redirected medially by the pterygoid hamulus	N. to medial pterygoid (CN V$_3$)	*Bilaterally:* tenses anterior portion of the soft palate and flattens its arch, separating the nasopharynx from oropharynx. Opens pharyngotympanic (auditory) tube. *Unilaterally:* deviates soft palate laterally.
Levator veli palatini	Vaginal process and petrous part of temporal bone (via a tendon, anterior to the carotid canal); it is connected to the inferior portion of the pharyngotympanic tube	Palatine aponeurosis (the two levators combine to form a muscular sling)	Vagus n. (CN X) via pharyngeal plexus	*Bilaterally:* pulls the posterior portion of the soft palate superoposteriorly, separating the nasopharynx from the oropharynx.
Uvular muscle (musculus uvulae)	Palatine bone (posterior nasal spine) and palatine aponeurosis (superior surface)	Mucosa of the uvula		Pulls the uvula posterosuperiorly, separating the nasopharynx from the oropharynx.
Palatoglossus (palatoglossal arch)	Palatine aponeurosis (oral surface)	Lateral tongue to dorsum or intrinsic transverse muscle		*Bilaterally:* pulls the root of the tongue superiorly narrowing the oropharngeal isthmus, separating the oral cavity from the oropharynx.

Sensory innervation: lesser palatine nn. (from CN V$_2$)
Blood supply: lesser palatine a. (from maxillary a.), ascending palatine a. (from facial a.), palatine branch of the ascending pharyngeal a. (from external carotid a.)
Venous drainage: greater and lesser palatine vv. to pterygoid plexus
Lymphatic drainage: submandibular nodes, retropharyngeal nodes

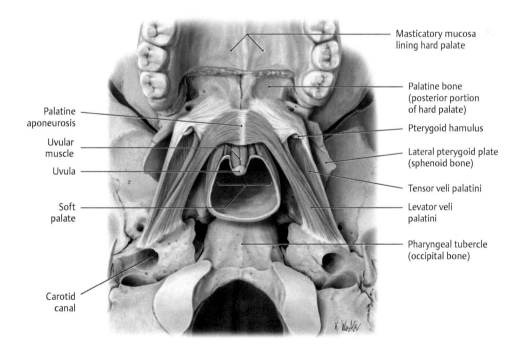

Fig. 8.47 Muscles of the soft palate and pharyngotympanic tube
Inferior view. The soft palate is the aponeurotic and muscular region hanging from the hard palate at the posterior portion of the oral cavity. It separates the oropharynx from the nasopharynx, particularly during swallowing when it is tensed. The palatoglossus restricts the communication between the oral cavity and oropharynx. The tensor veli palatini has a significant role in keeping open the pharyngotympanic (auditory) tube.

Pharynx: Divisions & Contents

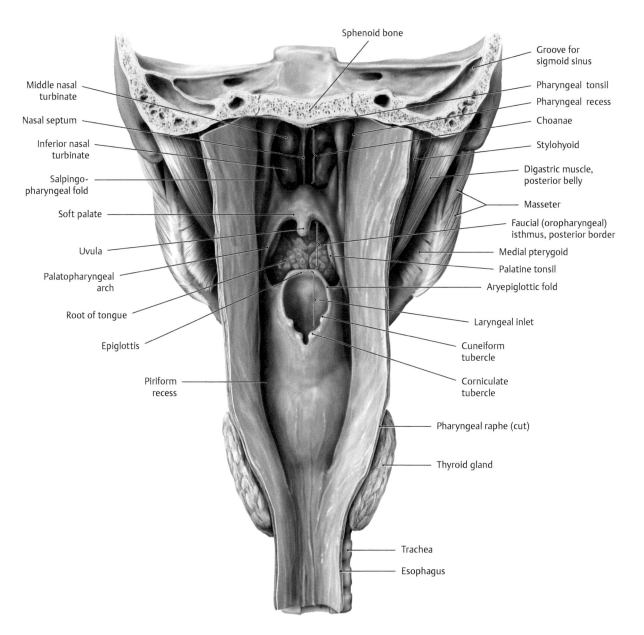

Fig. 8.48 Pharyngeal mucosa and musculature
Posterior view. **A** Mucosal lining. **B** Internal musculature. The muscular posterior wall of the pharynx has been divided along the midline (pharyngeal raphe) and spread open to demonstrate its mucosal anatomy.

Table 8.13 Levels of the pharynx

The anterior portion of the muscular pharyngeal tube communicates with three cavities (nasal, oral, and laryngeal). The three anterior openings divide the pharynx into three parts with corresponding vertebral levels.

Region	Level	Description	Communications	
Nasopharynx (Epipharynx)	C1	Upper portion, lying between the roof (formed by sphenoid and occipital bones) and the soft palate	Nasal cavity	Via choanae
			Tympanic cavity	Via pharyngotympanic tube
Oropharynx (Mesopharynx)	C2–C3	Middle portion, lying between the uvula and the epiglottis	Oral cavity	Via oropharyngeal isthmus (formed by the palatoglossal arch)
Laryngopharynx (Hypopharynx)	C4–C6	Lower portion, lying between the epiglottis and the inferior border of the cricoid cartilage	Larynx	Via laryngeal inlet
			Esophagus	Via cricopharyngeus (pharyngeal sphincter)

Fig. 8.49 Waldeyer's ring

Posterior view of the opened pharynx. Waldeyer's ring is composed of immunocompetent lymphatic tissue (tonsils and lymph follicles). The tonsils are "immunological sentinels" surrounding the passageways from the mouth and nasal cavity to the pharynx. The lymph follicles are distributed over all of the epithelium, showing marked regional variations. Waldeyer's ring consists of the following structures:

- Unpaired pharyngeal tonsil on the roof of the pharynx
- Paired palatine tonsils in the oropharynx between the anterior and posterior pillars (the palatoglossal arch and the palatopharyngeal arch)
- Lingual tonsil, the lymph nodes embedded in the postsulcal portion of the tongue
- Paired tubal tonsils (tonsillae tubariae), which may be thought of as lateral extensions of the pharyngeal tonsil
- Paired lateral bands in the salpingopharyngeal fold

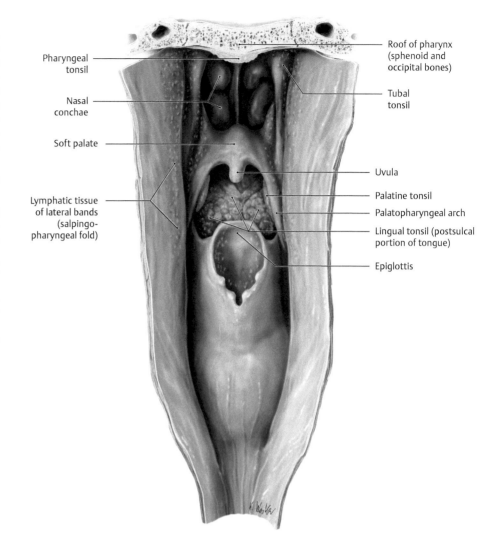

Pharyngeal tonsil

Nasal conchae

Soft palate

Lymphatic tissue of lateral bands (salpingopharyngeal fold)

Roof of pharynx (sphenoid and occipital bones)

Tubal tonsil

Uvula

Palatine tonsil

Palatopharyngeal arch

Lingual tonsil (postsulcal portion of tongue)

Epiglottis

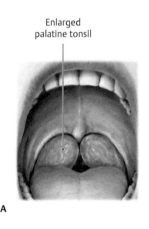

Enlarged palatine tonsil

A

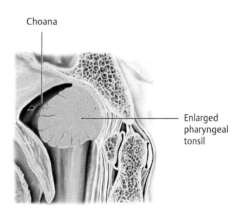

Choana

Enlarged pharyngeal tonsil

B

Fig. 8.50 Abnormal enlargement of the pharyngeal and palatine tonsils

A Anterior view of the oral cavity. **B** Sagittal section through the roof of the pharynx.

A Severe enlargement of the palatine tonsil (due to viral or bacterial infection, as in tonsillitis) may significantly narrow the outlet of the oral cavity, causing difficulty in swallowing (dysphagia). Tonsillectomy, surgical removal of the palatine tonsil from the tonsillar bed along with its accompanying fascia, may damage the glossopharyngeal nerve (CN IX), which lies on the lateral wall of the pharynx. This could result in loss of sensation and taste from the posterior one third of the tongue.

B An enlargement of the pharyngeal tonsil is very common in pre-school-aged children. Chronic recurrent nasopharyngeal infections at that age often evoke a heightened immune response in the lymphatic tissue, causing "adenoids" or "polyps." The enlarged pharyngeal tonsil blocks the choanae, obstructing the nasal airway and forcing the child to breathe through the mouth. Because the mouth is constantly open during respiration at rest, an experienced examiner can quickly diagnose the adenoidal condition by visual inspection.

Muscles of the Pharynx (I)

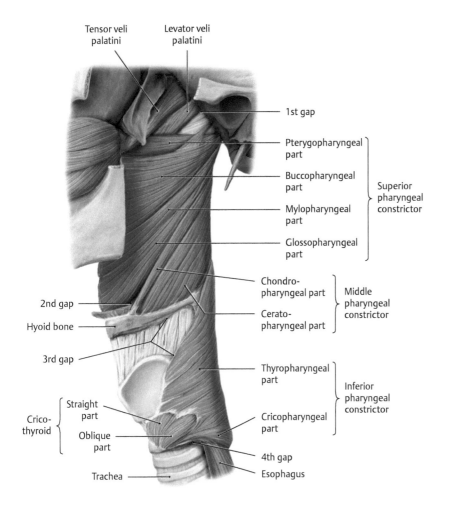

Fig. 8.51 Pharyngeal constrictors
Left lateral view.

Table 8.14 Pharyngeal gaps	
Gap	**Transmitted structures**
1st gap	Pharyngotympanic tube
	Levator veli palatini
2nd gap	Stylopharyngeus (inserts on larynx)
	Glossopharyngeal n. (CN IX)
3rd gap	Internal laryngeal n.
	Superior laryngeal a. and v.
4th gap	Recurrent laryngeal n.
	Inferior laryngeal a.

Table 8.15 Pharyngeal constrictors					
Muscle		**Origin**	**Insertion**	**Innervation**	**Action**
Superior pharyngeal constrictor	Pterygopharyngeus	Pterygoid hamulus (occasionally to the medial pterygoid plate)	Occipital bone (pharyngeal tubercle of basilar part, via median pharyngeal raphe)	Vagus n. (CN X) via pharyngeal plexus	Constricts the upper pharynx
	Buccopharyngeus	Pterygomandibular raphe			
	Mylopharyngeus	Mylohyoid line of mandible			
	Glossopharyngeus	Lateral tongue			
Middle pharyngeal constrictor	Chondropharyngeus	Hyoid (lesser horn) and stylohyoid ligament			Constricts the middle pharynx
	Ceratopharyngeus	Hyoid (greater horn)			
Inferior pharyngeal constrictor	Thyropharyngeus	Thyroid lamina and hyoid bone (inferior horn)			Constricts the lower pharynx
	Cricopharyngeus	Cricoid cartilage (lateral margin)		Recurrent laryngeal n. (CN X) and/or external laryngeal n.	Sphincter at intersection of laryngopharynx and esophagus

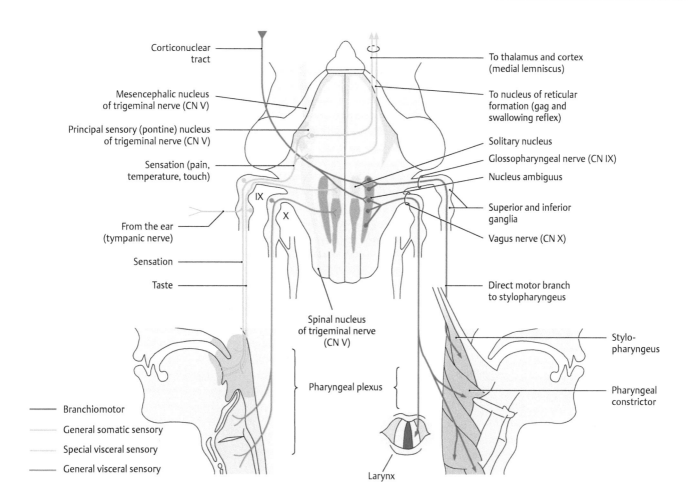

Fig. 8.52 Pharyngeal plexus

The pharynx receives sensory and motor innervation via the pharyngeal plexus, formed by both the glossopharyngeal (CN IX) and vagus (CN X) nerves, along with postganglionic sympathetic fibers from the superior cervical ganglion. *Note:* Only the vagus nerve contributes motor fibers to the plexus (the stylopharyngeus is supplied directly by CN IX).

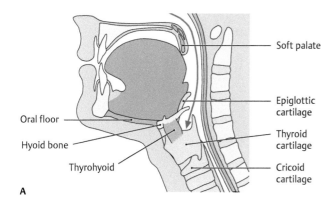

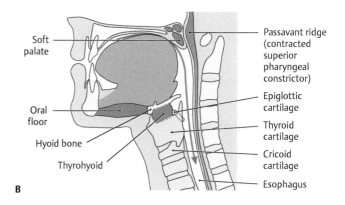

Fig. 8.53 Swallowing

The larynx, part of the airway, is located at the inlet to the digestive tract (**A**). During swallowing (**B**), the airway must be occluded to keep food from entering the larynx and the trachea (preventing choking). Swallowing consists of three phases:

1. Oral stage (voluntary initiation): The lingual muscles move the food bolus to the oropharyngeal isthmus, which first expands and then contracts.

2. Pharyngeal stage (reflex closure of airway): The longitudinal pharyngeal muscles elevate the larynx. The lower airway (laryngeal inlet) is covered by the epiglottis. Meanwhile, the soft palate is tensed and elevated against the posterior pharyngeal wall, sealing off the upper airway.

3. Pharyngoesophageal stage (reflex transport): The constrictors move the food bolus to the stomach.

Muscles of the Pharynx (II)

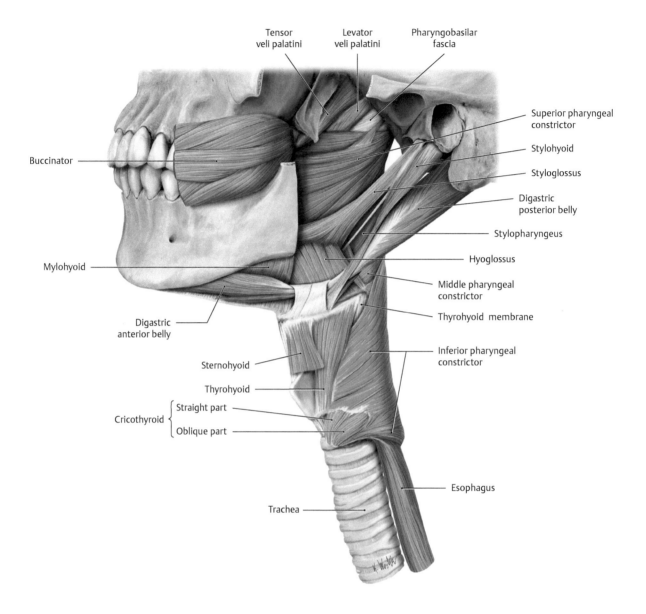

Fig. 8.54 Pharyngeal musculature
Left lateral view.

Table 8.16 Pharyngeal elevators

Muscle	Origin	Insertion	Innervation	Action
Palatopharyngeus (palatopharyngeal arch)	Palatine aponeurosis (superior surface) and posterior border of palatine bone	Thyroid cartilage (posterior border) or lateral pharynx	Vagus n. (CN X) via pharyngeal plexus	*Bilaterally:* Elevates the pharynx anteromedially.
Salpingopharyngeus	Cartilaginous pharyngotympanic tube (inferior surface)	Along salpingopharyngeal fold to palatopharyngeus		*Bilaterally:* Elevates the pharynx; may also open pharyngotympanic tube.
Stylopharyngeus	Styloid process (medial surface of base)	Lateral pharynx, mixing with pharyngeal constrictors, palatopharyngeus, and thyroid cartilage (posterior border)	Glossopharyngeal n. (CN IX)	*Bilaterally:* Elevates the pharynx and larynx.

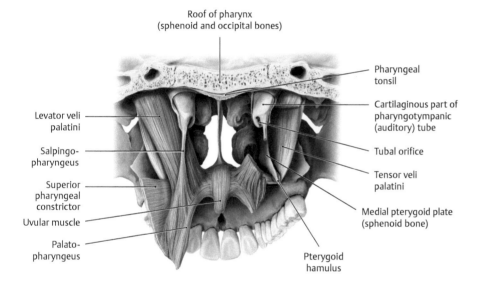

Roof of pharynx
(sphenoid and occipital bones)

Pharyngeal tonsil

Cartilaginous part of pharyngotympanic (auditory) tube

Levator veli palatini

Salpingo-pharyngeus

Superior pharyngeal constrictor

Uvular muscle

Palato-pharyngeus

Tubal orifice

Tensor veli palatini

Medial pterygoid plate (sphenoid bone)

Pterygoid hamulus

Fig. 8.55 Muscles of the soft palate and pharnygeal elevators
Posterior view.

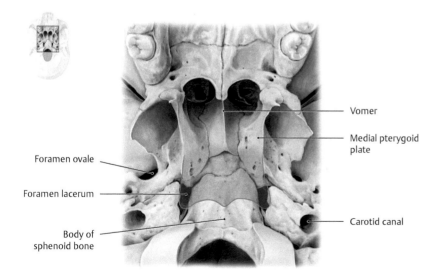

Vomer

Medial pterygoid plate

Foramen ovale

Foramen lacerum

Body of sphenoid bone

Carotid canal

Fig. 8.56 Pharyngobasilar fascia at the base of the skull
Inferior view. The pharyngeal musculature arises from the base of the skull by a thick sheet of connective tissue, the pharyngobasilar fascia its outline is (shown in red). The pharyngobasilar fascia ensures that the nasopharynx is always open.

235

Muscles of the Pharynx (III) & Innervation

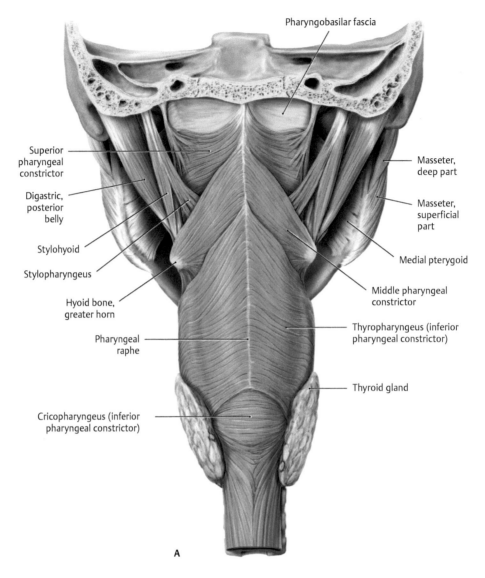

Pharyngobasilar fascia

Superior
pharyngeal
constrictor

Digastric,
posterior
belly

Stylohyoid

Stylopharyngeus

Hyoid bone,
greater horn

Pharyngeal
raphe

Cricopharyngeus (inferior
pharyngeal constrictor)

Masseter,
deep part

Masseter,
superficial
part

Medial pterygoid

Middle pharyngeal
constrictor

Thyropharyngeus (inferior
pharyngeal constrictor)

Thyroid gland

A

Fig. 8.57 Pharyngeal musculature
A Posterior view. **B** Internal musculature. The pharynx is a muscular tube composed of three *pharyngeal constrictors* (**Table 8.15**) and three *pharyngeal elevators* (**Table 8.16**).

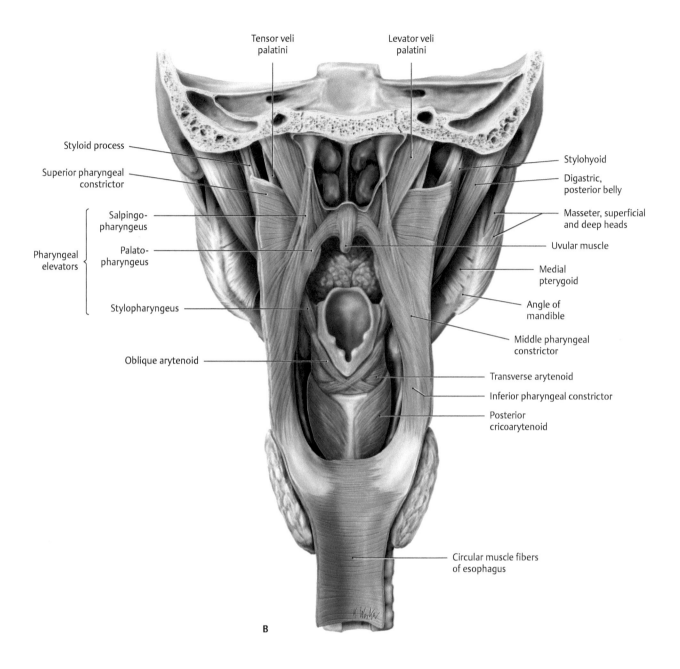

Tensor veli palatini

Levator veli palatini

Styloid process

Superior pharyngeal constrictor

Pharyngeal elevators

Salpingo-pharyngeus

Palato-pharyngeus

Stylopharyngeus

Oblique arytenoid

Stylohyoid

Digastric, posterior belly

Masseter, superficial and deep heads

Uvular muscle

Medial pterygoid

Angle of mandible

Middle pharyngeal constrictor

Transverse arytenoid

Inferior pharyngeal constrictor

Posterior cricoarytenoid

Circular muscle fibers of esophagus

B

Neurovascular Topography of the Pharynx

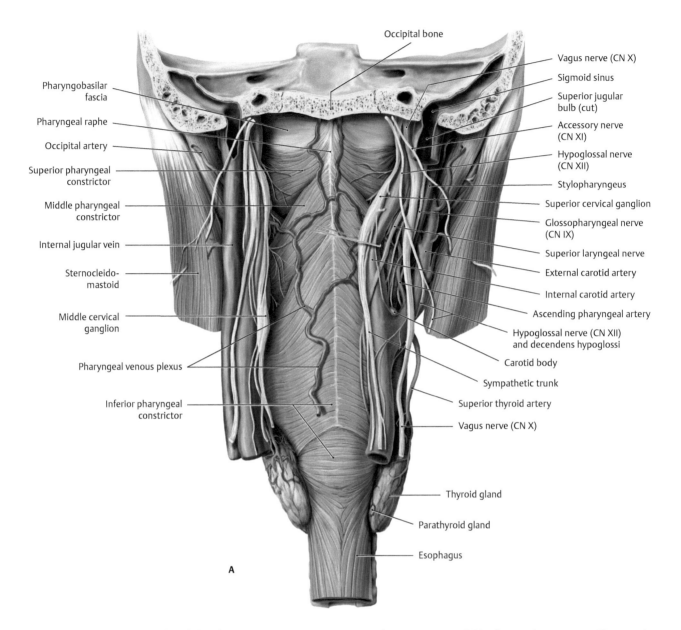

Occipital bone

Vagus nerve (CN X)

Sigmoid sinus

Superior jugular bulb (cut)

Accessory nerve (CN XI)

Hypoglossal nerve (CN XII)

Stylopharyngeus

Superior cervical ganglion

Glossopharyngeal nerve (CN IX)

Superior laryngeal nerve

External carotid artery

Internal carotid artery

Ascending pharyngeal artery

Hypoglossal nerve (CN XII) and decendens hypoglossi

Carotid body

Sympathetic trunk

Superior thyroid artery

Vagus nerve (CN X)

Thyroid gland

Parathyroid gland

Esophagus

Pharyngobasilar fascia

Pharyngeal raphe

Occipital artery

Superior pharyngeal constrictor

Middle pharyngeal constrictor

Internal jugular vein

Sternocleido-mastoid

Middle cervical ganglion

Pharyngeal venous plexus

Inferior pharyngeal constrictor

A

Fig. 8.58 Neurovascular topography of the pharynx
A Posterior view with fascia removed. **B** Posterior view with pharynx opened along pharyngeal raphe.

The majority of the pharyngeal muscles are supplied by motor fibers from the pharyngeal nerve plexus. Exceptions are the stylopharyngeus muscle, which is innervated by a motor branch from glossopharyngeal nerve (CN IX), and the cricopharyngeus muscle (the inferior head of the inferior constrictor), which is generally supplied by the recurrent laryngeal nerve and/or the external laryngeal nerve (occasionally by the pharyngeal plexus). The pharyngeal nerve plexus is composed of both motor and sensory fibers. The glossopharyngeal and vagus nerves (CN

IX and CN X, respectively) both contribute sensory fibers to the nerve plexus; only the vagus nerve distributes motor fibers to the pharyngeal plexus (some of these fibers may be considered to have originated from the spinal accessory nerve [CN XI]). Regardless of origin, they are distributed by the vagus nerve. The plexus also receives autonomic fibers from the cervical sympathetic chain.

Arteries in the region of the pharynx, primarily branches of the external carotid artery, contribute to the vascular supply of the pharyngeal structures. The venous drainage of the posterior wall of the pharynx is primarily into the pharyngeal venous plexus, which in turn drains into the internal jugular vein.

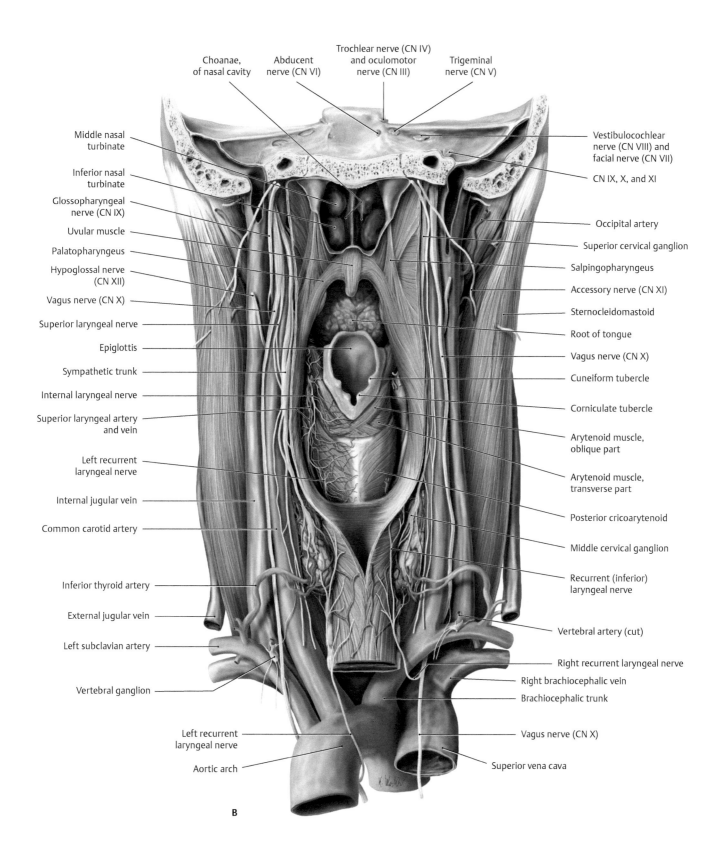

Middle nasal turbinate

Inferior nasal turbinate

Glossopharyngeal nerve (CN IX)

Uvular muscle

Palatopharyngeus

Hypoglossal nerve (CN XII)

Vagus nerve (CN X)

Superior laryngeal nerve

Epiglottis

Sympathetic trunk

Internal laryngeal nerve

Superior laryngeal artery and vein

Left recurrent laryngeal nerve

Internal jugular vein

Common carotid artery

Inferior thyroid artery

External jugular vein

Left subclavian artery

Vertebral ganglion

Left recurrent laryngeal nerve

Aortic arch

Choanae, of nasal cavity

Abducent nerve (CN VI)

Trochlear nerve (CN IV) and oculomotor nerve (CN III)

Trigeminal nerve (CN V)

Vestibulocochlear nerve (CN VIII) and facial nerve (CN VII)

CN IX, X, and XI

Occipital artery

Superior cervical ganglion

Salpingopharyngeus

Accessory nerve (CN XI)

Sternocleidomastoid

Root of tongue

Vagus nerve (CN X)

Cuneiform tubercle

Corniculate tubercle

Arytenoid muscle, oblique part

Arytenoid muscle, transverse part

Posterior cricoarytenoid

Middle cervical ganglion

Recurrent (inferior) laryngeal nerve

Vertebral artery (cut)

Right recurrent laryngeal nerve

Right brachiocephalic vein

Brachiocephalic trunk

Vagus nerve (CN X)

Superior vena cava

B

239

Potential Tissue Spaces in the Head & Spread of Dental Infections

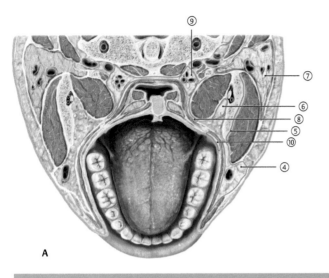

A

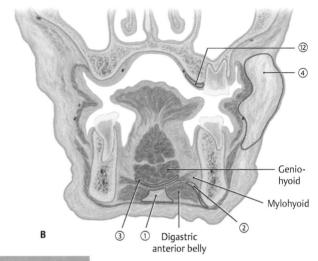

B

Genio-hyoid

Mylohyoid

Digastric
anterior belly

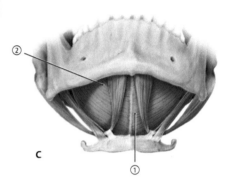

C

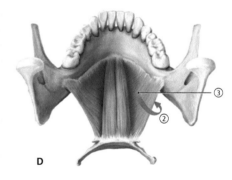

D

Fig. 8.59 Potential tissue spaces in the head

A Transverse section at the level of the occlusal plane of the mandibular teeth, superior view. **B** Coronal section through the molar region of the oral cavity. **C** Floor of the mouth, inferior oblique view. **D** Floor of the mouth, superior view.

Potential tissue spaces in the head become true spaces when they are infiltrated by bacterial products of infection, such as hyaluronidase, which break down the connective tissue in these spaces. These spaces, defined by the positions of bones, muscles, and fascia, initially confine an infection, but because of communication between spaces, infections can travel.

Table 8.17 Potential tissue spaces of the head		
Potential tissue space	**Is located**	**Communicates with**
Around mandible		
① Submental space	Below inferior border of mandible and beneath mylohyoid muscle, at midline of neck (corresponds to submental triangle region)	Submandibular spaces on both sides
② Submandibular space	Below inferior border of mandible and beneath mylohyoid muscle, bounded by anterior and posterior bellies of digastic muscle	Sublingual, submental, and parapharyngeal spaces
③ Sublingual space	Above mylohyoid muscle and below the tongue	Submandibular and paraphayngeal spaces
④ Buccal space	In cheek, lateral to buccinator muscle	Canine, submasseteric, and paraphayngeal spaces, and cavernous sinus
⑤ Submasseteric space	Between lateral surface of ramus of mandible and masseter muscle	Parapharyngeal spaces
⑥ Pterygomandibular space	Between medial surface of ramus and the medial pterygoid muscle	Buccal, infratemporal, parotid, submasseteric, paraphayngeal, and peritonsillar spaces
⑦ Parotid space	Behind ramus of mandible, in and around parotid gland	Parapharyngeal then retropharyngeal spaces with potential spread to mediastinum
⑧ Parapharyngeal space	Lateral to the pharynx in the suprahyoid region of neck	Continuous with retropharyngeal space
⑨ Retropharyngeal space	• Between buccopharyngeal fascia anteriorly and prevertebral fascia posteriorly • Extends from base of skull to retrovisceral space in infrahyoid region of neck	Parapharyngeal, submandibular, sublingual, submasseteric, and peritonsillar spaces, and mediastinum
⑩ Peritonsillar	Around palatine tonsils between pillars of fauces, bounded by the medial surface of the superior constrictor muscle	Submandibular and sublingual spaces
Around maxilla		
⑪ Canine space	Between levator anguli oris and levator labii superioris	Cavernous sinus
⑫ Palatal space	Between periosteum and mucosa of hard palate mucosa	None
⑬ Infratemporal space	Within infratemporal fossa	Pterygomandibular and buccal spaces, cavernous sinus (via pterygoid plexus)

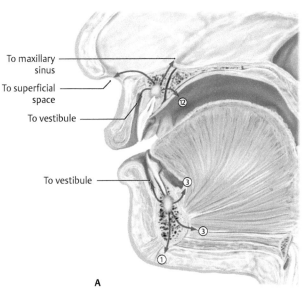

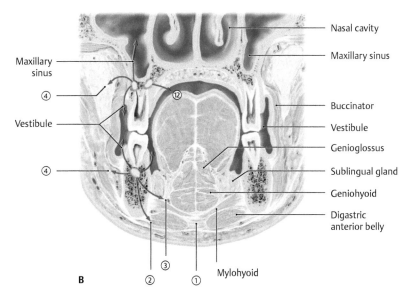

A

B

Table 8.18 Route of infection from dental source		
Source of infection	**Route of infection**	**Symptoms**
Mandibular anterior teeth	Below attachment of mylohoid to ① submental space	Swelling under chin
Mandibular molars	Below attachment of mylohyoid to ② submandibular space	Swelling in submandibular region, resulting in difficulty swallowing (dysphagia), difficulty breathing (dyspnea), and difficulty articulating speech (dysarthria), and neck pain and swelling, drooling, earache, and malaise (=Ludwig angina)
Mandibular premolars/molars	Below geniohyoid and above mylohyoid to ③ sublingual space	Swelling in floor of mouth, resulting in elevated tongue and difficulty speaking and swallowing
Maxillary or mandibular premolars/molars	Above (for maxillary teeth) or below (for mandibular teeth) the attachment of buccinators to ④ buccal space	Extensive swelling of cheek, which may extend to the upper lip or eye
Mandibular third molars	Posterolaterally between lateral aspect of ramus of mandible and masseter to ⑤ submassateric space	Pain, trismus,* swelling of tonsillar pillars
	Posteriorly between the medial aspect of ramus of mandible and medial pterygoid to ⑥ pterygomandibular space	Trismus,* intraoral swelling along the medial aspect of the mandible
Maxillary or mandibular molars	Posteromedially to enter ⑧ parapharyngeal space then to ⑨ retropharyngeal space	Pain, trismus,* swollen soft palate with deviated uvula, difficulty swallowing, difficulty breathing (airway obstruction could be life-threatening)
Maxillary anterior teeth (usually canines)	Above origin of levator anguli oris to ⑪ canine space	Swelling along lateral border of nose, which may extend to periorbital region; eyelids may become swollen shut
Maxillary premolars or molars	From the palatal root into ⑫ palatal space	Small, painful swelling of palate
Maxillary molars	Posteriorly to ⑬ infratemporal space	Severe trismus,* bulging of temporalis, intraoral swelling in region of maxillary tuberosity

* Trismus is spasm of the muscles of mastication that results in the inability to open the mouth.

Fig. 8.60 Potential routes for the spread of infection from apical dental abscesses

A Sagittal section through canines (anterior teeth). **B** Coronal section through molars (posterior teeth). **C** Transverse section of area posterior to the third molar tooth, superior view.

Apical dental infections may spread to a number of regions in the head and neck, including the superficial facial space, the palate, the vestibule, the maxillary sinus, and the sublingual, submandibular, and submental spaces. Infections entering into the sublingual and submandibular spaces may ultimately reach the mediastinum through their posterior communications with the parapharyngeal spaces; these spaces in turn communicate with the retropharyngeal space and the carotid sheaths. Infections in mandibular third molar teeth may spread to the buccal, submasseteric, pterygopalatine, and parapharyngeal spaces.

Bones of the Orbit

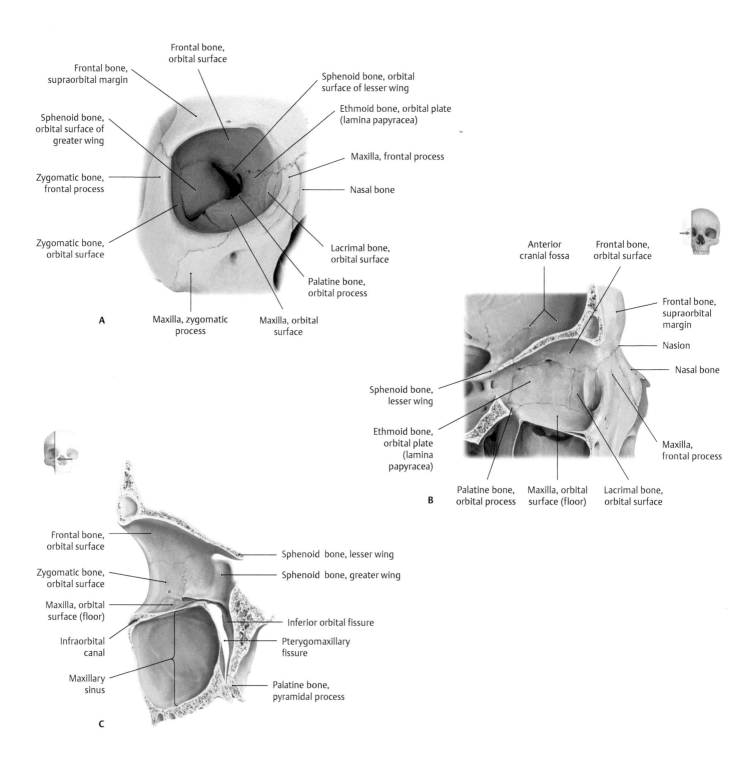

Fig. 9.1 Bones of the orbit
Right orbit. **A,D** Anterior view. **B,E** Lateral view with lateral orbital wall removed. **C,F** Medial view with medial orbit wall removed. The orbit is formed by seven bones: the frontal, zygomatic, ethmoid, sphenoid, lacrimal, and palatine bones, and the maxilla. The neurovascular structures of the orbit communicate with the surrounding spaces via several major passages (see **Table 9.1**): the superior and inferior orbital fissures, the optic canal, the anterior and posterior ethmoidal foramina, the infraorbital canal, and the nasolacrimal duct. The neurovascular structures of the orbit also communicate with the superficial face by passing through the orbital rim. *Note:* The exposed maxillary sinus can be seen in the medial and lateral views. The maxillary hiatus contains the ostium by which the maxillary sinus opens into the nasal cavity superior to the inferior nasal concha. The inferior orbital fissure is continuous inferoposteriorly with the pterygomaxillary fissure, which is the boundary between the infratemporal and pterygopalatine fossae. The infratemporal fossa is on the lateral side of the pterygomaxillary fissure; the pterygopalatine fossa is on the medial side.

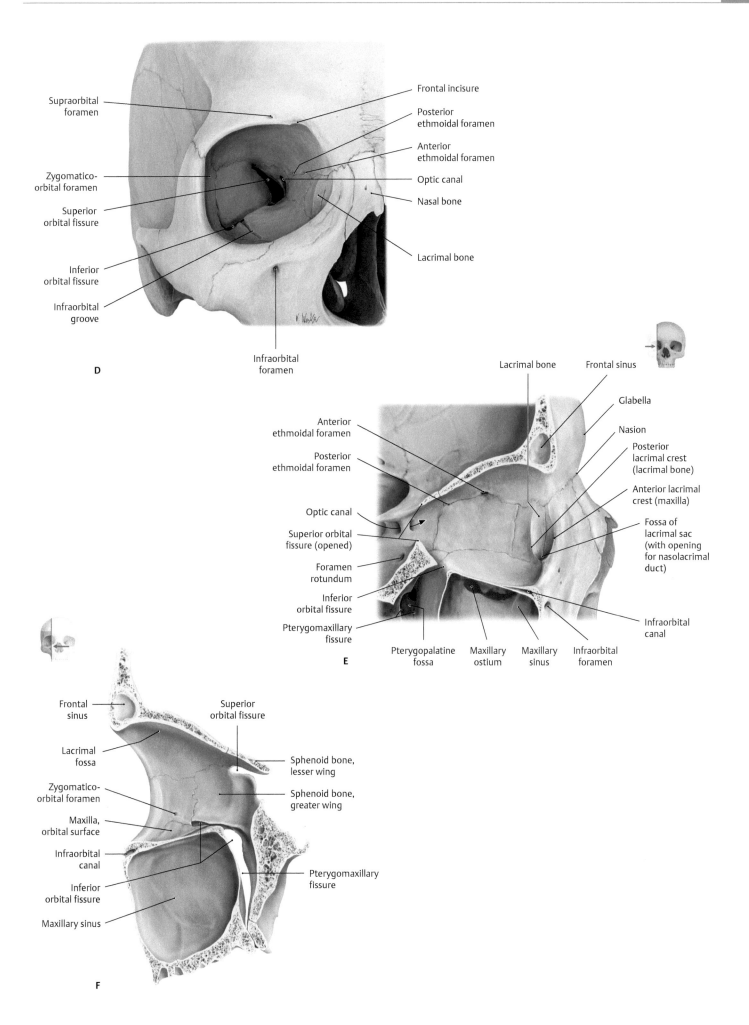

Supraorbital foramen

Frontal incisure

Posterior ethmoidal foramen

Anterior ethmoidal foramen

Zygomatico-orbital foramen

Optic canal

Superior orbital fissure

Nasal bone

Lacrimal bone

Inferior orbital fissure

Infraorbital groove

Infraorbital foramen

D

Lacrimal bone

Frontal sinus

Anterior ethmoidal foramen

Glabella

Posterior ethmoidal foramen

Nasion

Posterior lacrimal crest (lacrimal bone)

Optic canal

Anterior lacrimal crest (maxilla)

Superior orbital fissure (opened)

Fossa of lacrimal sac (with opening for nasolacrimal duct)

Foramen rotundum

Inferior orbital fissure

Pterygomaxillary fissure

Infraorbital canal

Pterygopalatine fossa

Maxillary ostium

Maxillary sinus

Infraorbital foramen

E

Frontal sinus

Superior orbital fissure

Lacrimal fossa

Sphenoid bone, lesser wing

Zygomatico-orbital foramen

Sphenoid bone, greater wing

Maxilla, orbital surface

Infraorbital canal

Pterygomaxillary fissure

Inferior orbital fissure

Maxillary sinus

F

Communications of the Orbit

Fig. 9.2 Bones of the orbit and adjacent cavities

Coronal section, anterior view. The bones of the orbit also form portions of the walls of neighboring cavities. Disease processes may originate in the orbit and spread to these cavities, or originate in these cavities and spread to the orbit.

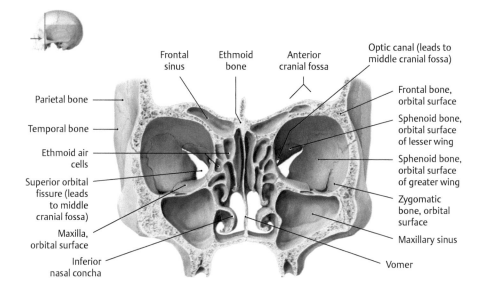

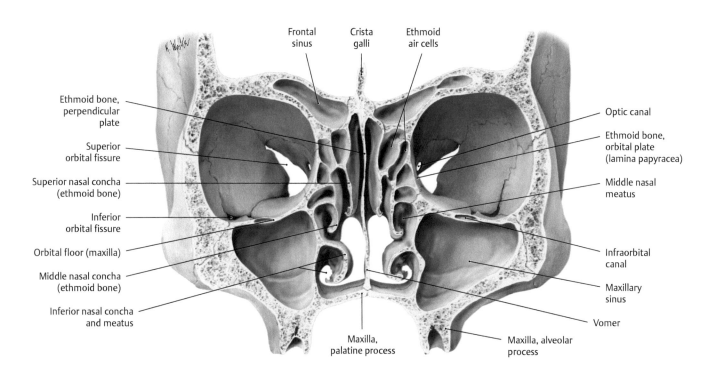

Fig. 9.3 Orbits and neighboring structures

Coronal section through both orbits, anterior view. The walls separating the orbit from the ethmoid air cells (0.3 mm, lamina papyracea) and from the maxillary sinus (0.5 mm, orbital floor) are very thin. Thus, both of these walls are susceptible to fractures and provide routes for the spread of tumors and inflammatory processes into or out of the orbit. The superior orbital fissure communicates with the middle cranial fossa, and so several structures that are not pictured here—the sphenoid sinus, pituitary gland, and optic chiasm—are also closely related to the orbit.

Table 9.1 Communications of the orbit

Structure	Communicates	Via	Neurovascular structures in canal/fissure
Frontal sinus and anterior ethmoid air cells	Superiorly	Unnamed canaliculi	• Sensory filaments
	Medially	Anterior ethmoidal canal	• Anterior ethmoidal a. (from ophthalmic a.) • Anterior ethmoidal v. (to superior ophthalmic v.) • Anterior ethmoidal n. (CN V$_1$)
Sphenoid sinus and posterior ethmoid air cells	Medially	Posterior ethmoidal canal	• Posterior ethmoidal a. (from ophthalmic a.) • Posterior ethmoidal v. (to superior ophthalmic v.) • Posterior ethmoidal n. (CN V$_1$)

Middle cranial fossa	Posteriorly	Superior orbital fissure	• Cranial nerves to the extraocular muscles (oculomotor n. [CN III], trochlear n. [CN IV], and abducent n. [CN VI])
			• Ophthalmic n. (CN V$_1$) and branches:
			  ◦ Lacrimal n.
			  ◦ Frontal n. (branches into supraorbital and supratrochlear nn.)
			  ◦ Nasociliary n. (branches into anterior and posterior ethmoidal nn. and infratrochlear n.)
			• Superior (and occasionally inferior) ophthalmic v. (to cavernous sinus)
			• Recurrent meningeal branch of lacrimal a. (anastomoses with middle meningeal a.)

	Posteriorly	Optic canal	• Optic n. (CN II) • Ophthalmic a. (from internal carotid a.)
Pterygopalatine fossa	Posteroinferiorly (medially)	Inferior orbital fissure*	• Infraorbital a. (from maxillary a.) • Infraorbital v. (to pterygoid plexus)* • Infraorbital n. (CN V$_2$)
Infratemporal fossa	Posteroinferiorly (laterally)		• Zygomatic n. (CN V$_2$) • Inferior ophthalmic v. (variable, to cavernous sinus)
Nasal cavity	Inferomedially	Nasolacrimal canal	• Nasolacrimal duct
Maxillary sinus	Inferiorly	Unnamed canaliculi	• Sensory filaments
Face and temporal fossa	Anteriorly	Zygomaticofacial canal	• Zygomaticofacial n. (CN V$_2$) • Anastomotic branch of lacrimal a. (to transverse facial and zygomatico-orbital aa.)
		Zygomaticotemporal canal	• Zygomaticotemporal n. (CN V$_2$) • Anastomotic branch of lacrimal a. (to deep temporal aa.)
Face	Anteriorly	Supraorbital foramen (notch)	• Supraorbital n., lateral branch (CN V$_1$) • Supraorbital a. (from ophthalmic a.) • Supraorbital v. (to angular v.)
		Frontal incisure	• Supratrochlear a. (from ophthalmic a.) • Supratrochlear n. (CN V$_1$) • Supraorbital n., medial branch (CN V$_1$)
		Orbital rim, medial aspect	• Infratrochlear n. (CN V$_1$) • Dorsal nasal a. (from ophthalmic a.) • Dorsal nasal v. (to angular v.)
		Orbital rim, lateral aspect	• Lacrimal n. (CN V$_1$) • Lacrimal a. (from ophthalmic a.) • Lacrimal v. (to superior ophthalmic v.)

* The infraorbital a., v., and n. travel in the infraorbital canal on the floor of the orbit and emerge at the inferior orbital fissure. The inferior orbital fissure is continuous inferiorly with the pterygomaxillary fissure, which is the boundary between the infratemporal and the pterygopalatine fossa. The infratemporal fossa lies on the lateral side of the pterygomaxillary fissure; the pterygopalatine fossa lies on the medial side.

Extraocular Muscles

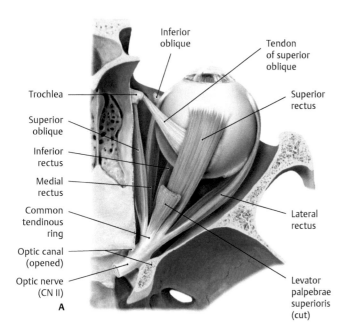

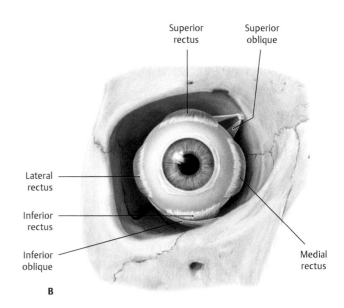

Fig. 9.4 Extraocular (extrinsic eye) muscles
Right eye. **A** Superior view. **B** Anterior view. The eyeball is moved in the orbit by four rectus muscles (superior, medial, inferior, lateral) and two oblique muscles (superior and inferior). The four rectus muscles arise from a tendinous ring around the optic canal (common tendinous ring, common annular tendon) and insert on the sclera of the eyeball. The superior and inferior obliques arise from the body of the sphenoid and the medial orbital margin of the maxilla, respectively. The superior oblique passes through a tendinous loop (trochlea) attached to the superomedial orbital margin (frontal bone); this redirects it at an acute angle to its insertion on the superior surface of the eyeball. The coordinated interaction of all six functionally competent extraocular muscles is necessary for directing both eyes toward the visual target. The brain then processes the two perceived retinal images in a way that provides binocular vision perception. Impaired function of one or more extraocular muscles causes deviation of the eye from its normal position, resulting in diplopia (double vision). This impaired function may be due to trauma to CN III, IV, and VI or due to diseases that affect nerves, e.g., multiple sclerosis (MS) or diabetes.

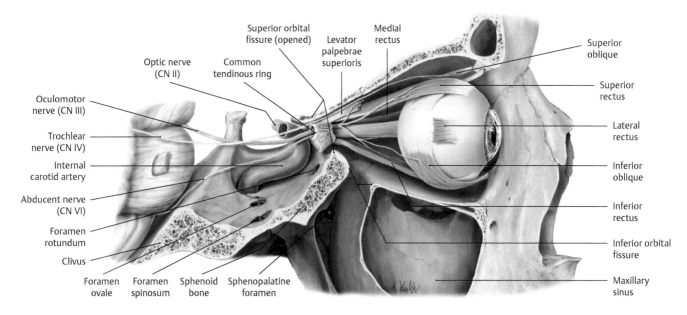

Fig. 9.5 Innervation of the extraocular muscles
Right eye, lateral view with the lateral wall of the orbit removed. The extraocular muscles are supplied by cranial nerves III, IV, and VI (see **Table 9.2**). *Note:* Levator palpebrae superioris is also supplied by CN III. After emerging from the brainstem, these cranial nerves first traverse the cavernous sinus, where they are in close proximity to the internal carotid artery. From there they pass through the superior orbital fissure to enter the orbit and supply their respective muscles. The optic nerve (CN II) enters the orbit via the more medially located optic canal (see **Fig. 9.1D**).

Fig. 9.6 **Actions of the extraocular muscles**

Right eye, superior view with orbital roof removed. Primary actions (red), secondary actions (blue).

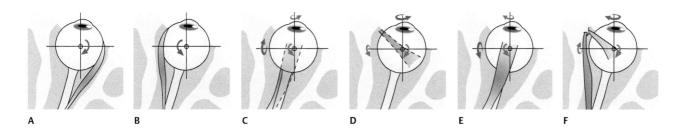

A   B   C   D   E   F

Muscle	Primary action	Secondary action	Innervation
A Lateral rectus	Abduction	–	Abducent n. (CN VI)
B Medial rectus	Adduction	–	Oculomotor n. (CN III), inferior branch
C Inferior rectus	Depression	Adduction and lateral rotation	
D Inferior oblique	Elevation and abduction	Lateral rotation	
E Superior rectus	Elevation	Adduction and medial rotation	Oculomotor n. (CN III), superior branch
F Superior oblique	Depression and abduction	Medial rotation	Trochlear n. (CN IV)

Table 9.2 **Actions and innervation of the extraocular muscles**

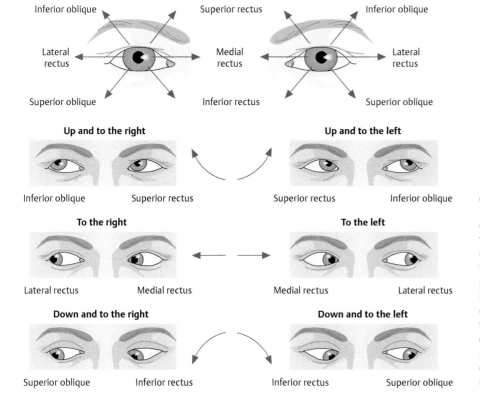

Fig. 9.7 **The six cardinal directions of gaze**

In the clinical evaluation of ocular motility to diagnose *oculomotor palsies,* six cardinal directions of gaze are tested (see arrows). Note that different muscles may be activated in each eye for any particular direction of gaze. For example, gaze to the right is effected by the combined actions of the lateral rectus of the right eye and the medial rectus of the left eye. These two muscles, moreover, are supplied by different cranial nerves (VI and III, respectively).

If one muscle is weak or paralyzed, deviation of the eye will be noted during certain ocular movements (see **Fig. 9.9**).

Innervation of the Extraocular Muscles (CN III, IV, & VI)

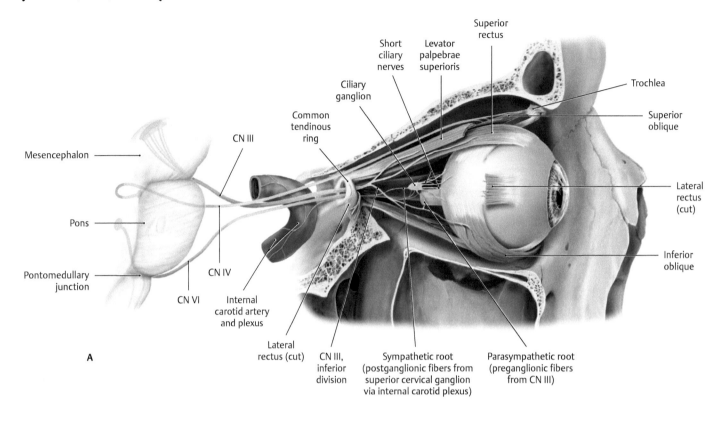

A

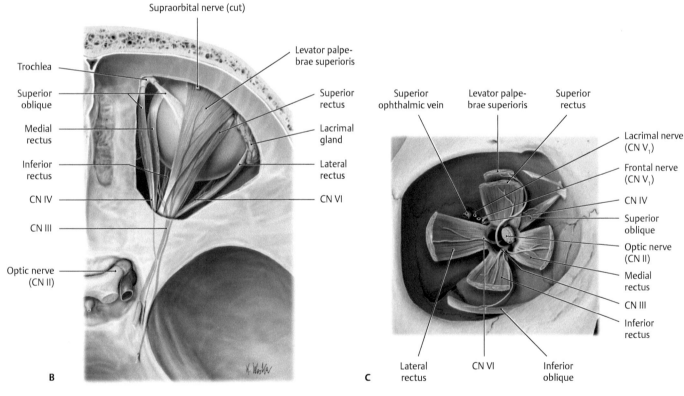

B

C

Fig. 9.8 Nerves supplying the ocular muscles

Right orbit. **A** Lateral view with temporal wall removed. **B** Superior view of opened orbit. **C** Anterior view. Cranial nerves III, IV, and VI enter the orbit through the superior orbital fissure, lateral to the optic canal (CN IV then passes lateral to the common tendinous ring, and CN III and VI pass through it). All three nerves supply somatomotor innervation to the extraocular muscles. See Chapter 4 for a full discussion of CN III, IV, and VI. Of the three, only the oculomotor nerve (CN III) contains both somatic and visceral fibers; it is also the only one that innervates multiple extraocular and intraocular muscles.

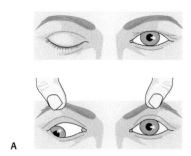
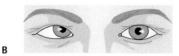
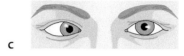

A   B   C

Fig. 9.9 Oculomotor palsies
Palsy of the right side shown during attempted straight-ahead gaze.
A Complete oculomotor palsy. **B** Trochlear palsy. **C** Abducent palsy.
Oculomotor palsies may result from lesions involving the cranial nerve nucleus, the course of the nerve, or the eye muscle itself. Depending on the involved muscle, symptoms may include deviated position of the affected eye and diplopia. The patient attempts to compensate for this by adjusting the position of the head.

A **Complete oculomotor (CN III) palsy:** Affects four extraocular muscles, two intraocular muscles (see **Table 9.3**), and the levator palpebrae superioris. Symptoms and affected muscle(s): Eyeball deviates toward lower outer quadrant = disabled superior, inferior, and medial recti and inferior oblique. Mydriasis (pupil dilation) = disabled pupillary sphincter. Loss of near accommodation = disabled ciliary muscle. Ptosis (drooping of eyelid) = disabled levator palpebrae superioris. The palpebral fissure cannot be opened during complete ptosis in which both the levator palpebrae superioris (CN III) and superior tarsus (sympathetic) muscles are paralyzed. Diplopia will therefore not be observed.

B **Trochlear nerve (CN IV) palsy:** Eye deviates slightly superomedially, causing diplopia = disabled superior oblique.

C **Abducent nerve (CN VI) palsy:** Eye deviates medially, causing diplopia = disabled lateral rectus.

Table 9.3 Cranial nerves of the extraocular muscles

Course*	Fibers	Nuclei	Function	Effects of nerve injury
Oculomotor nerve (CN III)				
Runs anteriorly from mesencephalon	Somatic efferent	Oculomotor nucleus	Innervates: • Levator palpebrae superioris • Superior, medial, and inferior rectus • Inferior oblique	Complete oculomotor palsy (paralysis of extra and intraocular muscles): • Ptosis (drooping of eyelid) • Downward and lateral gaze deviation • Diplopia (double vision) • Mydriasis (pupil dilation) • Accommodation difficulties (ciliary paralysis)
	Visceral efferent	Visceral oculomotor (Edinger-Westphal) nucleus	Synapse with neurons in ciliary ganglia. Innervates: • Pupillary sphincter • Ciliary muscle	
Trochlear nerve (CN IV)				
Emerges from posterior surface of brainstem near midline, courses anteriorly around the cerebral peduncle	Somatic efferent	Nucleus of the trochlear n.	Innervates: • Superior oblique	• Diplopia • Affected eye is higher and deviated medially (dominance of inferior oblique)
Abducent nerve (CN VI)				
Follows a long extradural path**	Somatic efferent	Nucleus of the abducent n.	Innervates: • Lateral rectus	• Diplopia • Medial strabismas (due to unopposed action of medial rectus)

* All three nerves enter the orbit through the superior orbital fissure; CN III and CN VI pass through the common tendinous ring of the extraocular muscles.
** The abducent nerve follows an extradural course; abducent nerve palsy may therefore develop in association with meningitis and subarachnoid hemorrhage.

Neurovasculature of the Orbit

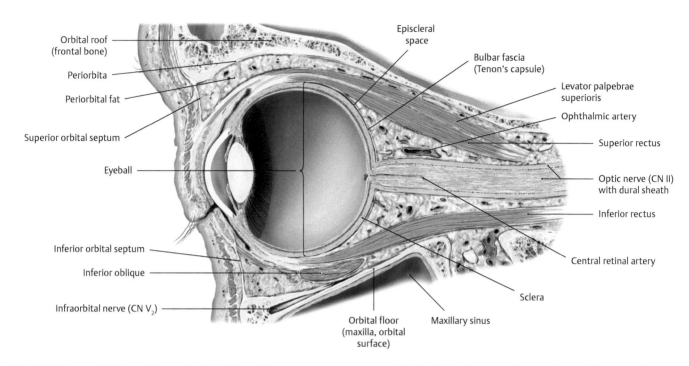

Fig. 9.10 Upper, middle, and lower levels of the orbit
Right orbit. Sagittal section viewed from the medial side. The orbit is lined with periosteum (periorbita) and filled with periorbital fat, which is bounded anteriorly by the orbital septa and toward the eyeball by a mobile sheath of connective tissue (bulbar fascia, Tenon's capsule). The narrow space between the bulbar fascia and sclera is called the episcleral space. Embedded in the periorbital fat are the eyeball, optic nerve, lacrimal gland, extraocular muscles, and associated neurovascular structures. Topographically, the orbit is divided into three levels:

- Upper level: orbital roof to levator palpebrae superioris
- Middle level: superior rectus to optic nerve
- Lower level: optic nerve to orbital floor

Table 9.4	Neurovascular contents of the orbit	
Orbital level	**Arteries and veins**	**Nerves**

Upper level	• Lacrimal a. (from ophthalmic a.)
	• Lacrimal v. (to superior ophthalmic v.)
	• Supraorbital a. (terminal branch of ophthalmic a.)
	• Supraorbital v. (forms angular v. with supratrochlear v.)
		• Lacrimal n. (CN V$_1$)
		• Frontal n. (CN V$_1$) and terminal branches:
		  ○ Supraorbital n.
		  ○ Supratrochlear n.
		• Trochlear n. (CN IV)

Middle level	• Ophthalmic a. (from internal carotid a.) and branches:
	  ○ Central retinal a.
	  ○ Posterior ciliary aa.
	• Superior ophthalmic v. (to cavernous sinus)
		• Nasociliary n. (CN V$_1$)
		• Abducent n. (CN VI)
		• Oculomotor n. (CN III), superior branch and fibers from inferior branch (to ciliary ganglion)
		• Optic n. (CN II)
		• Ciliary ganglion and roots:
		  ○ Parasympathetic root (presynaptic autonomic fibers from CN III)
		  ○ Sympathetic root (postsynaptic fibers from superior cervical ganglion)
		  ○ Sensory root (sensory fibers from eyeball to nasociliary n.)
		• Short ciliary nn. (fibers from/to ciliary ganglion)

Lower level	• Infraorbital a. (terminal branch of maxillary a.) • Inferior ophthalmic v. (to cavernous sinus and/or pterygoid plexus)	• Infraorbital n. (CN V$_2$) • Oculomotor n. (CN III), inferior branch

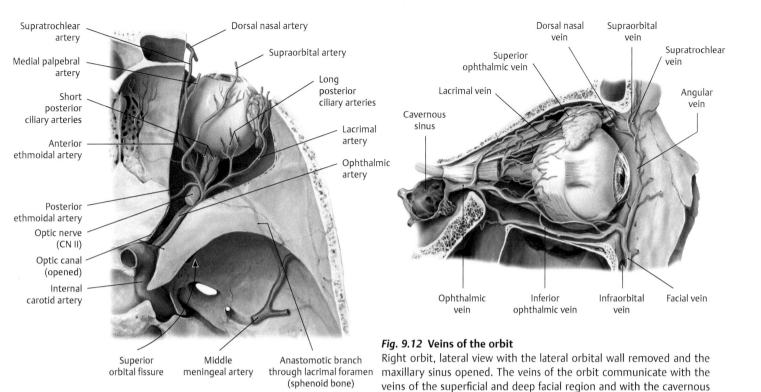

Fig. 9.11 Branches of the ophthalmic artery
Superior view of opened right orbit. While running below CN II in the optic canal, the ophthalmic artery gives off the central retinal artery, which pierces and travels with CN II. The ophthalmic artery then exits the canal and branches to supply the intraorbital structures (including the eyeball).

Fig. 9.12 Veins of the orbit
Right orbit, lateral view with the lateral orbital wall removed and the maxillary sinus opened. The veins of the orbit communicate with the veins of the superficial and deep facial region and with the cavernous sinus (potential spread of infectious pathogens, see **Fig. 3.23**).

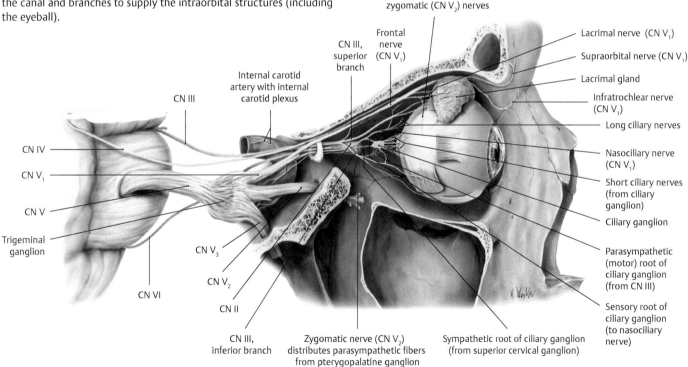

Fig. 9.13 Innervation of the orbit
Lateral view of opened right orbit. The extraocular muscles receive motor innervation from three cranial nerves: oculomotor (CN III), trochlear (CN IV), and abducent (CN VI). The ciliary ganglion distributes parasympathetic fibers to the intraocular muscles via the short ciliary nerves. Parasympathetic fibers reach the ganglion via the inferior branch of CN III. Sympathetic fibers from the superior cervical ganglion travel along the internal carotid artery to the superior orbital fissure. In the orbit, sympathetic fibers run with the nasociliary nerve (CN V₁) and/or ophthalmic artery and pass through the ciliary ganglion (the nasociliary nerve also gives off direct sensory branches, the long ciliary nerves, which may carry postganglionic sympathetic fibers). Sensory fibers from the eyeball pass through the ciliary ganglion to the nasociliary nerve (CN V₁). *Note:* Parasympathetic fibers to the lacrimal gland are distributed by the lacrimal nerve (CN V₁), which communicates with the zygomatic nerve (CN V₂) via a communicating branch from the zygomaticotemporal nerve. The zygomatic nerve distributes "hitchhiking" postganglionic fibers from the pterygopalatine ganglion (the preganglionic fibers arise from CN VII).

251

Topography of the Orbit (I)

Fig. 9.14 Intracavernous course of the cranial nerves that enter to the orbit

Anterior and middle cranial fossae on the right side, superior view. The lateral and superior walls of the cavernous sinus have been opened. The trigeminal ganglion has been retracted slightly laterally, the orbital roof has been removed, and the periorbita has been fenestrated. All three of the cranial nerves that supply the ocular muscles (oculomotor nerve, trochlear nerve, and abducent nerve) enter the cavernous sinus, where they come into close relationship with the first and second divisions of the trigeminal nerve and with the internal carotid artery. While the third and fourth cranial nerves course in the lateral wall of the cavernous sinus with the ophthalmic and maxillary divisions of the trigeminal nerve, the abducent nerve runs directly through the cavernous sinus in close proximity to the internal carotid artery. Because of this relationship, the abducent nerve may be damaged as a result of sinus thrombosis or an intracavernous aneurysm of the internal carotid artery.

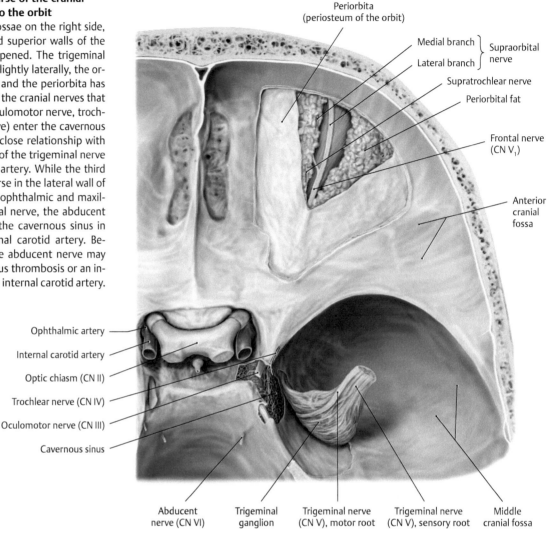

Fig. 9.15 Neurovasculature in the optic canal and superior orbital fissure

Right orbit, anterior view with most of the orbital contents removed.

Optic canal: optic nerve (CN II) and ophthalmic artery.

Superior orbital fissure (inside common tendinous ring): abducent (CN VI), nasociliary (CN V₁), and oculomotor (CN III) nerves.

Superior orbital fissure (outside common tendinous ring): superior and inferior ophthalmic veins, frontal (CN V₁), lacrimal (CN V₁), and trochlear (CN IV) nerves.

Inferior orbital fissure (contents not shown): zygomatic (CN V₂) nerve and branches, infraorbital artery, vein, and nerve in infraorbital canal.

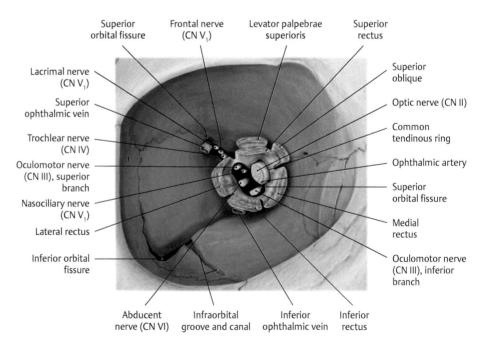

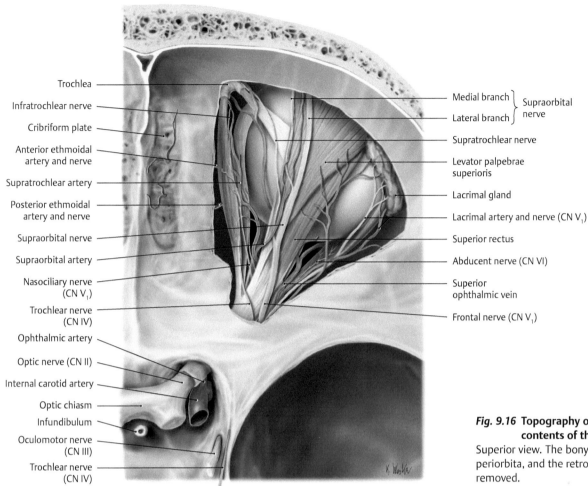

Trochlea

Infratrochlear nerve

Cribriform plate

Anterior ethmoidal artery and nerve

Supratrochlear artery

Posterior ethmoidal artery and nerve

Supraorbital nerve

Supraorbital artery

Nasociliary nerve (CN V₁)

Trochlear nerve (CN IV)

Ophthalmic artery

Optic nerve (CN II)

Internal carotid artery

Optic chiasm

Infundibulum

Oculomotor nerve (CN III)

Trochlear nerve (CN IV)

Medial branch ⎫ Supraorbital
Lateral branch ⎭ nerve

Supratrochlear nerve

Levator palpebrae superioris

Lacrimal gland

Lacrimal artery and nerve (CN V₁)

Superior rectus

Abducent nerve (CN VI)

Superior ophthalmic vein

Frontal nerve (CN V₁)

***Fig. 9.16* Topography of the right orbit: contents of the upper level**
Superior view. The bony roof of the orbit, the periorbita, and the retro-orbital fat have been removed.

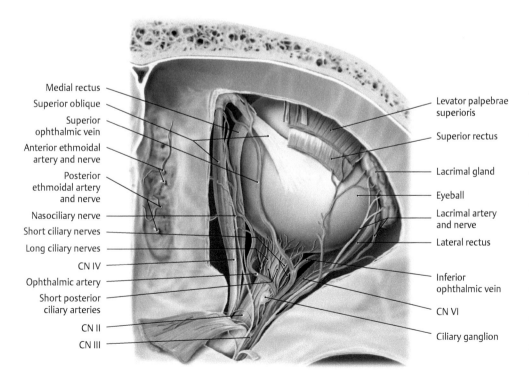

Medial rectus

Superior oblique

Superior ophthalmic vein

Anterior ethmoidal artery and nerve

Posterior ethmoidal artery and nerve

Nasociliary nerve

Short ciliary nerves

Long ciliary nerves

CN IV

Ophthalmic artery

Short posterior ciliary arteries

CN II

CN III

Levator palpebrae superioris

Superior rectus

Lacrimal gland

Eyeball

Lacrimal artery and nerve

Lateral rectus

Inferior ophthalmic vein

CN VI

Ciliary ganglion

***Fig. 9.17* Topography of the right orbit: contents of the middle level**
Superior view. The levator palpebrae superioris and the superior rectus have been divided and reflected backward, and all fatty tissue has been removed to better expose the optic nerve.
Note: The ciliary ganglion is approximately 2 mm in diameter and lies lateral to the optic nerve approximately 2 cm behind the eyeball. The ciliary ganglion relays parasympathetic fibers to the eye and intraocular muscles via the short ciliary nerves. The short ciliary nerves also contain sensory and sympathetic fibers (see **Fig. 9.13**).

253

Topography of the Orbit (II)

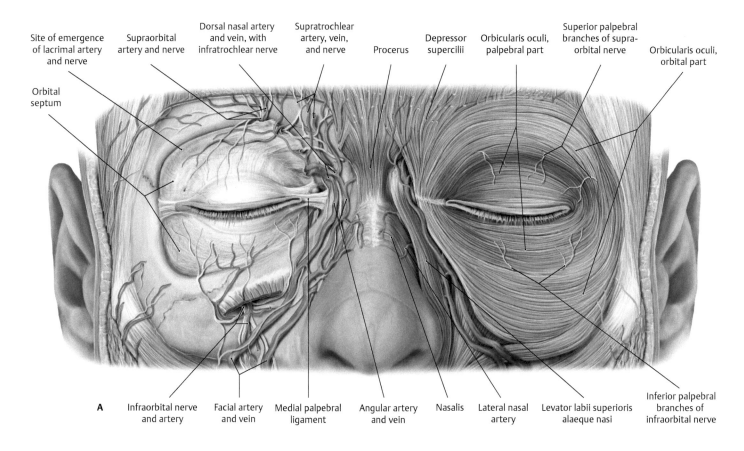

A

Labels (clockwise from top left):
- Site of emergence of lacrimal artery and nerve
- Supraorbital artery and nerve
- Dorsal nasal artery and vein, with infratrochlear nerve
- Supratrochlear artery, vein, and nerve
- Procerus
- Depressor supercilii
- Orbicularis oculi, palpebral part
- Superior palpebral branches of supraorbital nerve
- Orbicularis oculi, orbital part
- Orbital septum
- Infraorbital nerve and artery
- Facial artery and vein
- Medial palpebral ligament
- Angular artery and vein
- Nasalis
- Lateral nasal artery
- Levator labii superioris alaeque nasi
- Inferior palpebral branches of infraorbital nerve

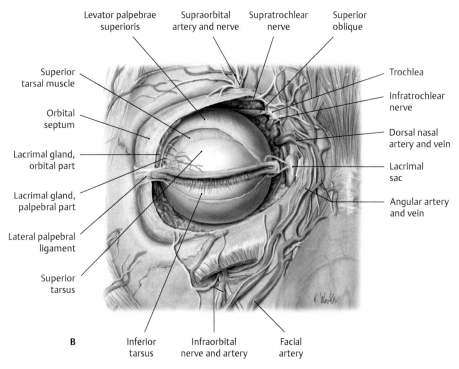

B

Labels:
- Levator palpebrae superioris
- Supraorbital artery and nerve
- Supratrochlear nerve
- Superior oblique
- Superior tarsal muscle
- Orbital septum
- Lacrimal gland, orbital part
- Lacrimal gland, palpebral part
- Lateral palpebral ligament
- Superior tarsus
- Trochlea
- Infratrochlear nerve
- Dorsal nasal artery and vein
- Lacrimal sac
- Angular artery and vein
- Inferior tarsus
- Infraorbital nerve and artery
- Facial artery

Fig. 9.18 Superficial and deep neurovascular structures of the orbital region

Right eye, anterior view.

A Superficial layer. The orbital septum on the right side has been exposed by removal of the orbicularis oculi. **B** Deep layer. Anterior orbital structures have been exposed by partial removal of the orbital septum.

The regions supplied by the *internal* carotid artery (supraorbital artery) and *external* carotid artery (infraorbital artery, facial artery) meet in this region. The extensive anastomosis between the angular vein (extracranial) and superior ophthalmic veins (intracranial) creates a portal of entry by which microorganisms may reach the cavernous sinus (risk of sinus thrombosis, meningitis, see p. 70). It is sometimes necessary to ligate this anastomosis in the orbital region, as in patients with extensive infections of the external facial region.

Note the passage of the supra- and infraorbital nerves (branches of CN V_1 and CN V_2) through the accordingly named foramina. The sensory function of these two trigeminal nerve divisions can be tested at these nerve exit points.

Fig. 9.19 Surface anatomy of the eye
Right eye, anterior view. The measurements indicate the width of the normal palpebral fissure. It is important to know these measurements because there are a number of diseases in which they are altered. For example, the palpebral fissure may be widened in peripheral facial paralysis or narrowed in ptosis (drooping of the eyelid) due to oculomotor palsy.

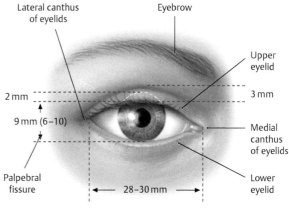

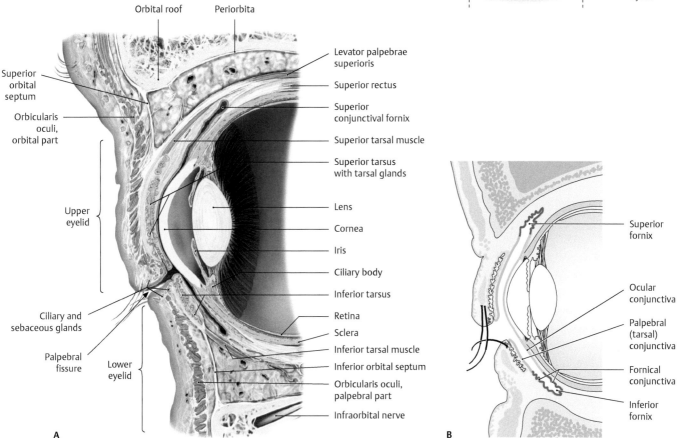

Fig. 9.20 Structure of the eyelids and conjunctiva
A Sagittal section through the anterior orbital cavity. **B** Anatomy of the conjunctiva.
The eyelid consists clinically of an outer and an inner layer with the following components:

- Outer layer: palpebral skin, sweat glands, ciliary glands (= modified sweat glands, Moll glands), sebaceous glands (Zeis glands), and two striated muscles, the orbicularis oculi and levator palpebrae (upper eyelid only), innervated by the facial nerve and the oculomotor nerve, respectively.
- Inner layer: the tarsus (fibrous tissue plate), the superior and inferior tarsal muscles (of Müller; *smooth* muscle innervated by sympathetic fibers), the tarsal or palpebral conjunctiva, and the tarsal glands (meibomian glands).

Regular blinking (20 to 30 times per minute) keeps the eyes from drying out by evenly distributing the lacrimal fluid and glandular secretions. Mechanical irritants (e.g., grains of sand) evoke the *blink reflex*, which also serves to protect the cornea and **conjunctiva**. The conjunctiva (tunica conjunctiva) is a vascularized, thin, glistening mucous membrane that is subdivided into the *palpebral conjunctiva* (green), *fornical conjunctiva* (red), and *ocular conjunctiva* (yellow). The ocular conjunctiva borders directly on the corneal surface and combines with it to form the **conjunctival sac**, whose functions include:

- facilitating ocular movements,
- enabling painless motion of the palpebral conjunctiva and ocular conjunctiva relative to each other (lubricated by lacrimal fluid), and
- protecting against infectious pathogens (collections of lymphocytes along the fornices).

The superior and inferior fornices are the sites where the conjunctiva is reflected from the upper and lower eyelid, respectively, onto the eyeball. They are convenient sites for the instillation of ophthalmic medications. *Inflammation of the conjunctiva* is common and causes a dilation of the conjunctival vessels resulting in "pink eye." Conversely, a deficiency of red blood cells (anemia) may lessen the prominence of vascular markings in the conjunctiva. This is why the conjunctiva should be routinely inspected in every clinical examination.

Lacrimal Apparatus

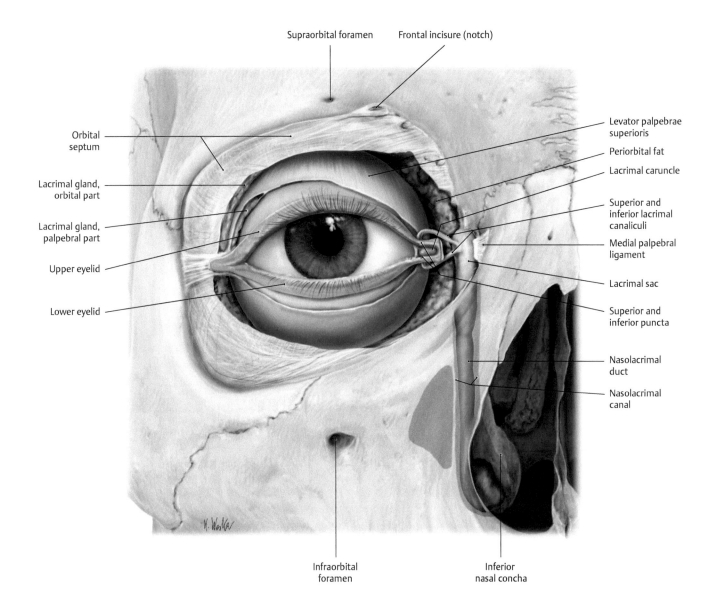

Fig. 9.21 Lacrimal apparatus
Right eye, anterior view. The orbital septum has been partially removed, and the tendon of insertion of the levator palpebrae superioris has been divided. The hazelnut-sized **lacrimal gland** is located in the lacrimal fossa of the frontal bone and produces most of the lacrimal fluid. Smaller *accessory lacrimal glands* (Krause or Wolfring glands) are also present. The tendon of levator palpebrae subdivides the lacrimal gland, which normally is not visible or palpable, into an *orbital lobe* (two thirds of gland) and a *palpebral lobe* (one third). The sympathetic fibers innervating the lacrimal gland originate from the superior cervical ganglion and travel along arteries to reach the lacrimal gland. Parasympathetic fibers reach the lacrimal gland via the lacrimal nerve (CN V$_1$). The lacrimal nerve communicates with the zygomatic nerve (CN V$_2$), which relays postganglionic parasympathetic fibers from the pterygopalatine ganglion. The preganglionic parasympathetic fibers that synapse in the pterygopalatine ganglion travel as the greater petrosal nerve, which arises from the genu of the facial nerve (CN VII) (see **Fig. 4.90**).

The **lacrimal apparatus** can be understood by tracing the flow of lacrimal fluid obliquely downward from the superolateral margin of the orbit (by the lacrimal gland) to the inferomedial margin (see **Fig. 9.23**). From the superior and inferior *puncta,* the lacrimal fluid enters the superior and inferior *lacrimal canaliculi,* which direct the fluid into the *lacrimal sac.* Finally, it drains through the *nasolacrimal duct* to an outlet below the inferior concha of the nose. "Watery eyes" are a typical cold symptom caused by obstruction of the inferior opening of the nasolacrimal duct. Dry eyes, on the other hand, is a symptom of Sjögren syndrome, an autoimmune disease causing keratoconjuctivitis sicca (diminished tear production) and xerostomia (dry mouth). It is associated with rheumatoid arthritis (in 50% of cases) and lupus. Lymphocytes and plasma cells infiltrate secretory glands and cause injury. Diminished tear production causes dry, itchy, gritty eyes, while diminshed saliva production makes swallowing difficult and increases the likelihood of development of dental caries. Rhematoid arthritis causes joint pain, swelling and stiffness.

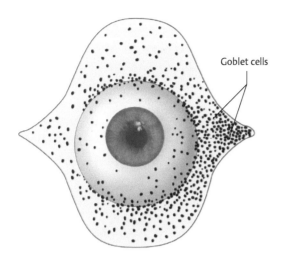

Fig. 9.22 Distribution of goblet cells in the conjunctiva
Goblet cells are mucus-secreting cells within an epithelial covering. Their secretions (mucins) are an important constituent of the lacrimal fluid. Mucins are also secreted by the main lacrimal gland.

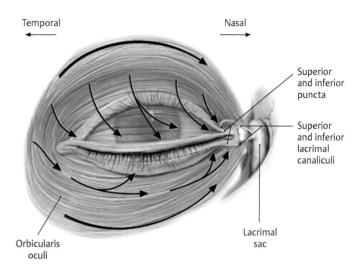

Fig. 9.23 Mechanical propulsion of the lacrimal fluid
During closure of the eyelids, contraction of the orbicularis oculi proceeds in a temporal-to-nasal direction. The successive contraction of these muscle fibers propels the lacrimal fluid toward the lacrimal passages. *Note:* Facial paralysis prevents closure of the eyelids, causing the eye to dry out.

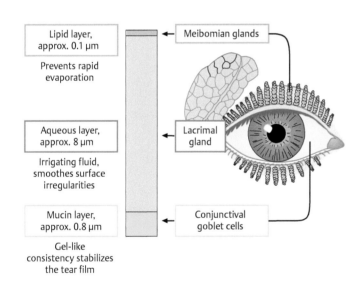

Fig. 9.24 Structure of the tear film
The tear film is a complex fluid with several morphologically distinct layers, whose components are produced by individual glands. The outer lipid layer, produced by the meibomian glands, protects the aqueous middle layer of the tear film from evaporating.

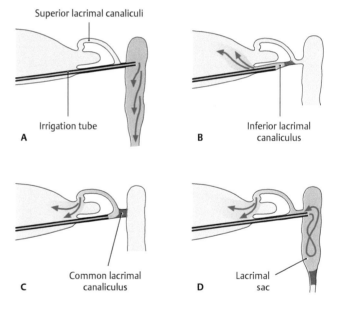

Fig. 9.25 Obstructions to lacrimal drainage
Sites of obstruction in the lacrimal drainage system can be located by irrigating the system with a special fluid.

A No obstruction to lacrimal drainage.
B,C Stenosis in the inferior or common lacrimal canaliculus. The stenosis causes a damming back of lacrimal fluid behind the obstructed site. In **B** the fluid refluxes through the inferior lacrimal canaliculus, and in **C** it flows through the superior lacrimal canaliculus.
D Stenosis below the level of the lacrimal sac (postlacrimal sac stenosis). When the entire lacrimal sac has filled with fluid, the fluid begins to reflux into the superior lacrimal canaliculus. In such cases, the lacrimal fluid often has a purulent, gelatinous appearance.

Eyeball

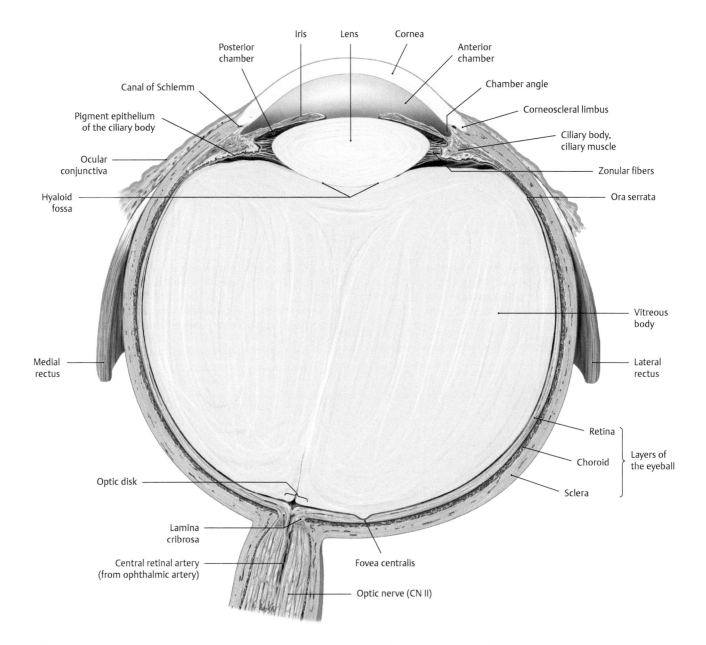

Fig. 9.26 Eyeball

Right eye, superior view of transverse section. Most of the eyeball is composed of three concentric layers surrounding vitreous humor: the sclera, the choroid, and the retina.

Posterior portion of the eyeball: The **sclera** is the posterior portion of the outer coat of the eyeball. It is a firm layer of connective tissue that gives attachment to the tendons of all the extraocular muscles. The middle layer of the eye, the **choroid**, is the most highly vascularized region in the body and serves to regulate the temperature of the eye and to supply blood to the outer layers of the retina. The inner layer of the eye, the **retina**, includes an inner layer of photosensitive cells (sensory retina) and an outer layer of retinal pigment epithelium. The axons of the optic nerve (CN II) pierce the lamina cribrosa of the sclera at the optic disk. The *fovea centralis* is a depressed area in the central retina approximately 4 mm temporal to the optic disk. Incident light is normally focused on the fovea centralis, the site of greatest visual acuity.

Anterior portion: The anterior portion of the eyeball has a different structure that is continuous with the posterior portion. The outer fibrous coat is the cornea, the "window of the eye," which bulges forward. At the corneoscleral limbus, the cornea is continuous with the less convex sclera. In the angle of the anterior chamber, the sclera forms the trabecular meshwork, which is connected to the canal of Schlemm. Beneath the sclera is the vascular coat of the eye, also called the uveal tract. It consists of three parts: the iris, ciliary body, and choroid. The iris shields the eye from excessive light and covers the lens. Its root is continuous with the ciliary body, which contains the ciliary muscle for visual accommodation (alters the refractive power of the lens). The epithelium of the ciliary body produces the aqueous humor. The ciliary body is continuous at the ora serrata with the choroid. The outer layer of the retina (pigment epithelium) is continued forward as the pigment epithelium of the ciliary body and the epithelium of the iris.

Globe rupture involves a full-thickness defect in the cornea and/or sclera. It may occur following penetrating or blunt trauma. It is a true ophthalmologic emergency that requires prompt surgical repair to prevent permanent loss of vision or poor eye functionality.

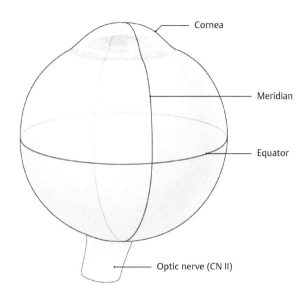

Fig. 9.27 Reference lines and points on the eye
The line marking the greatest circumference of the eyeball is the *equator*. Lines perpendicular to the equator are called *meridians*.

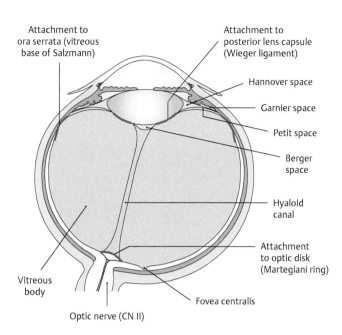

Fig. 9.28 Vitreous body (vitreous humor)
Right eye, transverse section, superior view. Sites where the vitreous body is attached to other ocular structures are shown in red, and adjacent spaces are shown in green. The vitreous body stabilizes the eyeball and protects against retinal detachment. Devoid of nerves and vessels, it consists of 98% water and 2% hyaluronic acid and collagen. The "hyaloid canal" is an embryological remnant of the hyaloid artery. For the treatment of some diseases, the vitreous body may be surgically removed (vitrectomy) and the resulting cavity filled with physiological saline solution.

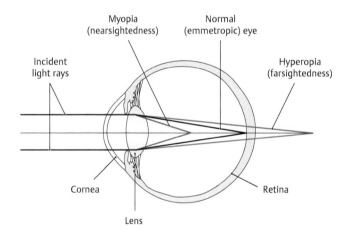

Fig. 9.29 Light refraction
In a normal (emmetropic) eye, parallel rays from a distant light source are refracted by the cornea and lens to a focal point on the retinal surface.

- In myopia (nearsightedness), the rays are focused to a point *in front* of the retina.
- In hyperopia (farsightedness), the rays are focused *behind* the retina.
- In astigmatism (asymmetrical lens curvature in the horizontal and vertical axes) some rays are focused in front of the retina and some behind.

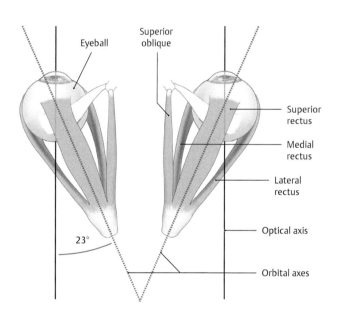

Fig. 9.30 Optical axis and orbital axis
Superior view of both eyes showing the medial, lateral, and superior recti and the superior oblique. The optical axis deviates from the orbital axis by 23 degrees. Because of this disparity, the point of maximum visual acuity, the fovea centralis, is lateral to the "blind spot" of the optic disk.

Eye: Blood Supply

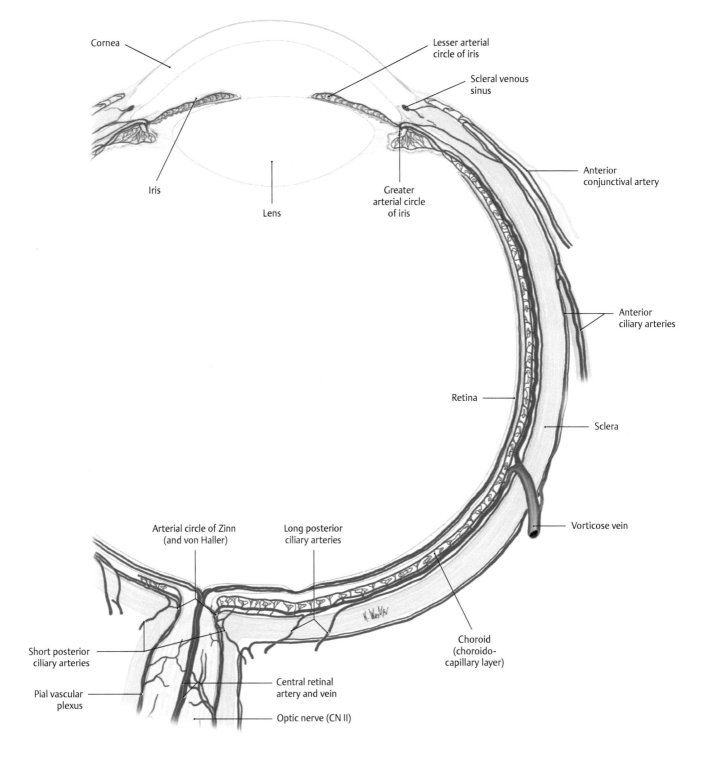

Fig. 9.31 Blood supply of the eye

Transverse section through the right eye at the level of the optic nerve, superior view. All of the arteries that supply the eye arise from the *ophthalmic artery,* a branch of the internal carotid artery. Its ocular branches are:

- Central retinal artery to the retina
- Short posterior ciliary arteries to the choroid
- Long posterior ciliary arteries to the ciliary body and iris, where they supply the greater and lesser arterial circles of the iris (see **Fig. 9.41**)

- Anterior ciliary arteries, which arise from the vessels of the rectus muscles of the eye and anastomose with the posterior ciliary vessels

Blood is drained from the eyeball by four to eight vorticose veins, which pierce the sclera behind the equator and open into the superior or inferior ophthalmic vein.

The superior ophthalmic vein communicates with cavernous sinus via the superior orbital fissure; the inferior ophthalmic vein communicates posteriorly with the pterygoid plexus of veins via the inferior orbital fissure and with the cavernous sinus.

Fig. 9.32 **Arteries of the optic nerve (CN II)**
Lateral view. The central retinal artery, the first branch of the ophthalmic artery, enters the optic nerve from below approximately 1 cm behind the eyeball and courses with it to the retina while giving off multiple small branches. The posterior ciliary artery also gives off several small branches that supply the optic nerve. The distal part of the optic nerve receives its arterial blood supply from an arterial ring (circle of Zinn and von Haller) formed by anastomoses among the side branches of the short posterior ciliary arteries and central retinal artery.

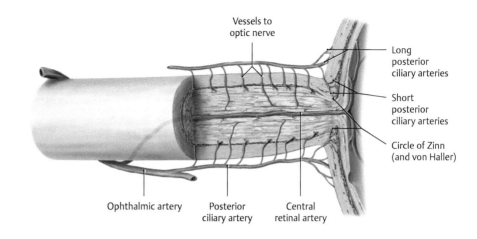

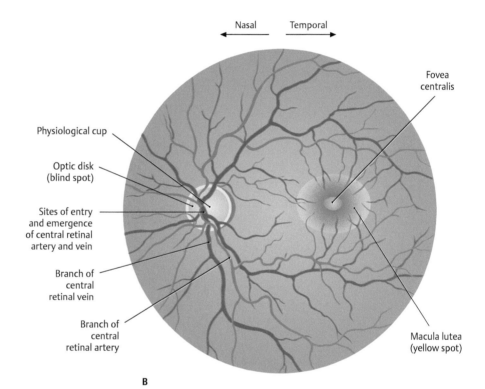

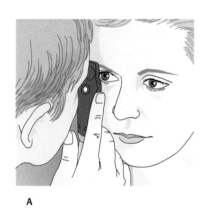

A

B

Fig. 9.33 **Ophthalmoscopic examination of the optic fundus**
A Examination technique (direct ophthalmoscopy). **B** Normal appearance of the optic fundus.
In direct ophthalmoscopy, the following structures of the optic fundus can be directly evaluated at approximately 16 × magnification:

- The condition of the retina
- The blood vessels (particularly the central retinal artery)
- The optic disk (where the optic nerve emerges from the eyeball)
- The macula lutea and fovea centralis

Because the retina is transparent, the color of the optic fundus is determined chiefly by the pigment epithelium and the blood vessels of the choroid. It is uniformly pale red in light-skinned persons and is considerably browner in dark-skinned persons. Abnormal detachment of the retina is usually associated with a loss of retinal transparency, and the retina assumes a yellowish white color. The central retinal artery and vein can be distinguished from each other by their color and caliber: arteries have a brighter red color and a smaller caliber than the veins.

This provides a means for the early detection of vascular changes (e.g., stenosis, wall thickening, microaneurysms), such as those occurring in diabetes mellitus (diabetic retinopathy) or hypertension. The *optic disk* normally has sharp margins, a yellow-orange color, and a central depression, the physiological cup. The disk is subject to changes in pathological conditions such as elevated intracranial pressure (papilledema with ill-defined disk margins). On examination of the *macula lutea,* which is 3 to 4 mm temporal to the optic disk, it can be seen that numerous branches of the central retinal artery radiate toward the macula but do not reach its center, the fovea centralis (the fovea receives its blood supply from the choroid). A common age-related disease of the macula lutea is macular degeneration. It is caused by the buildup of yellow deposits, or drusen, on the macula that damages the rods and cones. Symptoms are insidious and may affect one or both eyes. They include blurriness or loss of central vision, which may manifest as difficulty reading and difficulty recognizing faces, decreased color intensity, and decreased adaptation to dark environments.

Eye: Lens & Cornea

Fig. 9.34 Position of the lens and cornea

Transverse section through the cornea, lens, and suspensory apparatus of the lens. The normal lens is clear, transparent, and only 4 mm thick. It is suspended in the hyaloid fossa of the vitreous body. The lens is attached by rows of fibrils (zonular fibers) to the ciliary muscle, whose contractions alter the shape and focal length of the lens. Thus, the lens is a dynamic structure that can change its shape in response to visual requirements. The anterior chamber of the eye is situated in front of the lens, and the posterior chamber is located between the iris and the anterior epithelium of the lens. The lens, like the vitreous body, is devoid of nerves and blood vessels and is composed of elongated epithelial cells (lens fibers).

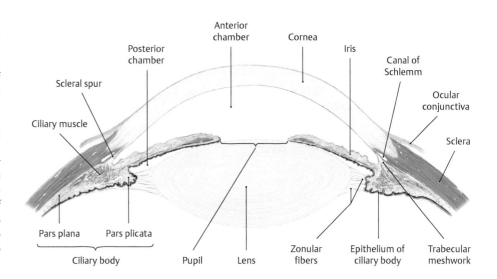

Fig. 9.35 Lens and ciliary body

Posterior view. The curvature of the lens is regulated by the muscle fibers of the annular ciliary body. The *ciliary body* lies between the ora serrata and the root of the iris and consists of a relatively flat part (pars plana) and a part that is raised into folds (pars plicata). The latter part is ridged by approximately 70 to 80 radially oriented ciliary processes, which surround the lens like a halo when viewed from behind. The ciliary processes contain large capillaries, and their epithelium secretes the aqueous humor. Very fine *zonular fibers* extend from the basal layer of the ciliary processes to the equator of the lens. These fibers and the spaces between them constitute the suspensory apparatus of the lens, called the *zonule*. Most of the ciliary body is occupied by

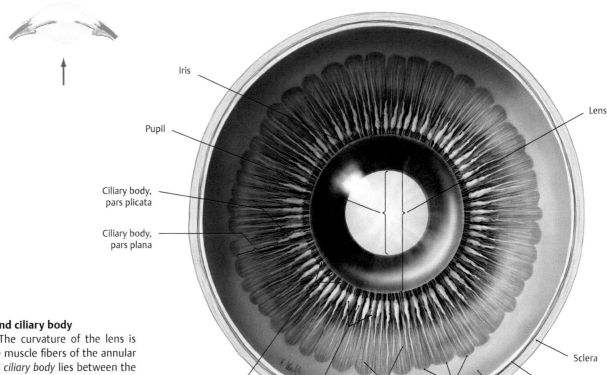

the ciliary muscle, a smooth muscle composed of meridional, radial, and circular fibers. It arises mainly from the scleral spur (a reinforcing ring of sclera just below the canal of Schlemm), and it attaches to structures including the Bruch membrane of the choroid and the inner surface of the sclera. When the ciliary muscle contracts, it pulls the choroid forward and relaxes the zonular fibers. As these fibers become lax, the intrinsic resilience of the lens causes it to assume the more convex relaxed shape that is necessary for near vision. This is the basic mechanism of visual accommodation.

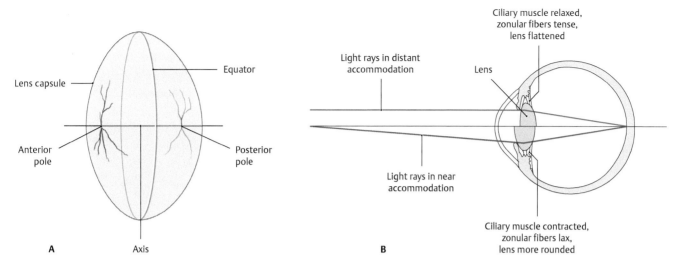

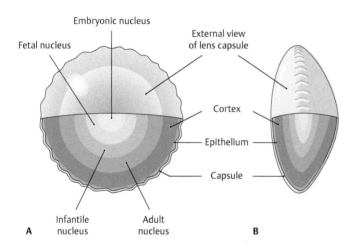

Fig. 9.36 Reference lines and dynamics, oblique lateral view of the lens

A Principal reference lines of the lens: The lens has an *anterior* and *posterior pole,* an *axis* passing between the poles, and an *equator.* The lens has a biconvex shape with a greater radius of curvature posteriorly (16 mm) than anteriorly (10 mm). Its function is to transmit light rays and make fine adjustments in refraction. Its refractive power ranges from 10 to 20 diopters, depending on the state of accommodation. The cornea has a considerably higher refractive power of 43 diopters.

B Light refraction and dynamics of the lens, sagittal section:
- Upper half of diagram: fine adjustment of the eye for *far vision.* Parallel light rays arrive from a distant source, and the lens is flattened.
- Lower half of diagram: For *near vision* (accommodation to objects less than 5 m from the eye), the lens assumes a more rounded shape. This is effected by contraction of the ciliary muscle (parasympathetic innervation from the oculomotor nerve), causing the zonular fibers to relax and allowing the lens to assume a more rounded shape because of its intrinsic resilience.

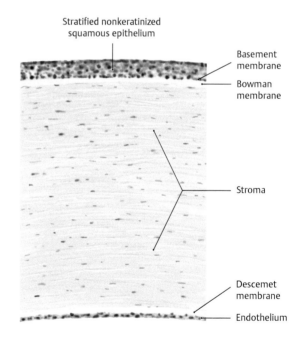

Fig. 9.37 Growth of the lens and zones of discontinuity
A Anterior view. **B** Lateral view.
The lens continues to grow throughout life, doing so in a manner opposite to that of other epithelial structures (i.e., the youngest cells are at the surface of the lens, whereas the oldest cells are deeper). Due to the constant proliferation of epithelial cells, which are all firmly incorporated in the lens capsule, the tissue of the lens becomes increasingly dense with age. A slit-lamp examination will demonstrate zones of varying cell density (zones of discontinuity). The zone of highest cell density, the *embryonic nucleus,* is at the center of the lens. With further growth, it becomes surrounded by the *fetal nucleus.* The *infantile nucleus* develops after birth, and finally the *adult nucleus* begins to form during the third decade of life. These zones are the basis for the morphological classification of cateracts, a structural alteration in the lens or its capsule, causing opacity, that is more or less normal in old age (present in 10% of all 80-year-olds). It produces blurred, cloudy vision.

Fig. 9.38 Structure of the cornea
The cornea is covered externally by stratified, nonkeratinized squamous epithelium whose basal lamina borders on the anterior limiting lamina (Bowman membrane). The stroma (substantia propria) makes up approximately 90% of the corneal thickness and is bounded on its deep surface by the posterior limiting lamina (Descemet membrane). Beneath is a single layer of corneal endothelium. The cornea does have a nerve supply (for corneal reflexes), but it is not vascularized and therefore has an immunologically privileged status: normally, a corneal transplant can be performed without fear of a host rejection response.

Eye: Iris & Ocular Chambers

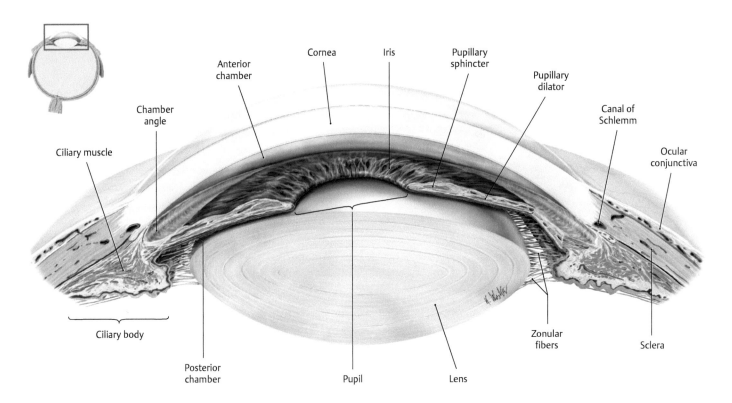

Fig. 9.39 **Iris and chambers of the eye**
Transverse section through the anterior segment of the eye, superior view. The iris, the choroid, and the ciliary body at the periphery of the iris are part of the uveal tract. In the iris, the pigments are formed that determine eye color. The iris is an optical diaphragm with a central aperture, the pupil, placed in front of the lens. The pupil is 1 to 8 mm in diameter; it constricts on contraction of the pupillary sphincter (*parasympathetic* innervation via the oculomotor nerve and ciliary ganglion) and dilates on contraction of the pupillary dilator (*sympathetic* innervation from the superior cervical ganglion via the internal carotid plexus). Together, the iris and lens separate the anterior chamber of the eye from the posterior chamber. The posterior chamber behind the iris is bounded posteriorly by the vitreous body, centrally by the lens, and laterally by the ciliary body. The anterior chamber is bounded anteriorly by the cornea and posteriorly by the iris and lens.

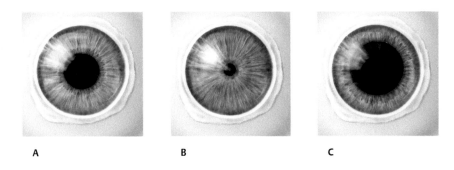

Fig. 9.40 **Pupil size**
A Normal pupil size. **B** Maximum constriction (miosis). **C** Maximum dilation (mydriasis).
The regulation of pupil size is aided by the two intraocular muscles, the pupillary sphincter and pupillary dilator. The pupillary sphincter (parasympathetic innervation) narrows the pupil, and the pupillary dilator (sympathetic innervation) enlarges the pupil. Pupil size is normally adjusted in response to incident light and serves mainly to optimize visual acuity.

Normally, the pupils are circular in shape and equal in size (3 to 5 mm). Various influences may cause the pupil size to vary over a range from 1.5 mm (miosis) to 8 mm (mydriasis). A greater than 1 mm discrepancy of pupil size between the right and left eyes is called *aniso-coria*. Mild anisocoria is physiological in some individuals. Pupillary reflexes such as convergence and the consensual light response are described on pp. 273 and 274.

Table 9.5 Changes in pupil size: causes	
Pupil constriction (parasympathetic)	**Pupil dilation (sympathetic)**
Light	Darkness
Sleep, fatigue	Pain, excitement
Miotic agents: • Parasympathomimetics (e.g., tear gas, VX and sarin, Alzheimer's drugs such as rivastigmine) • Sympatholytics (e.g., antihypertensives)	Mydriatic agents: • Parasympatholytics (e.g., atropine) • Sympathomimetics (e.g., epinephrine)
Horner syndrome (also causes ptosis and narrowing of palpebral fissure)	Oculomotor palsy
General anesthesia, morphine	Migraine attack, glaucoma attack

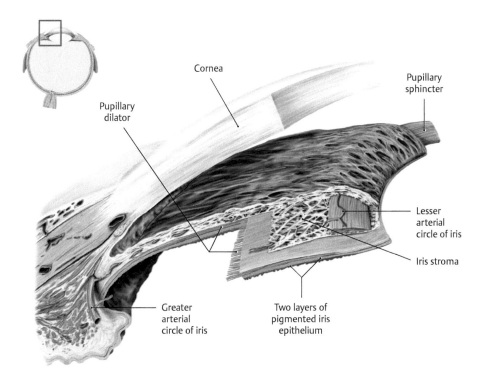

Fig. 9.41 Structure of the iris

Transverse and parasagittal section, superior view. The basic structural framework of the iris is the vascularized stroma, which is bounded on its deep surface by two layers of pigmented iris epithelium. The loose, collagen-containing stroma of the iris contains outer and inner vascular circles (greater and lesser arterial circles), which are interconnected by small anastomotic arteries. The pupillary sphincter is an annular muscle located in the stroma bordering the pupil. The radially disposed pupillary dilator is not located in the stroma; rather, it is composed of numerous myofibrils in the iris epithelium (myoepithelium). The stroma of the iris is permeated by pigmented connective tissue cells (melanocytes). When heavily pigmented, these melanocytes of the anterior border zone of the stroma render the iris brown or "black." Otherwise, the characteristics of the underlying stroma and epithelium determine eye color, in a manner that is not fully understood.

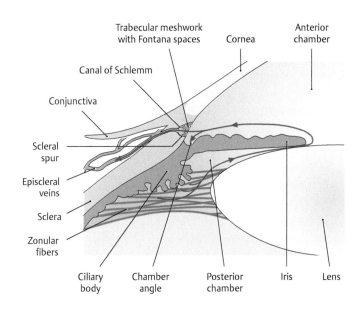

Fig. 9.42 Normal drainage of aqueous humor

The aqueous humor (approximately 0.3 mL per eye) is an important determinant of the intraocular pressure. It is produced by the non-pigmented ciliary epithelium of the ciliary processes in the *posterior* chamber (approximately 0.15 mL/hour) and passes through the pupil into the *anterior* chamber of the eye. The aqueous humor seeps through the spaces of the trabecular meshwork (Fontana spaces) in the chamber angle and enters the canal of Schlemm (venous sinus of the sclera), through which it drains to the episcleral veins. The draining aqueous humor flows toward the chamber angle along a pressure gradient (intraocular pressure = 15 mm Hg, pressure in the episcleral veins = 9 mm Hg) and must surmount a physiological resistance at two sites:

- *Pupillary resistance* (between the iris and lens)
- *Trabecular resistance* (narrow spaces in the trabecular meshwork)

Approximately 85% of the aqueous humor flows through the trabecular meshwork into the canal of Schlemm. Only 15% drains through the uveoscleral vascular system into the vortical veins (uveoscleral drainage route).

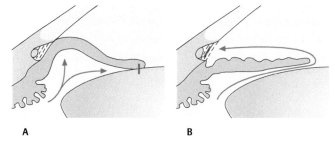

Fig. 9.43 Obstruction of aqueous drainage and glaucoma

Normal function of the optical system requires normal intraocular pressure (15 mm Hg in adults). This maintains a smooth curvature of the corneal surface and helps keep the photoreceptor cells in contact with the pigment epithelium. Obstruction of the normal drainage of aqueous humor causes an increase in intraocular pressure. This constricts the optic nerve at the lamina cribrosa, where it emerges from the eyeball through the sclera. Such constriction eventually leads to blindness. There are two types of glaucoma:

A Acute (closed-angle) glaucoma: The chamber angle is obstructed by iris tissue. Aqueous fluid cannot drain into the anterior chamber and pushes portions of the iris upward, blocking the chamber angle. This type of glaucoma often develops quickly.

B Chronic (open-angle) glaucoma: The chamber angle is open, but drainage through the trabecular meshwork is impaired. Ninety percent of all glaucomas are primary chronic open-angle glaucomas. This is increasingly prevalent after 40 years of age. Treatment options include parasympathomimetics (to induce sustained contraction of the ciliary muscle and pupillary sphincter), prostaglandin analogues (to improve aqueous drainage), and beta-adrenoceptor agonists (to decrease production of aqueous humor).

265

Eye: Retina

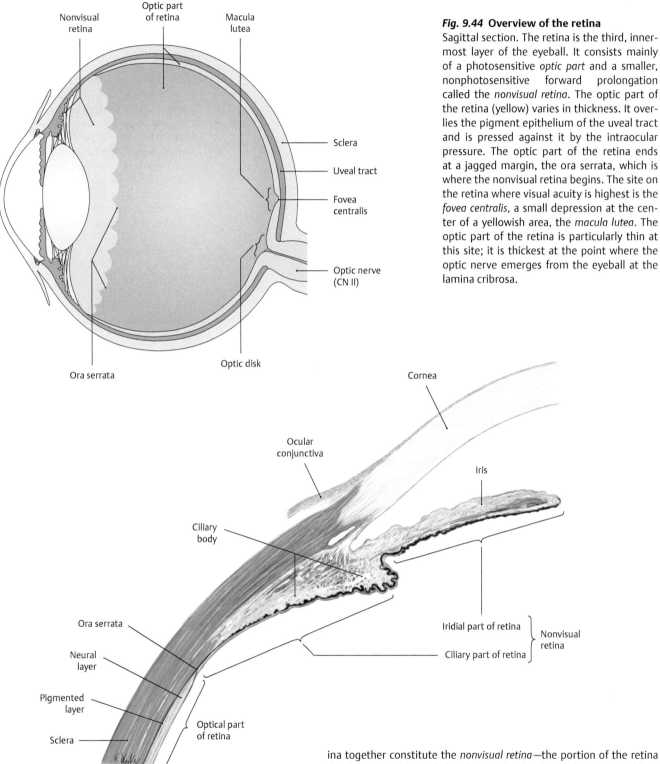

Fig. 9.44 Overview of the retina
Sagittal section. The retina is the third, innermost layer of the eyeball. It consists mainly of a photosensitive *optic part* and a smaller, nonphotosensitive forward prolongation called the *nonvisual retina*. The optic part of the retina (yellow) varies in thickness. It overlies the pigment epithelium of the uveal tract and is pressed against it by the intraocular pressure. The optic part of the retina ends at a jagged margin, the ora serrata, which is where the nonvisual retina begins. The site on the retina where visual acuity is highest is the *fovea centralis,* a small depression at the center of a yellowish area, the *macula lutea.* The optic part of the retina is particularly thin at this site; it is thickest at the point where the optic nerve emerges from the eyeball at the lamina cribrosa.

Fig. 9.45 Parts of the retina
Transverse section, superior view. The posterior surface of the iris bears a double layer of pigment epithelium, the *iridial part* of the retina. Just peripheral to it is the *ciliary part* of the retina, also formed by a *double* layer of epithelium (one of which is pigmented) and covering the posterior surface of the ciliary body. The iridial and ciliary parts of the retina together constitute the *nonvisual retina*—the portion of the retina that is not sensitive to light. The nonvisual retina ends at a jagged line, the ora serrata, where the light-sensitive *optic part* of the retina begins. Consistent with the development of the retina from the embryonic optic cup, two layers can be distinguished within the optic part:

- An outer layer nearer the sclera: the *pigmented layer,* consisting of a single layer of pigmented retinal epithelium.
- An inner layer nearer the vitreous body: the *neural layer,* comprising a system of receptor cells, interneurons, and ganglion cells.

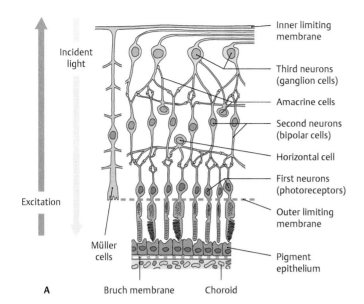

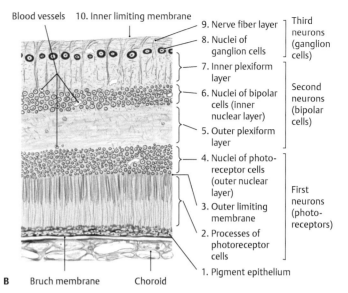

Fig. 9.46 Structure of the retina

A Retinal neurons of the visual pathway. **B** Anatomical layers of the retina. Light passes through all the layers of the retina to be received by the photoreceptors on the outermost surface of the retina. Sensory information is then transmitted via three retinal neurons of the visual pathway to the optic disk:

- First neurons (pink): Photoreceptor cells (light-sensitive sensory cells) that transform light stimuli (photons) into electrochemical signals. The two types of photoreceptors are rods and cones, named for the shape of their receptor segment. The retina contains 100 million to 125 million rods, which are responsible for twilight and night vision, but only about 6 million to 7 million cones. Different cones are specialized for the perception of red, green, and blue. The processes and nuclei of the first neurons compose anatomical layers 2 to 4 (see **B**).
- Second neurons (yellow): Bipolar cells that receive impulses from the photoreceptors and relay them to the ganglion cells. These neurons compose anatomical layers 5 to 7.

- Third neurons (green): Retinal ganglion cells whose axons converge at the optic disk to form the optic nerve (CN II) and reach the lateral geniculate and superior colliculus. These neurons compose anatomical layers 8 to 10. There are approximately 1 million retinal ganglion axons per eye.

Support cells: Müller cells (blue) are glial cells that span the neural layer radially from the inner to the outer limiting membranes, creating a supporting framework for the neurons. In addition to the vertical connections, horizontal and amacrine cells (gray) function as interneurons that establish lateral connections. Impulses transmitted by the receptor cells are thereby processed and organized within the retina (signal convergence).
Pigment epithelium: The outer layer of the retina (the pigment epithelium, brown) is attached to the Bruch membrane, which contains elastic fibers and collagen fibrils and mediates the exchange of substances between the adjacent choroid (choriocapillaris) and the photoreceptor cells. *Note:* The photoreceptors are in contact with the pigment epithelium but are not attached to it. The retina may become detached (if untreated, this leads to blindness).

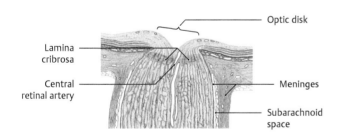

Fig. 9.47 Optic disk ("blind spot") and lamina cribrosa

The unmyelinated axons of the third neurons (retinal ganglion cells) pass to a collecting point at the posterior pole of the eye. There they unite to form the optic nerve and leave the retina through numerous perforations in the sclera (lamina cribrosa). (*Note:* The optic disk has no photoreceptors and is therefore the physiological blind spot.) In the optic nerve, these axons are myelinated by oligodendrocytes. The optic nerve (CN II) is an extension of the diencephalon and therefore has all the coverings of the brain (dura mater, arachnoid, and pia mater). It is surrounded by a subarachnoid space that contains cerebrospinal fluid (CSF) and communicates with the subarachnoid spaces of the brain and spinal cord.

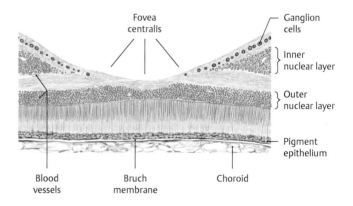

Fig. 9.48 Macula lutea and fovea centralis

Temporal to the optic disk is the macula lutea. At its center is a funnel-shaped depression approximately 1.5 mm in diameter, the fovea centralis, which is the site of maximum visual acuity. At this site the inner retinal layers are heaped toward the margin of the depression, so that the cells of the photoreceptors (just cones, no rods) are directly exposed to the incident light. Furthermore blood vessels detour around the fovea. This arrangement significantly reduces scattering of the light rays.

267

Visual System (I): Overview & Geniculate Part

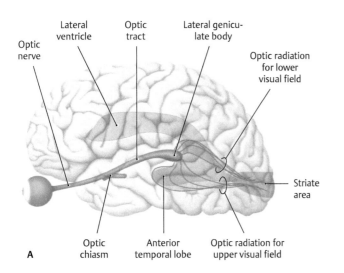

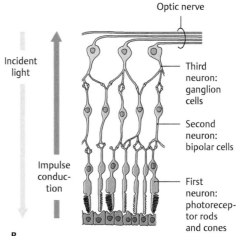

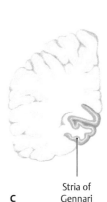

A — Optic nerve, Lateral ventricle, Optic tract, Lateral geniculate body, Optic radiation for lower visual field, Striate area, Optic chiasm, Anterior temporal lobe, Optic radiation for upper visual field

B — Incident light, Impulse conduction, Optic nerve, Third neuron: ganglion cells, Second neuron: bipolar cells, First neuron: photoreceptor rods and cones

C — Stria of Gennari

Fig. 9.49 Overview of the visual pathway
Left lateral view. The visual pathway extends from the eye, an anterior prolongation of the diencephalon, back to the occipital pole. Thus, it encompasses almost the entire longitudinal axis of the brain. The principal stations are as follows:
Retina: The first three neurons of the visual pathway (**B**):

- First neuron: photoreceptor rods and cones, located on the deep retinal surface opposite the direction of the incoming light ("inversion of the retina").
- Second neuron: bipolar cells.
- Third neuron: ganglion cells whose axons are collected to form the optic nerve.

Optic nerve (CN II), optic chiasm, and optic tract: This neural portion of the visual pathway is part of the central nervous system and is surrounded by meninges. Thus, the optic nerve is actually a tract rather than a true nerve. The optic nerves join below the base of the diencephalon to form the optic chiasm, which then divides into the two optic tracts. Each of these tracts divides in turn into a lateral and medial root.

Lateral geniculate body: Ninety percent of the axons of the third neuron (= 90 % of the optic nerve fibers) terminate in the lateral geniculate body on neurons that project to the striate area (visual cortex, see below). This is the *geniculate part of the visual pathway*. It is concerned with *conscious* visual perception and is conveyed by the lateral root of the optic tract. The remaining 10% of the third-neuron axons in the visual pathway do not terminate in the lateral geniculate body. This is the *nongeniculate part of the visual pathway* (medial root, see **Fig. 9.54**), and its signals are not consciously perceived.

Optic radiation and visual cortex (striate area): The optic radiation begins in the lateral geniculate body, forms a band that winds around the inferior and posterior horns of the lateral ventricles, and terminates in the visual cortex or striate area (= Brodmann area 17). Located in the occipital lobe, the visual cortex can be grossly identified by a prominent stripe of white matter in the otherwise gray cerebral cortex (the stria of Gennari, see **C**). This white stripe runs parallel to the brain surface and is shown in the inset, where the gray matter of the visual cortex is shaded light red.

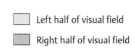

Left half of visual field

Right half of visual field

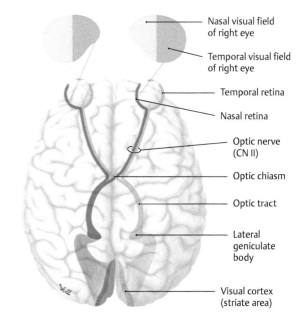

Nasal visual field of right eye

Temporal visual field of right eye

Temporal retina

Nasal retina

Optic nerve (CN II)

Optic chiasm

Optic tract

Lateral geniculate body

Visual cortex (striate area)

Fig. 9.50 Representation of each visual field in the contralateral visual cortex
Superior view. The light rays in the *nasal* part of each visual field are projected to the *temporal* half of the retina, and those from the temporal part are projected to the nasal half. Because of this arrangement, the left half of the visual field projects to the visual cortex of the right occipital pole, and the right half projects to the visual cortex of the left occipital pole. For clarity, each visual field in the diagram is divided into two halves. *Note:* The axonal fibers from the nasal half of each retina cross to the opposite side at the optic chiasm and then travel with the uncrossed fibers from the temporal half of each retina.

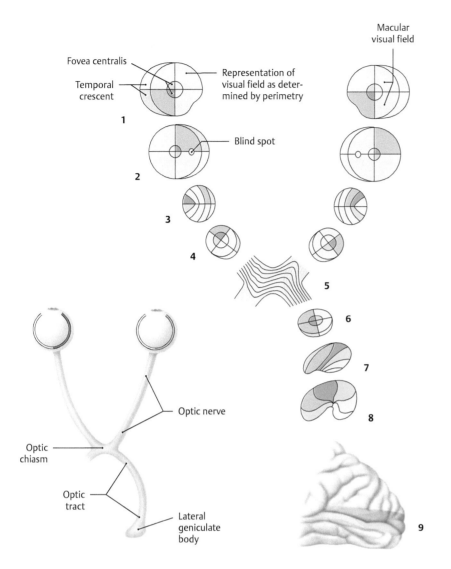

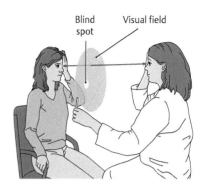

Fig. 9.52 Informal visual field examination with the confrontation test

The visual field examination is an essential step in the examination of lesions of the visual pathway (see **Fig. 9.53**). The **confrontation test** is an *informal* test in which the examiner (with an intact visual field) and the patient sit face-to-face, cover one eye, and each fixes their gaze on the other's open eye, creating identical visual axes. The examiner then moves his or her index finger from the outer edge of the visual field toward the center until the patient signals that he or she can see the finger. With this test the examiner can make a gross assessment as to the presence and approximate location of a possible visual field defect. The *precise* location and extent of a visual field defect can be determined by **perimetry**, in which points of light replace the examiner's finger. The results of the test are entered in charts that resemble the small diagrams in **Fig. 9.53**.

Fig. 9.51 Geniculate part of visual pathway: topographic organization

The visual field is divided into four quadrants: upper temporal, upper nasal, lower nasal, and lower temporal. The lower nasal quadrant is indented by the nose. The representation of this subdivision is continued into the visual cortex. *Note:* Only the left visual hemifield (blue) is shown here (compare to **Fig. 9.50**).

1 Visual hemifield: Each visual hemifield is divided into three zones (indicated by color shading):

- Fovea centralis: The smallest and darkest zone is at the center of the visual field. It corresponds to the fovea centralis, the point of maximum visual acuity on the retina. The fovea centralis has a high receptor density; accordingly, a great many axons pass centrally from its receptors. It is therefore represented by a disproportionately large area in the visual cortex.
- Macular visual field: The largest zone in the visual hemisphere; it also contains the blind spot.
- Temporal crescent: The temporal, monocular part of the visual field. This corresponds to more peripheral portions of the retina that contain fewer receptors and therefore fewer axons, resulting in a smaller representational area in the visual cortex.

2 Retinal projection: All light that reaches the retina must pass through the narrow pupil, which functions like the aperture of a camera. Up/down and nasal/temporal are therefore reversed when the image is projected on the retina.

3,4 Optic nerve: In the distal part of the optic nerve, the fibers that represent the macular visual field initially occupy a lateral position (**3**), then move increasingly toward the center of the nerve (**4**).

5 Optic chiasm: While traversing the optic chiasm, the fibers of the nasal retina of the optic nerve cross the midline to the opposite side.

6 Start of the optic tract: Fibers from the corresponding halves of the retinas unite (e.g., right halves of the left and right retinas in the right optic tract). The impulses from the left visual field (right retinal half) will therefore terminate in the right striate area.

7 End of the optic tract: Fibers are collected to form a wedge before entering the lateral geniculate body.

8 Lateral geniculate body: Macular fibers occupy almost half of the wedge. After the fibers are relayed to the fourth neuron, they project to the posterior end of the occipital pole (= visual cortex).

9 Visual cortex: There exists a point-to-point (retinotopic) correlation between the number of axons in the retina and the number of axons in the visual cortex (e.g., the central part of the visual field is represented by the largest area in the visual cortex, due to the large number of axons concentrated in the fovea centralis). The central lower half of the visual field is represented by a large area on the occipital pole above the calcarine sulcus; the central upper half of the visual field is represented below the sulcus.

Visual System (II): Lesions & Nongeniculate Part

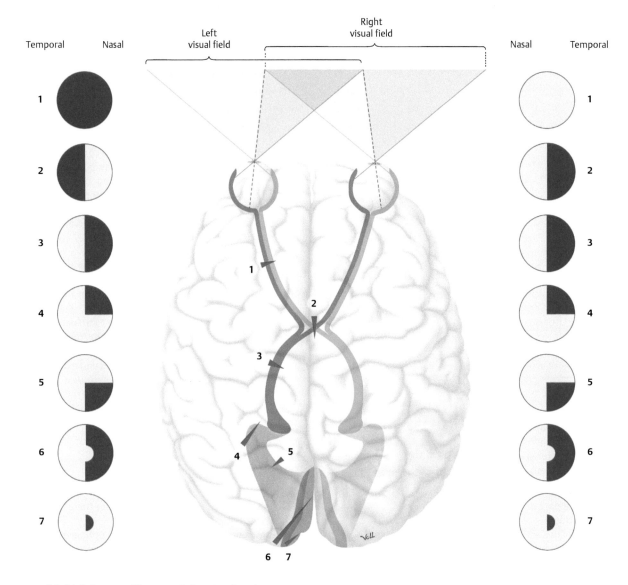

Fig. 9.53 Visual field defects and lesions of the visual pathway
Circles represent the perceived visual disturbances (scotomas, or areas of darkness) in the left and right eyes. These characteristic visual field defects (anopias) result from lesions at specific sites along the visual pathway. Lesion sites are illustrated in the left visual pathway as red wedges. The nature of the visual field defect often points to the location of the lesion. *Note:* Lesions past the optic chiasm will all be homonymous (same visual field in both eyes).

1 Unilateral optic nerve lesion: Blindness (amaurosis) in the affected eye.
2 Lesion of optic chiasm: Bitemporal hemianopia (think of a horse wearing blinders). Only fibers from the nasal portions of the retina (representing the temporal visual field) cross in the optic chiasm.
3 Unilateral optic tract lesion: Contralateral homonymous hemianopia. The lesion interrupts fibers from the temporal portion of the retina on the ipsilateral side and nasal portions of the retina on the contralateral side. The patient therefore has visual impairment of the same visual hemisphere in both eyes.

4 Unilateral lesion of the optic radiation in the anterior temporal lobe: Contralateral upper quadrantanopia ("pie in the sky" deficit). Lesions in the anterior temporal lobe affect only those fibers winding under the inferior horn of the lateral ventricle (see **Fig. 9.49**). These fibers represent only the upper half of the visual field (in this case the nasal portion).
5 Unilateral lesion of the optic radiation in the parietal lobe: Contralateral lower quadrantanopia. Fibers from the lower half of the visual field course superior to the lateral ventricle in the parietal lobe.
6 Occipital lobe lesion: Homonymous hemianopia. The lesion affects the optic radiations from both the upper and lower visual fields. However, as the optic radiation fans out widely before entering the visual cortex, foveal vision is often spared. These lesions are most commonly due to intracerebral hemorrhage; the visual field defects vary considerably with the size of the hemorrhage.
7 Occipital pole lesion (confined to cortical area): Homonymous hemianopic central scotoma. The cortical areas of the occipital pole represent the macula.

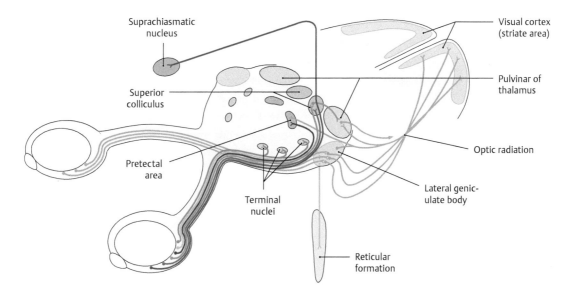

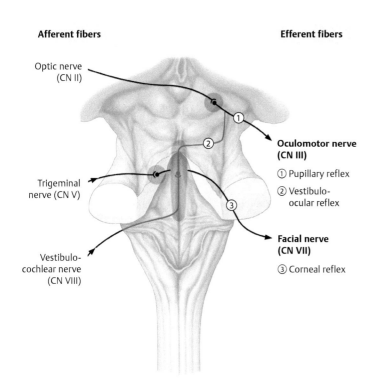

Fig. 9.54 Nongeniculate part of the visual pathway
Approximately 10% of the axons of the optic nerve do not terminate on neurons in the lateral geniculate body for projection to the visual cortex. They continue along the medial root of the optic tract, forming the *nongeniculate part* of the visual pathway. The information from these fibers is not processed at a conscious level but plays an important role in the unconscious regulation of various vision-related processes and in visually mediated reflexes (e.g., the afferent limb of the pupillary light reflex). Axons from the nongeniculate part of the visual pathway terminate in the following regions:

• Axons to the superior colliculus transmit kinetic information that is necessary for tracking moving objects by unconscious eye and head movements (retinotectal system).
• Axons to the pretectal area transmit afferents for pupillary responses and accommodation reflexes (retinopretectal system). Subdivision

into specific nuclei has not yet been accomplished in humans, and so the term "area" is used.
• Axons to the suprachiasmatic nucleus of the hypothalamus influence circadian rhythms.
• Axons to the thalamic nuclei (optic tract) in the tegmentum of the mesencephalon and to the vestibular nuclei transmit afferent fibers for optokinetic nystagmus (=jerky, physiological eye movements during the tracking of fast-moving objects). This has also been called the "accessory visual system."
• Axons to the pulvinar of the thalamus form the visual association cortex for oculomotor function (neurons are relayed in the superior colliculus).
• Axons to the parvocellular nucleus of the reticular formation function during arousal.

Fig. 9.55 Brainstem reflexes
Brainstem reflexes are important in the examination of comatose patients. Loss of all brainstem reflexes is considered evidence of brain death. Three of these reflexes are described below:
Pupillary reflex: The pupillary reflex relies on the nongeniculate parts of the visual pathway (see **Fig. 9.57**). The afferent fibers for this reflex come from the optic nerve, which is an extension of the diencephalon. The efferents for the pupillary reflex come from the accessory nucleus of the oculomotor nerve (CN III), which is located in the brainstem. Loss of the pupillary reflex may signify a lesion of the diencephalon (interbrain) or mesencephalon (midbrain).
Vestibulo-ocular reflex: Irrigating the ear canal with cold water in a normal individual evokes nystagmus that beats toward the opposite side (afferent fibers are conveyed in the vestibulocochlear nerve [CN VIII], efferent fibers in the oculomotor nerve [CN III]). When the vestibulo-ocular reflex is absent in a comatose patient, it is considered a poor sign because this reflex is the most reliable clinical test of brainstem function.
Corneal reflex: This reflex is not mediated by the visual pathway. The afferent fibers for the reflex (elicited by stimulation of the cornea, as by touching it with a sterile cotton wisp) are conveyed in the trigeminal nerve (CN VI) and the efferent fibers (contraction of the orbicularis oculi in response to corneal irritation) in the facial nerve (CN VII). The relay center for the corneal reflex is located in the pontine region of the brainstem. Loss of the corneal reflex can be due to sensory loss in CN V_1, weakness or paralysis of the facial nerve (CN VII), or to brainstem disease.

Visual System (III): Reflexes

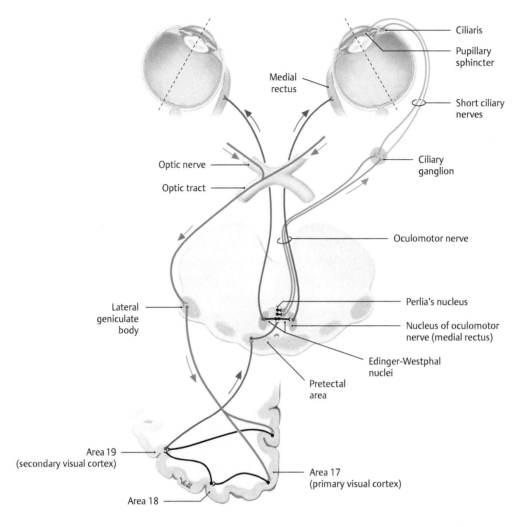

Fig. 9.56 Pathways for convergence and accommodation
When the distance between the eyes and an object decreases, three processes must occur in order to produce a sharp, three-dimensional visual impression (the first two are simultaneous):

1. Convergence (red): The visual axes of the eyes move closer together. The two medial rectus muscles contract to move the ocular axis medially. This keeps the image of the approaching object on the fovea centralis.
2. Accommodation: The lenses adjust their focal length. The curvature of the lens is increased to keep the image of the object sharply focused on the retina. The ciliary muscle contracts, which relaxes the tension on the lenticular fibers. The intrinsic pressure of the lens then causes it to assume a more rounded shape. (*Note:* The lens is flattened by the contraction of the lenticular fibers, which are attached to the ciliary muscle.)
3. Pupillary constriction: The pupil is constricted by the pupillary sphincter to increase visual acuity.

Convergence and accommodation may be conscious (fixing the gaze on a near object) or unconscious (fixing the gaze on an approaching automobile).
Pathways: The pathways can be broken into three components:

1. Geniculate visual pathway (purple): Axons of the first neurons (photoreceptors) and second neurons (bipolar cells) relay sensory information to the third neurons (retinal ganglion cells), which course in the optic nerve (CN II) to the lateral geniculate body. There they

synapse with the fourth neuron, whose axons project to the primary visual cortex (area 17).
2. Visual cortexes to cranial nerve nuclei: Interneurons (black) connect the primary (area 17) and secondary (area 19) visual cortexes. Synaptic relays (red) connect area 19 to the pretectal area and ultimately Perlia's nucleus (yellow), located between the two Edinger-Westphal (visceral oculomotor) nuclei (green).
3. Cranial nerves: At Perlia's nucleus, the pathway for convergence diverges with the pathways for accommodation and pupillary constriction:

   • Convergence: Neurons relay impulses to the somatomotor nucleus of the oculomotor nerve, whose axons pass directly to the medial rectus muscle via the oculomotor nerve (CN III).
   • Accommodation and pupillary constriction: Neurons relay impulses to the Edinger-Westphal nucleus, whose preganglionic parasympathetic axons project to the ciliary ganglion. After synapsing in the ciliary ganglion, the postganglionic axons pass either to the ciliary muscle (accommodation) or the pupillary sphincter (pupillary constriction) via the short ciliary nerves.

Note: The pupillary sphincter light response is abolished in tertiary syphilis, while accommodation (ciliary muscle) and convergence (medial rectus) are preserved. This phenomenon, called an Argyll Robertson pupil, indicates that the connections to the ciliary and pupillary sphincter muscles are mediated by different tracts, although the anatomy of these tracts is not yet fully understood.

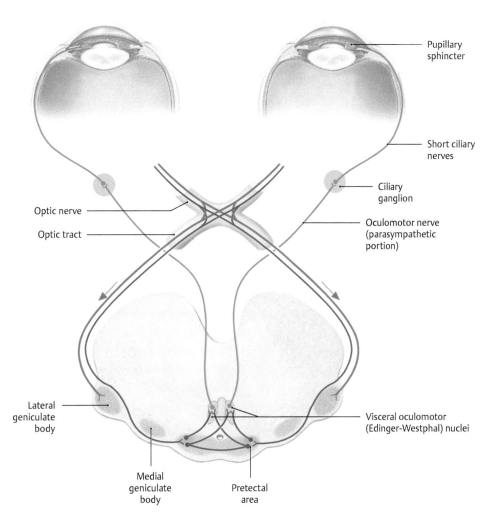

Fig. 9.57 Pupillary light reflex
The pupillary light reflex enables the eye to adapt to varying levels of brightness. When a large amount of light enters the eye (e.g., beam of a headlight), the pupil constricts to protect the photoreceptors in the retina; when the light fades, the pupil dilates. This reflexive pathway takes place without conscious input via the nongeniculate part of the visual pathway. The reflex can be broken into components:

1. Afferent limb: The first (photoreceptor) and second (bipolar) neurons relay sensory information to the third (retinal ganglion) neurons, which combine to form the optic nerve (CN II). Most third neurons (purple) synapse at the lateral geniculate body (geniculate part of the visual pathway). The third neurons responsible for the light reflex (blue) synapse at the pretectal area in the medial root of the optic tract (nongeniculate part of the visual pathway). Fourth neurons from the pretectal area pass to the parasympathetic Edinger-Westphal nuclei. *Note:* Because both nuclei are innervated, a consensual light response can occur (contraction of one pupil will cause contraction of the other).
2. Efferent limb: Fifth neurons from the Edinger-Westphal nuclei (preganglionic parasympathetic neurons) synapse in the ciliary ganglion. Sixth neurons (postganglionic parasympathetic neurons) pass to the pupillary sphincter via the short ciliary nerves.

Loss of light response: Because fourth neurons from the pretectal area pass to both Edinger-Westphal nuclei, a consensual light response can occur (contraction of one pupil will cause contraction of the other). The light response must therefore be tested both directly and indirectly:

- Direct light response: Tested by covering both eyes of the conscious, cooperative patient and then uncovering one eye. After a short latency period, the pupil of the light-exposed eye will contract.
- Indirect light response: Tested by placing the examiner's hand on the bridge of the patient's nose, shading one eye from the beam of a flashlight while shining it into the other eye. The object is to test whether shining the light into one eye will cause the pupil of the shaded eye to contract as well (consensual light response).

Lesions can occur all along the pathway for the pupillary light reflex. The direct and indirect light responses can be used to determine the level:

- Unilateral optic nerve lesion: This produces blindness on the affected side. If the patient is unconscious or uncooperative, the light responses can determine the lesion, as the afferent limb of the pupillary light reflex is lost. Affected side: No direct light response and no consensual light response on the opposite side. Unaffected side: Direct light response and consensual light response on the opposite (affected) side. Because the efferent limb of the reflex is not mediated by the optic nerve, the functional afferent limb can bypass the impaired afferent limb.
- Lesion of the parasympathetic Edinger-Westphal nucleus or the ciliary ganglion: The efferent limb of the pupillary light reflex is lost. Affected side: No direct or indirect pupillary light response on the opposite side. Unaffected side: Direct light response, no indirect light response on the opposite (affected) side.
- Lesion of the optic radiation or visual cortex (geniculate part of the visual pathway): Intact pupillary reflex (direct and indirect light response on both sides).

273

Visual System (IV): Coordination of Eye Movement

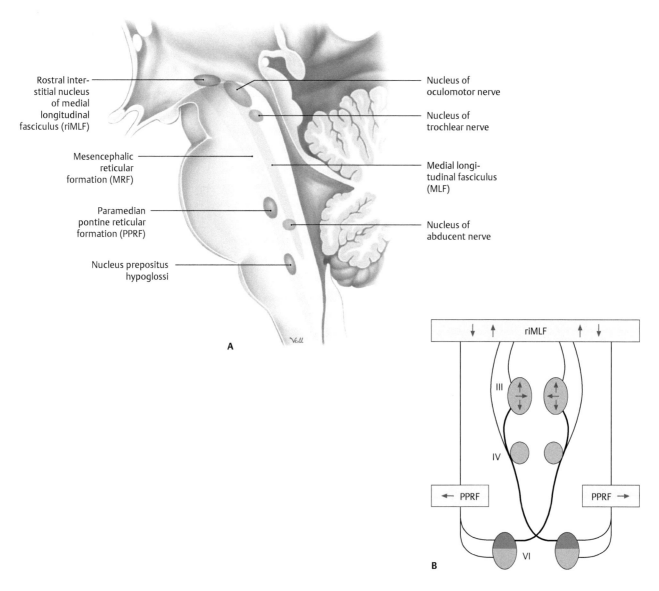

Fig. 9.58 Oculomotor nuclei and connections in the brainstem
A Midsagittal section viewed from left side. **B** Circuit diagram showing the supranuclear organization of eye movements.

The extraocular muscles receive motor innervation from the oculomotor (CN III), trochlear (CN IV), and abducent (CN VI) nerves. The concerted movement of the extraocular muscles allows for shifting of gaze, the swift movement of the visual axis toward the intended target. These rapid, precise, "ballistic" eye movements are called *saccades*. They are preprogrammed and, once initiated, cannot be altered until the end of the saccadic movement. The nuclei of CN III, IV, and VI (red) are involved in these saccadic movements. They are interconnected for this purpose by the medial longitudinal fasciculus (MLF, blue). Because these complex movements involve all the extraocular muscles and their associated nerves, the activity of the nuclei must be coordinated at a higher, or supranuclear, level. For example, gazing to the right requires four concerted movements:

- Contract right lateral rectus (CN VI nucleus activated)
- Relax right medial rectus (CN III nucleus inhibited)
- Relax left lateral rectus (CN VI nucleus inhibited)
- Contract left medial rectus (CN III nucleus activated)

These conjugate eye movements are coordinated by premotor nuclei (purple) in the mesencephalic reticular formation (green). Horizontal gaze movements are programmed in the nuclear region of the paramedian pontine reticular formation (PPRF). Vertical gaze movements are programmed in the rostral interstitial nucleus of the medial longitudinal fasciculus (riMLF). Both gaze centers establish bilateral connections with the nuclei of CN III, IV, and VI. The tonic signals for maintaining the new eye position originate from the nucleus prepositus hypoglossi.

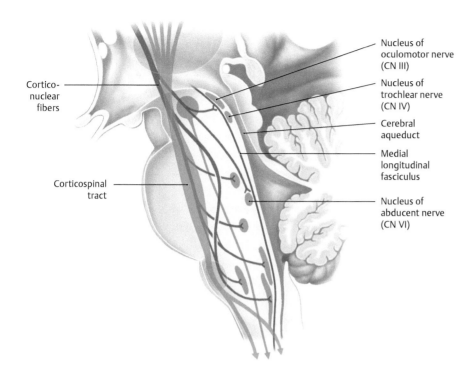

Corticonuclear fibers

Corticospinal tract

Nucleus of oculomotor nerve (CN III)

Nucleus of trochlear nerve (CN IV)

Cerebral aqueduct

Medial longitudinal fasciculus

Nucleus of abducent nerve (CN VI)

Fig. 9.59 Course of the medial longitudinal fasciculus in the brainstem
Midsagittal section viewed from the left side. The medial longitudinal fasciculus (MLF) runs anterior to the cerebral aqueduct on both sides and continues from the mesencephalon to the cervical spinal cord. It transmits fibers for the coordination of conjugate eye movements. A lesion of the MLF results in internuclear ophthalmoplegia (see **Fig. 9.60**).

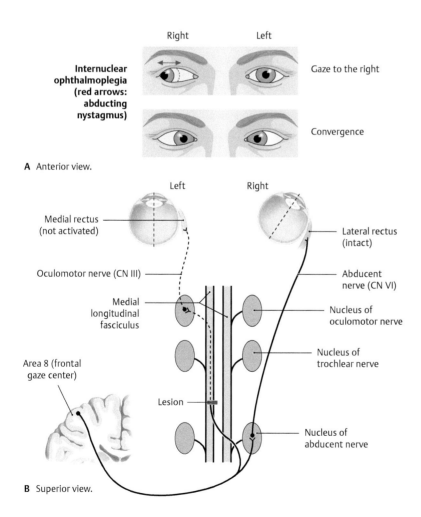

Internuclear ophthalmoplegia (red arrows: abducting nystagmus)

Right Left

Gaze to the right

Convergence

A Anterior view.

Left Right

Medial rectus (not activated)

Oculomotor nerve (CN III)

Medial longitudinal fasciculus

Area 8 (frontal gaze center)

Lesion

Lateral rectus (intact)

Abducent nerve (CN VI)

Nucleus of oculomotor nerve

Nucleus of trochlear nerve

Nucleus of abducent nerve

B Superior view.

Fig. 9.60 Internuclear ophthalmoplegia
The medial longitudinal fasciculus (MLF) interconnects the oculomotor nuclei and also connects them with the opposite side. When this "information highway" is interrupted, internuclear ophthalmoplegia develops. This type of lesion most commonly occurs between the nuclei of the abducent and the oculomotor nerves. It may be unilateral or bilateral. Typical causes are multiple sclerosis and diminished blood flow. The lesion is manifested by the loss of conjugate eye movements. With a lesion of the left MLF, as shown here, the left medial rectus muscle is no longer activated during gaze to the right. The eye cannot be moved *inward* on the side of the lesion (loss of the medial rectus), and the opposite eye goes into an abducting nystagmus (lateral rectus is intact and innervated by the abducent nerve). Reflex movements such as convergence are not impaired, as there is no peripheral or nuclear lesion, and this reaction is not mediated by the MLF.

Radiographs of the Orbit

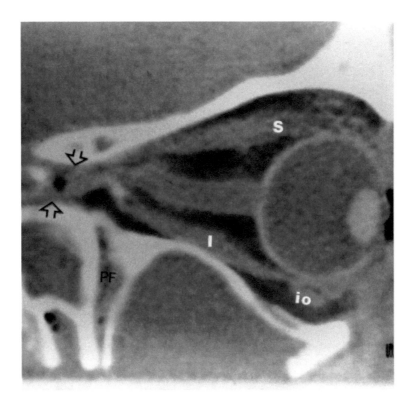

Fig. 9.61 **Orbital CT anatomy**
Parasagittal CT scan of a cadaver head shows globe; optic nerve; superior rectus muscle (S), inferior rectus muscle (I), inferior oblique muscle (IO); common tendon of Zinn (arrows); and pterygomaxillary fissure (PF). The orbital periosteum, the so-called periorbita, lines the bony orbit as orbital fascia and is relatively loosely attached to the bony orbit. The periosteum is connected with the dura mater and sheath of the optic nerve at the optic canal. Normally, periosteum cannot be dif-ferentiated from adjacent soft tissues. The periosteum is continuous with the periosteum of the bones of the face and is continuous with the periosteal layer of dura at the superior orbital fissure. Note continuity of the periorbita with the periosteum of the pterygopalatine fossa and pterygomaxillary fissure (PF). CT scan courtesy of FW Zonneveld, PhD. Reproduced from Mafee MF, et al. Orbital space-occupying lesions: role of CT and MRI: an analysis of 145 cases. Radiol Clin North Am 1987; 25:529. With permission.

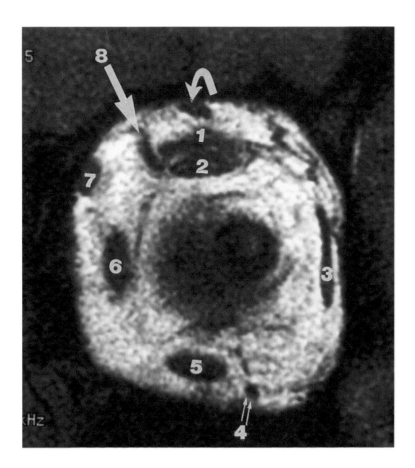

Fig. 9.62
Coronal T1W MR scan, taken with 3 inch surface coil (450/28, TR/TE, FOV: 8×8, 256×256, 3 mm slice thickness, 0.0 spacing), showing the levator palpebrae superioris (1), superior rectus muscle (2), lateral rectus muscle (3), inferior ophthalmic vein (4), inferior rectus muscle (5), medial rectus muscle (6), superior oblique muscle (7), superior oph-

thalmic vein (8), and frontal nerve (curved arrow). Note numerous connective-tissue septa within the fat cushion of the orbit, giving the appearance of a fatty reticulum. As seen, the connective-tissue septa are present within the central orbital fat as well as between the orbital walls, the muscles, and partially volumed globe.

Overview & External Ear (I)

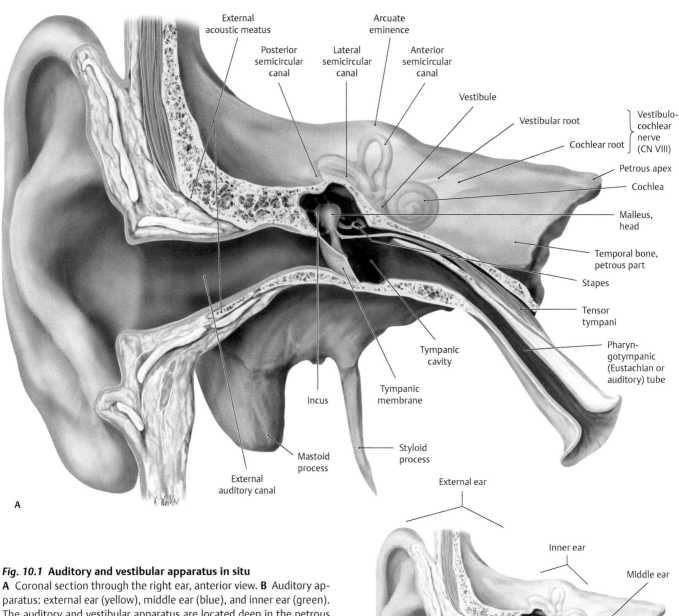

Fig. 10.1 Auditory and vestibular apparatus in situ
A Coronal section through the right ear, anterior view. **B** Auditory apparatus: external ear (yellow), middle ear (blue), and inner ear (green). The auditory and vestibular apparatus are located deep in the petrous part of the temporal bone. The **auditory apparatus** consists of the external ear, middle ear, and inner ear. Sound waves are captured by the auricle and travel through the external auditory canal to the tympanic membrane (the lateral boundary of the middle ear). The sound waves set the tympanic membrane into motion, and these mechanical vibrations are transmitted by the chain of auditory ossicles in the middle ear to the oval window, which leads into the inner ear. The ossicular chain induces vibrations in the membrane covering the oval window, and these in turn cause a fluid column in the inner ear to vibrate, setting receptor cells in motion. The transformation of sound waves into electrical impulses takes place in the inner ear, which is the actual organ of hearing. The external ear and middle ear, on the other hand, constitute the *sound conduction apparatus*. The organ of balance is the **vestibular apparatus**, which is also located in the inner ear. It contains the *semicircular canals* for the perception of angular acceleration (rotational head movements) and the *saccule* and *utricle* for the perception of linear acceleration. Diseases of the vestibular apparatus produce dizziness (vertigo).

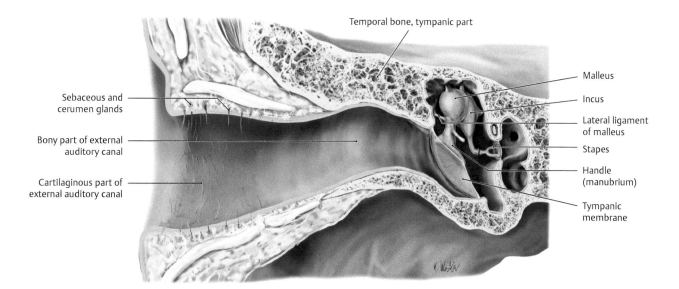

Temporal bone, tympanic part

Malleus

Incus

Lateral ligament of malleus

Stapes

Handle (manubrium)

Tympanic membrane

Sebaceous and cerumen glands

Bony part of external auditory canal

Cartilaginous part of external auditory canal

Fig. 10.2 External auditory canal, tympanic membrane, and tympanic cavity
Coronal section, right ear, anterior view. The tympanic membrane (eardrum) separates the external auditory canal from the tympanic cavity of the middle ear. The external auditory canal is an S-shaped tunnel that is approximately 3 cm long with an average diameter of 0.6 cm. The outer third of the ear canal is cartilaginous. The inner two thirds of the canal are osseous, the wall being formed by the tympanic part of the temporal bone. The cartilaginous part in particular bears numerous sebaceous and cerumen glands beneath the keratinized stratified squamous epithelium. The cerumen glands produce a watery secretion that combines with the sebum and sloughed epithelial cells to form a protective barrier (cerumen, "earwax") that screens out foreign bodies and keeps the epithelium from drying out. If the cerumen absorbs water (e.g., after swimming), it may obstruct the ear canal (cerumen impaction), temporarily causing a partial loss of hearing.

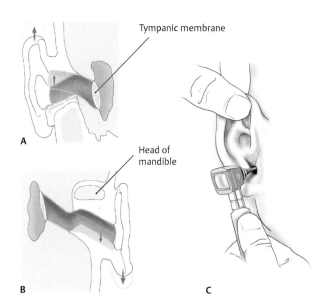

Tympanic membrane

Head of mandible

A

B

C

Fig. 10.3 Curvature of the external auditory canal
Right ear, anterior view (**A**) and transverse section (**B**).
The external auditory canal is most curved in its cartilaginous portion. When the tympanic membrane is inspected with an otoscope, the auricle should be pulled backward and upward in order to straighten the cartilaginous part of the ear canal so that the speculum of the otoscope can be introduced (**C**).
Note the proximity of the cartilaginous anterior wall of the external auditory canal to the temporomandibular joint (TM). This allows the examiner to palpate movements of the head of the mandible within the TMJ by inserting the small finger into the outer part of the ear canal.

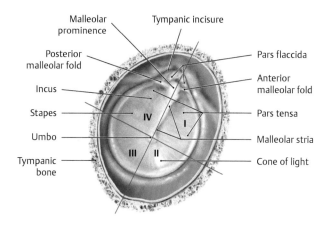

Malleolar prominence

Tympanic incisure

Posterior malleolar fold

Pars flaccida

Anterior malleolar fold

Incus

Stapes

Pars tensa

Umbo

Malleolar stria

Tympanic bone

Cone of light

IV

I

III

II

Fig. 10.4 Tympanic membrane
Right tympanic membrane, lateral view. The healthy tympanic membrane has a pearly gray color and an oval shape with an average surface area of approximately 75 mm². It consists of a lax portion, the *pars flaccida* (Shrapnell membrane), and a larger taut portion, the *pars tensa*, which is drawn inward at its center to form the umbo ("navel"). The umbo marks the lower tip of the handle (manubrium) of the malleus, which is attached to the tympanic membrane all along its length. It is visible through the pars tensa as a light-colored streak (malleolar stria). The tympanic membrane is divided into four quadrants in a clockwise direction: anterosuperior (I), anteroinferior (II), posteroinferior (III), posterosuperior (IV). The boundary lines of the quadrants are the malleolar stria and a line intersecting it perpendicularly at the umbo. The quadrants of the tympanic membrane are clinically important because they are used in describing the location of lesions. A triangular area of reflected light can be seen in the anteroinferior quadrant of a normal tympanic membrane. The location of this "cone of light" is helpful in evaluating the tension of the tympanic membrane.

279

External Ear (II): Auricle

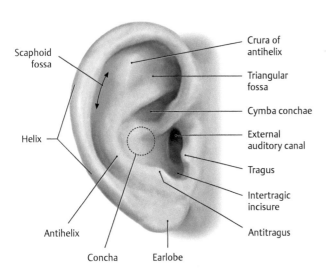

Fig. 10.5 Right auricle
The auricle of the ear encloses a cartilaginous framework (auricular cartilage) that forms a funnel-shaped receptor for acoustic vibrations.

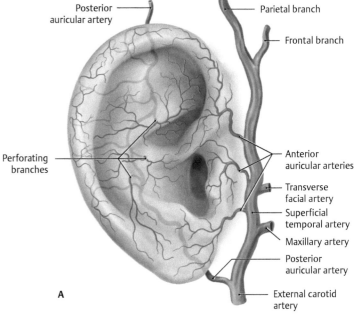

Fig. 10.7 Arterial supply of the auricle
Lateral view (**A**) and posterior view (**B**) of right auricle.
The proximal and medial portions of the laterally directed anterior surface of the ear are supplied by the anterior auricular arteries, which arise from the superficial temporal artery. The other parts of the auricle are supplied by branches of the posterior auricular artery, which arises from the external carotid artery. These vessels are linked by extensive anastomoses, so operations on the external ear are unlikely to compromise the auricular blood supply. The copious blood flow through the auricle contributes to temperature regulation: dilation of the vessels helps dissipate heat through the skin. The lack of insulating fat predisposes the ear to frostbite, which is particularly common in the upper third of the auricle. The auricular arteries have corresponding veins that drain to the superficial temporal vein.

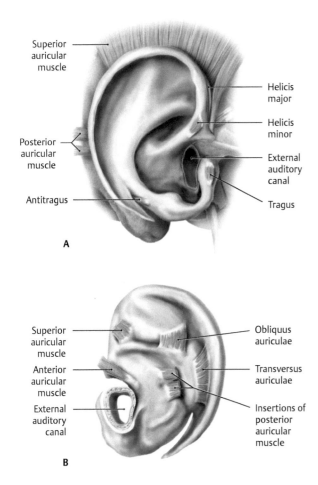

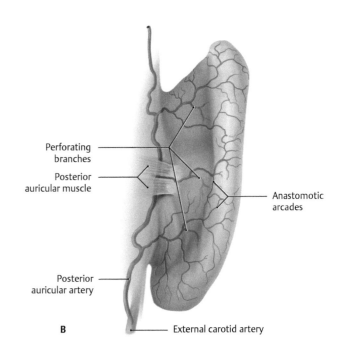

Fig. 10.6 Cartilage and muscles of the auricle
A Lateral view of the external surface. **B** Medial view of the posterior surface of the right ear.
The skin (removed here) is closely applied to the elastic cartilage of the auricle (light blue). The muscles of the ear are classified as muscles of facial expression and, like the other members of this group, are supplied by the facial nerve (CN VII). Prominent in other mammals, the auricular muscles are vestigial in humans, with no significant function.

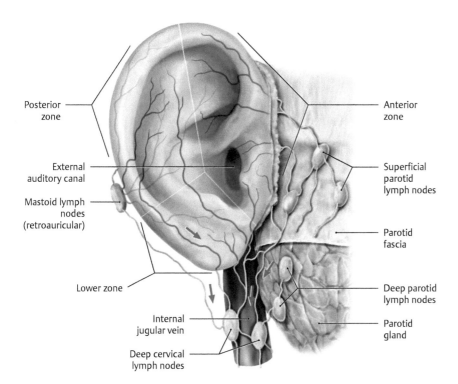

Fig. 10.8 Auricle and external auditory canal: lymphatic drainage

Right ear, oblique lateral view. The lymphatic drainage of the ear is divided into three zones, all of which drain directly or indirectly into the deep cervical lymph nodes along the internal jugular vein. The lower zone drains directly into the deep cervical lymph nodes. The anterior zone first drains into the parotid lymph nodes, the posterior zone into the mastoid lymph nodes.

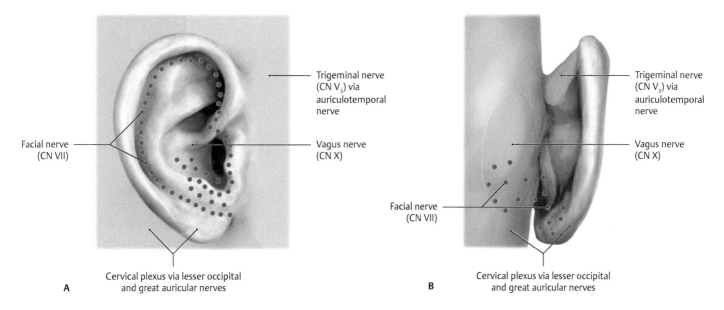

Fig. 10.9 Sensory innervation of the auricle

Right ear, lateral view (**A**) and posterior view (**B**). The auricular region has a complex nerve supply because, developmentally, it is located at the boundary between the cranial nerves (pharyngeal arch nerves) and branches of the cervical plexus. Three cranial nerves contribute to the innervation of the auricle:

- Trigeminal nerve (CN V₃)
- Facial nerve (CN VII; the skin area that receives sensory innervation from the facial nerve is not precisely known)
- Vagus nerve (CN X)

Two branches of the **cervical plexus** are involved:

- Lesser occipital nerve (C 2)
- Great auricular nerve (C 2, C 3)

Note: Because the vagus nerve contributes to the innervation of the external auditory canal (auricular branch), mechanical cleaning of the ear canal (by inserting an aural speculum or by irrigating the ear) may evoke coughing and nausea. The auricular branch of the vagus nerve passes through the mastoid canaliculus and through a space between the mastoid process and the tympanic part of the temporal bone (tympanomastoid fissure, see p. 33) to the external ear and external auditory canal.

281

Middle Ear (I): Tympanic Cavity & Pharyngotympanic Tube

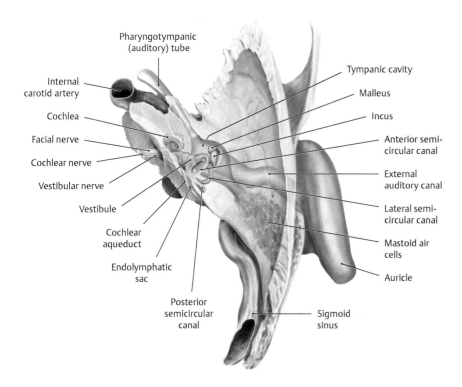

Pharyngotympanic
(auditory) tube

Internal
carotid artery

Cochlea

Facial nerve

Cochlear nerve

Vestibular nerve

Vestibule

Cochlear
aqueduct

Endolymphatic
sac

Posterior
semicircular
canal

Tympanic cavity

Malleus

Incus

Anterior semi-
circular canal

External
auditory canal

Lateral semi-
circular canal

Mastoid air
cells

Auricle

Sigmoid
sinus

Fig. 10.10 Middle ear and associated structures
Right petrous temporal bone, superior view. The middle ear (light blue) is located within the petrous part of the temporal bone between the external ear (yellow) and inner ear (green). The tympanic cavity of the middle ear contains the chain of auditory ossicles, of which the malleus (hammer) and incus (anvil) are visible here. The tympanic cavity communicates anteriorly with the nasopharynx via the pharyngotympanic (auditory) tube and posteriorly with the mastoid air cells. Infections can spread from the nasopharynx to the mastoid air cells by this route.

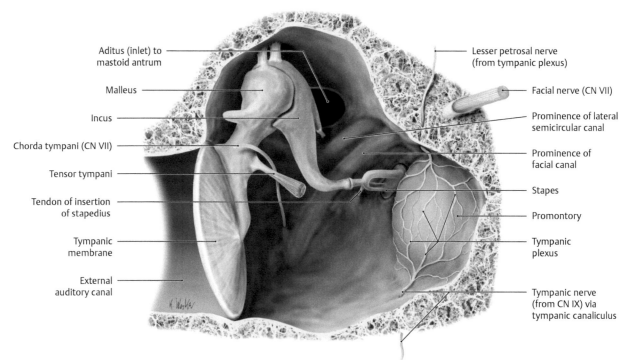

Aditus (inlet) to
mastoid antrum

Malleus

Incus

Chorda tympani (CN VII)

Tensor tympani

Tendon of insertion
of stapedius

Tympanic
membrane

External
auditory canal

Lesser petrosal nerve
(from tympanic plexus)

Facial nerve (CN VII)

Prominence of lateral
semicircular canal

Prominence of
facial canal

Stapes

Promontory

Tympanic
plexus

Tympanic nerve
(from CN IX) via
tympanic canaliculus

Fig. 10.11 Walls of the tympanic cavity
Coronal section anterior view with the anterior wall removed. The tympanic cavity is a slightly oblique space that is bounded by six walls:

- Lateral (membranous) wall: boundary with the external ear; formed largely by the tympanic membrane.
- Medial (labyrinthine) wall: boundary with the inner ear; formed largely by the promontory, or the bony eminence, overlying the basal turn of the cochlea.
- Inferior (jugular) wall: forms the floor of the tympanic cavity and borders on the bulb of the jugular vein.

- Posterior (mastoid) wall: borders on the air cells of the mastoid process, communicating with the cells through the aditus (inlet) of the mastoid antrum.
- Superior (tegmental) wall: forms the roof of the tympanic cavity.
- Anterior (carotid) wall (removed here): includes the opening to the pharyngotympanic (auditory) tube and borders on the carotid canal.

The lateral side of the tympanic membrane is innervated by three cranial nerves: CN V_3 (auriculotemporal nerve), CN VII (posterior auricular nerve; pathway uncertain), and CN X (auricular branch). The medial side of the tympanic membrane is innervated by CN IX (tympanic branch).

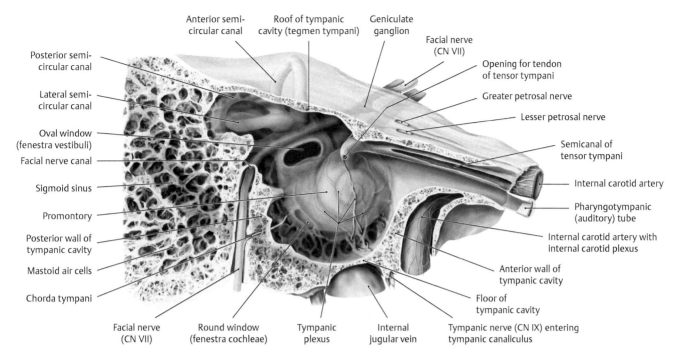

Fig. 10.12 Nerves in the petrous bone

Oblique sagittal section showing the medial wall of the tympanic cavity (see **Fig. 10.11**). The tympanic nerve branches from CN IX as it passes through the jugular foramen, and conveys sensory and preganglionic parasympathetic fibers into the tympanic cavity by passing through the tympanic canaliculus. The fibers from the tympanic plexus provide sensory innervation to the tympanic cavity (including the medial surface of the tympanic membrane), mastoid air cells, and part of the pharyngotympanic tube. *Note:* The lateral surface of the tympanic membrane receives sensory innervation from branches of CN V₃, CN VII, and CN X (see **Fig. 10.11**).

The preganglionic parasympathetic fibers of the tympanic nerve are reformed from the tympanic plexus as the lesser petrosal nerve. These fibers synapse in the otic ganglion; the postganglionic parasympathetic fibers travel with the auriculotemporal nerve (a branch of CN V₃) to supply the parotid gland.

In the facial canal, the facial nerve (CN VII) gives off a number of branches: the greater petrosal nerve, the nerve to the stapedius, the chorda tympani, and an auricular branch. The greater petrosal nerve and the chorda tympani both carry taste fibers and preganglionic parasympathetic fibers. The greater petrosal nerve joins with the deep petrosal nerve (postganglionic sympathetic) to form the nerve of the pterygoid canal (vidian nerve). The preganglionic parasympathetic fibers in the nerve of the pterygoid canal synapse at the pterygopalatine ganglion. The postganglionic parasympathetic fibers are then distributed by branches of the maxillary nerve to the lacrimal gland, palatine glands, superior labial glands, and mucosa of the paranasal sinuses and nasal cavity. The preganglionic parasympathetic fibers of the chorda tympani synapse at the submandibular ganglion, and the postganglionic fibers are distributed to the submandibular and sublingual glands.

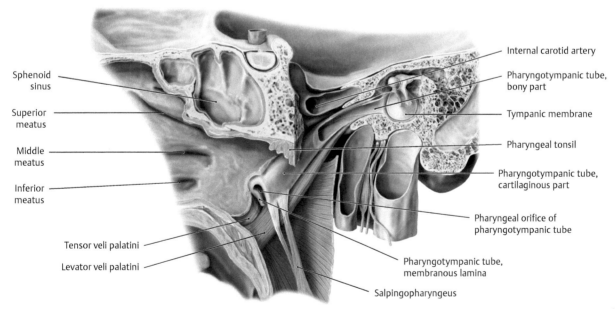

Fig. 10.13 Pharyngotympanic (Eustachian or auditory) tube

Medial view of right nasal cavity. The pharyngotympanic tube creates an open channel between the middle ear and nasopharynx. Air passing through the tube serves to equalize the air pressure on the two sides of the tympanic membrane. This equalization is essential for maintaining normal tympanic membrane mobility, necessary for normal hearing. One third of the tube is bony (in the petrous bone). The cartilaginous two thirds continue toward the nasopharynx, expanding to form a

hook (hamulus) that is attached to a membranous lamina. The fibers of the tensor veli palatini arise from this lamina; when they tense the soft palate (during swallowing), these fibers open the pharyngotympanic tube. The tube is also opened by the salpingopharyngeus and levator veli palatini. The tube is lined with ciliated respiratory epithelium: the cilia beat toward the pharynx, inhibiting the passage of microorganisms into the middle ear.

Middle Ear (II): Auditory Ossicles & Tympanic Cavity

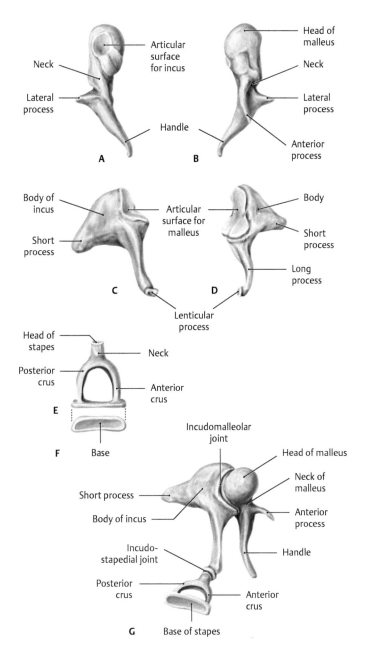

Fig. 10.14 Auditory ossicles

Auditory ossicles of the left ear. The ossicular chain (**G**) of the middle ear establishes an articular connection between the tympanic membrane and the oval window. It consists of three small bones:

- Malleus ("hammer"): **A** Posterior view. **B** Anterior view.
- Incus ("anvil"): **C** Medial view. **D** Anterolateral view.
- Stapes ("stirrup"): **E** Superior view. **F** Medial view.

Note the synovial joint articulations between the malleus and incus (incudomalleolar joint) and the incus and stapes (incudostapedial joint).

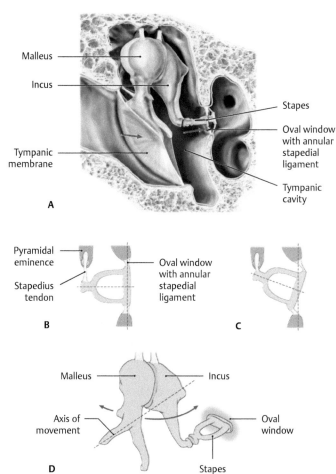

Fig. 10.15 Function of the ossicular chain

Anterior view.

A Sound waves (periodic pressure fluctuations in the air) set the tympanic membrane into vibration. The ossicular chain transmits the vibrations of the tympanic membrane (and thus the sound waves) to the oval window, which in turn communicates them to an aqueous medium (perilymph). Conductive deafness occurs when there is impaired transmission of sound waves. Although sound waves encounter very little resistance in air, they encounter considerably higher impedance when they reach the fluid interface of the inner ear. The sound waves must therefore be amplified ("impedance matching"). The difference in surface area between the tympanic membrane and oval window increases the sound pressure by a factor of 17. This is augmented by the 1.3-fold mechanical advantage of the lever action of the ossicular chain. Thus, in passing from the tympanic membrane to the inner ear, the sound pressure is amplified by a factor of 22. If the ossicular chain fails to transform the sound pressure between the tympanic membrane and stapes base (footplate), the patient will experience conductive hearing loss of magnitude approximately 20 dB.

B, C Sound waves impinging on the tympanic membrane induce motion in the ossicular chain, causing a tilting movement of the stapes (**B** normal position, **C** tilted position). The movements of the stapes base against the membrane of the oval window (stapedial membrane) induce corresponding waves in the fluid column in the inner ear.

D The movements of the ossicular chain are essentially rocking movements (the dashed line indicates the axis of the movements, the arrows indicate their direction). Two muscles affect the mobility of the ossicular chain: the tensor tympani and the stapedius (see **Fig. 10.16**).

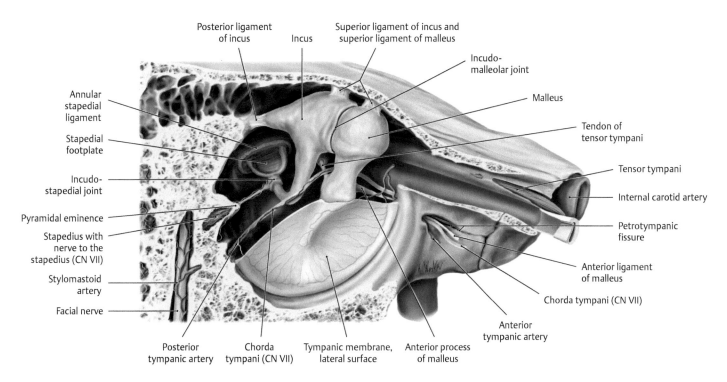

Posterior ligament
of incus

Incus

Superior ligament of incus and
superior ligament of malleus

Incudo-
malleolar joint

Malleus

Annular
stapedial
ligament

Stapedial
footplate

Tendon of
tensor tympani

Incudo-
stapedial joint

Tensor tympani

Internal carotid artery

Pyramidal eminence

Petrotympanic
fissure

Stapedius with
nerve to the
stapedius (CN VII)

Stylomastoid
artery

Anterior ligament
of malleus

Facial nerve

Chorda tympani (CN VII)

Posterior
tympanic artery

Chorda
tympani (CN VII)

Tympanic membrane,
lateral surface

Anterior process
of malleus

Anterior
tympanic artery

Fig. 10.16 Ossicular chain in the tympanic cavity
Lateral view of the right ear. The joints and their stabilizing ligaments can be seen with the two muscles of the middle ear—the stapedius and tensor tympani. The *stapedius* (innervated by the stapedial branch of the facial nerve) inserts on the stapes. When it contracts, it stiffens the sound conduction apparatus and dampens sound transmission to the inner ear. This filtering function is believed to be particularly important at high sound frequencies ("high-pass filter"). When sound is transmitted into the middle ear through a probe placed in the external

ear canal, one can measure the action of the stapedius (stapedius reflex test, p. 293 by measuring the change in acoustic impedance (i.e., the amplification of the sound waves). Contraction of the *tensor tympani* (innervated by the trigeminal nerve CN V_3 via the medial pterygoid nerve) stiffens the tympanic membrane, thereby reducing the transmission of sound. Both muscles undergo a reflex contraction in response to loud acoustic stimuli. *Note:* The chorda tympani (from CN VII) passes through the middle ear without a bony covering (making it susceptible to injury during otological surgery).

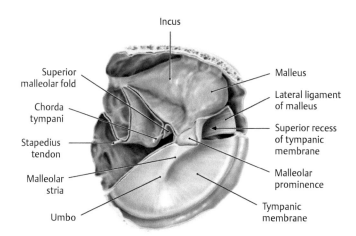

Incus

Superior
malleolar fold

Malleus

Chorda
tympani

Lateral ligament
of malleus

Stapedius
tendon

Superior recess
of tympanic
membrane

Malleolar
stria

Malleolar
prominence

Umbo

Tympanic
membrane

Fig. 10.17 Mucosal lining of the tympanic cavity
Posterolateral view with the tympanic membrane partially removed. The tympanic cavity and the structures it contains (ossicular chain, tendons, nerves) are covered with mucosa. The epithelium consists mainly of a simple squamous type, with areas of ciliated columnar cells and goblet cells. Because the tympanic cavity communicates directly with the respiratory tract (nasopharynx) through the pharyngotympanic tube, it can also be interpreted as a specialized paranasal sinus. Like the sinuses, it is susceptible to frequent infections (otitis media), which may cause ear pain, a hearing deficit, a purulent discharge from the ear, and balance problems.

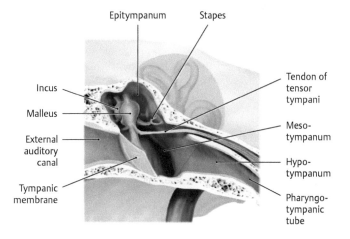

Epitympanum

Stapes

Incus

Malleus

Tendon of
tensor
tympani

External
auditory
canal

Meso-
tympanum

Tympanic
membrane

Hypo-
tympanum

Pharyngo-
tympanic
tube

Fig. 10.18 Clinically important levels of the tympanic cavity
The tympanic cavity is divided into three levels in relation to the tympanic membrane:

- Epitympanum (epitympanic recess, attic) above the tympanic membrane
- Mesotympanum medial to the tympanic membrane
- Hypotympanum (hypotympanic recess) below the tympanic membrane

The epitympanum communicates with the mastoid air cells, and the hypotympanum communicates with the pharyngotympanic tube.

285

Inner Ear (I): Overview & Innervation (CN VIII)

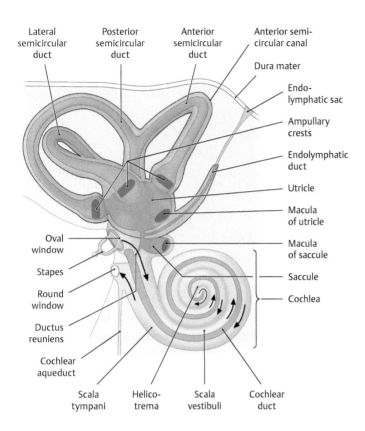

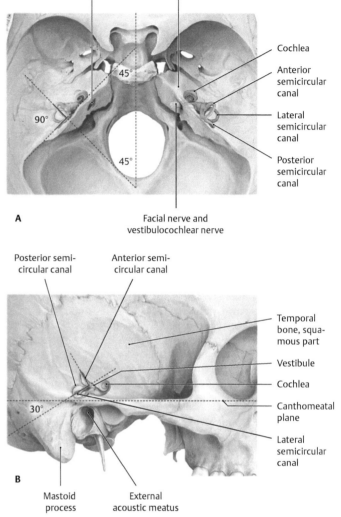

Fig. 10.19 Inner ear

The inner ear, embedded within the petrous part of the temporal bone, is formed by a membranous labyrinth, which floats within a similarly shaped bony labyrinth, loosely attached by connective tissue fibers. **Membranous labyrinth (blue):** The membranous labyrinth is filled with endolymph. This endolymphatic space (blue) communicates with the endolymphatic sac, an epidural pouch on the posterior surface of the petrous bone via the endolymphatic duct. *Note:* The auditory and vestibular endolymphatic spaces are connected by the ductus reuniens. **Bony labyrinth (beige):** The bony labyrinth is filled with perilymph. This perilymphatic space (beige) is connected to the subarachnoid space by the cochlear aqueduct (perilymphatic duct), which ends at the posterior surface of the petrous part of the temporal bone, inferior to the internal acoustic meatus.

The inner ear contains the auditory apparatus (hearing) and the vestibular apparatus (balance). **Auditory apparatus (see pp. 290–291):** The sensory epithelium of the auditory apparatus (organ of Corti) is found in the cochlea. The cochlea consists of the membranous cochlear duct and bony cochlear labyrinth. Damage to the cochlea or cochlear nerve, which combines with the vestibular nerve to form CN VIII, leads to sensineural deafness. **Vestibular apparatus (see pp. 294–295):** The sensory epithelium of the vestibular apparatus is found in the saccule, the utricle, and the three membranous semicircular ducts. The saccule and utricle are enclosed in the bony vestibule, and the ducts are enclosed in bony semicircular canals.

Fig. 10.20 Projection of the inner ear onto the bony skull

A Superior view of the petrous part of the temporal bone. **B** Right lateral view of the squamous part of the temporal bone.

The apex of the cochlea is directed anteriorly and laterally—not upward as one might intuitively expect. The bony semicircular canals are oriented at an approximately 45-degree angle to the cardinal body planes (coronal, transverse, and sagittal). It is important to know this arrangement when interpreting thin-slice CT scans of the petrous bone. *Note:* The location of the semicircular canals is of clinical importance in thermal function tests of the vestibular apparatus. The lateral (horizontal) semicircular canal is directed 30 degrees forward and upward. If the head of the *supine* patient is elevated by 30 degrees, the horizontal semicircular canal will assume a vertical alignment. Because warm fluids tend to rise, irrigating the auditory canal with warm (44°C) or cool (30°C) water (relative to the normal body temperature) can induce a thermal current in the endolymph of the semicircular canal, causing the patient to manifest vestibular nystagmus (jerky eye movements, vestibulo-ocular reflex). Because head movements always stimulate both vestibular apparatuses, caloric testing is the only method of *separately* testing the function of each vestibular apparatus (important in the diagnosis of unexplained vertigo).

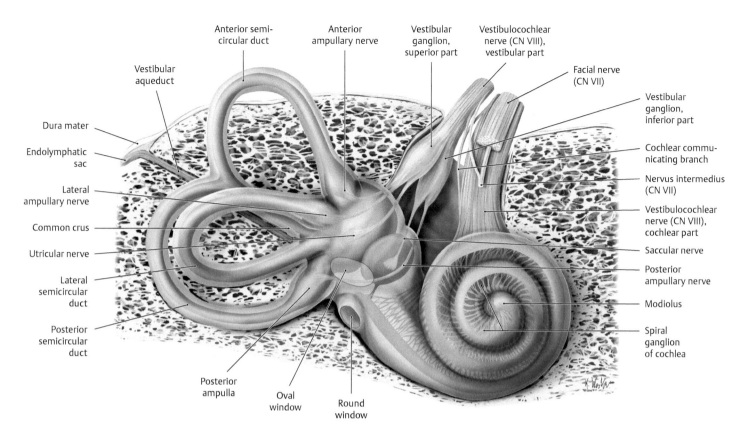

Fig. 10.21 Innervation of the membranous labyrinth
Right ear, anterior view. Afferent impulses from the vestibular and auditory membranous labyrinths are relayed via dentritic processes to cell bodies in the *vestibular* and *spiral ganglia*, respectively. The central processes of the vestibular and spiral ganglia form the vestibular and cochlear parts of the vestibulocochlear nerve (CN VIII), respectively (see pp. 140–141 for a full discussion of CN VIII). CN VIII relays afferent impulses to the brainstem through the internal acoustic meatus and cerebellopontine angle. *Vestibular ganglion:* The cell bodies of afferent neurons (bipolar ganglion cells) in the superior part of the vestibular ganglion receive afferent impulses from the anterior and lateral semicircular canals and the saccule; cell bodies in the inferior part receive afferent impulses from the posterior semicircular canal and utricle. *Spiral ganglia:* Located in the central bony core of the cochlea (modiolus), the cell bodies of bipolar ganglion cells in the spiral ganglia receive afferent impulses from the auditory apparatus via their dentritic processes.

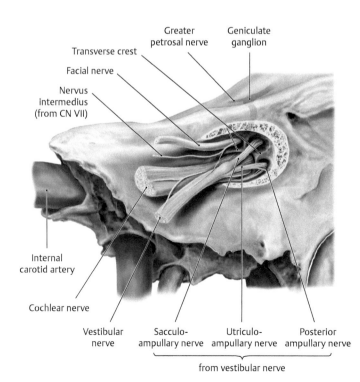

Fig. 10.22 Cranial nerves in the right internal acoustic meatus
Posterior oblique view of the fundus of the internal acoustic meatus. The approximately 1 cm-long internal auditory canal begins at the internal acoustic meatus on the posterior wall of the petrous bone. It contains:

- Vestibulocochlear nerve (CN VIII) with its cochlear and vestibular parts
- Facial nerve (CN VII), along with its parasympathetic and taste fibers (nervus intermedius)
- Labyrinthine artery and vein (not shown)

Given the close proximity of the vestibulocochlear nerve and facial nerve in the bony canal, a tumor of the vestibulocochlear nerve (*acoustic neuroma*) may exert pressure on the facial nerve, leading to peripheral facial paralysis. Acoustic neuroma is a benign tumor that originates from the Schwann cells of vestibular fibers, so it would be more accurate to call it a *vestibular schwannoma*. Tumor growth always begins in the internal auditory canal; as the tumor enlarges, it may grow into the cerebellopontine angle (see p. 140). Acute, unilateral inner ear dysfunction with hearing loss (sudden sensorineural hearing loss), often accompanied by tinnitus (ringing in the ears), typically reflects an underlying vascular disturbance (vasospasm of the labyrinthine artery causing decreased blood flow).

Arteries & Veins of the Middle & Inner Ear

The structures of the external and middle ear are supplied primarily by branches of the external carotid artery. (*Note:* The caroticotympanic arteries arise from the internal carotid artery.) The inner ear is supplied by the labyrinthine artery, which arises from the basilar artery. Venous drainage of the auricle is to the superficial temporal vein (via auricular veins), whereas drainage of the external ear is to the external jugular and maxillary veins and the pterygoid plexus. The veins of the tympanic cavity drain to the pterygoid plexus and superior petrosal sinus; the inner ear drains to the labyrinthine vein, which empties into the superior petrosal or transverse sinuses.

Table 10.1 Arteries of the ear

Artery	Origin	Distribution
Caroticotympanic aa.	Internal carotid a.	Pharyngotympanic (auditory) tube and anterior wall of tympanic cavity
Stylomastoid a.	Posterior auricular a. or occipital a.	Tympanic cavity, mastoid air cells and antrum, stapedius muscle, stapes
Inferior tympanic a.	Ascending pharyngeal a.	Medial wall of tympanic cavity, promontory
Deep auricular a.	Maxillary a.	External surface of tympanic membrane
Posterior tympanic a.	Stylomastoid a.	Chorda tympani, tympanic membrane, malleus
Superior tympanic a.	Middle meningeal a.	Tensor tympani, roof of tympanic cavity, stapes
Anterior tympanic a.	Maxillary a.	Tympanic membrane, mastoid antrum, malleus, incus
Tubal a.	Ascending pharyngeal a.	Pharyngotympanic tube and anterior tympanic cavity
Tympanic branches	A. of pterygoid canal	Tympanic cavity and pharyngotympanic tube
(Superficial) petrosal a.	Middle meningeal a.	Facial n. in facial canal and tympanic cavity
Labyrinthine a. (internal auditory a.)	Basilar a. directly or via its anterior inferior cerebellar branch	Cochlea and vestibular system

Note: The arteries supplying the tympanic cavity and its contents form a rich arterial anastomotic network within the middle ear. The venous drainage of the middle ear is primarily into the pterygoid plexus of veins located in the infratemporal fossa or into dural venous sinuses.

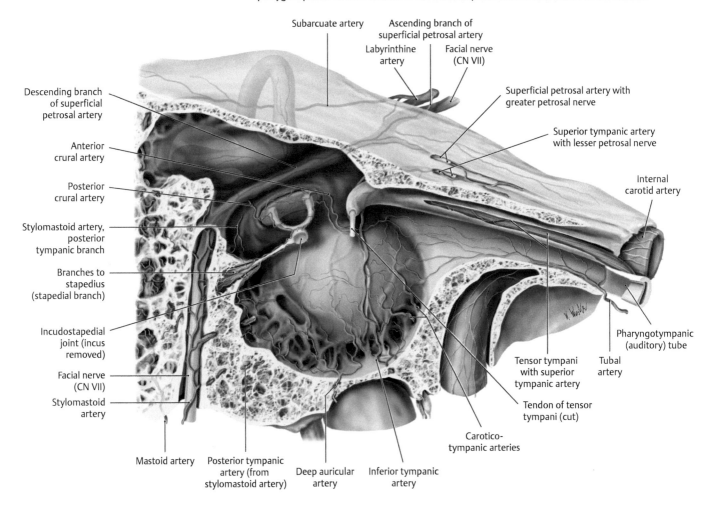

Fig. 10.23 Arteries of the tympanic cavity and mastoid air cells
Right petrous bone, anterior view. The malleus, incus, chorda tympani, and anterior tympanic artery have been removed (see **Fig. 10.24**).

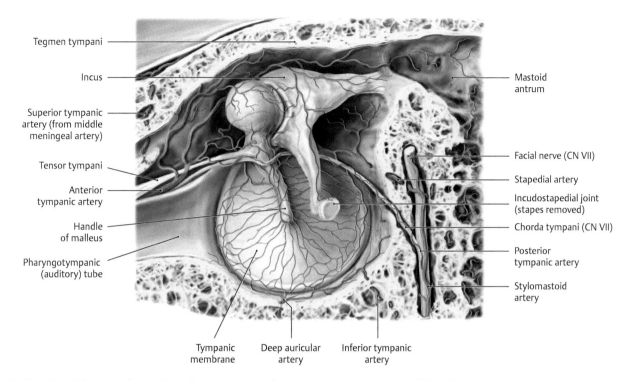

Tegmen tympani

Incus

Superior tympanic artery (from middle meningeal artery)

Tensor tympani

Anterior tympanic artery

Handle of malleus

Pharyngotympanic (auditory) tube

Mastoid antrum

Facial nerve (CN VII)

Stapedial artery

Incudostapedial joint (stapes removed)

Chorda tympani (CN VII)

Posterior tympanic artery

Stylomastoid artery

Tympanic membrane

Deep auricular artery

Inferior tympanic artery

Fig. 10.24 Arteries of the ossicular chain and tympanic membrane
Medial view of the right tympanic membrane (see **Fig. 10.13** for orientation). This region receives most of its blood supply from the anterior tympanic artery. With inflammation of the tympanic membrane, the arteries may become so dilated that their course in the tympanic membrane can be seen, as illustrated here.

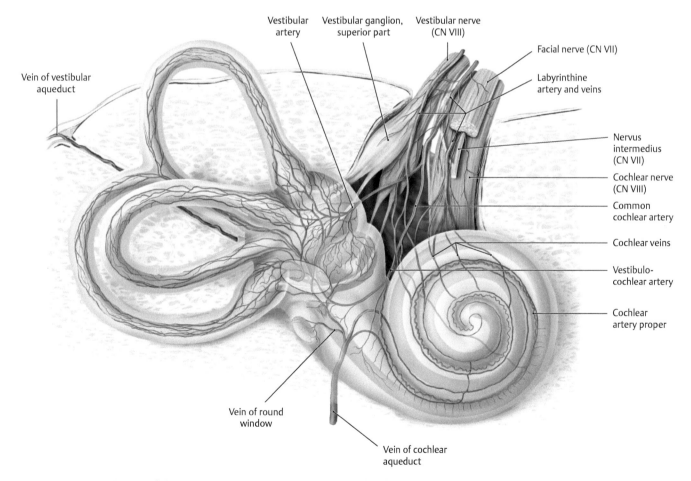

Vestibular artery

Vestibular ganglion, superior part

Vestibular nerve (CN VIII)

Vein of vestibular aqueduct

Facial nerve (CN VII)

Labyrinthine artery and veins

Nervus intermedius (CN VII)

Cochlear nerve (CN VIII)

Common cochlear artery

Cochlear veins

Vestibulo-cochlear artery

Cochlear artery proper

Vein of round window

Vein of cochlear aqueduct

Fig. 10.25 Arteries and veins of the inner ear
Right anterior view. The labyrinth receives its arterial blood supply from the labyrinthine (internal auditory) artery, which generally arises directly from the basilar artery, but may arise from the anterior inferior cerebellar artery. Venous blood drains to the labyrinthine vein and into the inferior petrosal sinus or the transverse sinuses.

289

Inner Ear (II): Auditory Apparatus

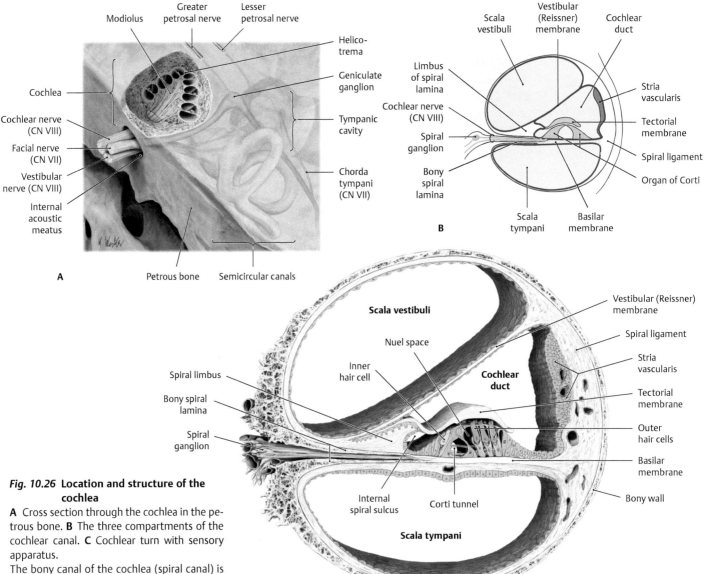

Fig. 10.26 **Location and structure of the cochlea**

A Cross section through the cochlea in the petrous bone. **B** The three compartments of the cochlear canal. **C** Cochlear turn with sensory apparatus.

The bony canal of the cochlea (spiral canal) is approximately 30 to 35 mm long in the adult. It makes two and a half turns around its bony axis, the *modiolus,* which is permeated by branched cavities and contains the spiral ganglion (perikarya of the afferent neurons). The base of the cochlea is directed toward the internal acoustic meatus (**A**). A cross section through the cochlear canal displays three membranous compartments arranged in three levels (**B**). The upper and lower compartments, the *scala vestibuli* and *scala tympani,* each contain perilymph; the middle level, the *cochlear duct* (scala media), contains endolymph. The perilymphatic spaces are interconnected at the apex by the *helicotrema,* and the endolymphatic space ends blindly at the apex. The cochlear duct, which is triangular in cross section, is separated from the scala vestibuli by the *vestibular (Reissner) membrane* and from the scala tympani by the *basilar membrane.* The basilar membrane represents a bony projection of the modiolus (*spiral lamina*) and

widens steadily from the base of the cochlea to the apex. High frequencies (up to 20,000 Hz) are perceived by the narrow portions of the basilar membrane, whereas low frequencies (down to about 200 Hz) are perceived by its broader portions (*tonotopic organization*). The basilar membrane and bony spiral lamina thus form the floor of the cochlear duct, upon which the actual organ of hearing, the organ of Corti, is located. This organ consists of a system of sensory cells and supporting cells covered by an acellular gelatinous flap, the *tectorial membrane.* The sensory cells (inner and outer hair cells) are the receptors of the organ of Corti (**C**). These cells bear approximately 50 to 100 stereocilia, and on their apical surface synapse on their basal side with the endings of afferent and efferent neurons. They

have the ability to transform mechanical energy into electrochemical potentials. A magnified cross-sectional view of a cochlear turn (**C**) also reveals the *stria vascularis,* a layer of vascularized epithelium in which the endolymph is formed. This endolymph fills the membranous labyrinth (appearing here as the cochlear duct, which is part of the labyrinth). The organ of Corti is located on the basilar membrane. It transforms the energy of the acoustic traveling wave into electrical impulses, which are then carried to the brain by the cochlear nerve. The principal cell of signal transduction is the inner hair cell. The function of the basilar membrane is to transmit acoustic waves to the inner hair cell, which transforms them into impulses that are received and relayed by the cochlear ganglion.

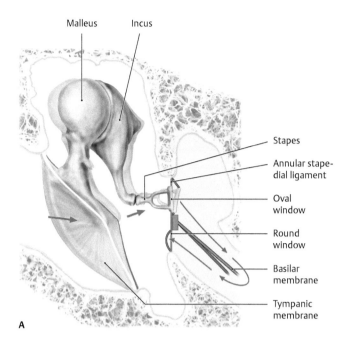

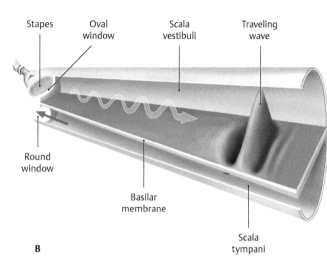

A

B

Fig. 10.27 Sound conduction during hearing

A Sound conduction from the middle ear to the inner ear: Sound waves in the air deflect the tympanic membrane, whose vibrations are conducted by the ossicular chain to the oval window. The sound pressure induces motion of the oval window membrane, whose vibrations are, in turn, transmitted through the perilymph to the basilar membrane of the inner ear (see **B**). The round window equalizes pressures between the middle and inner ear.

B Formation of a traveling wave in the cochlea: The sound wave begins at the oval window and travels up the scala vestibuli to the apex of the cochlea ("traveling wave"). The amplitude of the traveling wave gradually increases as a function of the sound frequency and reaches a maximum value at particular sites (shown greatly exaggerated in the drawing). These are the sites where the receptors of the organ of Corti are stimulated and signal transduction occurs. To understand this process, one must first grasp the structure of the organ of Corti (the actual organ of hearing), which is depicted in **Fig. 10.28**.

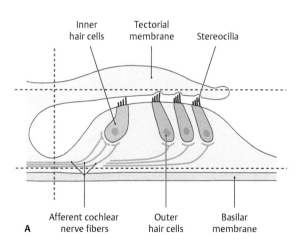

A

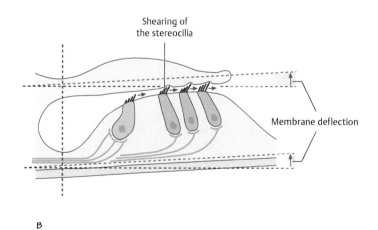

B

Fig. 10.28 Organ of Corti at rest (A) and deflected by a traveling wave (B)

The traveling wave is generated by vibrations of the oval window membrane. At each site that is associated with a particular sound frequency, the traveling wave causes a maximum deflection of the basilar membrane and thus of the tectorial membrane, setting up shearing movements between the two membranes. These shearing movements

cause the stereocilia on the *outer* hair cells to bend. In response, the hair cells actively change their length, thereby increasing the local amplitude of the traveling wave. This additionally bends the stereocilia of the *inner* hair cells, stimulating the release of glutamate at their basal pole. The release of this substance generates an excitatory potential on the afferent nerve fibers, which is transmitted to the brain.

Auditory Pathway

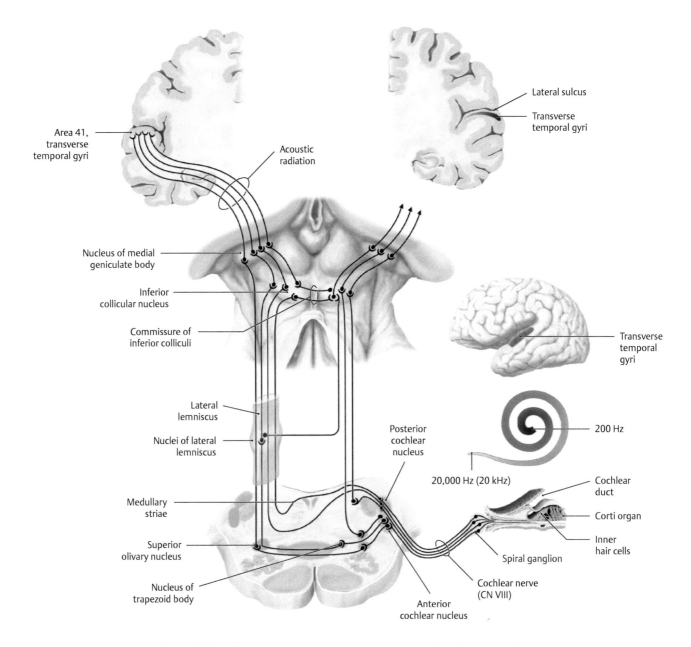

Fig. 10.29 Afferent auditory pathway of the left ear

The receptors of the auditory pathway are the inner hair cells of the organ of Corti. Because they lack neural processes, they are called *secondary sensory cells.* They are located in the cochlear duct of the basilar membrane and are studded with stereocilia, which are exposed to shearing forces from the tectorial membrane in response to a traveling wave. This causes bowing of the stereocilia (see **Fig. 10.28**). These bowing movements act as a stimulus to evoke cascades of neural signals. Dendritic processes of the bipolar neurons in the spiral ganglion pick up the stimulus. The bipolar neurons then transmit impulses via their axons, which are collected to form the cochlear nerve, to the anterior and posterior cochlear nuclei. In these nuclei the signals are relayed to the second neuron of the auditory pathway. Information from the cochlear nuclei is then transmitted via four to six nuclei to the primary auditory cortex, where the auditory information is consciously perceived (analogous to the visual cortex). The primary auditory cortex is located in the transverse temporal gyri (Heschl gyri, Brodmann area 41). The auditory pathway thus contains the following key stations:

- Inner hair cells in the organ of Corti
- Spiral ganglion
- Anterior and posterior cochlear nuclei
- Nucleus of the trapezoid body and superior olivary nucleus
- Nucleus of the lateral lemniscus
- Inferior collicular nucleus
- Nucleus of the medial geniculate body
- Primary auditory cortex in the temporal lobe (transverse temporal gyri = Heschl gyri or Brodmann area 41)

The individual parts of the cochlea are correlated with specific areas in the auditory cortex and its relay stations. This is known as the *tonotopic organization of the auditory pathway.* This organizational principle is similar to that in the visual pathway. Binaural processing of the auditory information (= stereo hearing) first occurs at the level of the superior olivary nucleus. At all further stages of the auditory pathway there are also interconnections between the right and left sides of the auditory pathway (for clarity, these are not shown here). A cochlea that has ceased to function can sometimes be replaced with a cochlear implant.

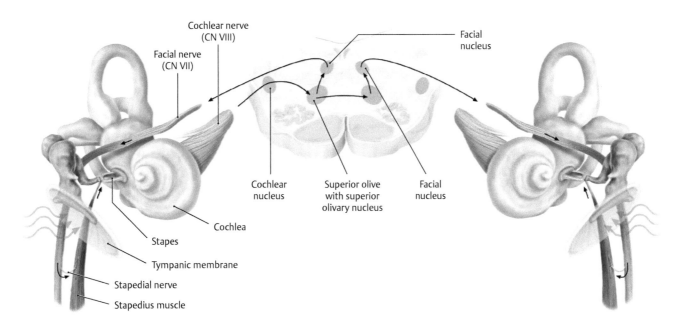

Fig. 10.30 The stapedius reflex
When the volume of an acoustic signal reaches a certain threshold, the stapedius reflex triggers a contraction of the stapedius muscle. This reflex can be utilized to test hearing without the patient's cooperation ("objective" auditory testing). The test is done by introducing a sonic probe into the ear canal and presenting a test noise to the tympanic membrane. When the noise volume reaches a certain threshold, it evokes the stapedius reflex, and the tympanic membrane stiffens. The change in the resistance of the tympanic membrane is then measured and recorded. The *afferent* limb of this reflex is in the cochlear nerve. Information is conveyed to the facial nucleus on each side by way of the superior olivary nucleus. The *efferent* limb of this reflex is formed by branchiomotor (visceromotor) fibers of the facial nerve.

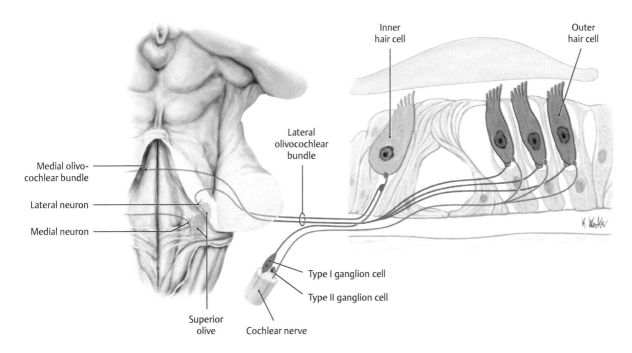

Fig. 10.31 Efferent fibers from the olive to the Corti organ
Besides the afferent (sensory) fibers from (blue) the organ of Corti, which form the vestibulocochlear nerve, there are also efferent (motor) fibers (red) that pass to the organ of Corti in the inner ear and are concerned with the active preprocessing of sound ("cochlear amplifier") and acoustic protection. The efferent fibers arise from neurons that are located in either the lateral or medial part of the superior olive and project from there to the cochlea (lateral or medial olivocochlear bun- dle). The fibers of the lateral neurons pass *uncrossed* to the dendrites of the *inner* hair cells, whereas the fibers of the medial neurons *cross* to the opposite side and terminate at the base of the *outer* hair cells, whose activity they influence. When stimulated, the outer hair cells can actively amplify the traveling wave. This increases the sensitivity of the inner hair cells (the actual receptor cells). The activity of the efferents from the olive can be recorded as otoacoustic emissions (OAE). This test can be used to screen for hearing abnormalities in newborns.

Inner Ear (III): Vestibular Apparatus

Fig. 10.32 Structure of the vestibular apparatus

The vestibular apparatus is the organ of balance. It consists of the membranous semicircular ducts, which contain sensory ridges (ampullary crests) in their dilated portions (ampullae), and of the saccule and utricle with their macular organs. The sensory organs in the semicircular ducts respond to angular acceleration; the macular organs, which have an approximately vertical and horizontal orientation, respond to horizontal (utricular macula) and vertical (saccular macula) linear acceleration, as well as to gravitational forces.

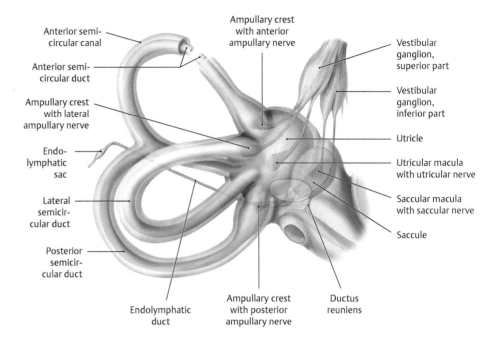

Fig. 10.33 Structure of the ampulla and ampullary crest

Cross section through the ampulla of a semicircular canal. Each canal has a bulbous expansion at one end (ampulla) that is traversed by a connective tissue ridge with sensory epithelium (ampullary crest). Extending above the ampullary crest is a gelatinous cupula, which is attached to the roof of the ampulla. Each of the sensory cells of the ampullary crest (approximately 7000 in all) bears on its apical pole one long kinocilium and approximately 80 shorter stereocilia, which project into the cupula. When the head is rotated in the plane of a particular semicircular canal, the inertial lag of the endolymph causes a deflection of the cupula, which in turn causes a bowing of the stereocilia. The sensory cells are either depolarized (excitation) or hyperpolarized (inhibition), depending on the direction of ciliary displacement.

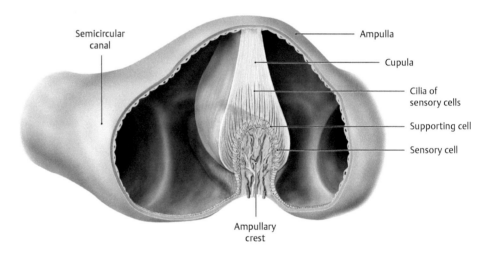

Fig. 10.34 Structure of the utricular and saccular maculae

The maculae are thickened oval areas in the epithelial lining of the utricle and saccule, each averaging 2 mm in diameter and containing arrays of sensory and supporting cells. Like the sensory cells of the ampullary crest, the sensory cells of the macular organs bear specialized stereocilia, which project into an otolithic membrane. The latter consists of a gelatinous layer, similar to the cupula, but it has calcium carbonate crystals or otoliths (*statoliths*) embedded in its surface. With their high specific gravity, these crystals exert traction on the gelatinous mass in response to linear acceleration, and this induces shearing movements of the cilia. The sensory cells are either depolarized or hyperpolarized by the movement, depending on the orientation of the cilia. There are two distinct categories of vestibular hair cells (type I and type II); type I cells (light red) are goblet shaped.

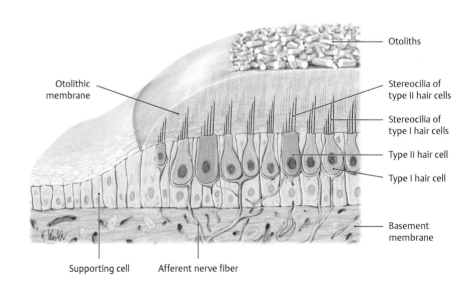

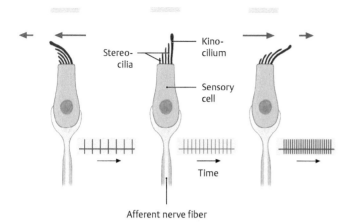

Fig. 10.35 Stimulus transduction in the vestibular sensory cells
Each of the sensory cells of the maculae and ampullary crest bears on its apical surface one long kinocilium and approximately 80 stereocilia of graduated lengths, forming an array that resembles a pipe organ. This arrangement results in a polar differentiation of the sensory cells. The cilia are straight while in a resting state. When the stereocilia are deflected toward the kinocilium, the sensory cell depolarizes, and the frequency of action potentials (discharge rate of impulses) is increased (right side of diagram). When the stereocilia are deflected away from the kinocilium, the cell hyperpolarizes, and the discharge rate is decreased (left side of diagram). This mechanism regulates the release of the transmitter glutamate at the basal pole of the sensory cell, thereby controlling the activation of the afferent nerve fiber (depolarization stimulates glutamate release, and hyperpolarization inhibits it). In this way the brain receives information on the magnitude and direction of movements and changes of position.

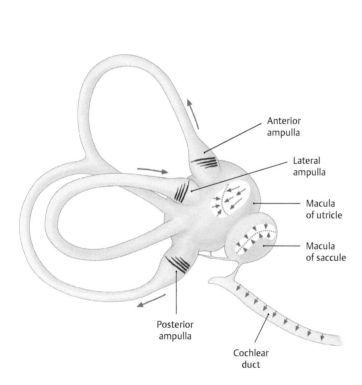

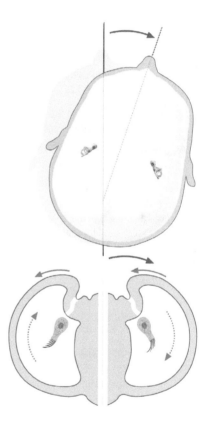

Fig. 10.36 Specialized orientations of the stereocilia in the vestibular apparatus (ampullary crest and maculae)
Because the stimulation of the sensory cells by deflection of the stereocilia *away from* or *toward* the kinocilium is what initiates signal transduction, the spatial orientation of the cilia must be specialized to ensure that every position in space and every movement of the head stimulates or inhibits certain receptors. The ciliary arrangement shown here ensures that every direction in space will correlate with the maximum sensitivity of a particular receptor field. The arrows indicate the polarity of the cilia (i.e., each of the arrowheads points in the direction of the kinocilium in that particular field).
Note that the sensory cells show an opposite, reciprocal arrangement in the sensory fields of the utricle and saccule.

Fig. 10.37 Interaction of contralateral semicircular canals during head rotation
When the head rotates to the right (red arrow), the endolymph flows to the left because of its inertial mass (solid blue arrow, taking the head as the reference point). Owing to the alignment of the stereocilia, the left and right semicircular canals are stimulated in opposite fashion. On the right side, the stereocilia are deflected toward the kinocilium (dotted arrow; the discharge rate increases). On the left side, the stereocilia are deflected away from the kinocilium (dotted arrow; the discharge rate decreases). This arrangement heightens the sensitivity to stimuli by increasing the stimulus contrast between the two sides. In other words, the difference between the decreased firing rate on one side and the increased firing rate on the other side enhances the perception of the kinetic stimulus.

Vestibular Pathway

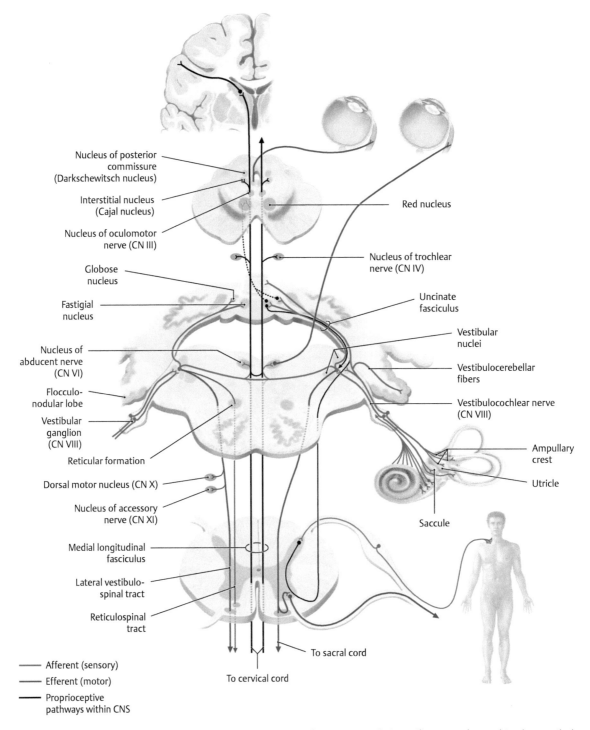

Nucleus of posterior commissure (Darkschewitsch nucleus)

Interstitial nucleus (Cajal nucleus)

Nucleus of oculomotor nerve (CN III)

Globose nucleus

Fastigial nucleus

Nucleus of abducent nerve (CN VI)

Flocculo- nodular lobe

Vestibular ganglion (CN VIII)

Reticular formation

Dorsal motor nucleus (CN X)

Nucleus of accessory nerve (CN XI)

Medial longitudinal fasciculus

Lateral vestibulo- spinal tract

Reticulospinal tract

Red nucleus

Nucleus of trochlear nerve (CN IV)

Uncinate fasciculus

Vestibular nuclei

Vestibulocerebellar fibers

Vestibulocochlear nerve (CN VIII)

Ampullary crest

Utricle

Saccule

To sacral cord

To cervical cord

—— Afferent (sensory)
—— Efferent (motor)
—— Proprioceptive pathways within CNS

Fig. 10.38 Central connections of the vestibular nerve (CN VIII)
Three systems are involved in the regulation of human balance:

- Vestibular system
- Proprioceptive system
- Visual system

The peripheral receptors of the *vestibular system* are located in the membranous labyrinth, which consists of the utricle and saccule and the ampullae of the three semicircular ducts. The maculae of the utri- cle and saccule respond to linear acceleration, and the semicircular duct organs in the ampullary crests respond to angular (rotational) acceleration. Like the hair cells of the inner ear, the receptors of the vestibular system are *secondary* sensory cells. The basal portions of the secondary sensory cells are surrounded by dendritic processes of bi-

polar neurons. Their perikarya are located in the vestibular ganglion. The axons from these neurons form the vestibular nerve and terminate in the four vestibular nuclei. Besides input from the vestibular appara- tus, these nuclei also receive sensory input (see **Fig. 10.39**). The ves- tibular nuclei show a topographical organization (see **Fig. 10.40**) and distribute their efferent fibers to three targets:

- Motor neurons in the spinal cord via the lateral vestibulospinal tract. These motor neurons help to maintain an upright stance, mainly by increasing the tone of extensor muscles.
- Flocculonodular lobe of the cerebellum (archicerebellum) via vestib- ulocerebellar fibers.
- Ipsilateral and contralateral oculomotor nuclei via the ascending part of the medial longitudinal fasciculus.

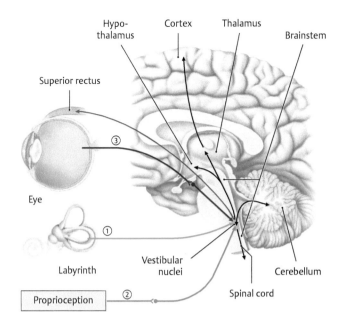

Fig. 10.39 Role of the vestibular nuclei in the maintenance of balance

The vestibular nuclei receive afferent input from the vestibular system ①, proprioceptive system ② (position sense, muscles, and joints), and visual system ③. They then distribute efferent fibers to nuclei that control the motor systems important for balance. These nuclei are located in the:

- Spinal cord (motor support)
- Cerebellum (fine control of motor function)
- Brainstem (oculomotor nuclei for oculomotor function)

Efferents from the vestibular nuclei are also distributed to the following regions:

- Thalamus and cortex (spatial sense)
- Hypothalamus (autonomic regulation: vomiting in response to vertigo)

Note: Acute failure of the vestibular system is manifested by rotary vertigo.

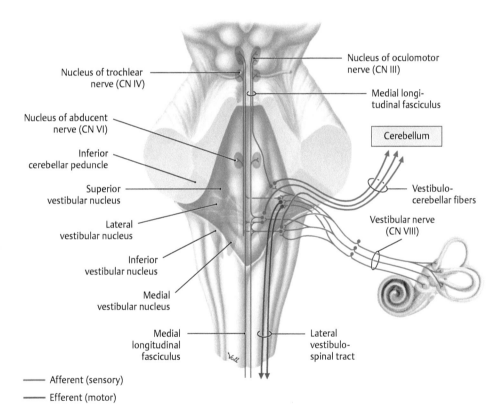

—— Afferent (sensory)
—— Efferent (motor)

Fig. 10.40 Vestibular nuclei: topographic organization and central connections

Four nuclei are distinguished:

- Superior vestibular nucleus (of Bechterew)
- Lateral vestibular nucleus (of Deiters)
- Medial vestibular nucleus (of Schwalbe)
- Inferior vestibular nucleus (of Roller)

The vestibular system has a topographic organization:

- Afferent fibers of the saccular macula terminate in the inferior vestibular nucleus and lateral vestibular nucleus.
- Afferent fibers of the utricular macula terminate in the medial part of the inferior vestibular nucleus, the lateral part of the medial vestibular nucleus, and the lateral vestibular nucleus.

- Afferent fibers from the ampullary crests of the semicircular canals terminate in the superior vestibular nucleus, the upper part of the inferior vestibular nucleus, and the lateral vestibular nucleus.

The efferent fibers from the lateral vestibular nucleus pass to the lateral vestibulospinal tract. This tract extends to the sacral part of the spinal cord, its axons terminating on motor neurons. Functionally, it is concerned with keeping the body upright, chiefly by increasing the tone of the extensor muscles. The vestibulocerebellar fibers from the other three nuclei act through the cerebellum to modulate muscular tone. All four vestibular nuclei distribute ipsilateral and contralateral axons via the medial longitudinal fasciculus to the three motor nuclei of the nerves to the extraocular muscles (i.e., the nuclei of the oculomotor [CN III], trochlear [CN IV], and abducent [CN VI] nerves).

Radiographs of the Ear

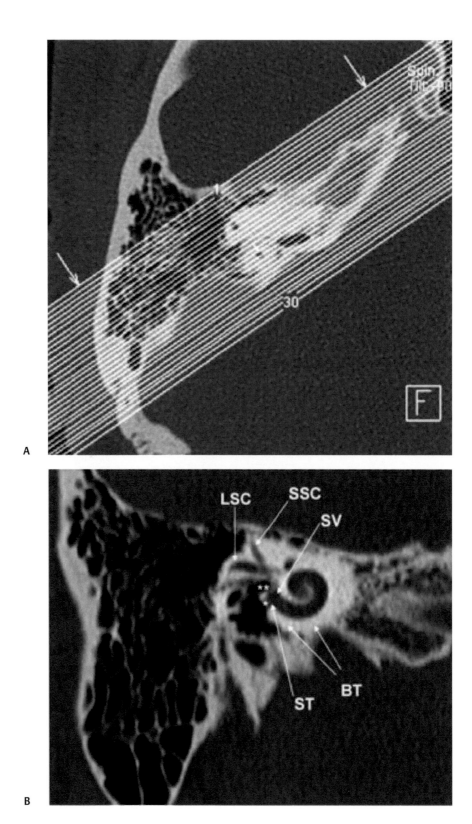

Fig. 10.41 Stenver computed tomography image.
A Plane of section for Stenver's projection. **B** Stenver's view reveals oval window niche (******) leading to the scala vestibule (SV) of the basilar turn of the cochlea. Round window niche (*) leads to the scala tympani (ST) of basilar turn of the cochlea (BT). This image plane is useful in evaluating the postoperative appearance of the cochlear implant, which is inserted into the scala tympani via either the round window or the adjacent cochleostomy. LSC, lateral semicircular canal; SSC, superior semicircular canal.

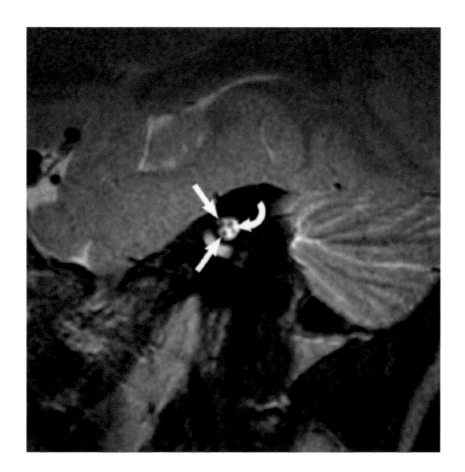

Fig. 10.42 Normal nerves at the internal auditory canal (IAC) fundus.
Oblique sagittal T2-weighted magnetic resonance image demonstrates the four nerves at the fundus of the IAC: the facial nerve superiorly and anteriorly, the cochlear nerve anteroinferiorly, and the superior and inferior vestibular nerves posteriorly (curved arrow).

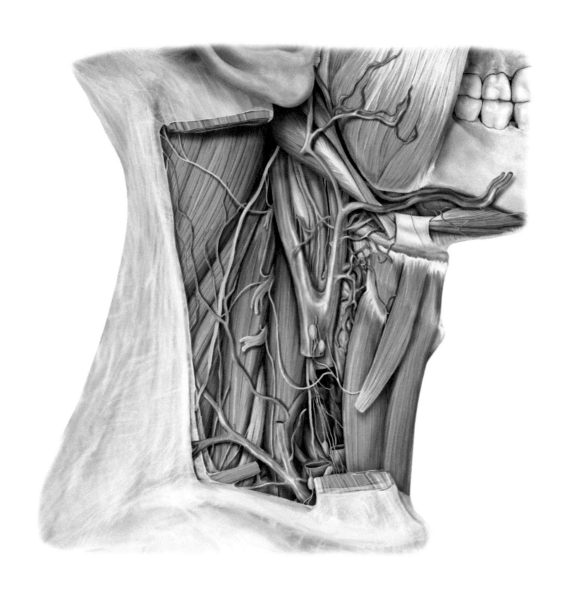

Neck

Vertebral Column & Vertebrae

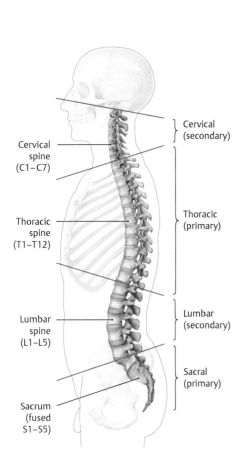

Fig. 11.1 Spinal curvature

Left lateral view. The spinal (vertebral) column is divided into four regions: the cervical, thoracic, lumbar, and sacral spines. In the neonate, all regions demonstrate an anteriorly concave curvature. This single concave curvature in the neonate is referred to as the primary curvature of the vertebral column.

During development, the cervical and lumbar regions of the vertebral column develop anteriorly convex curvatures. These changes are referred to as secondary curvatures. The cervical secondary curvature develops as infants begin to hold up their heads. The lumbar secondary curvatures are the result of upright bipedal locomotion.

Kyphosis is a pathological condition where the thoracic primary curvature is abnormally exaggerated (hunchback, rounded back). Lordosis is a pathological condition where the secondary curvatures are exaggerated. Lordosis may occur in either the cervical or lumbar regions (swayback) of the vertebral column. Differing from the abnormal development of primary and secondary curvatures, scoliosis is an abnormal lateral deviation of the vertebral column.

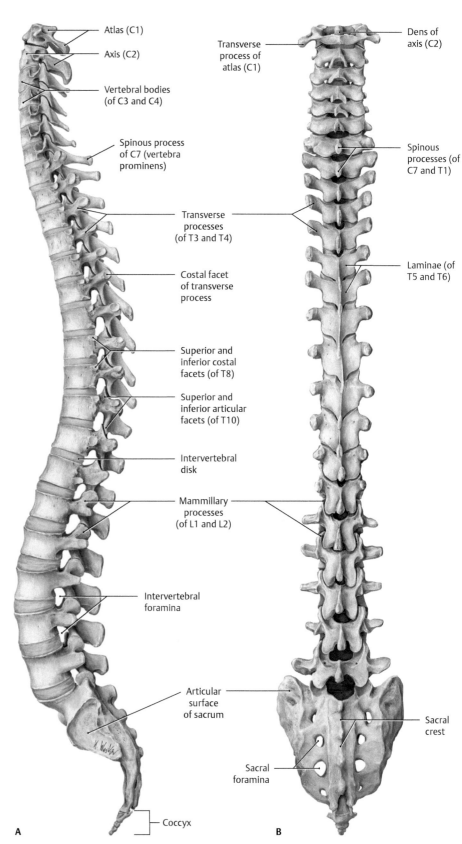

Fig. 11.2 Vertebral column

A Left lateral view. **B** Posterior view. The vertebral column is divided into four regions: cervical, thoracic, lumbar, and sacral. Each vertebra consists of a vertebral body and vertebral (neural) arch. The vertebral bodies (with intervening intervertebral disks) form the load-bearing component of the vertebral column. The vertebral (neural) arches enclose the vertebral canal, protecting the spinal cord.

Fig. 11.3 **Structure of vertebrae**
Schematic, left oblique posterosuperior view. Each vertebra consists of a load-bearing body and an arch that encloses the vertebral foramen. The arch is divided into the pedicle and lamina. Vertebrae have transverse and spinous processes that provide sites of attachment for muscles. Vertebrae articulate at facets on the superior and inferior articular processes. Thoracic vertebrae articulate with ribs at costal facets.

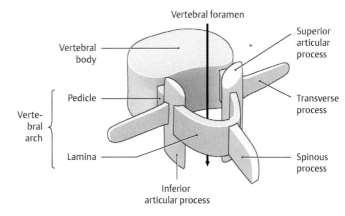

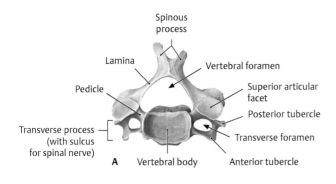

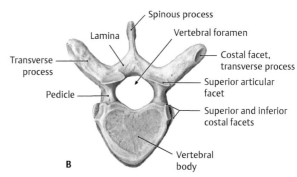

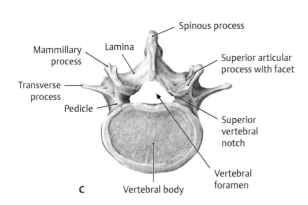

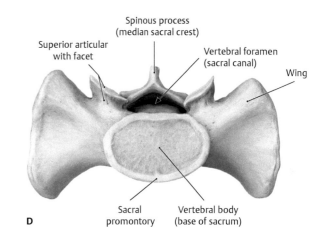

Fig. 11.4 **Typical vertebrae**
Superior view. **A** Cervical vertebra (C4). **B** Thoracic vertebra (T6). **C** Lumbar vertebra (L4). **D** Sacrum. The vertebral bodies increase in size cranially to caudally.

Table 11.1 **Structural elements of vertebrae**

Each vertebra consists of a body and an arch that enclose the vertebral foramen. The types of vertebrae can be distinguished particularly easily by examining their transverse processes. The sacrum has structures that are analogous to the other vertebrae.

Vertebrae	Body	Foramen	Transverse process	Spinous process
Cervical vertebrae C3–C7	Small (kidney-shaped)	Large (triangular)	Transverse foramina	C3–C5: short C7: long C3–C6: bifid
Thoracic vertebrae T1–T12	Medium (heart-shaped) with costal facets	Small (circular)	Costal facets	Long
Lumbar vertebrae L1–L5	Large (kidney-shaped)	Medium (triangular)	Mammillary processes	Short and broad
Sacrum (fused S1–S5)	Large to small (decreases from base to apex)	Sacral canal (triangular)	Fused (forms wing of sacrum)	Short (median sacral crest)

Cervical Spine

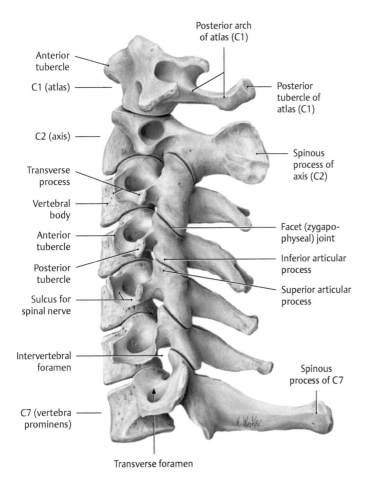

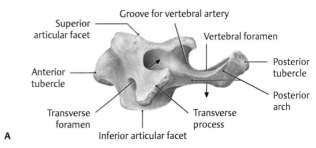

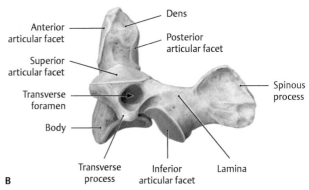

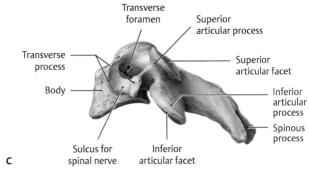

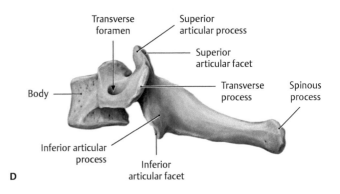

Fig. 11.5 Cervical spine (C1–C7)
Left lateral view. The cervical spine consists of seven vertebrae. C1 and C2 are atypical and are discussed individually.

Typical cervical vertebrae (C3–C7): Typical cervical vertebrae have relatively small, kidney-shaped bodies. The superior and inferior articular processes are broad and flat; their facets are flat and inclined at approximately 45 degrees from the horizontal. The vertebral arches enclose a large, triangular vertebral foramen. Spinal nerves emerge from the vertebral canal via the intervertebral foramina formed between the pedicles of adjacent vertebrae. The transverse processes of cervical vertebrae are furrowed to accommodate the emerging nerve (sulcus for spinal nerve). The transverse processes also consist of an anterior and a posterior portion that enclose a transverse foramen. The transverse foramina allow the vertebral artery to ascend to the base of the skull. The spinous processes of C3–C6 are short and bifid. The spinous process of C7 (vertebra prominens) is longer and thicker; it is the first spinous process that is palpable through the skin.

Atlas (C1) and axis (C2): The atlas and axis are specialized for bearing the weight of the head and allowing it to move in all directions. The body of the axis contains a vertical prominence (dens) around which the atlas turns. The atlas does not have a vertebral body: it consists of an anterior and a posterior arch that allow the head to rotate in the horizontal plane.

Fig. 11.6 Left lateral view of cervical vertebrae
A Atlas (C1). **B** Axis (C2). **C** Typical cervical vertebra (C4). **D** Vertebra prominens (C7).

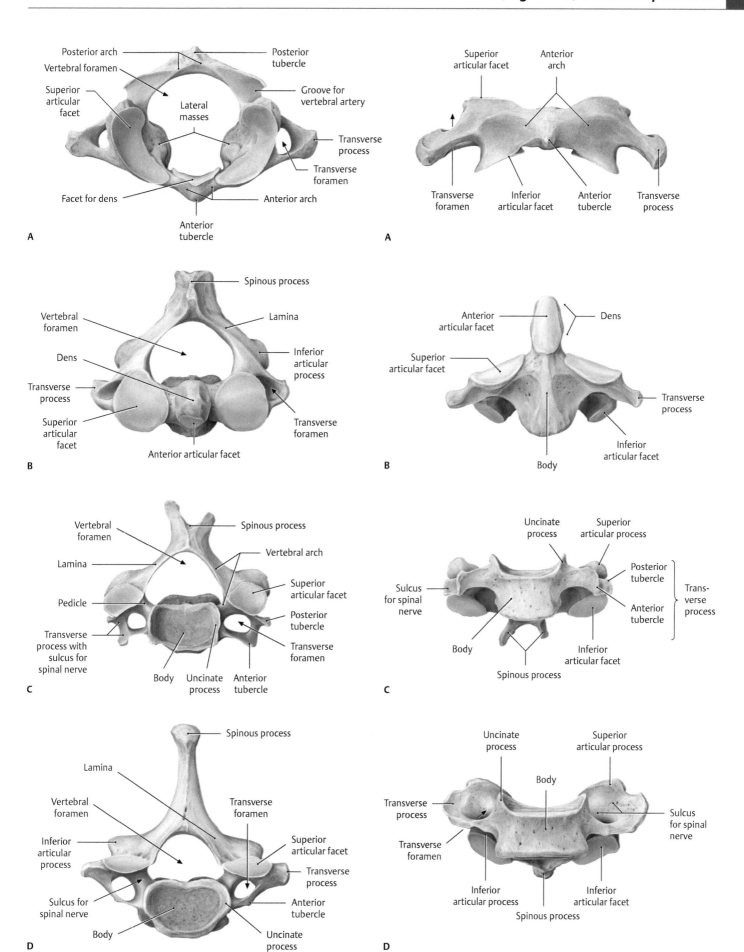

Fig. 11.7 Superior view of cervical vertebrae
A Atlas (C1). **B** Axis (C2). **C** Typical cervical vertebra (C4). **D** Vertebra prominens (C7).

Fig. 11.8 Anterior view of cervical vertebrae
A Atlas (C1). **B** Axis (C2). **C** Typical cervical vertebra (C4). **D** Vertebra prominens (C7).

Joints of the Cervical Spine

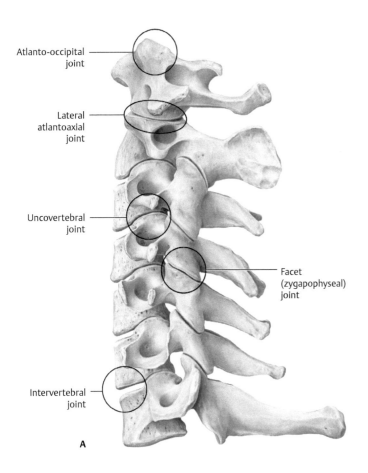

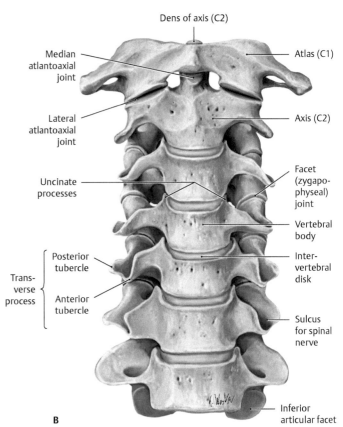

A

B

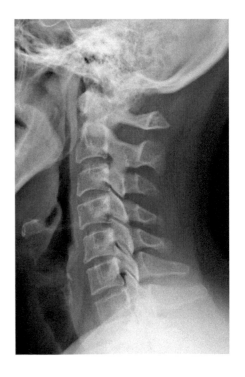

C

Fig. 11.9 **Joints of the cervical spine**
A Left lateral view. **B** Anterior view. **C** Radiograph of the cervical spine, left lateral view.

The cervical spine has five types of joints. Two joints (intervertebral and facet) are common to all regions of the spine, and three are specialized joints of the cervical spine.

Joints of the vertebral column: Adjacent vertebrae articulate at two points: vertebral bodies and articular processes. The bodies of adjacent vertebrae articulate at roughly horizontal intervertebral joints (via intervertebral disks). The articular processes of adjacent vertebrae articulate at facet (zygapophyseal) joints. In the cervical spine, the intervertebral joints are angled slightly anteroinferiorly, and the facet (zygapophyseal) joints are angled posteroinferiorly (roughly 45 degrees below horizontal).

Joints of the cervical spine: There are two types of joints that are particular to the cervical spine:

1. Uncovertebral joints: Upward protrusions of the lateral margins of cervical vertebral bodies form uncinate processes. These processes may articulate with the inferolateral margin of the adjacent superior vertebra, forming uncovertebral joints.
2. Craniovertebral joints (atlanto-occipital and atlantoaxial joints): The atlas (C1) and axis (C2) are specialized to bear the weight of the head and facilitate movement in all directions. This is made possible by craniovertebral joints (see **Fig. 11.10**).

Laxity of the cervical spine makes it prone to hyperextension injuries, such as "whiplash," the excessive and often violent backward movement of the head, resulting in fractures of the dens of the axis and traumatic spondylolisthesis (anterior or posterior displacement of a vertebra in relation to the one below it). Patient prognosis is largely dependent on the spinal level of the injuries.

306

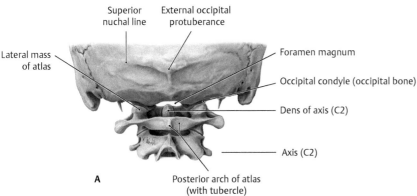

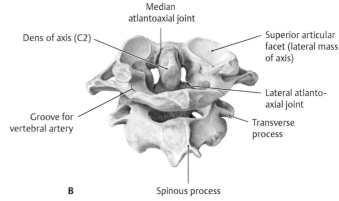

Fig. 11.10 Craniovertebral joints

A Posterior view. **B** Left oblique posterosuperior view.

There are five craniovertebral joints. The paired atlanto-occipital joints are articulations between the concave superior articular facets of the atlas (C1) and the convex occipital condyle of the occipital bone. These allow the head to rock back and forth in the sagittal plane. The atlantoaxial joints (two lateral and one medial) allow the atlas to rotate in the horizontal plane around the dens of the axis. The lateral atlantoaxial joints are the paired articulations between the inferior and superior articular facets of the atlas and axis, respectively. The median atlantoaxial joint is the unpaired articulation between the dens of the axis and the fovea of the atlas. *Note:* While only the atlanto-occipital joints are direct articulations between the cranium and vertebral column, the atlantoaxial joints are generally classified as craniovertebral joints as well.

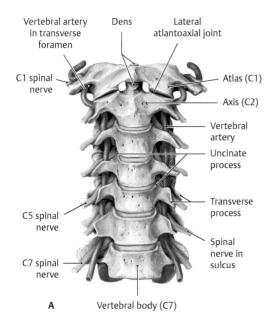

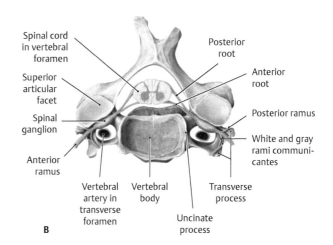

Fig. 11.11 Neurovasculature of the cervical spine

A Anterior view. **B** Superior view.

The transverse processes of the cervical vertebrae are extremely important in communicating neurovascular structures. Spinal nerves arise from the spinal cord in the vertebral canal. They exit via the intervertebral foramina formed by the pedicles of adjacent vertebrae.

The transverse processes of cervical vertebrae contain grooves (sulci) through which the spinal nerves pass. The transverse processes also contain transverse foramina that allow the vertebral artery to ascend from the subclavian artery and enter the skull via the foramen magnum. Injury to the cervical spine can compress the neurovascular structures as they emerge and ascend from the vertebral column.

307

Ligaments of the Vertebral Column

***Fig. 11.12* Ligaments of the vertebral column**

The ligaments of the vertebral column bind the vertebrae to one another and enable the spine to withstand high mechanical loads and shearing stresses. The ligaments are divided into ligaments of the vertebral bodies and arches (**Table 11.2**).

A Ligaments of the vertebral column. Left lateral view of T11–L3 with T11 and T12 sectioned midsagittally.
B Ligaments of the vertebral body (anterior and posterior longitudinal ligaments, and intervertebral disk), schematic.
C Ligamenta flava, schematic.
D Interspinous ligaments and ligamenta flava, schematic.
E Complete ligaments of the vertebral column, schematic.

Table 11.2 Ligaments of the vertebral column
Vertebral body ligaments
Anterior longitudinal ligament (along anterior surface of vertebral bodies)
Posterior longitudinal ligament (along posterior surface of vertebral bodies, i.e., anterior surface of vertebral canal)
Intervertebral disk (between adjacent vertebral bodies; the anulus fibrosus limits rotation, and the nucleus pulposus absorbs compressive forces)
Vertebral (neural) arch ligaments
Ligamenta flava (between laminae)
Interspinous ligaments (between spinous processes)
Supraspinous ligaments (along posterior border of spinous processes; in the cervical spine, the supraspinous ligament is broadened into the nuchal ligament)
Intertransverse ligaments (between transverse processes)
Facet joint capsules (enclose the articulation between the facets of the superior and inferior articular processes of adjacent vertebrae)

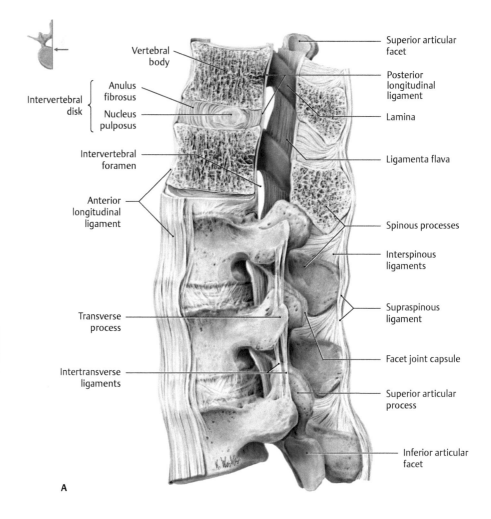

A

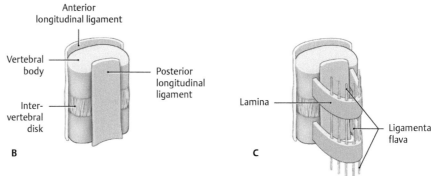

B   **C**

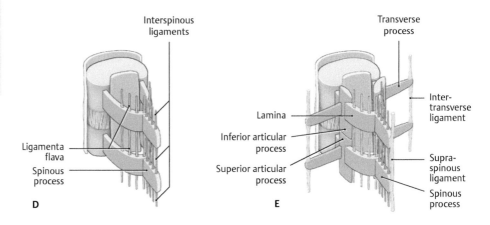

D   **E**

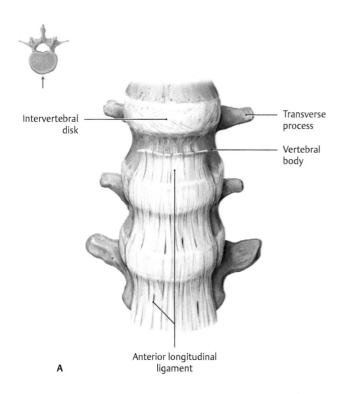

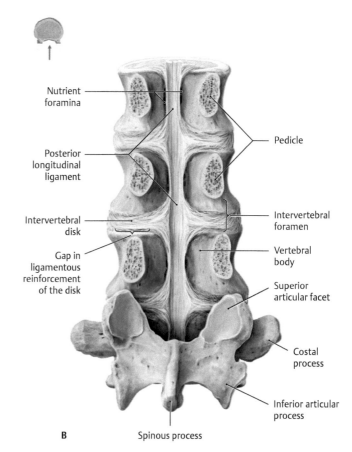

Fig. 11.13 Individual ligaments of the vertebral column

The anterior and posterior longitudinal ligaments and ligamenta flava maintain the normal curvature of the spine.

A Anterior longitudinal ligament. Anterior view. The anterior longitudinal ligament runs broadly on the anterior side of the vertebral bodies from the skull base to the sacrum. Its deep collagenous fibers bind adjacent vertebral bodies together (they are firmly attached to vertebral bodies and loosely attached to intervertebral disks). Its superficial fibers span multiple vertebrae.

B Posterior longitudinal ligament. Posterior view with vertebral canal windowed (vertebral arches removed). The thinner posterior longitudinal ligament descends from the clivus along the posterior surface of the vertebral bodies, passing into the sacral canal. The ligament broadens at the level of the intervertebral disk (to which it is attached by tapered lateral extensions). It narrows again while passing the vertebral body (to which it is attached at the superior and inferior margins).

C Ligamenta flava and intertransverse ligaments. Anterior view with vertebral canal windowed (vertebral bodies removed). The ligamentum flavum is a thick, powerful ligament that connects adjacent laminae and reinforces the wall of the vertebral canal posterior to the intervertebral foramina. The ligament consists mainly of elastic fibers that produce the characteristic yellow color. When the spinal column is erect, the ligamenta flava are tensed, stabilizing the spine in the sagittal plane. The ligamenta flava also limit forward flexion of the spine. *Note:* The tips of the transverse processes are connected by interspinous ligaments that limit the rocking movements of vertebrae upon one another.

A — Intervertebral disk, Transverse process, Vertebral body, Anterior longitudinal ligament

B — Nutrient foramina, Posterior longitudinal ligament, Intervertebral disk, Gap in ligamentous reinforcement of the disk, Pedicle, Intervertebral foramen, Vertebral body, Superior articular facet, Costal process, Inferior articular process, Spinous process

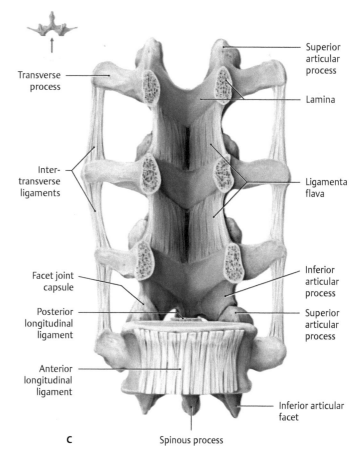

C — Transverse process, Intertransverse ligaments, Facet joint capsule, Posterior longitudinal ligament, Anterior longitudinal ligament, Superior articular process, Lamina, Ligamenta flava, Inferior articular process, Superior articular process, Inferior articular facet, Spinous process

309

Ligaments of the Cervical Spine

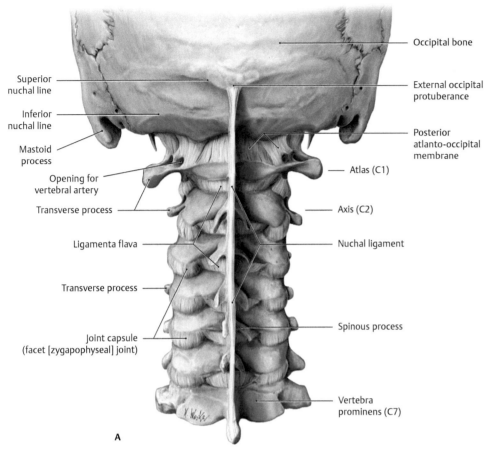

Occipital bone

External occipital protuberance

Posterior atlanto-occipital membrane

Superior nuchal line

Inferior nuchal line

Mastoid process

Opening for vertebral artery

Transverse process

Ligamenta flava

Transverse process

Joint capsule (facet [zygapophyseal] joint)

Atlas (C1)

Axis (C2)

Nuchal ligament

Spinous process

Vertebra prominens (C7)

A

Fig. 11.14 Ligaments of the cervical spine
A Posterior view.
B Anterior view after removal of the anterior skull base.
C Midsagittal section, left lateral view. The nuchal ligament is the broadened, sagittally oriented part of the supraspinous ligament that extends from the vertebra prominens (C7) to the external occipital protuberance.

B → ← A

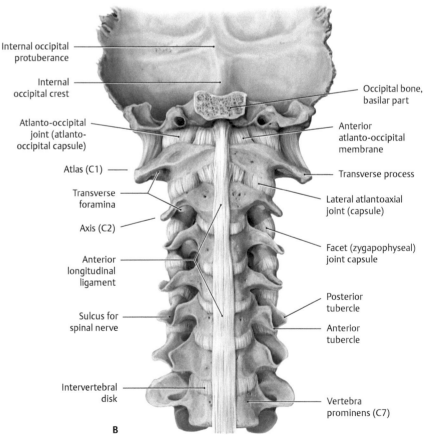

Internal occipital protuberance

Internal occipital crest

Atlanto-occipital joint (atlanto-occipital capsule)

Atlas (C1)

Transverse foramina

Axis (C2)

Anterior longitudinal ligament

Sulcus for spinal nerve

Intervertebral disk

Occipital bone, basilar part

Anterior atlanto-occipital membrane

Transverse process

Lateral atlantoaxial joint (capsule)

Facet (zygapophyseal) joint capsule

Posterior tubercle

Anterior tubercle

Vertebra prominens (C7)

B

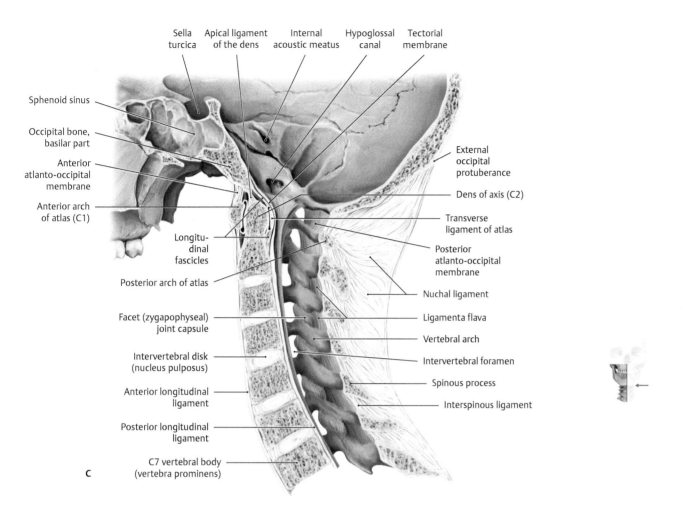

Sella turcica
Apical ligament of the dens
Internal acoustic meatus
Hypoglossal canal
Tectorial membrane

Sphenoid sinus

Occipital bone, basilar part

Anterior atlanto-occipital membrane

Anterior arch of atlas (C1)

Longitu-dinal fascicles

Posterior arch of atlas

Facet (zygapophyseal) joint capsule

Intervertebral disk (nucleus pulposus)

Anterior longitudinal ligament

Posterior longitudinal ligament

C7 vertebral body (vertebra prominens)

External occipital protuberance

Dens of axis (C2)

Transverse ligament of atlas

Posterior atlanto-occipital membrane

Nuchal ligament

Ligamenta flava

Vertebral arch

Intervertebral foramen

Spinous process

Interspinous ligament

C

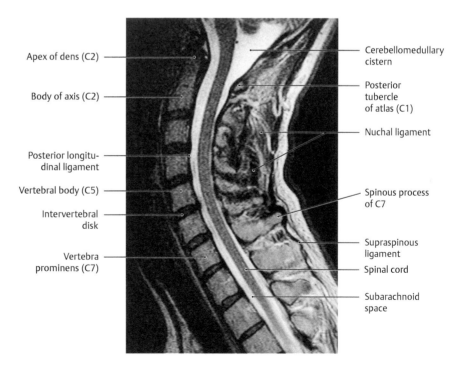

Apex of dens (C2)

Body of axis (C2)

Posterior longitu-dinal ligament

Vertebral body (C5)

Intervertebral disk

Vertebra prominens (C7)

Cerebellomedullary cistern

Posterior tubercle of atlas (C1)

Nuchal ligament

Spinous process of C7

Supraspinous ligament

Spinal cord

Subarachnoid space

Fig. 11.15 Magnetic resonance image of the cervical spine
Midsagittal section, left lateral view, T2-weighted TSE sequence.
(From Vahlensieck M, Reiser M. MRT des Bewegungsapparates. 2nd ed.
Stuttgart: Thieme; 2001.)

Ligaments of the Craniovertebral Joints

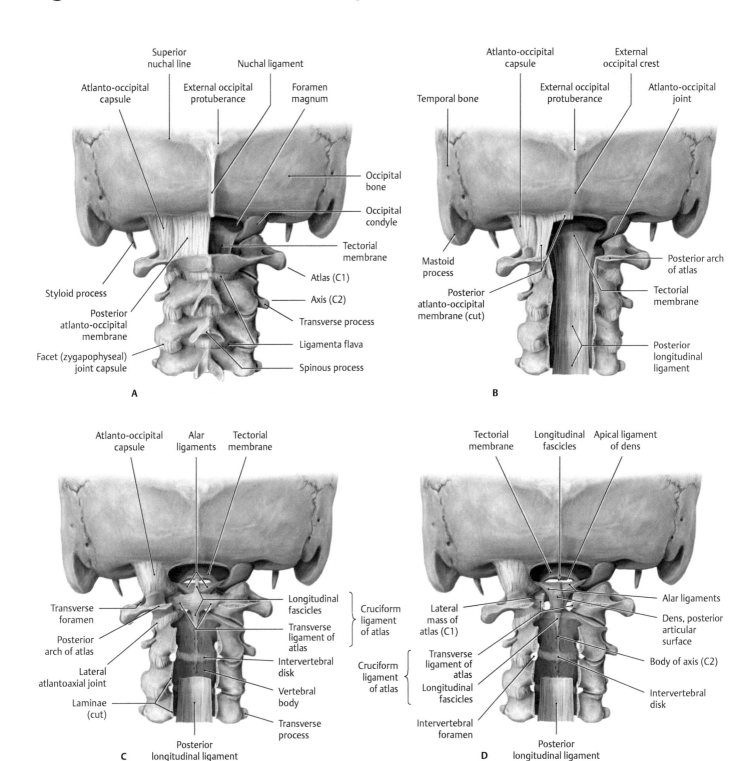

Fig. 11.16 Ligaments of the craniovertebral joints and cervical spine

Skull and upper cervical spine, posterior view.

A The posterior atlanto-occipital membrane stretches from the posterior arch of the atlas to the posterior rim of the foramen magnum. This membrane has been removed on the right side.

B With the vertebral canal opened and the spinal cord removed, the tectorial membrane, a broadened expansion of the posterior longitudinal ligament, is seen to form the anterior boundary of the vertebral canal at the level of the craniovertebral joints.

C With the tectorial membrane removed, the cruciform ligament of the atlas can be seen. The transverse ligament of the atlas forms the thick horizontal bar of the cross, and the longitudinal fascicles form the thinner vertical bar.

D The transverse ligament of the atlas and longitudinal fascicles have been partially removed to demonstrate the paired alar ligaments, which extend from the lateral surfaces of the dens to the corresponding inner surfaces of the occipital condyles, and the unpaired apical ligament of the dens, which passes from the tip of the dens to the anterior rim of the foramen magnum.

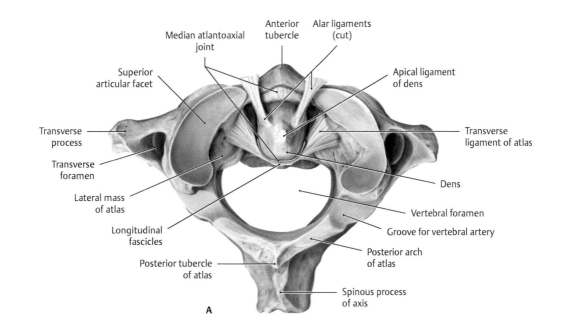

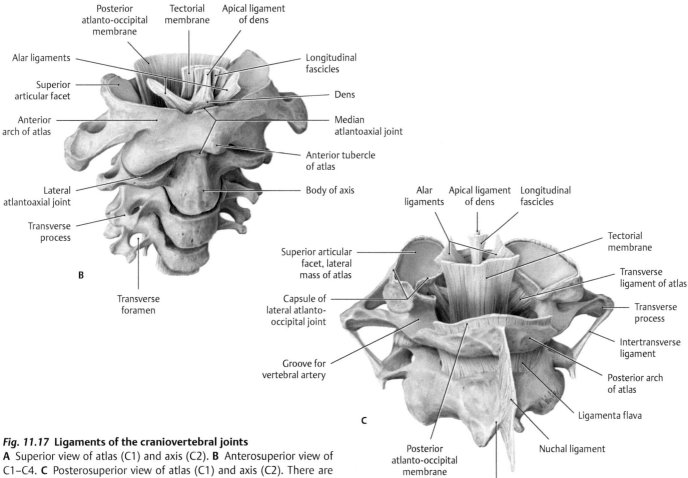

Fig. 11.17 **Ligaments of the craniovertebral joints**
A Superior view of atlas (C1) and axis (C2). **B** Anterosuperior view of C1–C4. **C** Posterosuperior view of atlas (C1) and axis (C2). There are five craniovertebral joints. The paired atlanto-occipital joints are articulations between the concave superior articular facets of the atlas and the convex occipital condyles of the occipital bone. The joints are stabilized by the atlanto-occipital joint capsule and the posterior atlanto-occipital membrane (the equivalent of the ligamenta flava). The paired lateral atlantoaxial and unpaired median atlantoaxial joints allow the atlas to rotate in the horizontal plane around the dens of the axis. They are stabilized by the alar ligaments, the apical ligament of the dens, and the cruciform ligament of the atlas (transverse ligament and longitudinal fascicles).

Muscles of the Neck: Overview

Fig. 11.18 Sternocleidomastoid and trapezius
A Sternocleidomastoid, right lateral view.
B Trapezius, posterior view.

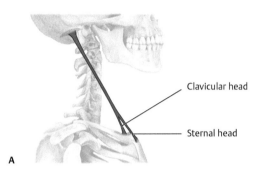

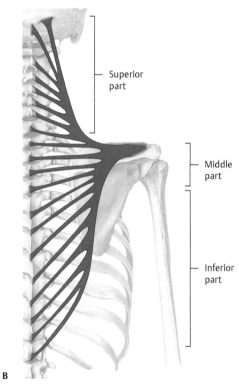

Table 11.3 Muscles of the neck

The muscles of the neck lie at the intersection of the skull, vertebral column, and upper limb. They can therefore be classified in multiple ways based on location and function. In the pages that follow, the neck muscles are grouped as follows:

Superficial neck muscles

Muscles that lie superficial to the deep layer (lamina) of the deep cervical fascia and are innervated by the anterior rami of spinal nerves

Posterior neck muscles (intrinsic back muscles)

Muscles that insert on the cervical spine and are innervated by the posterior rami of spinal nerves
• Intrinsic back muscles (including nuchal muscles)
  ◦ Short nuchal/craniovertebral muscles

Anterior neck muscles

Muscles that insert on the anterior cervical spine and are innervated by the anterior rami of spinal nerves
• Anterior vertebral (prevertebral) muscles
• Lateral vertebral muscles (scalenes)

Muscles that do not insert on the cervical spine
• Suprahyoid muscles
• Infrahyoid muscles

Fig. 11.19 Superficial neck muscles
A Left lateral view. **B** Anterior view of sternocleidomastoid and trapezius. Unlike the rest of the neck muscles, the superficial neck muscles are located superficial to the prevertebral layer of the deep cervical fascia and are innervated by the anterior rami of the spinal nerves.

Platysma: The platysma, like the muscles of facial expression, is not enveloped in its own fascial sheath, but is instead directly associated with (and in parts inserted into) the skin. (*Note:* It is innervated by the same nerve as the muscles of facial expression, the facial nerve.) The platysma is highly variable in size — its fibers may reach from the lower face to the upper thorax.

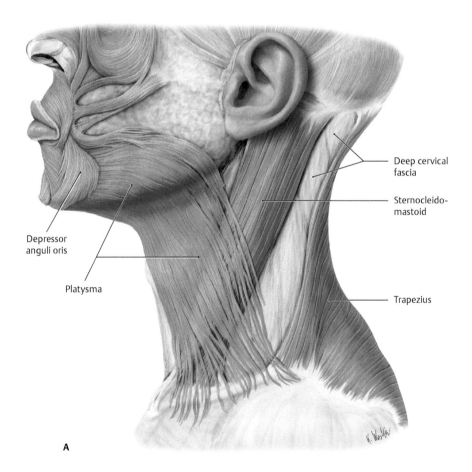

Table 11.4 Superficial neck muscles

Muscle	Origin	Insertion	Innervation	Action
Platysma	Mandible (inferior border); skin of lower face and angle of mouth	Skin over lower neck and superior and lateral thorax	Facial n. (CN VII), cervical branch	Depresses and wrinkles skin of lower face and mouth; tenses skin of neck; aids forced depression of mandible
Sternocleidomastoid	Occipital bone (superior nuchal line); temporal bone (mastoid process)	Sternal head: sternum (manubrium) Clavicular head: clavicle (medial ⅓)	Accessory n. (CN IX), spinal part	*Unilateral:* Moves chin up and out (tilts head to same side and rotates head to opposite side) *Bilateral:* Extends head; aids in respiration when head is fixed
Trapezius, superior part*	Occipital bone; C1–C7 (spinous processes)	Clavicle (lateral ⅓)		Draws scapula obliquely upward; rotates glenoid cavity inferiorly
Rhomboid minor (see **Fig. 11.20**)	Nuchal ligament (inferior part), C7–T1 (spinous processes)	Medial (vertebral) border of the scapula, superior to the intersection with the scapular spine	C4–C5 anterior rami (C5 fibers are from the dorsal scapular n.)	Scapular movements (e.g., retraction and rotation)
Levator scapulae (see **Fig. 11.20**)	C1–C4 (posterior tubercles of transverse processes)	Scapula (medial to superior angle)	C3–C5 anterior rami (C5 fibers are from the dorsal scapular n.)	Scapular movements (e.g., elevation, retraction, and rotation)
Serratus posterior superior (see **Fig. 11.22**)	Nuchal ligament (inferior part), C7–T3 (spinous processes)	Ribs 2–5	Anterior rami of thoracic spinal nn. (intercostal nn.)	Postulated to be an accessory muscle of respiration; assists in elevating ribs

*The middle and inferior parts are not described here.

Sternocleidomastoid and trapezius: The trapezius lies between the superficial and prevertebral layers of the deep cervical fascia. The superficial layer splits to enclose the sternocleidomastoid and the trapezius.

Congenital torticollis (wryneck) is a condition in which shortening of the sternocleidomastoid muscle causes the head to tilt to one side with the chin pointing upward to the opposite side. This shortening is thought to be the result of trauma at birth causing bleeding and swelling within the muscle and subsequent scar tissue which renders the muscle unable to lengthen in the growing neck. It is often associated with hip dysplasia. Symptoms that appear in infancy include abnormal posturing of the head and chin, limited range of motion in the neck, and one side of the face and head may flatten as the child sleeps on one side only.

B

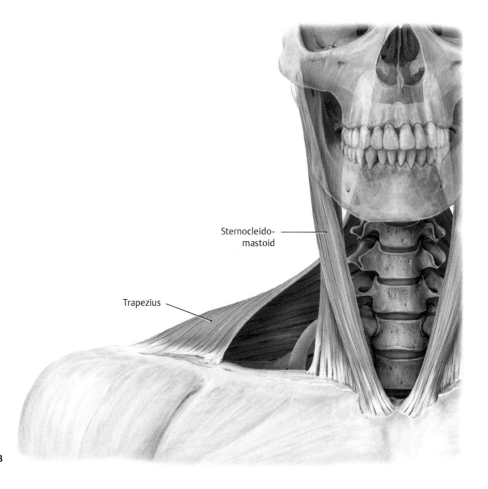

Sternocleido-mastoid

Trapezius

Muscles of the Neck & Back (I)

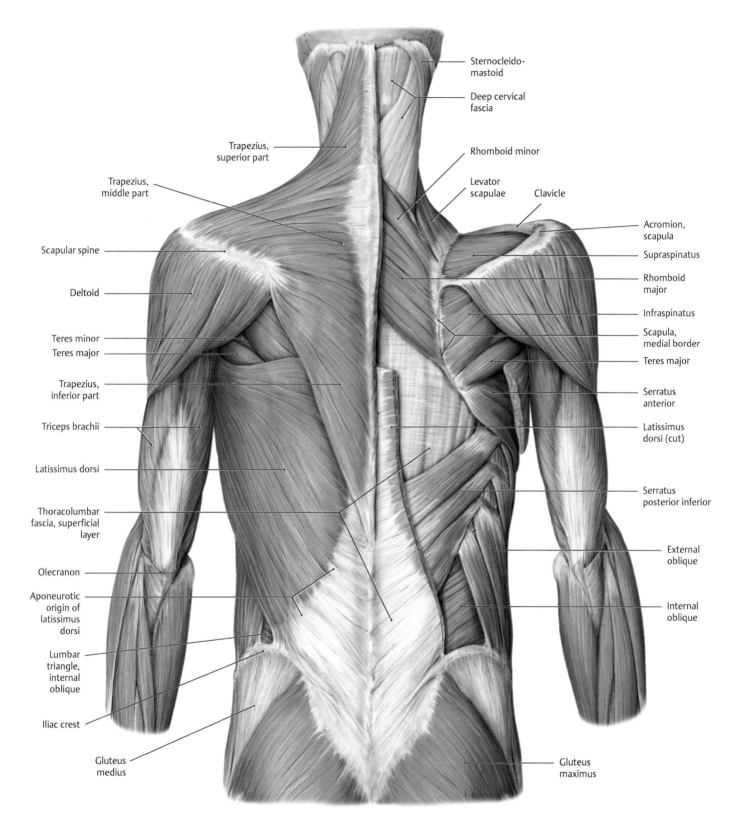

Fig. 11.20 Muscles of the neck and back
Posterior view with trapezius and latissimus dorsi cut on right side. The extrinsic back muscles lie superficial to the thoracolumbar and deep cervical fascia. They are muscles of the upper limb (derived from the limb buds) that have migrated to the back. The intrinsic back muscles lie between the thoracolumbar and deep cervical fascia. They are derived from epaxial muscle. Because of their different embryonic origins, the intrinsic back muscles are innervated by the posterior rami of the spinal nerves, and the extrinsic back muscles are innervated by the anterior rami. Note: The trapezius and sternocleidomastoid are innervated by the accessory nerve (CN XI).

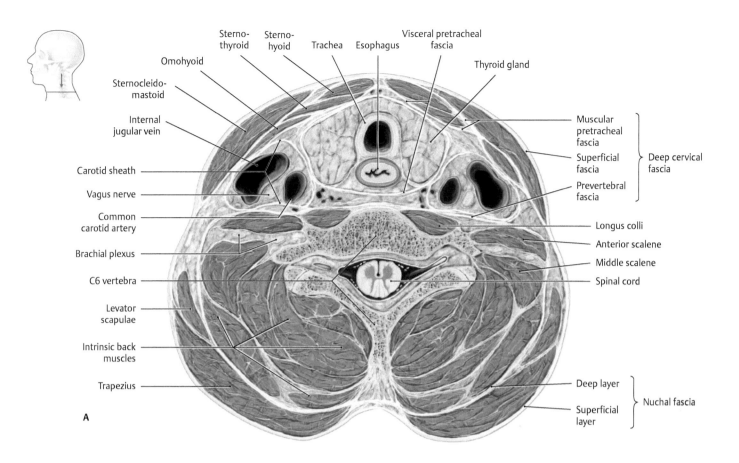

Sterno-thyroid | Sterno-hyoid | Trachea | Esophagus | Visceral pretracheal fascia | Thyroid gland

Omohyoid

Sternocleido-mastoid

Internal jugular vein

Carotid sheath

Vagus nerve

Common carotid artery

Brachial plexus

C6 vertebra

Levator scapulae

Intrinsic back muscles

Trapezius

Muscular pretracheal fascia
Superficial fascia
} Deep cervical fascia
Prevertebral fascia

Longus colli
Anterior scalene
Middle scalene
Spinal cord

Deep layer
} Nuchal fascia
Superficial layer

A

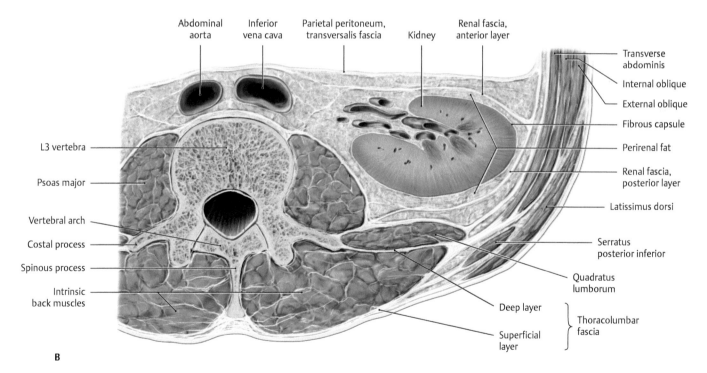

Abdominal aorta | Inferior vena cava | Parietal peritoneum, transversalis fascia | Kidney | Renal fascia, anterior layer

L3 vertebra

Psoas major

Vertebral arch

Costal process

Spinous process

Intrinsic back muscles

Transverse abdominis
Internal oblique
External oblique
Fibrous capsule
Perirenal fat
Renal fascia, posterior layer
Latissimus dorsi
Serratus posterior inferior
Quadratus lumborum

Deep layer
} Thoracolumbar fascia
Superficial layer

B

Fig. 11.21 Fascial planes
Transverse sections, superior view.
A Neck at the level of the C6 vertebra.
B Posterior trunk wall at the level of the L3 vertebra (with cauda equina removed from vertebral canal).
The muscles of the neck and back are separated by layers of deep fascia. The outermost layer, the superficial layer of the deep cervical fascia, encloses all muscles with the exception of the platysma (this is located in the superficial fascia, not to be confused with the superficial layer of the deep cervical fascia). The deep cervical fascia, located

in the anterior neck, is continuous posteriorly with the nuchal fascia in the posterior neck. The superficial layer of the nuchal fascia is continuous inferiorly with the superficial layer of the thoracolumbar fascia. The intrinsic muscles of the neck and back lie within the deep layer of the nuchal fascia, which is continuous with the prevertebral fascia (anteriorly) and thoracolumbar fascia (inferiorly). The muscles and structures of the anterior neck are enclosed in individual fascial sheaths (i.e., the visceral pretracheal fascia, muscular pretracheal fascia, and carotid sheath).

Muscles of the Neck & Back (II)

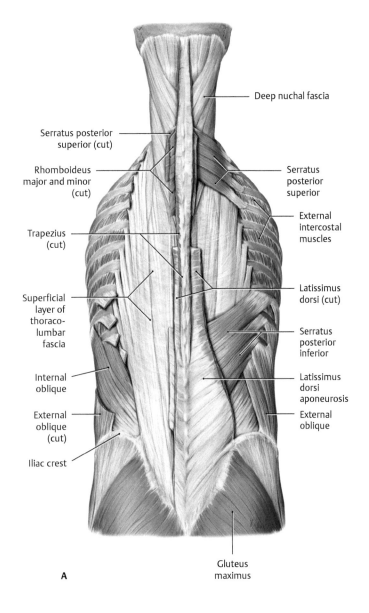

Serratus posterior superior (cut)

Rhomboideus major and minor (cut)

Trapezius (cut)

Superficial layer of thoraco-lumbar fascia

Internal oblique

External oblique (cut)

Iliac crest

Deep nuchal fascia

Serratus posterior superior

External intercostal muscles

Latissimus dorsi (cut)

Serratus posterior inferior

Latissimus dorsi aponeurosis

External oblique

Gluteus maximus

A

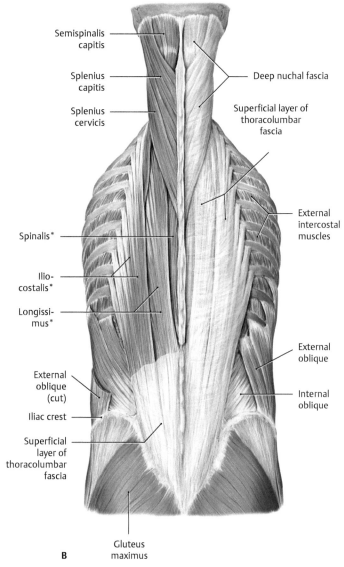

Semispinalis capitis

Splenius capitis

Splenius cervicis

Spinalis*

Ilio-costalis*

Longissi-mus*

External oblique (cut)

Iliac crest

Superficial layer of thoracolumbar fascia

Deep nuchal fascia

Superficial layer of thoracolumbar fascia

External intercostal muscles

External oblique

Internal oblique

Gluteus maximus

B

Fig. 11.22 Extrinsic and intrinsic back muscles
Posterior view. These dissections demonstrate the distinction between the intrinsic back muscles and the surrounding extrinsic back muscles and trunk muscles. The intrinsic back muscles lie within the deep nuchal fascia, which is continuous inferiorly with the superficial layer of the thoracolumbar fascia. They are derived from epaxial muscles and therefore innervated by the posterior rami of spinal nerves. The muscles of the trunk are derived from hypaxial muscle and therefore innervated by the anterior rami of spinal nerves. The visible trunk muscles are the abdominal muscles (internal and external obliques) and the thoracic muscles (external intercostals).

A *Removed:* Extrinsic back muscles (with the exception of the serratus posterior and the aponeurotic origin of the latissimus dorsi on the right side).
B *Removed:* All extrinsic back muscles and portions of the fascial covering (deep nuchal and superficial layers of the thoracolumbar fasciae).

*The spinalis, iliocostalis, and longissimus are collectively known as the erector spinae.

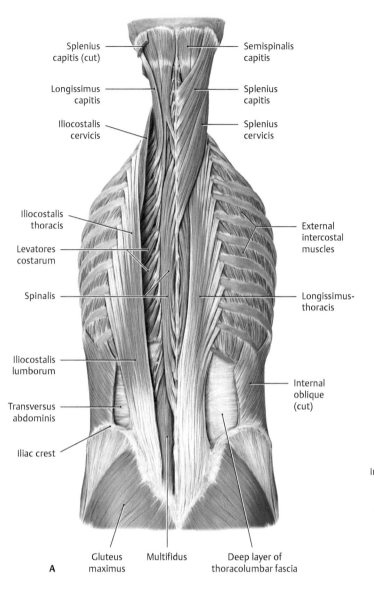

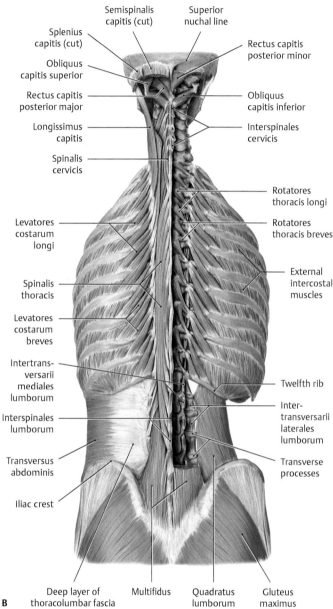

***Fig. 11.23* Intrinsic back muscles**

Posterior view. These dissections reveal the layers of intrinsic back muscles. The iliocostalis, longissimus, and spinalis collectively form the erector spinae. They lie deep to the superficial layer of the thoracolumbar fascia and cover the other intrinsic back muscles.

A *Removed on left side:* Longissimus (except cervical portion), splenius capitis and cervicis. *Removed on right side:* Iliocostalis. Note the deep layer of the thoracolumbar fascia, which gives origin to the internal oblique and transversus abdominis.

B *Removed on left side:* Iliocostalis, longissimus, and internal oblique. *Removed on right side:* Erector spinae, multifidus, transversus abdominis, splenius capitis, and semispinalis capitis.

Muscles of the Posterior Neck

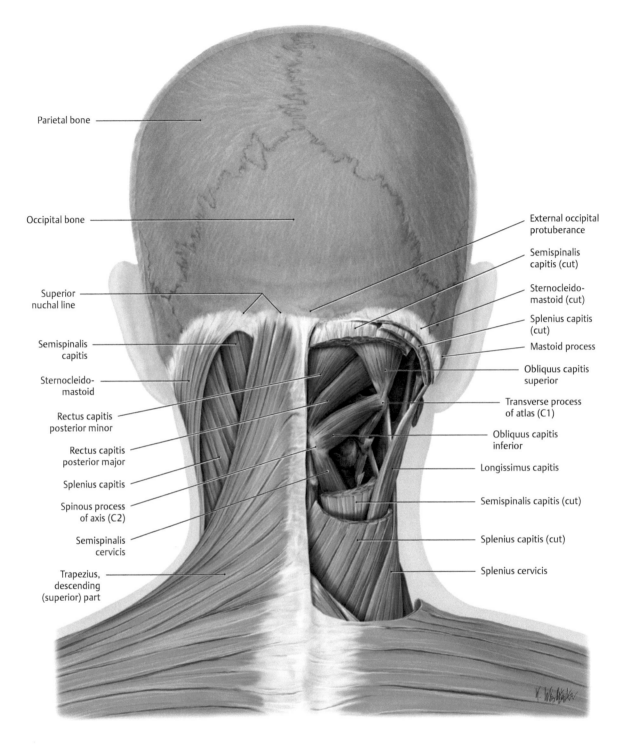

Parietal bone

Occipital bone

Superior
nuchal line

Semispinalis
capitis

Sternocleido-
mastoid

Rectus capitis
posterior minor

Rectus capitis
posterior major

Splenius capitis

Spinous process
of axis (C2)

Semispinalis
cervicis

Trapezius,
descending
(superior) part

External occipital
protuberance

Semispinalis
capitis (cut)

Sternocleido-
mastoid (cut)

Splenius capitis
(cut)

Mastoid process

Obliquus capitis
superior

Transverse process
of atlas (C1)

Obliquus capitis
inferior

Longissimus capitis

Semispinalis capitis (cut)

Splenius capitis (cut)

Splenius cervicis

Fig. 11.24 Muscles in the nuchal region

Posterior view of nuchal region. As the neck is at the intersection of the trunk, head, and upper limb, its muscles can be divided according to embryonic origin, function, or location. Those muscles (extrinsic and intrinsic) located in the posterior neck are often referred to as the nuchal muscles. The nuchal muscles are further divided into short nu-chal muscles, which are intrinsic back muscles innervated by the posterior rami of cervical spinal nerves. Based on location, the short nuchal muscles may also be referred to as suboccipital muscles. The anterior and posterior vertebral muscles collectively move the craniovertebral joints.

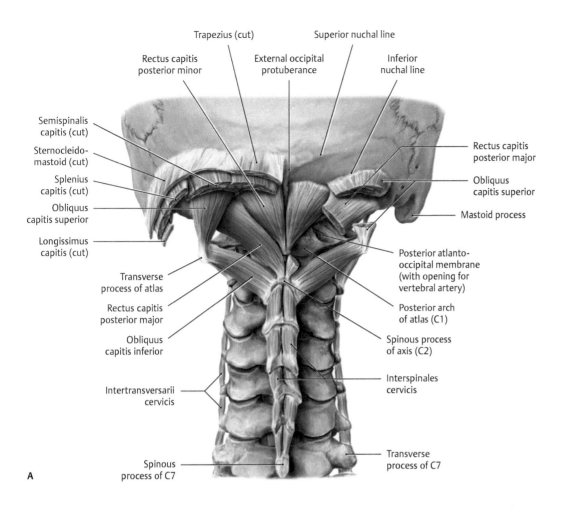

Trapezius (cut)

Rectus capitis posterior minor

Superior nuchal line

External occipital protuberance

Inferior nuchal line

Semispinalis capitis (cut)

Sternocleido-mastoid (cut)

Splenius capitis (cut)

Obliquus capitis superior

Longissimus capitis (cut)

Transverse process of atlas

Rectus capitis posterior major

Obliquus capitis inferior

Intertransversarii cervicis

Spinous process of C7

Rectus capitis posterior major

Obliquus capitis superior

Mastoid process

Posterior atlanto-occipital membrane (with opening for vertebral artery)

Posterior arch of atlas (C1)

Spinous process of axis (C2)

Interspinales cervicis

Transverse process of C7

A

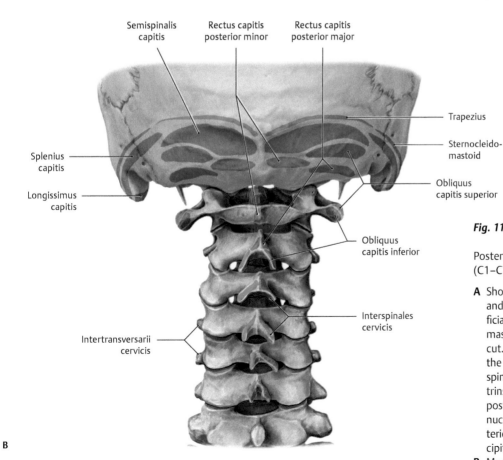

Semispinalis capitis

Rectus capitis posterior minor

Rectus capitis posterior major

Splenius capitis

Longissimus capitis

Intertransversarii cervicis

Trapezius

Sternocleido-mastoid

Obliquus capitis superior

Obliquus capitis inferior

Interspinales cervicis

B

Fig. 11.25 **Muscle attachments in the nuchal region**

Posterior view of skull and cervical spine (C1–C7).

A Short nuchal muscles with interspinales and intertransversarii cervicis. The superficial muscles (trapezius and sternocleidomastoid, innervated by CN XI) have been cut. The intrinsic back muscles inserting on the skull (splenius, longissimus, and semispinalis capitis) have also been cut. The intrinsic back muscles are all innervated by posterior rami of spinal nerves. The short nuchal muscles are innervated by the posterior rami of the first spinal nerve (suboccipital nerve).

B Muscle origins (red) and insertions (blue).

321

Intrinsic Back Muscles (I): Erector Spinae & Interspinales

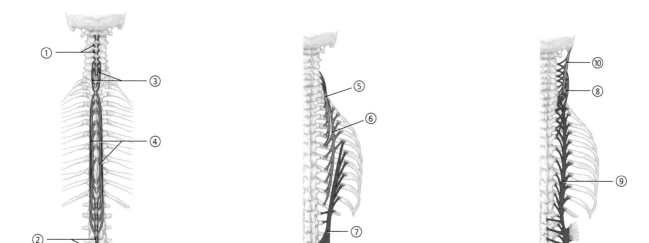

Fig. 11.26 Interspinales and erector spinae
Schematic, posterior view.
A Interspinales and spinalis. **B** Iliocostalis. **C** Longissimus.

Table 11.5 Erector spinae and interspinales

Like all intrinsic back muscles, these muscles are innervated by posterior rami of spinal nerves. The erector spinae and interspinales are innervated by lateral branches of the posterior rami. The longissimus is innervated by spinal nerves C1–L5, the iliocostalis by C8–L1.

Muscle		Origin	Insertion	Action
Interspinales	① I. cervicis	C1–C7 (between spinous processes of adjacent vertebrae)		Extends cervical spine
	② I. lumborum	L1–L5 (between spinous processes of adjacent vertebrae)		Extends lumbar spine
Spinalis*	③ S. cervicis	C5–T2 (spinous processes)	C2–C5 (spinous processes)	*Bilateral:* Extends spine *Unilateral:* Bends laterally to same side
	④ S. thoracis	T10–L3 (spinous processes, lateral surface)	T2–T8 (spinous processes, lateral surface)	
Iliocostalis*	⑤ I. cervicis	3rd–7th ribs	C4–C6 (transverse processes)	
	⑥ I. thoracis	7th–12th ribs	1st–6th ribs	
	⑦ I. lumborum	Sacrum; iliac crest; superficial layer of thoracolumbar fascia	6th–12th ribs; deep layer of thoracolumbar fascia; upper lumbar vertebrae (costal processes)	
Longissimus*	⑧ L. cervicis	T1–T6 (transverse processes)	C2–C5 (transverse processes)	
	⑨ L. thoracis	Sacrum; iliac crest; L1–L5 (spinous processes); lower thoracic vertebrae (transverse processes)	2nd–12th ribs; T1–T12 (transverse processes) ; L1–L5 (costal processes)	
	⑩ L. capitis	T1–T3 (transverse processes); C4–C7 (transverse and articular processes)	Temporal bone (mastoid process)	*Bilateral:* Extends head *Unilateral:* Flexes and rotates head to same side

*The spinalis, iliocostalis, and longissimus are collectively known as the erector spinae. *Note:* The iliocostalis and longissimus extend the entire spine. The spinalis acts only on the cervical and thoracic spines.

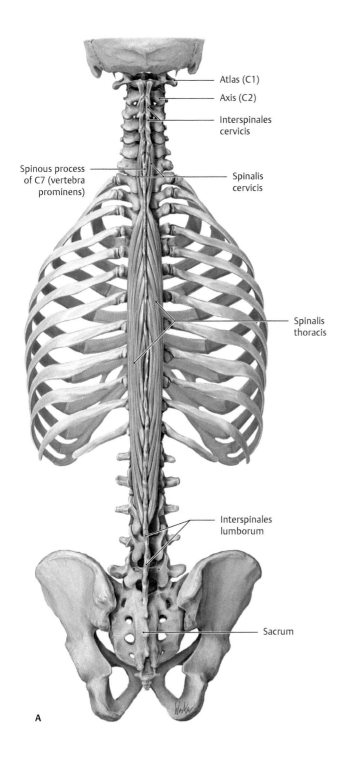

Atlas (C1)

Axis (C2)

Interspinales cervicis

Spinous process of C7 (vertebra prominens)

Spinalis cervicis

Spinalis thoracis

Interspinales lumborum

Sacrum

A

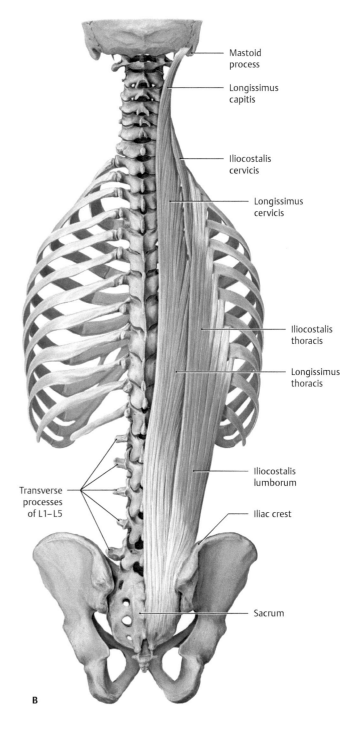

Mastoid process

Longissimus capitis

Iliocostalis cervicis

Longissimus cervicis

Iliocostalis thoracis

Longissimus thoracis

Iliocostalis lumborum

Iliac crest

Transverse processes of L1–L5

Sacrum

B

***Fig. 11.27* Interspinales and erector spinae muscles**
The spinalis, iliocostalis, and longissimus are collectively known as the erector spinae.
A Interspinales and spinalis. **B** Iliocostalis and longissimus.

Intrinsic Back Muscles (II)

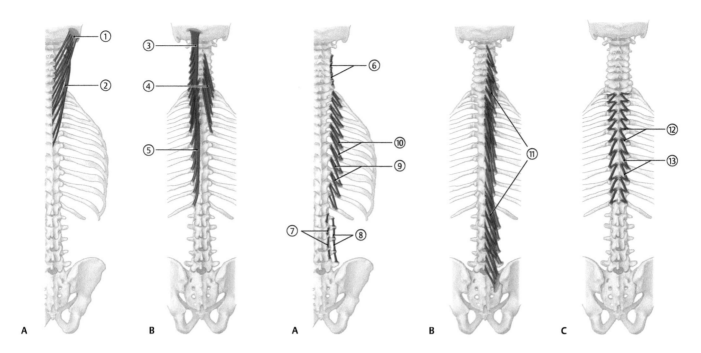

Fig. 11.28 Splenius and semispinalis
Schematic, posterior view. **A** Splenius.
B Semispinalis.

Fig. 11.29 Intertransversarii, levatores costarum, multifidus, and rotatores
Schematic, posterior view. **A** Intertransversarii and levatores costarum. **B** Multifidus.
C Rotatores.

Table 11.6 Splenius, semispinalis, intertransversarii, levatores costarum, multifidus, and rotatores				
All intrinsic back muscles are innervated by the posterior rami of the spinal nerves except for the intertransversii posteriores cervicis, which are innervated by the anterior rami of the spinal nerves. The splenius is innervated by spinal nerves C1–C6.				
Muscle		**Origin**	**Insertion**	**Action**
Splenius	① S. capitis	C7–T3 (spinous processes)	Occipital bone (lateral superior nuchal line); temporal bone (mastoid process)	*Bilateral:* Extends cervical spine and head *Unilateral:* Flexes and rotates head to same side
	② S. cervicis	T3–T6 (spinous processes)	C1–C2 (transverse processes)	
Semispinalis	③ S. capitis	C3–T6 (transverse processes)	Occipital bone (between superior and inferior nuchal lines)	*Bilateral:* Extends cervical and thoracic spine and head (stabilizes craniovertebral joints) *Unilateral:* Bends head and cervical and thoracic spine to same side, rotates them to opposite side
	④ S. cervicis	T1–T6 (transverse processes)	C2–C7 (spinous processes)	
	⑤ S. thoracis	T6–T12 (transverse processes)	C6–T4 (spinous processes)	
Inter-transversarii	I. anteriores cervicis	C2–C7 (between anterior tubercles of adjacent vertebrae)		*Bilateral:* Stabilizes and extends cervical and lumbar spine *Unilateral:* Bends cervical and lumbar spine laterally to same side
	⑥ I. posteriores cervicis	C2–C7 (between posterior tubercles of adjacent vertebrae)		
	⑦ I. mediales lumborum	L1–L5 (between mammillary processes of adjacent vertebrae)		
	⑧ I. laterales lumborum	L1–L5 (between costal processes of adjacent vertebrae)		
Levatores costarum	⑨ L.c. brevis	C7–T11 (transverse processes)	Costal angle of next lower rib	*Bilateral:* Extends thoracic spine *Unilateral:* Bends thoracic spine to same side, rotates thoracic spine to opposite side
	⑩ L.c. longi		Costal angle of second lower rib	
⑪ Multifidus			C4–T4 (transverse and articular processes), L1–L5 (mammillary processes), ilium, and sacrum superomedially to spinous process of vertbra two to four levels higher	*Bilateral:* Extends spine *Unilateral:* Flexes spine to same side, rotates spine to opposite side
Rotatores	⑫ R. breves	T1–T12 (between transverse process and spinous processes of next higher vertebra)		*Bilateral:* Extends thoracic spine *Unilateral:* Flexes spine to same side, rotates spine to opposite side
	⑬ R. longi	T1–T12 (between transverse process and spinous process of vertebra two levels higher)		

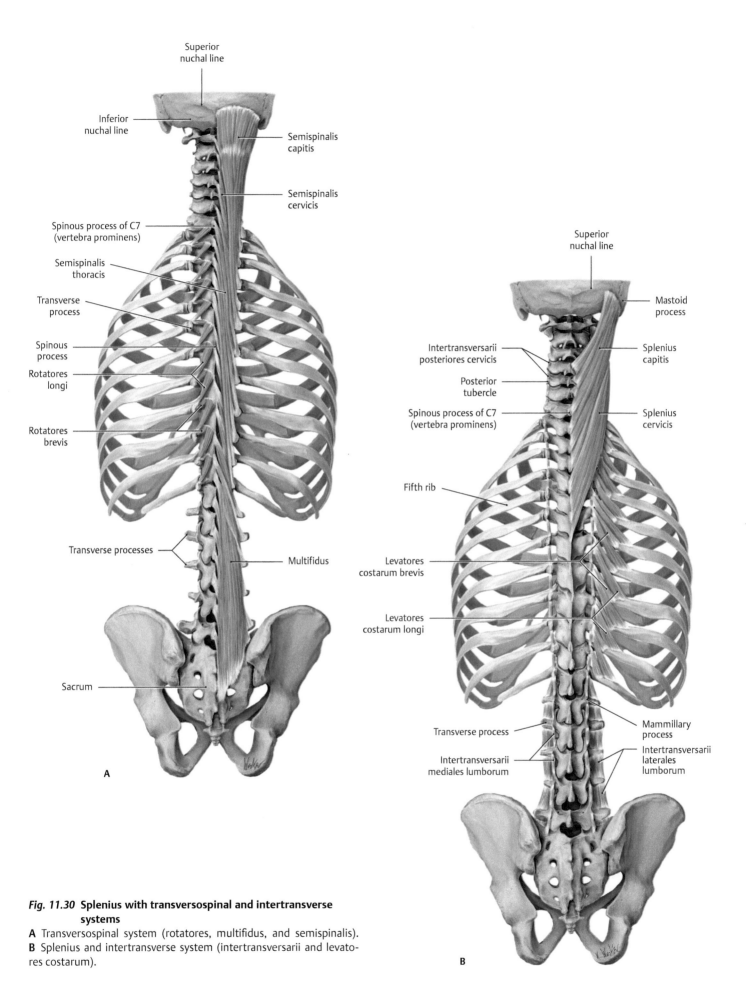

Fig. 11.30 Splenius with transversospinal and intertransverse systems

A Transversospinal system (rotatores, multifidus, and semispinalis).
B Splenius and intertransverse system (intertransversarii and levatores costarum).

Intrinsic Back Muscles (III): Short Nuchal & Craniovertebral Joint Muscles

Fig. 11.31 Short nuchal and craniovertebral joint muscles
Schematic, posterior view. The short nuchal and craniovertebral joint muscles are intrinsic back muscles that are innervated by the posterior ramus of the first spinal nerve (suboccipital nerve). These muscles contribute to the extension of the atlanto-occipital joint and rotation about the atlantoaxial joint.

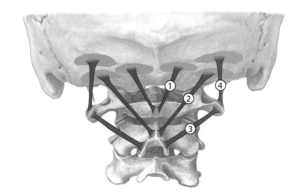

Table 11.7 Short nuchal muscles					
Muscle		**Origin**	**Insertion**	**Innervation**	**Action**
Rectus capitis posterior	① R.c.p. minor	C1 (posterior tubercle)	Inferior nuchal line (inner ⅓)	C1 spinal nerve (suboccipital n.), posterior ramus	*Bilateral:* Extends head *Unilateral:* Rotates head to same side
	② R.c.p. major	C2 (spinous process)	Inferior nuchal line (middle ⅓)		
Obliquus capitis	③ O.c. inferior	C2 (spinous process)	C1 (transverse process)		
	④ O.c. superior	C1 (transverse process)	Above the insertion of the rectus capitis posterior major or inferior nuchal line (middle ⅓)		*Bilateral:* Extends head *Unilateral:* Tilts head to same side; rotates head to opposite side

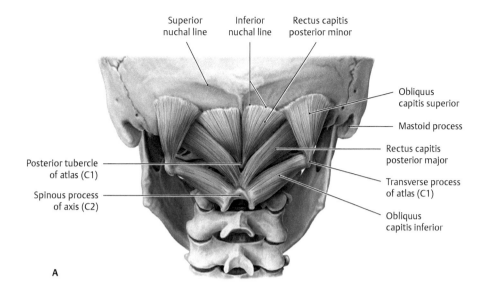

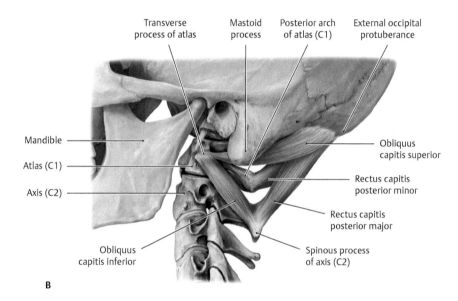

***Fig. 11.32* Suboccipital muscles**
A Posterior view. **B** Left lateral view.
The suboccipital muscles collectively act on the craniovertebral joints. The suboccipital muscles are the rectus capitis posterior major, rectus capitis posterior minor, obliquus capitis inferior, and obliquus capitis

superior. The posterior ramus of the first cervical spinal nerve innervates all four suboccipital muscles. Note: The suboccipital triangle is located between the rectus capitis posterior major, the obliquus capitis superior, and the obliquus capitis inferior.

Prevertebral & Scalene Muscles

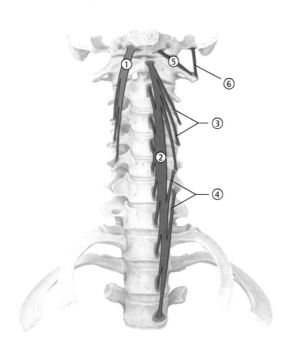

Fig. 11.33 Prevertebral muscles
Schematic, anterior view.

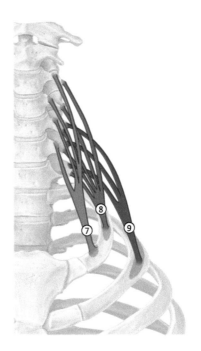

Fig. 11.34 Scalene muscles
Schematic, anterior view.

Table 11.8 Prevertebral and scalene muscles					
Muscle		**Origin**	**Insertion**	**Innervation**	**Action**
① Longus capitis		C3–C6 (anterior tubercles)	Occipital bone, basilar part	Cervical plexus, direct branches (C1–C3)	*Bilateral:* Flexes head *Unilateral:* Tilts and slightly rotates head to same side
Longus colli medial	② Vertical (cervicis) part	C5–T3 (anterior surfaces of vertebral bodies)	C2–C4 (anterior surfaces)	Anterior rami of C2–C6 spinal nn.	*Bilateral:* Flexes cervical spine *Unilateral:* Tilts and slightly rotates cervical spine to same side
	③ Superior oblique part	C3–C5 (anterior tubercles)	C1 (anterior tubercle)		
	④ Inferior oblique part	T1–T3 (anterior surfaces of vertebral bodies)	C5–C6 (anterior tubercles)		
Rectus capitis	⑤ R.c. anterior	C1 (lateral mass)	Occipital bone (basilar part)	Anterior ramus of C1 spinal n. (suboccipital n.)	*Bilateral:* Flexion at atlanto-occipital joint *Unilateral:* Lateral flexion at atlanto-occipital joint
	⑥ R.c. lateralis	C1 (transverse process)	Occipital bone (basilar part, lateral to occipital condyles)		
Scalenes	⑦ Anterior scalene	C3–C6 (anterior tubercles)	1st rib (scalene tubercle)	Anterior rami of cervical spinal nn.	*With ribs mobile:* Elevate upper ribs (in inspiration) *With ribs fixed:* Bend cervical spine to same side (unilateral contraction); flex cervical spine (bilateral contraction)
	⑧ Middle scalene	C1 and C2 (transverse processes); C3–C7 (posterior tubercles)	1st rib (posterior to groove for subclavian a.)		
	⑨ Posterior scalene	C5–C7 (posterior tubercles)	2nd rib (outer surface)		

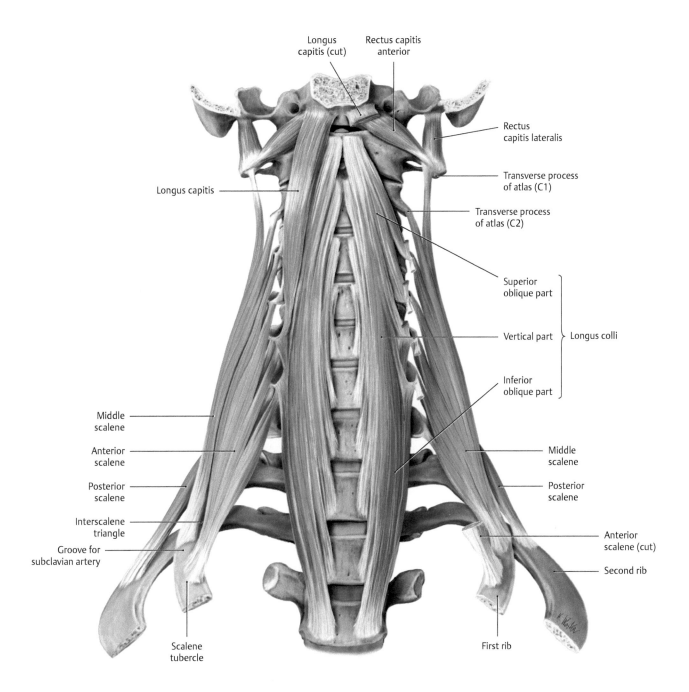

Longus
capitis (cut)

Rectus capitis
anterior

Rectus
capitis lateralis

Longus capitis

Transverse process
of atlas (C1)

Transverse process
of atlas (C2)

Superior
oblique part

Vertical part ⎱ Longus colli

Inferior
oblique part

Middle
scalene

Anterior
scalene

Posterior
scalene

Interscalene
triangle

Groove for
subclavian artery

Middle
scalene

Posterior
scalene

Anterior
scalene (cut)

Second rib

Scalene
tubercle

First rib

Fig. 11.35 Prevertebral and scalene muscles

Anterior view. *Removed on left side:* Longus capitis and anterior scalene. The prevertebral (anterior vertebral) muscles are the longus colli, longus capitis, rectus capitis lateralis, and rectus capitis anterior. The an- terior, middle, and posterior scalenes are the lateral vertebral muscles. The anterior and lateral vertebral muscles are innervated by the anterior rami of the cervical spinal nerves.

Suprahyoid & Infrahyoid Muscles

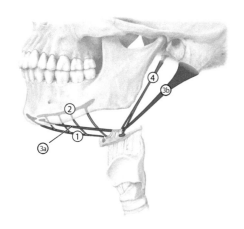

Fig. 11.36 Suprahyoid muscles
Schematic, left lateral view.

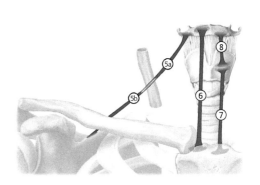

Fig. 11.37 Infrahyoid muscles
Schematic, anterior view.

Table 11.9 Suprahyoid and infrahyoid muscles				
Muscle	**Origin**	**Insertion**	**Innervation**	**Action**
Suprahyoid muscles				
① Geniohyoid	Mandible (inferior mental spine)	Hyoid bone	Anterior ramus of C1 via hypoglossal n. (CN XII)*	Draws hyoid bone forward (during swallowing); assists in opening mandible
② Mylohyoid	Mandible (mylohyoid line)	Hyoid bone (via median tendon of insertion, the mylohyoid raphe)	Mylohyoid n. (from CN V₃)	Tightens and elevates oral floor; draws hyoid bone forward (during swallowing); assists in opening mandible and moving it side to side (mastication)
③ⓐ Digastric, anterior belly	Mandible (digastric fossa)	Hyoid bone (via an intermediate tendon with a fibrous loop)	Facial n. (CN VII)	Elevates hyoid bone (during swallowing); assists in opening mandible
③ⓑ Digastric, posterior belly	Temporal bone (mastoid notch, medial to mastoid process)			
④ Stylohyoid	Temporal bone (styloid process)	Hyoid bone (via a split tendon)		
Infrahyoid muscles				
⑤ⓐ Omohyoid, superior belly	Intermediate tendon of omohyoid	Hyoid bone	Ansa cervicalis of cervical plexus (C1–C3)	Depresses (fixes) hyoid; draws larynx and hyoid down for phonation and terminal phases of swallowing**
⑤ⓑ Omohyoid, inferior belly	Scapula (superior border, medial to suprascapular notch)	Intermediate tendon of omohyoid		
⑥ Sternohyoid	Manubrium and sternoclavicular joint (posterior surface)	Hyoid bone		
⑦ Sternothyroid	Manubrium (posterior surface)	Thyroid cartilage (oblique line)	Ansa cervicalis C2, C3	
⑧ Thyrohyoid	Thyroid cartilage (oblique line)	Hyoid bone	Anterior ramus of C1 via hypoglossal n. (CN XII)	Depresses and fixes hyoid; raises the larynx during swallowing

*C1 anterior ramus fibers travel with the hypoglossal nerve for part of its pathway to target muscles.

**The omohyoid also tenses the cervical fascia (with an intermediate tendon). The intermediate tendon is attached to the clavicle, pulling the omohyoid into a more pronounced triangle.

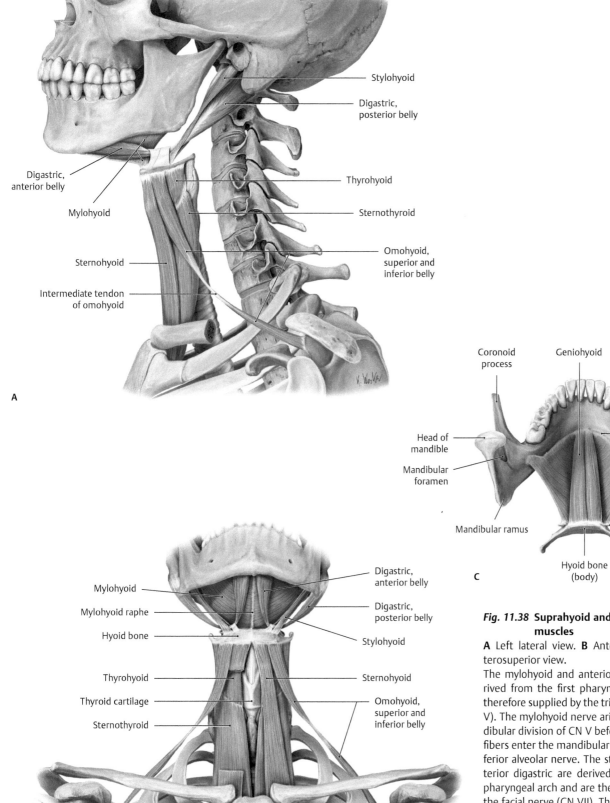

A Left lateral view.

- Stylohyoid
- Digastric, posterior belly
- Thyrohyoid
- Sternothyroid
- Omohyoid, superior and inferior belly
- Digastric, anterior belly
- Mylohyoid
- Sternohyoid
- Intermediate tendon of omohyoid

B

- Mylohyoid
- Mylohyoid raphe
- Hyoid bone
- Thyrohyoid
- Thyroid cartilage
- Sternothyroid
- Digastric, anterior belly
- Digastric, posterior belly
- Stylohyoid
- Sternohyoid
- Omohyoid, superior and inferior belly

C

- Coronoid process
- Geniohyoid
- Mylohyoid line
- Head of mandible
- Mandibular foramen
- Mandibular ramus
- Mylohyoid
- Lesser horn
- Greater horn
- Hyoid bone (body)

***Fig. 11.38* Suprahyoid and infrahyoid muscles**

A Left lateral view. **B** Anterior view. **C** Posterosuperior view.

The mylohyoid and anterior digastric are derived from the first pharyngeal arch and are therefore supplied by the trigeminal nerve (CN V). The mylohyoid nerve arises from the mandibular division of CN V before the majority of fibers enter the mandibular foramen as the inferior alveolar nerve. The stylohyoid and posterior digastric are derived from the second pharyngeal arch and are therefore supplied by the facial nerve (CN VII). The remainder of the suprahyoid and infrahyoid muscles are supplied by the anterior rami of the cervical spinal nerves. Fibers from the anterior ramus of C1 travel with the hypoglossal nerve (CN XII) to the geniohyoid and thyrohyoid. Fibers from the anterior rami of C1–C3 combine to form the ansa cervicalis, which gives off branches to the omohyoid, sternohyoid, and sternothyroid.

Radiographs of Bones & Muscles of the Neck

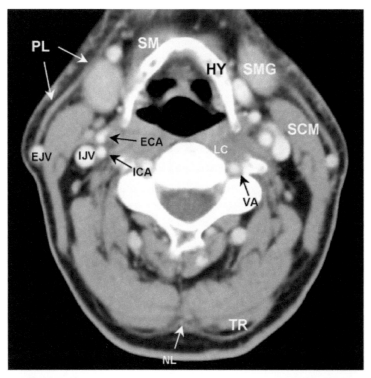

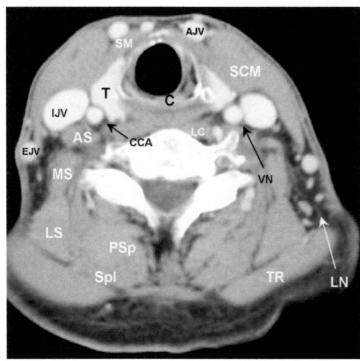

Fig. 11.39

Axial CT anatomy of the neck as seen at the level of the hyoid bone (**A**), cricoid ring (**B**), thyroid gland (**C**), and clavicles (**D**).

AJV = anterior jugular vein; AS = anterior scalene muscle; BPl brachial plexus; C = cricoid; CCA = common carotid artery; CL = clavicle; ECA = external carotid artery; EJV = external jugular vein; ES = esophagus; HY = hyoid bone; ICA = internal carotid artery; IJV = internal jugular vein; ITA = inferior thyroid artery; LC = longus colli muscle; LN = normal lymph nodes; LS = levator scapulae muscle; NL = nuchal ligament; MS = middle scalene muscle; PhrN = phrenic nerve; PL = platysma; PS = posterior scalene muscle; PSp = paraspinal muscles; RLN = recurrent laryngeal nerve; SCA = subclavian artery; SCLV = subclavian vein; SCM = sternocleidomastoid muscle; SM = strap muscles; SMG = submandibular gland; Spl = splenius capitis muscle; T = thyroid gland; Th1 = first thoracic vertebra; TR = trapezius muscle; VA = vertebral artery; VN = vagus nerve. (Source: Becker M. Anatomy. In: Valvassori G, Mafee M, Becker M, ed. Imaging of the Head and Neck. 2nd edition. Stuttgart: Thieme; 2004.)

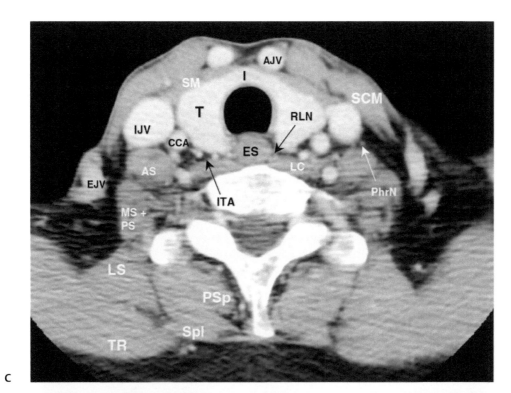

C

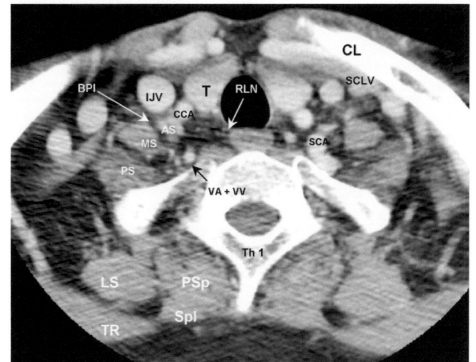

D

Arteries & Veins of the Neck

Fig. 12.1 Arteries of the neck

Left lateral view. The structures of the neck are supplied by branches of the external carotid artery and the subclavian artery (the internal carotid artery gives off no branches in the neck). The common carotid artery is enclosed in a fascial sheath (carotid sheath) along with the internal jugular vein and vagus nerve. The vertebral artery ascends through the transverse foramina of the cervical vertebrae (C6–C1).

The internal carotid artery is often affected by atherosclerosis, a hardening of the arterial walls due to plaque formation. These plaques can cause stenosis, thrombosis, and embolization, which could result in vision loss, transient ischemic attacks (TIAs), or stroke.

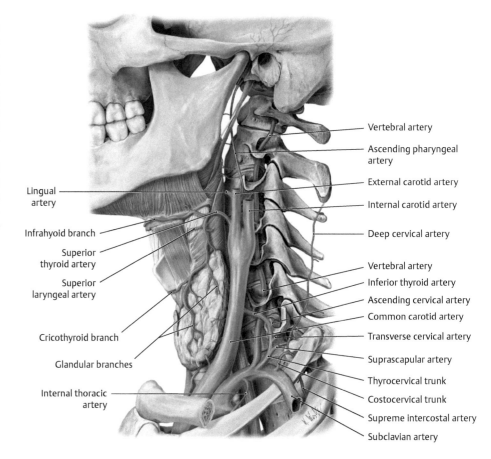

Table 12.1 **Arteries of the neck**

For a complete treatment of the arteries of the head and neck, see **Chapter 3**.

Artery	Branches	Secondary branches*	
External carotid a.	Superior thyroid a.	Superior laryngeal, cricothyroid, infrahyoid, and sternocleidomastoid aa.	
	Ascending pharyngeal a.	Pharyngeal, palatine, prevertebral, inferior tympanic, and meningeal aa.	
	Lingual a.	Suprahyoid, dorsal lingual, deep lingual, and sublingual aa.	
	Facial a.	Ascending palatine, tonsillar, glandular, and submental aa.	
	Occipital a.	Sternocleidomastoid, descending, mastoid, auricular, and meningeal aa.	
	Posterior auricular a.	Stylomastoid and auricular aa.	
	Superficial temporal a.	(Branching occurs on the face [see p. 162])	
	Maxillary a.	(Branches within the infratemporal fossa [see p. 180])	
Subclavian a.	Vertebral a.	Spinal aa. and muscular aa.	
	Thyrocervical trunk	Inferior thyroid a.	Inferior laryngeal, tracheal, esophageal, and ascending cervical aa.
		Suprascapular a.	
		Transverse cervical a.	Superficial and deep branches
	Internal thoracic a.	(Branching occurs within the thorax)	
	Descending (dorsal) scapular a.	(When present, it supplies the territory of the deep branch of the transverse cervical a.)	
	Costocervical trunk	Deep cervical a.	
		Supreme intercostal a.	

*Only branches that arise in the neck are listed here.

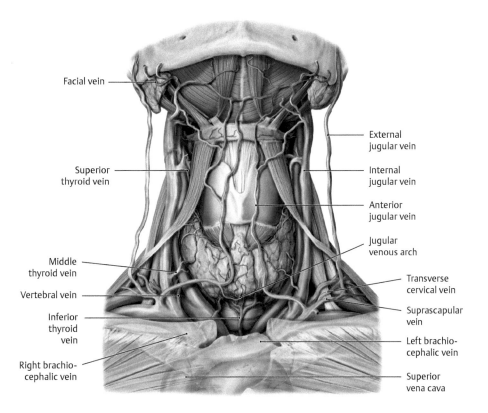

Fig. 12.2 Veins of the neck
Anterior view. The veins of the head and neck drain to the superior vena cava via the right and left brachiocephalic veins. The large internal jugular vein combines with the subclavian vein to form the brachioce- phalic vein on each side. The internal jugular vein is located within the carotid sheath. It receives blood from the anterior neck and the interior of the skull. The subclavian vein receives blood from the neck via the external and anterior jugular veins, which are located within the super- ficial cervical fascia. *Note:* The thyroid venous plexus and vertebral veins typically drain directly into the brachiocephalic veins.

Table 12.2 Veins of the neck			
For a complete treatment of the veins of the head and neck, see **Chapter 3**.			
Right and left brachiocephalic vv.*	Internal jugular v.	Sigmoid sinus, inferior petrosal sinus, pharyngeal vv., occipital, (common) facial, lingual, and superior and middle thyroid vv.	
	Subclavian v.	External jugular v.	Posterior external jugular, anterior jugular, transverse cervical, and suprascapular vv.**
	Vertebral v.	Internal and external vertebral venous plexuses; ascending cervical (anterior vertebral) and deep cervical vv.	
	Inferior thyroid vv.	Thyroid venous plexus	

*The brachiocephalic vein is formed by the joining of its two primary tributaries, the internal jugular vein and the subclavian vein. Only tributaries within the neck are listed above.
**The tributaries of the external jugular vein may on occasion drain directly into the subclavian vein.

Cervical Plexus

The neck receives innervation from the cervical spinal nerves as well as three cranial nerves: glossopharyngeal nerve (CN IX), vagus nerve (CN X), and accessory nerve (CN XI). CN IX and X innervate the pharynx and larynx; CN XI provides motor innervation to the trapezius and sternocleidomastoid. The course and distribution of the cranial nerves are described in **Chapter 4**.

Fig. 12.3 **Cervical plexus**
The anterior rami of spinal nerves C1–C4 emerge from the intervertebral foramina along the transverse processes of the cervical vertebrae. They emerge between the anterior and posterior scalenes and give off short direct branches to the scalenes and rectii capitis anterioris before coursing anteriorly to form the cervical plexus.
Motor fibers: Motor fibers from C1 course with the hypoglossal nerve (CN XII). Certain fibers continue with the nerve to innervate the thyrohyoid and geniohyoid. The remainder leave CN XII to form the superior root of the ansa cervicalis. The inferior root is formed by motor fibers from C2 and C3. The ansa cervicalis innervates the omohyoid, sternothyroid, and sternohyoid. Most motor fibers from C4 descend as the phrenic nerve, which innervates the diaphragm.
Sensory fibers: The sensory fibers of C2–C4 emerge from the cervical plexus as peripheral nerves. (*Note:* The sensory fibers of C1 go to the meninges.) These peripheral sensory nerves emerge from Erb's point and provide sensory innervation to the anterolateral neck.

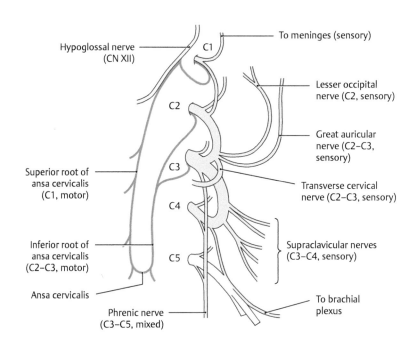

Table 12.3 **Branches of the cervical plexus**

	Sensory branches	Sensory function	Motor branches	Motor function
C1	—	—	Forms ansa cervicalis (motor part of cervical plexus) and separate motor branches of CI	Ansa cervicalis innervates infrahyoid muscles (except thyrohyoid). CI innervates thyrohyoid and geniohyoid in separate branches traveling with CN XII
C2	Lesser occipital n.	Form sensory part of cervical plexus; innervate anterior and lateral neck		
C2–C3	Great auricular n.			
	Transverse cervical n.			
C3–C4	Supraclavicular nn.		Contribute to phrenic n.*	Innervate diaphragm and pericardium*

* The anterior rami of C3–C5 combine to form the phrenic nerve.

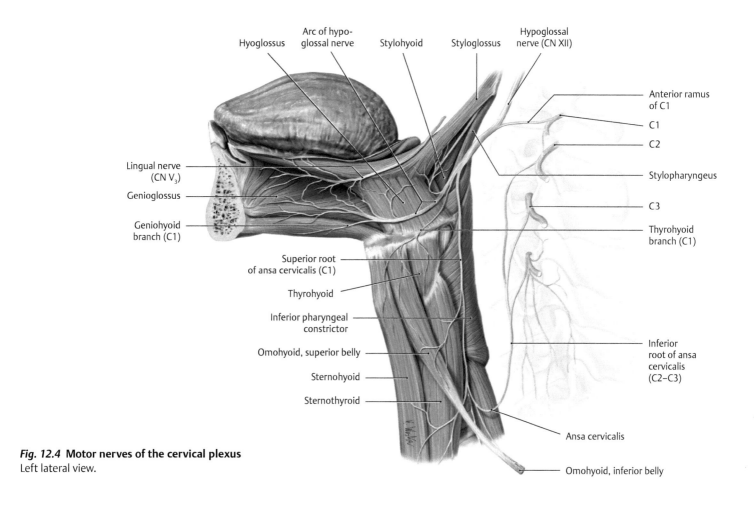

Fig. 12.4 Motor nerves of the cervical plexus
Left lateral view.

Hyoglossus

Arc of hypo-glossal nerve

Stylohyoid

Styloglossus

Hypoglossal nerve (CN XII)

Anterior ramus of C1

C1

C2

Stylopharyngeus

C3

Thyrohyoid branch (C1)

Lingual nerve (CN V₃)

Genioglossus

Geniohyoid branch (C1)

Superior root of ansa cervicalis (C1)

Thyrohyoid

Inferior pharyngeal constrictor

Omohyoid, superior belly

Sternohyoid

Sternothyroid

Inferior root of ansa cervicalis (C2–C3)

Ansa cervicalis

Omohyoid, inferior belly

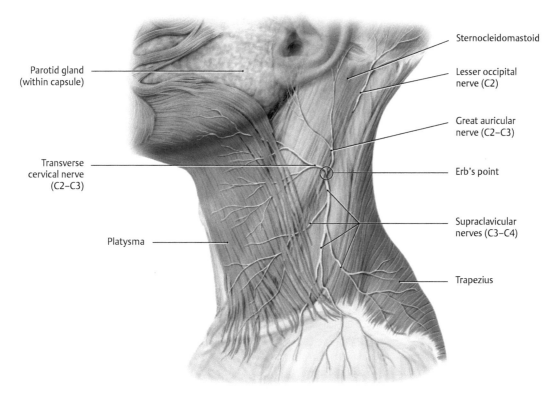

Fig. 12.5 Sensory nerves of the cervical plexus
Left lateral view.

Parotid gland (within capsule)

Transverse cervical nerve (C2–C3)

Platysma

Sternocleidomastoid

Lesser occipital nerve (C2)

Great auricular nerve (C2–C3)

Erb's point

Supraclavicular nerves (C3–C4)

Trapezius

Cervical Regions (Triangles)

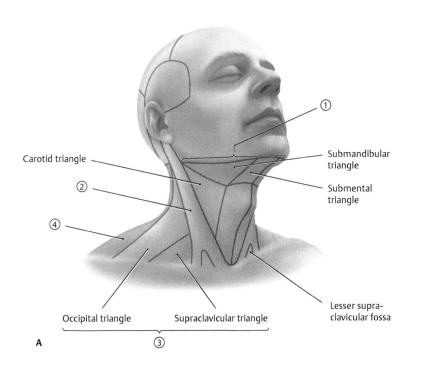

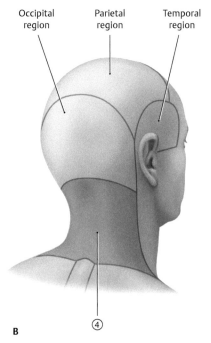

Fig. 12.6 Cervical regions
A Right lateral oblique view. **B** Left posterior oblique view.
For descriptive purposes, the anterolateral neck is divided into an anterior and a posterior cervical triangle, separated by the sternocleido-mastoid. The posterior portion of the neck is referred to as the nuchal region.

Table 12.4 Cervical regions	
Region	**Subdivision**
① Anterior cervical region (anterior cervical triangle): Bounded by the midline, mandible, and sternocleidomastoid.	Submandibular (digastric) triangle: Bounded by the mandible and the bellies of the digastric muscle.
	Carotid triangle: Bounded by the sternocleidomastoid, superior belly of the omohyoid, and posterior belly of the digastric.
	Muscular triangle: Bounded by the sternocleidomastoid, superior omohyoid, and sternohyoid.
	Submental triangle: Bounded by the anterior bellies of the digastric, the hyoid bone, and the mandible.
② Sternocleidomastoid region: The region lying under the sternocleidomastoid muscle.	
③ Lateral cervical region (posterior cervical triangle): Bounded by the sternocleidomastoid, trapezius, and clavicle.	Supraclavicular (omoclavicular or subclavian) triangle: Bounded by the inferior belly of the omohyoid, the clavicle, and the sternocleidomastoid.
	Occipital triangle: Bounded by the inferior belly of the omohyoid, the trapezius, and the sternocleidomastoid.
④ Posterior cervical region (nuchal region): Region lying under the trapezius muscle inferior to its insertion at the superior nuchal line and superior to the vertebra prominens (C7).	

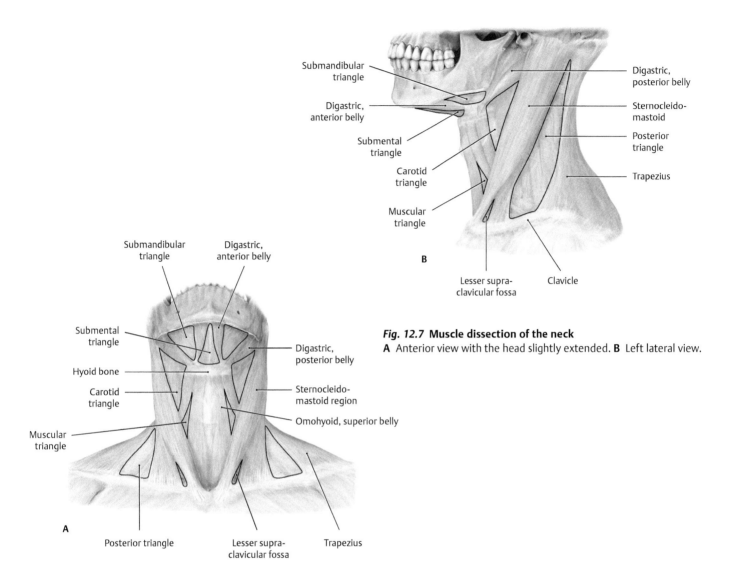

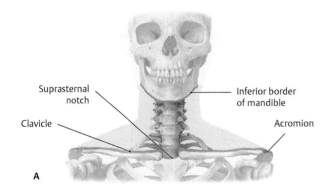

Fig. 12.7 Muscle dissection of the neck
A Anterior view with the head slightly extended. **B** Left lateral view.

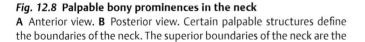

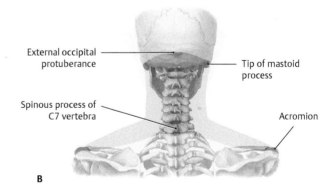

Fig. 12.8 Palpable bony prominences in the neck
A Anterior view. **B** Posterior view. Certain palpable structures define the boundaries of the neck are the inferior border of the mandible, tip of the mastoid process, and external occipital protuberance. The inferior boundaries are the suprasternal notch, clavicle, acromion, and spinous process of the C7 vertebra.

Cervical Fasciae

Fig. 12.9 Cervical fasciae

The structures of the neck are enclosed by multiple layers of cervical fasciae, sheets of connective tissue that subdivide the neck into compartments. The fascial layers are separated by interfascial spaces. There are four major fascial spaces in the neck: pretracheal, retropharyngeal, prevertebral, and carotid. These spaces are not prominent under normal conditions (the fasciae lie flat against each other). However, the spaces may provide routes for the spread of inflammatory processes (e.g., tonsillar infections in the infratemporal fossa) from regions of the head and neck into the mediastinum.

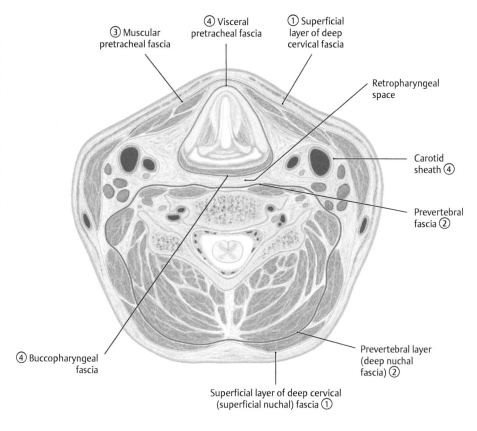

③ Muscular pretracheal fascia

④ Visceral pretracheal fascia

① Superficial layer of deep cervical fascia

Retropharyngeal space

Carotid sheath ④

Prevertebral fascia ②

Prevertebral layer (deep nuchal fascia) ②

④ Buccopharyngeal fascia

Superficial layer of deep cervical (superficial nuchal) fascia ①

Table 12.5 Cervical fasciae and fascial spaces

Despite generally being continuous, many of the fascial layers bear different names in different regions of the neck relative to the structures they enclose.

Fascial layer	Description	Contents
Superficial cervical fascia (not shown)	Subcutaneous tissue that lies deep to the skin and contains the platysma anterolaterally.	Platysma
① Superficial layer of deep cervical fascia (yellow) = Deep cervical fascia + Superficial nuchal fascia	Envelops the entire neck and is continuous with the nuchal ligament posteriorly.	Splits around the trapezius and sternocleidomastoid
② Prevertebral layer of deep cervical fascia (purple) = Prevertebral fascia + Deep nuchal fascia	Attaches superiorly to the skull base and continues inferiorly into the superior mediastinum, merging with the anterior longitudinal ligament. Continues along the subclavian artery and brachial plexus, becoming continuous with the axillary sheath. • The prevertebral fascia splits into an anterior (alar) and a posterior layer (the "danger space" is located between these layers).	Intrinsic back muscles and prevertebral muscles
Pretracheal fascia (green)	③ Muscular portion (light green)	Infrahyoid muscles
	④ Visceral portion (dark green): Attaches to the cricoid cartilage and is continuous posteriorly with the buccopharyngeal fascia. Continues inferiorly into the superior mediastinum, eventually merging with the fibrous pericardium.	Thyroid gland, trachea, esophagus, and pharynx
Carotid sheath (blue). Derived from deep, prevertebral, and pretracheal layers.	Consisting of loose areolar tissue, the sheath extends from the base of the skull (from the external opening of the carotid canal) to the aortic arch.	Common and internal carotid arteries, internal jugular vein, and vagus nerve (CN X); in addition, CN IX, CN XI, and CN XII briefly pass through the most superior part of the carotid sheath.

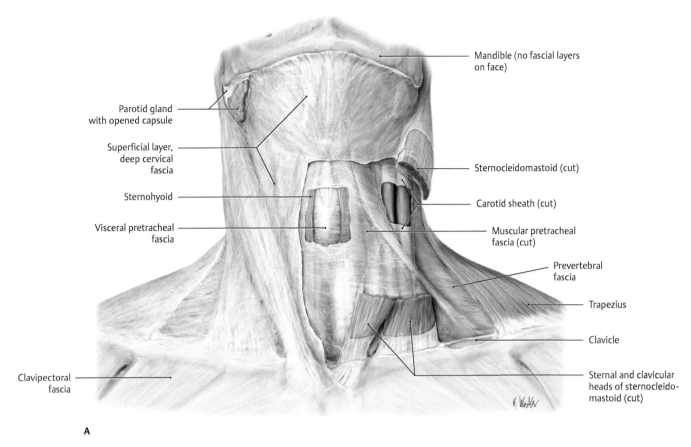

Parotid gland
with opened capsule

Superficial layer,
deep cervical
fascia

Sternohyoid

Visceral pretracheal
fascia

Clavipectoral
fascia

Mandible (no fascial layers
on face)

Sternocleidomastoid (cut)

Carotid sheath (cut)

Muscular pretracheal
fascia (cut)

Prevertebral
fascia

Trapezius

Clavicle

Sternal and clavicular
heads of sternocleido-
mastoid (cut)

A

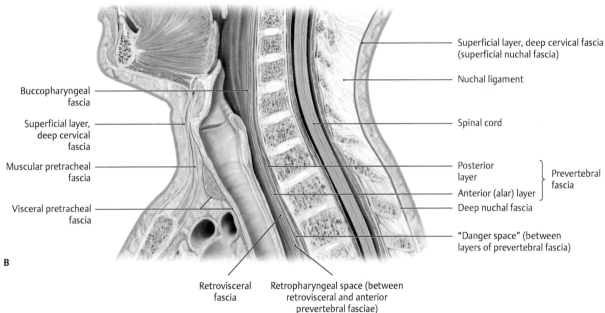

Buccopharyngeal
fascia

Superficial layer,
deep cervical
fascia

Muscular pretracheal
fascia

Visceral pretracheal
fascia

Superficial layer, deep cervical
fascia (superficial nuchal fascia)

Nuchal ligament

Spinal cord

Posterior
layer

Anterior (alar) layer

Prevertebral
fascia

Deep nuchal fascia

"Danger space" (between
layers of prevertebral fascia)

B

Retrovisceral
fascia

Retropharyngeal space (between
retrovisceral and anterior
prevertebral fasciae)

Fig. 12.10 **Fascial relationships in the neck**

A Anterior view with skin, superficial cervical fascia, and platysma removed. **B** Left lateral view of midsagittal section.

The superficial cervical fascia (not shown) lies just deep to the skin and contains the cutaneous muscle of the neck (platysma). The superficial layer of the deep cervical fascia contains the remainder of the structures in the neck. The deep cervical fascia attaches to the inferior border of the mandible and is continuous inferiorly with the clavipectoral fascia (anteriorly) and the superficial nuchal fascia and the thoracolumbar fascia (posteriorly). The superficial layer of the deep cervical fascia splits to enclose the parotid gland in a capsule (**A**, swelling of the parotid gland results in pain due to constriction by the capsule). It also splits to enclose the sternocleidomastoid and trapezius. In the anterior neck, the pretracheal layer lies just deep to the superficial layer of the deep cervical fascia. It consists of a muscular portion and a visceral portion, which collectively enclose the structures of the anterior neck, including the pharynx, trachea, and esophagus. The portion of the pretracheal fascia posterior to the esophagus is known as the retrovisceral fascia and is a continuation inferiorly of the buccopharyngeal fascia. (**B**). It is separated from the prevertebral fascia by the retropharyngeal space. Inferior to the laryngeal inlet, the prevertebral fascia splits into an anterior (alar) and a posterior layer, which are separated by the "danger space" — a potential route for the spread of infection from the pharynx into the superior mediastinum. With tuberculous osteomyelitis of the cervical spine, a retrophyarngeal abscess may develop in the "danger space" along the prevertebral fascia. Both prevertebral layers are continuous posteriorly with the deep nuchal fascia. *Note:* The laterally located carotid sheath (**A**) does not appear in the midsagittal section.

Anterior Neck

Fig. 12.11 Anterior neck

Anterior view. Left neck: Superficial cervical fascia removed to expose platysma. Right neck: Platysma removed to expose the deep cervical fascia. The superficial layer of the deep cervical fascia lies just deep to the cutaneous platysma muscle, which is innervated by the cervical branch of the facial nerve (CN VII). It attaches to the inferior border of the mandible and is continuous inferiorly with the clavipectoral fascia. The superficial layer splits to form a capsule around the parotid gland. Inflammation of the parotid gland (e.g., mumps) causes conspicuous facial swelling and deformity in this region ("hamster cheeks" with prominent earlobes). The superficial layer also divides into a deep and a posterior lamina to enclose the sternocleidomastoid. The superficial layer has been cut around the midline to expose the muscular pretracheal fascia, which encloses the infrahyoid muscles.

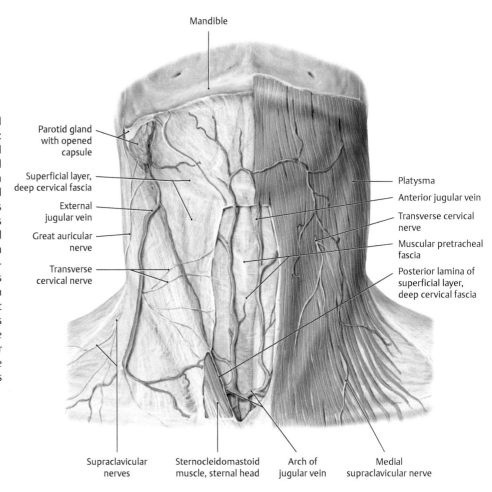

Fig. 12.12 Anterior cervical triangle

Anterior view. The pretracheal fascia has been removed to expose the anterior cervical triangle, bounded by the mandible and the anterior borders of the sternocleidomastoid muscles. The infrahyoid muscles are enclosed by the muscular pretracheal fascia (removed). The thyroid gland and larynx are enclosed by the visceral pretracheal fascia (removed). The anterior cervical triangle contains neurovasculature of the larynx and thyroid gland, including the first branch of the external carotid artery (the superior thyroid artery). The internal and external laryngeal nerves (from the superior laryngeal branch of CN X) are visible. C1 motor fibers run with the hypoglossal nerve (CN XII) to the thyrohyoid and geniohyoid (not shown). Certain C1 motor fibers leave CN XII to form the superior root of the ansa cervicalis. The inferior root is formed by motor fibers from C2 and C3. The ansa cervicalis innervates the omohyoid, sternothyroid, and sternohyoid.

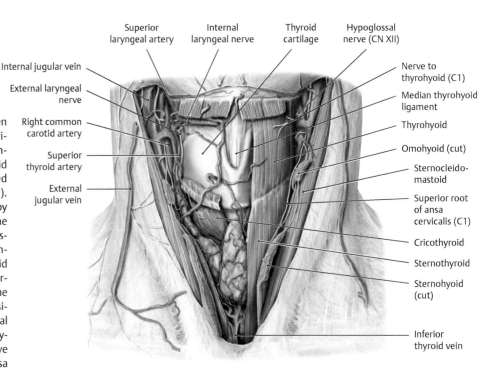

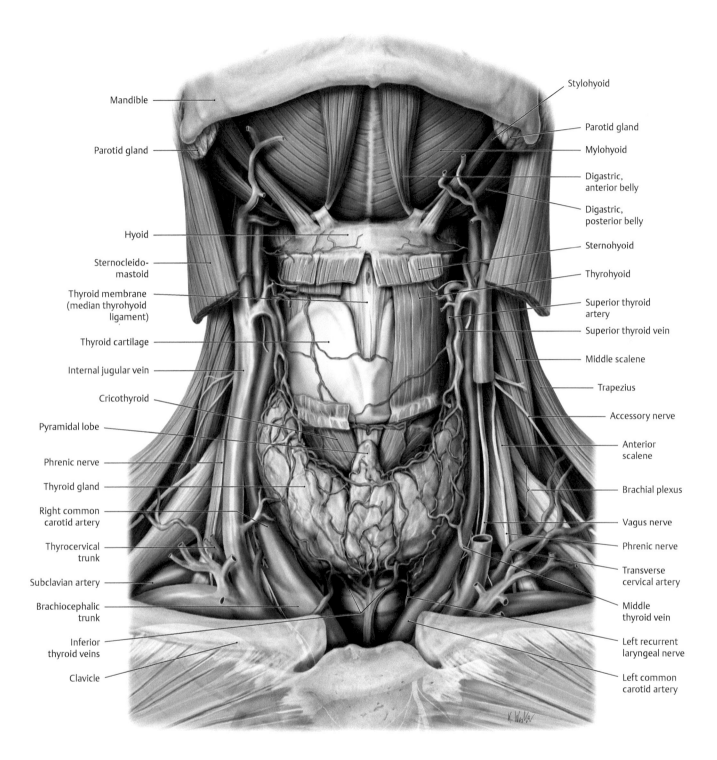

Mandible

Parotid gland

Hyoid

Sternocleido-mastoid

Thyroid membrane (median thyrohyoid ligament)

Thyroid cartilage

Internal jugular vein

Cricothyroid

Pyramidal lobe

Phrenic nerve

Thyroid gland

Right common carotid artery

Thyrocervical trunk

Subclavian artery

Brachiocephalic trunk

Inferior thyroid veins

Clavicle

Stylohyoid

Parotid gland

Mylohyoid

Digastric, anterior belly

Digastric, posterior belly

Sternohyoid

Thyrohyoid

Superior thyroid artery

Superior thyroid vein

Middle scalene

Trapezius

Accessory nerve

Anterior scalene

Brachial plexus

Vagus nerve

Phrenic nerve

Transverse cervical artery

Middle thyroid vein

Left recurrent laryngeal nerve

Left common carotid artery

Fig. 12.13 Root of the neck (thoracic inlet)
Anterior view. The root of the neck contains numerous structures, including the common carotid artery, subclavian artery, subclavian vein, internal jugular vein, inferior thyroid vein, vagus nerve, phrenic nerve, and recurrent laryngeal nerve. A goiter enlarging the inferior pole of the thyroid gland can easily compress neurovascular structures at the thoracic inlet.

343

Root of the Neck

Fig. 12.14 Root of the neck

Anterior view of left neck. *Removed:* Clavicle (sternal end), first rib, manubrium sterni, and thyroid gland. The left common carotid artery has been cut to expose sympathetic ganglia and the ascent of the left recurrent laryngeal nerve from the aortic arch (where it arises from CN X). The brachial plexus can be seen emerging from the interscalene space between the anterior and middle scalenes. It courses with the subclavian artery and vein into the axilla. The phrenic nerve descends on the anterior scalene into the mediastinum, where it innervates the diaphragm. The thoracic duct terminates at the jugulosubclavian venous junction on the left. It receives lymph from the entire body with the exception of the right upper quadrant, which drains to the right lymphatic duct. The anterior scalene muscle serves as landmark for structures at the root of the neck: the phrenic nerve and subclavian vein are anterior to the anterior scalene, while the brachial plexus and subclavian artery are posterior to it.

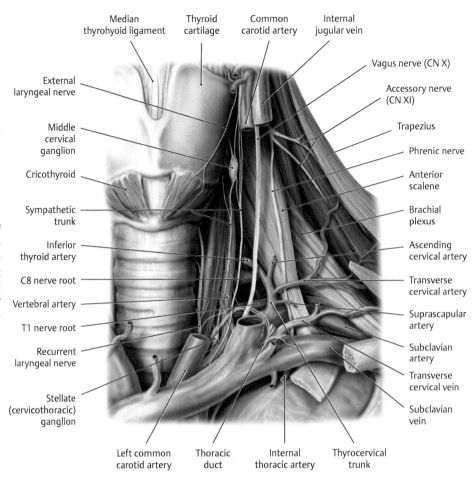

Fig. 12.15 Variants of the carotid arteries (after Faller and Poisel-Golth)

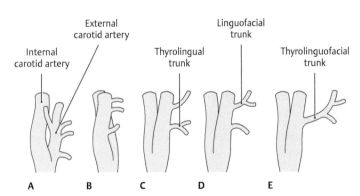

The internal carotid artery may arise from the common carotid artery posterolateral (49%, **A**) or anteromedial (9%, **B**) to the external carotid artery, or at other intermediate sites.

The external carotid artery may give off a thyrolingual trunk (4%, **C**), linguofacial trunk (23%, **D**), or thyrolinguofacial trunk (0.6%, **E**).

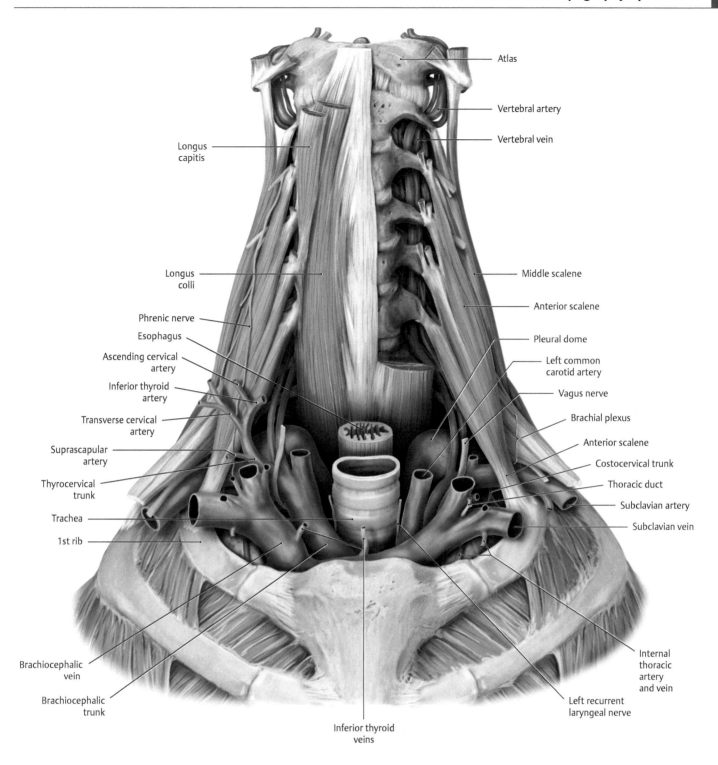

Fig. 12.16 Deepest Layer of the Neck, Anterior View

The larynx, thyroid, trachea, and esophagus have been removed to expose the prevertebral muscles and vertebral column of the neck. The two large vessels (the common carotid artery and the internal jugular vein) have been cut away on both sides, so the deeper lying vertebral artery is visible on the left; on the right it is hidden by the prevertebral muscles. The vertebral artery runs through the transverse foramina of the cervical vertebrae, from C6 upward. It continues over the arch of the atlas and enters the skull, where contributes to the blood supply to the brain and spinal cord. Also visible is the cervical plexus and the phrenic nerve, the latter extending down over the anterior scalene muscle to enter the thorax. It then passes anterior to the root of the lung and is found sandwiched between the mediastinal pleura and fibrous pericardium layer of the pericardial sac. The phrenic nerve supplies motor innervation to the muscle of the diaphragm and receives sensory innervation from the diaphragmatic and mediastinal pleura. Also seen in this dissection are the two bilateral arterial trunks with their branches:

- on the right, the thyrocervical trunk is shown with:
  – the inferior thyroid artery,
  – the transverse cervical artery with deep and superficial branches, and
  – the suprascapular artery;
  – Ascending cervical a.
- on the left, the costocervical trunk is shown. See **Fig. 12.1** for its branches:
  – the deep cervical artery, and the supreme intercostal artery.

The brachial plexus and the subclavian artery emerge from the gap between the anterior and middle scalene muscle; the subclavian vein passes anterior to the anterior scalene muscle. The thoracic duct enters the junction of the internal jugular and subclavian veins on the left after draining lymph from three quarters of the body.

345

Lateral Neck

Fig. 12.17 Lateral neck

Right lateral view. *Removed:* Superficial cervical fascia, platysma, and parotid capsule (superficial layer of the deep cervical fascia). The superficial layer of the deep cervical fascia encloses all the structures of the neck with the exception of the platysma. It splits to enclose the parotid gland in a capsule. The capsule has been opened to show the emergence of the cervical branch of the facial nerve (CN VII) from the parotid plexus. The cervical branch provides motor innervation to the platysma. The sensory nerves of the anterolateral neck (lesser occipital, great auricular, transverse cervical, and supraclavicular) arise from the cervical plexus, formed by the anterior rami of C1–C4. They pierce the investing layer at or near Erb's point, midway down the posterior border of the sternocleidomastoid. *Note:* The transverse cervical nerve (sensory) courses deep to the external jugular vein and forms a mixed anastomosis with the cervical branch (motor) of CN VII.

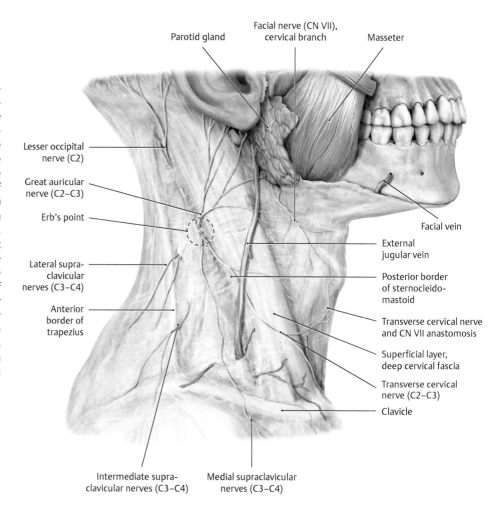

Fig. 12.18 Posterior cervical triangle

Right lateral view. **A** Superficial layer of the deep cervical fascia removed. **B** Pretracheal fascia removed. **C** Prevertebral fascia removed.

The superficial layer of the deep cervical fascia splits into anterior and a posterior lamina to enclose the sternocleidomastoid and trapezius, both of which are innervated by the accessory nerve (CN XI). (*Note:* The accessory nerve may be injured during lymph node biopsy.) Removing the superficial layer between the sternocleidomastoid and trapezius reveals the posterior cervical triangle (bounded inferiorly by the clavicle). This exposes the prevertebral fascia, which encloses the intrinsic and deep muscles of the neck. The prevertebral fascia is fused to the pretracheal fascia, which envelops the omohyoid (**B**). Removing the prevertebral fascia exposes the phrenic nerve (**C**), which arises from the cervical plexus and descends to innervate the diaphragm. The brachial plexus (**C**) is also visible at its point of emergence between the anterior and middle scalenes.

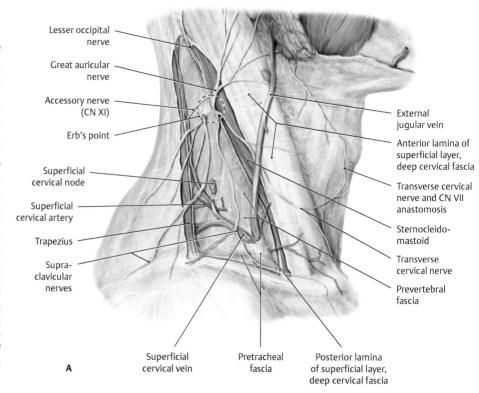

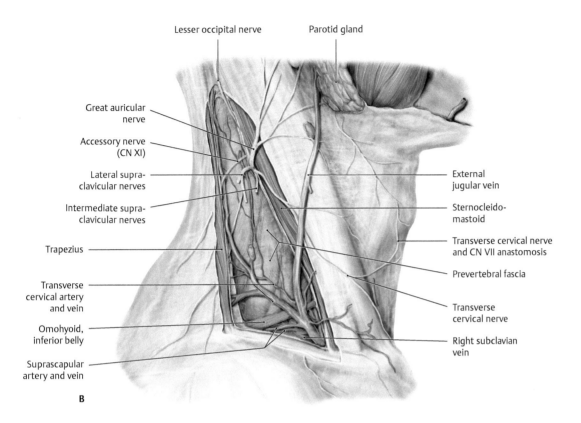

Lesser occipital nerve

Parotid gland

Great auricular
nerve

Accessory nerve
(CN XI)

Lateral supra-
clavicular nerves

Intermediate supra-
clavicular nerves

Trapezius

Transverse
cervical artery
and vein

Omohyoid,
inferior belly

Suprascapular
artery and vein

External
jugular vein

Sternocleido-
mastoid

Transverse cervical nerve
and CN VII anastomosis

Prevertebral fascia

Transverse
cervical nerve

Right subclavian
vein

B

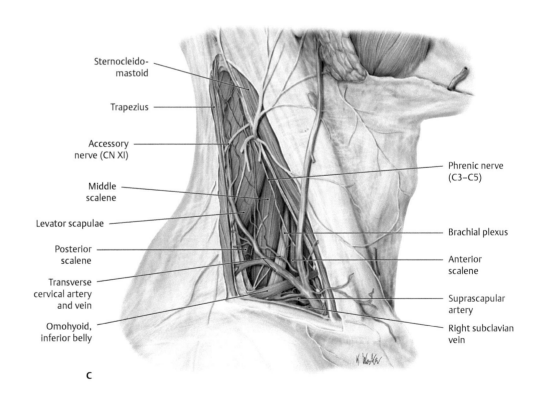

Sternocleido-
mastoid

Trapezius

Accessory
nerve (CN XI)

Middle
scalene

Levator scapulae

Posterior
scalene

Transverse
cervical artery
and vein

Omohyoid,
inferior belly

Phrenic nerve
(C3–C5)

Brachial plexus

Anterior
scalene

Suprascapular
artery

Right subclavian
vein

C

Deep Lateral Neck

Fig. 12.19 Carotid triangle

Right lateral view. The superficial layer of the deep cervical fascia has been removed to expose the carotid triangle, a subdivision of the anterior cervical triangle bounded by the sternocleidomastoid, superior belly of the omohyoid, and posterior belly of the digastric. The prevertebral and pretracheal fasciae have also been removed to expose the contents of the carotid triangle, which include the internal and external carotid arteries and the tributaries of the internal jugular vein. The sympathetic trunk runs between the major blood vessels along with the vagus nerve (CN X). C1 motor fibers course with the hypoglossal nerve (CN XII) to the thyrohyoid and geniohyoid. Certain C1 motor fibers leave to form the superior root of the ansa cervicalis (the inferior root is formed from C2–C3 fibers). The ansa cervicalis innervates the omohyoid, sternohyoid, and sternothyroid.

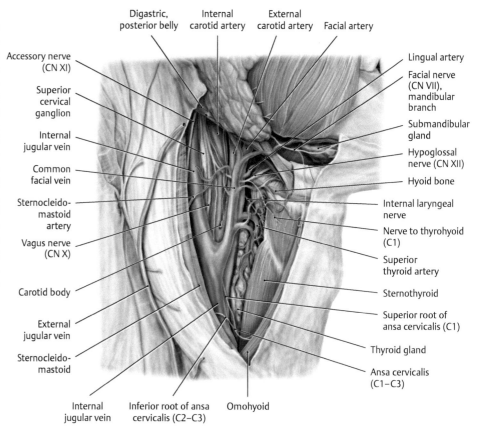

Fig. 12.20 Impeded blood flow and veins of the neck

When clinical factors (e.g., chronic lung disease, mediastinal tumors, or infections) impede the flow of blood to the right heart, blood dams up in the superior vena cava and, consequently, the external jugular vein (**A**). This causes conspicuous swelling in the external jugular (and sometimes more minor) veins (**B**).

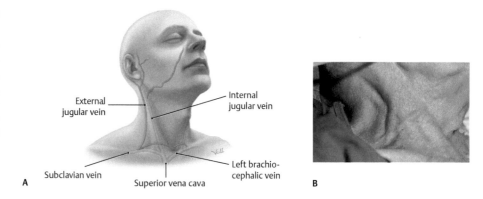

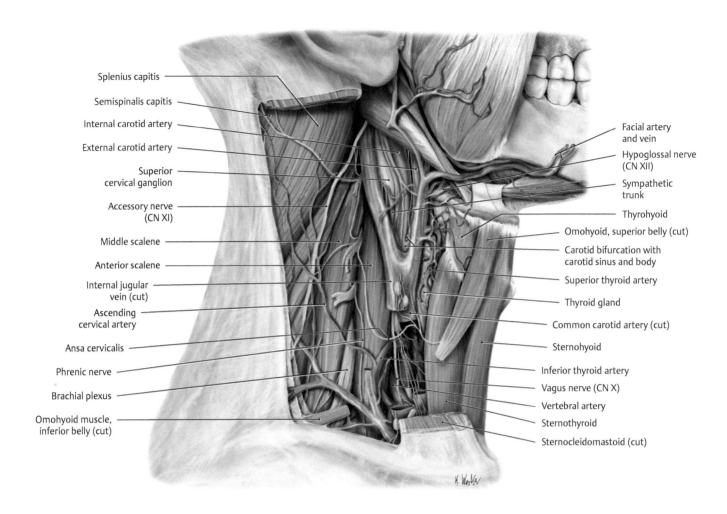

Splenius capitis
Semispinalis capitis
Internal carotid artery
External carotid artery
Superior cervical ganglion
Accessory nerve (CN XI)
Middle scalene
Anterior scalene
Internal jugular vein (cut)
Ascending cervical artery
Ansa cervicalis
Phrenic nerve
Brachial plexus
Omohyoid muscle, inferior belly (cut)

Facial artery and vein
Hypoglossal nerve (CN XII)
Sympathetic trunk
Thyrohyoid
Omohyoid, superior belly (cut)
Carotid bifurcation with carotid sinus and body
Superior thyroid artery
Thyroid gland
Common carotid artery (cut)
Sternohyoid
Inferior thyroid artery
Vagus nerve (CN X)
Vertebral artery
Sternothyroid
Sternocleidomastoid (cut)

Fig. 12.21 Deep lateral cervical region
Right lateral view. The sternocleidomastoid region and carotid triangle have been dissected along with adjacent portions of the posterior and anterior cervical triangles. The carotid sheath has been removed in this dissection along with the cervical fasciae and omohyoid muscle to demonstrate important neurovascular structures in the neck:

- Common carotid artery with internal and external carotid arteries
- Superior and inferior thyroid arteries
- Internal jugular vein
- Deep cervical lymph nodes along the internal jugular vein
- Sympathetic trunk, including ganglia
- Vagus nerve (CN X)
- Accessory nerve (CN XI)
- Hypoglossal nerve (CN XII)
- Brachial plexus
- Phrenic nerve

Massage of the carotid sinus slows heart rate via the baroreceptor reflex: increased stretch of baroreceptors in the carotid sinus increases the rate of firing of action potentials in the carotid sinus nerve (a branch of the glossopharnygeal nerve [CN IX]). Impulses are relayed to the vasomotor center in the medulla oblongata, which then decreases sympathetic outflow and increases parasympathetic outflow (via the vagus nerve) to the heart and blood vessels. This results in decreased heart rate, contractility, and cardiac output. It also causes dilation of vessels. This noninvasive technique is useful for termination of supra ventricular tachycardia (SVT).

The phrenic nerve (C3–C5) originates from the cervical plexus and the brachial plexus. The muscular landmark for locating the phrenic nerve is the anterior scalene, along which the nerve descends in the neck. The interscalene triangle is located between the anterior and middle scalene muscles and the first rib and is traversed by the brachial plexus and subclavian artery. The subclavian vein passes anterior to the anterior scalene.

Damage to the sympathetic chain, for example, due to a tumor at the apex of the lung ("Pancoast" tumor), thyrocervical venous dilation, or trauma, causes disruption of the sympathetic supply to the face. This is known as Horner syndrome and results in ipsilateral miosis (pupillary constriction), enophthalmos (a sunken eye), ptosis (drooping of the upper eyelid), and anhydrosis (loss of sweating) on the affected side.

Posterior Neck

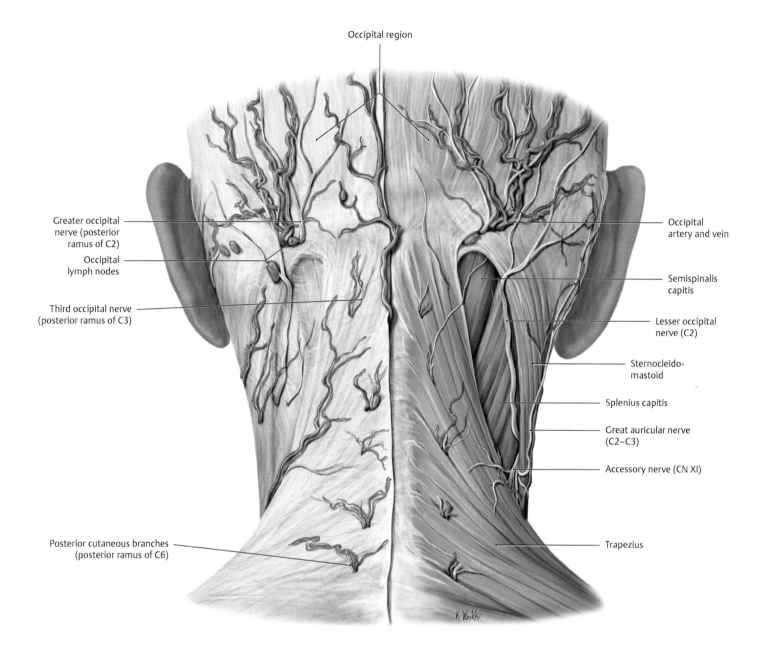

Occipital region

Greater occipital nerve (posterior ramus of C2)

Occipital lymph nodes

Third occipital nerve (posterior ramus of C3)

Posterior cutaneous branches (posterior ramus of C6)

Occipital artery and vein

Semispinalis capitis

Lesser occipital nerve (C2)

Sternocleido-mastoid

Splenius capitis

Great auricular nerve (C2–C3)

Accessory nerve (CN XI)

Trapezius

Fig. 12.22 Posterior cervical (nuchal) region

Posterior view. Left side: Superficial layer of superficial nuchal fascia. Right side: All fascia removed (superficial cervical fascia, superficial layer of the deep cervical fascia, prevertebral fascia).

The posterior cervical region is bounded superiorly by the superior nuchal line (the attachment of the trapezius and sternocleidomastoid to the occipital bone) and inferiorly by the palpable spinous process of the last cervical vertebra, the vertebra prominens (C7). The posterior cervical region, like the rest of the neck, is completely enveloped in superficial nuchal fascia (left side). The superficial layer of the deep cervical fascia envelops the trapezius and splits to enclose the sternocleidomastoid.

Both muscles are innervated by the accessory nerve (CN XI). The deep nuchal fascia (the posterior continuation of the prevertebral fascia) lies deep to the trapezius and sternocleidomastoid and encloses the intrinsic back muscles (here: semispinalis and splenius capitis). The intrinsic back muscles receive motor and sensory innervation from the posterior rami of the spinal nerves (see **Fig. 12.25**). The great auricular and lesser occipital nerves are also visible in this dissection. They are sensory nerves arising from the cervical plexus (formed by the anterior rami of C1–C4). The major artery of the occipital region is the occipital artery, a posterior branch of the external carotid artery.

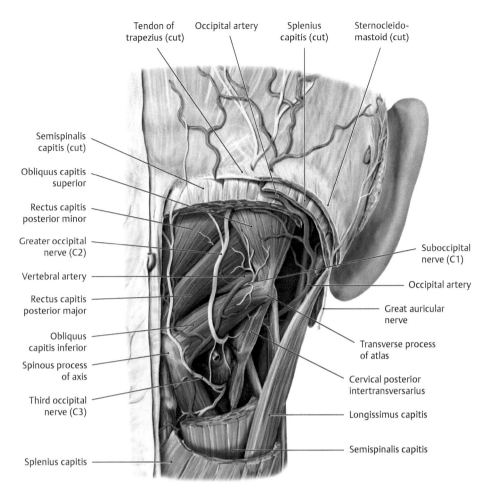

Tendon of trapezius (cut) — Occipital artery — Splenius capitis (cut) — Sternocleido-mastoid (cut)

Semispinalis capitis (cut)

Obliquus capitis superior

Rectus capitis posterior minor

Greater occipital nerve (C2)

Vertebral artery

Rectus capitis posterior major

Obliquus capitis inferior

Spinous process of axis

Third occipital nerve (C3)

Splenius capitis

Suboccipital nerve (C1)

Occipital artery

Great auricular nerve

Transverse process of atlas

Cervical posterior intertransversarius

Longissimus capitis

Semispinalis capitis

Fig. 12.23 Suboccipital triangle

Posterior view of right side. The suboccipital triangle is a muscular triangle lying deep to the trapezius, splenius capitis, and semi-spinalis capitis. It is bounded superiorly by the rectus capitis posterior major, laterally by the obliquus capitis superior, and inferiorly by the obliquus capitis inferior. A short segment of the vertebral artery runs through the deep part of the triangle after leaving the transverse foramen of the atlas. It gives off branches to the surrounding short nuchal muscles before exiting the suboccipital triangle by perforating the posterior atlanto-occipital membrane. The vertebral arteries unite intra-cranially to form the basilar artery, a major contributor to cerebral blood flow.

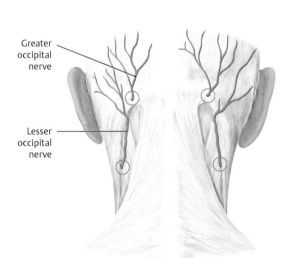

Greater occipital nerve

Lesser occipital nerve

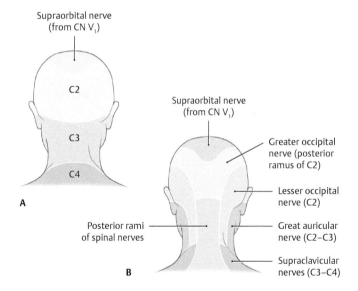

Supraorbital nerve (from CN V₁)

C2

C3

C4

A

Supraorbital nerve (from CN V₁)

Greater occipital nerve (posterior ramus of C2)

Lesser occipital nerve (C2)

Great auricular nerve (C2–C3)

Posterior rami of spinal nerves

Supraclavicular nerves (C3–C4)

B

Fig. 12.24 Sites of emergence of the occipital nerves

Posterior view. The sites where the lesser and greater occipital nerves emerge from the fascia into the subcutaneous connective tissue are clinically important because they are tender to palpation in certain diseases (e. g., meningitis). The examiner tests the sensation of these nerves by pressing lightly on the circled points with the thumb. If these points (but not their surroundings) are painful, the clinician should suspect meningitis.

Fig. 12.25 Cutaneous innervation of the posterior neck

Posterior view. **A** Segmental innervation (dermatomes). **B** Peripheral cutaneous nerves.

The occiput and nuchal regions derive most of their segmental innervation from the C2 and C3 spinal nerves. Of the specific cutaneous nerves, the greater occipital nerve is a branch of the posterior ramus of C2; the lesser occipital, great auricular, and supraclavicular nerves are branches of the cervical plexus (formed from the anterior rami of C1–C4).

Peripharyngeal Space (I)

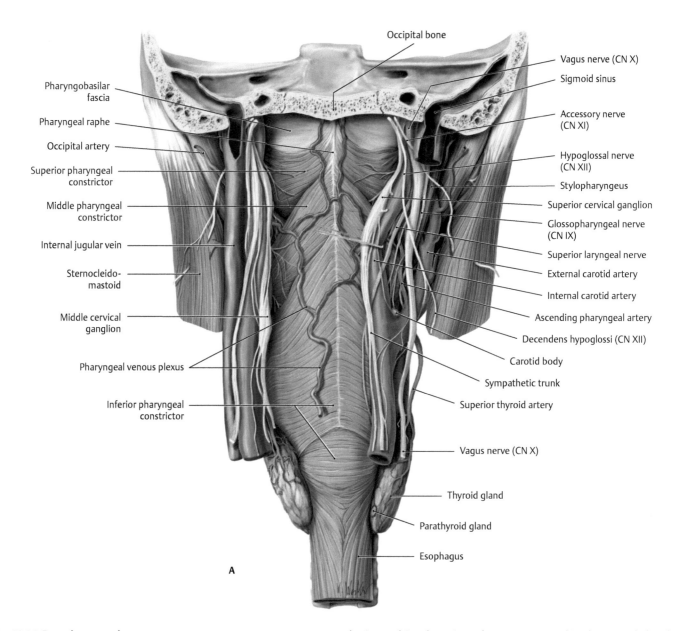

Occipital bone

Vagus nerve (CN X)

Sigmoid sinus

Accessory nerve (CN XI)

Hypoglossal nerve (CN XII)

Stylopharyngeus

Superior cervical ganglion

Glossopharyngeal nerve (CN IX)

Superior laryngeal nerve

External carotid artery

Internal carotid artery

Ascending pharyngeal artery

Decendens hypoglossi (CN XII)

Carotid body

Sympathetic trunk

Superior thyroid artery

Vagus nerve (CN X)

Thyroid gland

Parathyroid gland

Esophagus

Pharyngobasilar fascia

Pharyngeal raphe

Occipital artery

Superior pharyngeal constrictor

Middle pharyngeal constrictor

Internal jugular vein

Sternocleido-mastoid

Middle cervical ganglion

Pharyngeal venous plexus

Inferior pharyngeal constrictor

A

Fig. 12.26 Parapharyngeal space
Posterior view. **A** *Removed:* Fascial layers. **B** Pharynx opened along pharyngeal raphe. The common and internal carotid arteries travel with the internal jugular vein and vagus nerve within the carotid sheath, which attaches to the skull base.

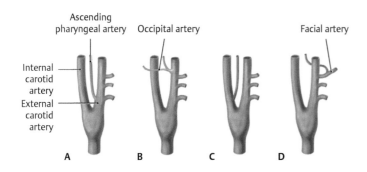

Ascending pharyngeal artery

Occipital artery

Facial artery

Internal carotid artery

External carotid artery

A   B   C   D

Fig. 12.27 Ascending pharyngeal artery: variants (after Tillmann, Lippert, and Pabst)
Left lateral view. The main arterial vessel supplying the upper and middle pharynx is the ascending pharyngeal artery. In 70% of cases (**A**) it arises from the posteroinferior surface of the external carotid artery. In approximately 20% of cases it arises from the occipital artery (**B**). Occasionally (8%) it originates from the internal carotid artery or carotid bifurcation (**C**), and in 2% of cases it arises from the facial artery (**D**).

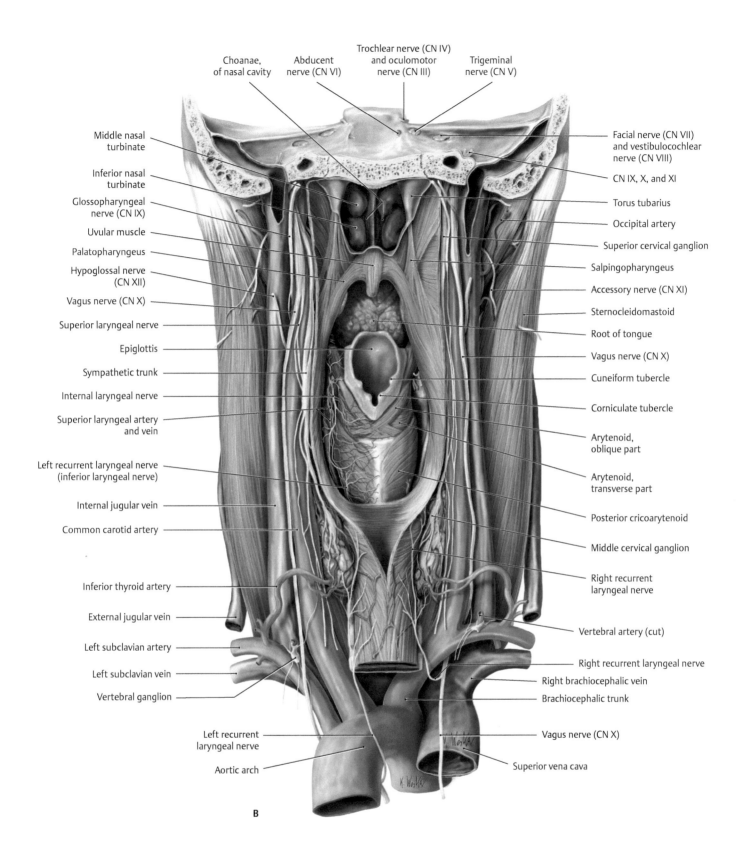

Middle nasal turbinate

Inferior nasal turbinate

Glossopharyngeal nerve (CN IX)

Uvular muscle

Palatopharyngeus

Hypoglossal nerve (CN XII)

Vagus nerve (CN X)

Superior laryngeal nerve

Epiglottis

Sympathetic trunk

Internal laryngeal nerve

Superior laryngeal artery and vein

Left recurrent laryngeal nerve (inferior laryngeal nerve)

Internal jugular vein

Common carotid artery

Inferior thyroid artery

External jugular vein

Left subclavian artery

Left subclavian vein

Vertebral ganglion

Left recurrent laryngeal nerve

Aortic arch

Choanae, of nasal cavity

Abducent nerve (CN VI)

Trochlear nerve (CN IV) and oculomotor nerve (CN III)

Trigeminal nerve (CN V)

Facial nerve (CN VII) and vestibulocochlear nerve (CN VIII)

CN IX, X, and XI

Torus tubarius

Occipital artery

Superior cervical ganglion

Salpingopharyngeus

Accessory nerve (CN XI)

Sternocleidomastoid

Root of tongue

Vagus nerve (CN X)

Cuneiform tubercle

Corniculate tubercle

Arytenoid, oblique part

Arytenoid, transverse part

Posterior cricoarytenoid

Middle cervical ganglion

Right recurrent laryngeal nerve

Vertebral artery (cut)

Right recurrent laryngeal nerve

Right brachiocephalic vein

Brachiocephalic trunk

Vagus nerve (CN X)

Superior vena cava

B

Peripharyngeal Space (II)

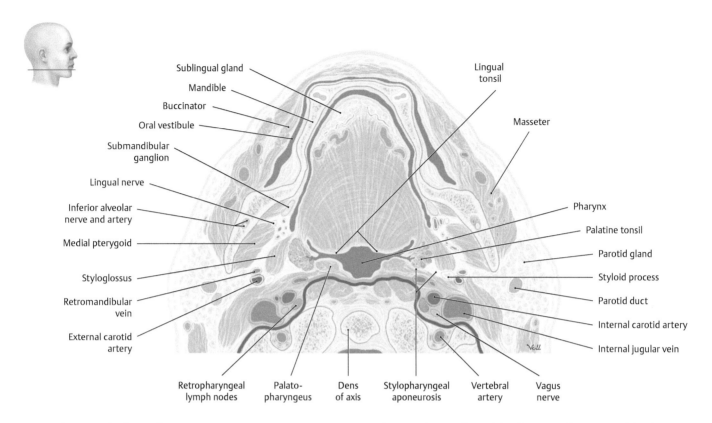

Fig. 12.28 Spaces in the neck

Transverse section, superior view. The pharynx, larynx, and thyroid gland are enclosed by the pretracheal fascia. The posterior portion of the pretracheal fascia that is in direct contact with the pharynx is called the buccopharyngeal fascia. The fascial space surrounding the pharynx (peripharyngeal space) is divided into a posterior (retropharyngeal) space and a lateral (parapharyngeal) space. The retro-

pharyngeal space (green) lies between the anterior (alar) layer of the prevertebral fascia (red) and the buccopharyngeal fascia, the posterior portion of the pretracheal fascia. The parapharyngeal space is divided by the stylopharyngeal aponeurosis into an anterior and a posterior part. The anterior part (yellow) is contained within the pretracheal fascia in the neck (this section is through the oral cavity). The posterior part (orange) is contained within the carotid sheath.

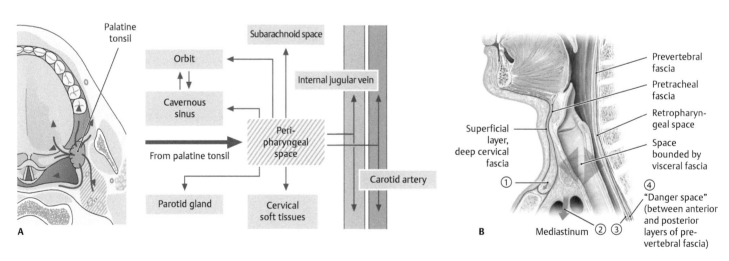

Fig. 12.29 Role of the peripharyngeal space in the spread of infection (after Becker, Naumann, and Pfaltz)

Bacteria and inflammatory processes from the oral and nasal cavities (e.g., tonsillitis, dental infections) may invade the peripharyngeal space. From there, they may spread in various directions (**A**). Invasion of the internal jugular vein may lead to bacteremia and sepsis. Invasion of the subarachnoid space poses a risk of meningitis. Inflammatory processes may also track downward into the mediastinum (gravita-

tion abscess), causing mediastinitus (**B**). These may spread anteriorly in the spaces between the superficial layer of the deep cervical fascia and muscular pretracheal fascia ① or in the space within the pretracheal fascia ②. They may also spread posteriorly in the retropharyngeal space ③ between the buccopharyngeal anterior fascia and the (alar) layer of the prevertebral fascia. Infections that enter the "danger space" ④ between the anterior and posterior layers of the prevertebral fascia may spread directly into the mediastinum.

354

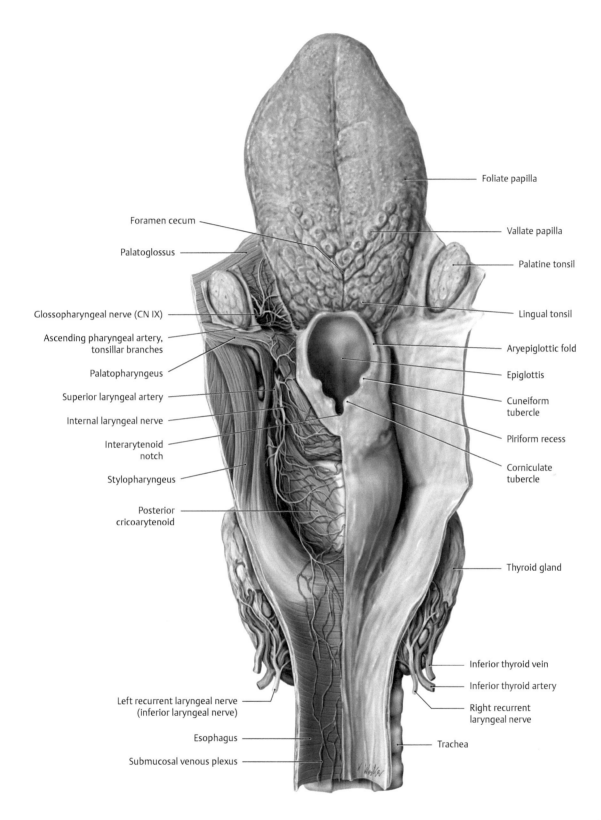

Foliate papilla

Foramen cecum

Vallate papilla

Palatoglossus

Palatine tonsil

Glossopharyngeal nerve (CN IX)

Lingual tonsil

Ascending pharyngeal artery, tonsillar branches

Aryepiglottic fold

Palatopharyngeus

Epiglottis

Superior laryngeal artery

Cuneiform tubercle

Internal laryngeal nerve

Interarytenoid notch

Piriform recess

Stylopharyngeus

Corniculate tubercle

Posterior cricoarytenoid

Thyroid gland

Inferior thyroid vein

Inferior thyroid artery

Left recurrent laryngeal nerve (inferior laryngeal nerve)

Right recurrent laryngeal nerve

Esophagus

Trachea

Submucosal venous plexus

Fig. 12.30 Neurovascular structures of the peripharyngeal space
Posterior view of an en bloc specimen composed of the tongue, larynx, esophagus, and thyroid gland, as it would be resected at autopsy for pathologic evaluation of the neck. This dissection clearly demonstrates the branching pattern of the neurovascular structures that occupy the plane between the pharyngeal muscles.

Note the vascular supply to the palatine tonsil and its proximity to the neurovascular bundle, which creates a risk of hemorrhage during tonsillectomy.

Radiographs of the Neurovascular Topography of the Neck

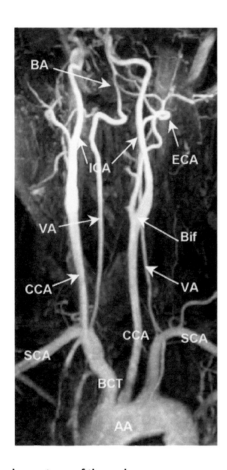

A

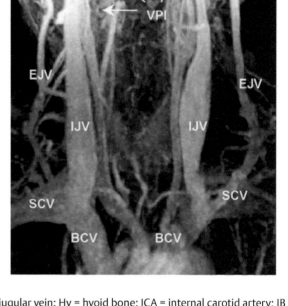

B

Fig. 12.31 Vascular anatomy of the neck
A MR angiography, coronal projection.
B MR phlebography, coronal projection.
C 3D reconstruction of cervical vessels from a CT volumetric data set obtained after administration of contrast material.

AA = aortic arch; BA = basilar artery; BCT = brachiocephalic trunk; BCV = brachiocephalic vein; Bif = carotid bifurcation; CCA = common carotid artery; Cl = clavicle; ECA = external carotid artery; EJV = external jugular vein; Hy = hyoid bone; ICA = internal carotid artery; JB = jugular bulb; M = manubrium; OV = occipital vein; S = scapula; SCA = subclavian artery; SCV = subclavian vein; SiS = sigmoid sinus; Thy = thyroid cartilage (ossified portions); VA = vertebral artery; VPl = vertebral venous plexus. (Source: Becker M. Anatomy. In: Valvassori G, Mafee M, Becker M, ed. Imaging of the Head and Neck. 2nd edition. Stuttgart: Thieme; 2004.)

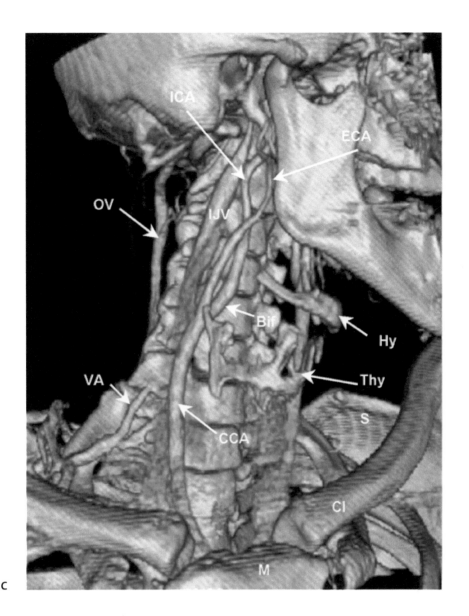

c

Larynx

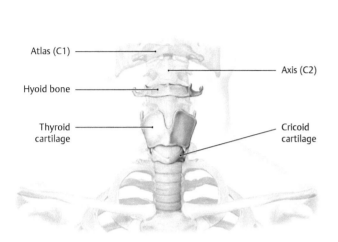

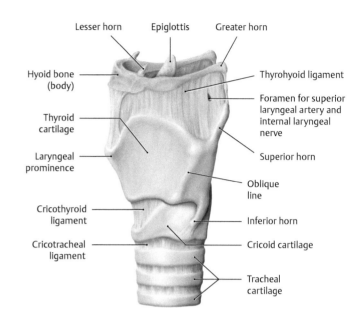

Fig. 13.1 Location of the larynx
Anterior view. The bony structures of the neck have characteristic vertebral levels (shown for upright adult male):

- Hyoid bone: C3
- Thyroid cartilage (superior border): C4
- Laryngotracheal junction: C6–C7

These structures are a half vertebra higher in women and children. The thyroid cartilage is especially prominent in males, forming the laryngeal prominence ("Adam's apple").

Fig. 13.2 Larynx: overview
Oblique left anterolateral view. The larynx consists of five cartilages: two external cartilages (thyroid and cricoid) and three internal cartilages (epiglottic, arytenoid, and corniculate). Elastic ligaments connect these cartilages to each other as well as to the trachea and hyoid bone. This allows laryngeal motion during swallowing. The thyroid, cricoid, and arytenoid cartilages are hyaline, and the epiglottis and corniculate cartilages are elastic cartilage.

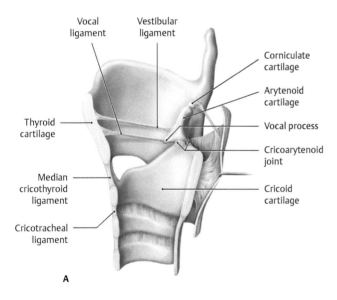

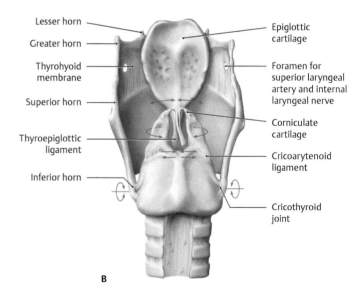

Fig. 13.3 Laryngeal cartilages and ligaments
A Left medial view of sagittal section. **B** Posterior view. Arrows indicate movement in the various joints.
The large thyroid cartilage encloses most of the other cartilages. It articulates with the cricoid cartilage inferiorly at the paired crico-

thyroid joints, allowing it to tilt relative to the cricoid cartilage. The arytenoid cartilages move during phonation: their bases can translate or rotate relative to the cricoid cartilage at the cricoarytenoid joint.

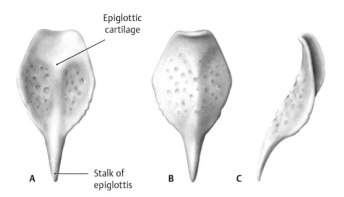

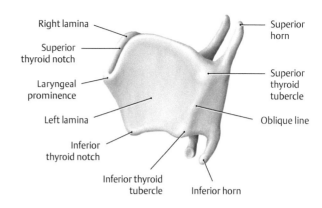

Fig. 13.4 Epiglottic cartilage
A Laryngeal (posteroinferior) view. **B** Lingual (anterosuperior) view. **C** Left lateral view.
The elastic epiglottic cartilage regulates the entrance of material into the larynx. During breathing, it is angled posterosuperiorly, allowing air to enter the larynx and trachea. During swallowing, the larynx is elevated relative to the hyoid bone. The epiglottis assumes a more horizontal position, preventing food from entering the airway.

Fig. 13.5 Thyroid cartilage
Oblique left lateral view. The hyaline thyroid cartilage consists of two quadrilateral plates (laminae) that are joined at the anterior midline. The superior portion of this junction is the laryngeal prominence ("Adam's apple"). The posterior ends of the laminae are prolonged forming the superior and inferior horns, which serve as anchors for ligaments.

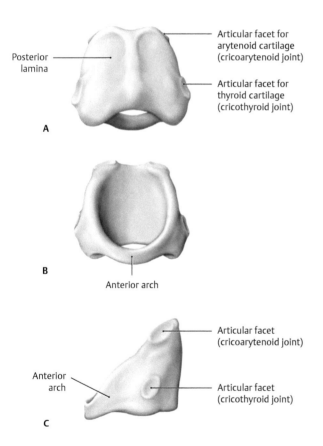

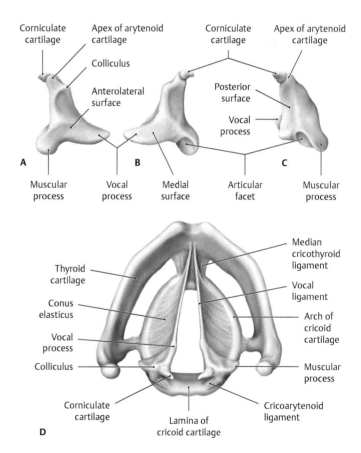

Fig. 13.6 Cricoid cartilage
A Posterior view. **B** Anterior view. **C** Left lateral view. The hyaline cricoid cartilage is a ring that is connected inferiorly to the highest tracheal cartilage by the cricotracheal ligament. The cricoid ring is expanded posteriorly to form a lamina. The laminae each have an upper and lower articular facet for the arytenoid cartilage (cricoarytenoid joint) and thyroid cartilage (cricothyroid joint), respectively.

Fig. 13.7 Arytenoid and corniculate cartilages
Right cartilages. **A** Right lateral view. **B** Left lateral (medial) view. **C** Posterior view. **D** Superior view.
The arytenoid cartilages alter the positions of the vocal cords during phonation. The pyramid shaped hyaline cartilages have three surfaces (anterolateral, medial, and posterior), an apex, and a base with vocal and muscular processes. The apex articulates with the tiny corniculate cartilages, which are composed of elastic cartilage.

Laryngeal Muscles

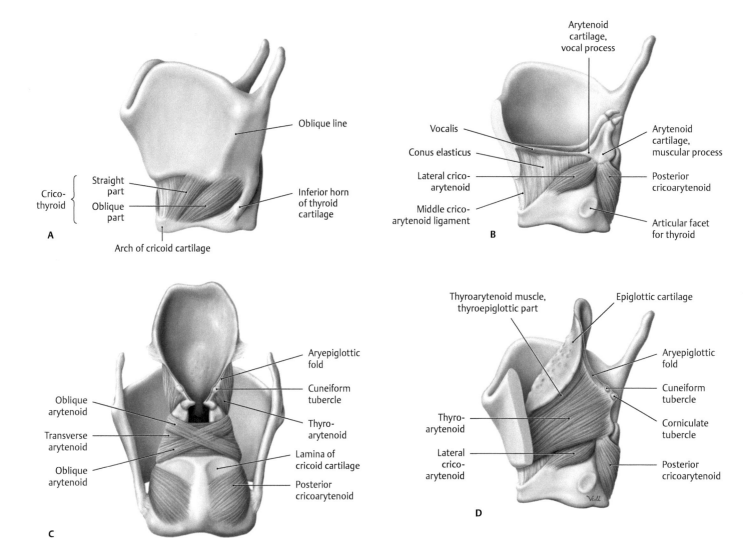

A — Crico-thyroid: Straight part, Oblique part — Oblique line — Inferior horn of thyroid cartilage — Arch of cricoid cartilage

B — Vocalis — Conus elasticus — Lateral crico-arytenoid — Middle crico-arytenoid ligament — Arytenoid cartilage, vocal process — Arytenoid cartilage, muscular process — Posterior cricoarytenoid — Articular facet for thyroid

C — Oblique arytenoid — Transverse arytenoid — Oblique arytenoid — Aryepiglottic fold — Cuneiform tubercle — Thyro-arytenoid — Lamina of cricoid cartilage — Posterior cricoarytenoid

D — Thyroarytenoid muscle, thyroepiglottic part — Thyro-arytenoid — Lateral crico-arytenoid — Epiglottic cartilage — Aryepiglottic fold — Cuneiform tubercle — Corniculate tubercle — Posterior cricoarytenoid

Table 13.1 Laryngeal muscles

The laryngeal muscles move the laryngeal cartilages relative to one another and affect the tension and/or position of the vocal folds. Numerous muscles move the larynx as a whole (infrahyoids, suprahyoids, pharyngeal constrictors, stylopharyngeus, etc.).

Muscle	Innervation	Action	Vocal folds	Rima glottidis
Posterior cricoarytenoid	Recurrent laryngeal n.**	Rotates arytenoid cartilage outward and slightly to the side	Abducts	Opens
Lateral cricoarytenoid*		Rotates arytenoid cartilage inward	Adducts	Closes
Transverse arytenoid		Moves arytenoids toward each other		
Thyroarytenoid		Rotates arytenoid cartilage inward	Relaxes	Closes
Vocalis***		Regulates tension of vocal folds	Relaxes	None
Cricothyroid	External laryngeal n.	Tilts cricoid cartilage forward, acting on the vocalis muscle to increase tension in the vocal folds	Lengthens	None

*The lateral cricoarytenoid is called the muscle of phonation as it initiates speech production.

**Unilateral loss of the recurrent laryngeal nerve (e.g., due to nodal metastases from a hilar bronchial carcinoma of the left lung) leads to ipsilateral palsy of the posterior cricoarytenoid. This prevents complete abduction of the vocal folds, causing hoarseness. Bilateral nerve loss (e.g., due to thyroid surgery) may cause asphyxiation.

***The vocalis is derived from the inferior fibers of the thyroarytenoid muscle. These fibers connect the arytenoid cartilage with the vocal ligament.

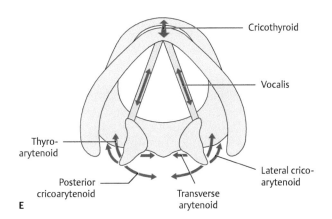

E

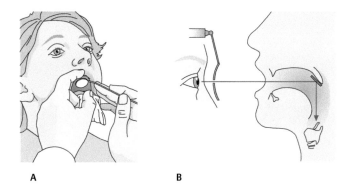

A   B

Fig. 13.8 Laryngeal muscles

A Left lateral oblique view of extrinsic laryngeal muscles. **B** Left lateral view of intrinsic laryngeal muscles (left thyroid lamina and epiglottis removed). **C** Posterior view. **D** Left lateral view. **E** Actions (arrows indicate directions of pull).

Fig. 13.9 Indirect laryngoscopy technique

A **Mirror examination of the larynx** from the perspective of the examiner. The larynx is not accessible to direct inspection but can be viewed with the aid of a small mirror. The examiner depresses the tongue with one hand while introducing the laryngeal mirror (or endoscope) with the other hand.

A Optical path: The laryngeal mirror is held in front of the uvula, directing light from the examiner's head mirror down toward the larynx. The image seen by the examiner is shown in **Fig. 13.10**.

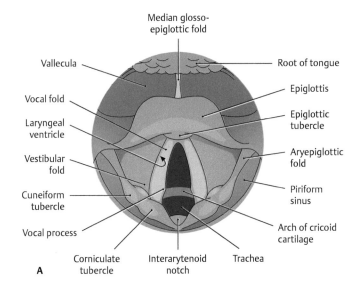

A

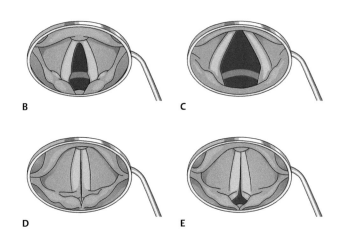

B   C

D   E

Fig. 13.10 Indirect laryngoscopy and vocal fold position

A Laryngoscopic mirror image. **B** Normal respiration. **C** Vigorous respiration. **D** Phonation position (vocal folds completely adducted). **E** Whispered speech (vocal folds slightly abducted).

Indirect laryngoscopy produces a virtual image of the larynx in which the right vocal fold appears on the right side of the mirror image and anterior structures (e.g., tongue base, valleculae, and epiglottis) appear at the top of the image. The vocal folds appear as smooth-edged bands (there are no blood vessels or submucosa below the stratified, nonkeratinized squamous epithelium of the vocal folds). They are therefore markedly lighter than the highly vascularized surrounding mucosa. The glottis can be evaluated in closed (respiratory) and opened (phonation) position by having the patient alternately inhale and sing "hee." The clinician can then determine pathoanatomical changes (e.g., redness, swelling, and ulceration) and functional changes (e.g., to vocal fold position).

Larynx: Neurovasculature

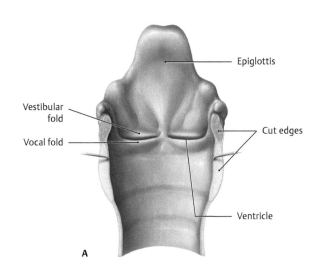

A

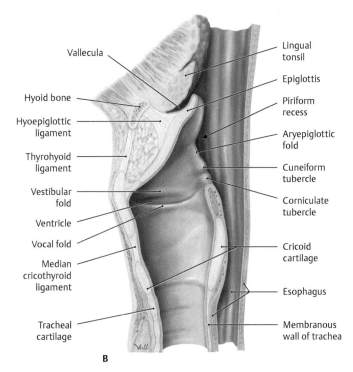

B

Fig. 13.11 Laryngeal mucosa

A Posterior view with pharynx and esophagus cut along the midline and spread open. **B** Left lateral view of midsagittal section. **C** Posterior view with laryngeal levels.

The larynx lies anterior to the laryngopharynx. Air enters through the laryngeal inlet formed by the epiglottis and aryepiglottic folds. Lateral to the aryepiglottic folds are pear-shaped mucosal fossae (piriform recesses), which channel food past the larynx and into the laryngopharynx and on into the esophagus. The interior of the larynx is lined with mucous membrane that is loosely applied to its underlying tissue (except at the vocal folds). The laryngeal cavity can be further subdivided with respect to the vestibular and vocal folds (**Table 13.2**).

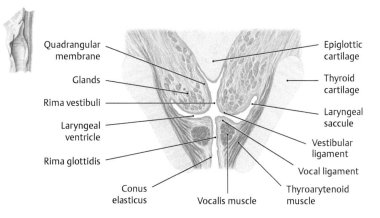

Fig. 13.12 Vestibular and vocal folds

Coronal histologic section. The vestibular and vocal folds are the mucosal coverings of underlying ligaments. The vocal folds ("vocal cords") contain the vocal ligament and vocalis muscle. The fissure between the vocal folds is the rima glottidis (glottis). The vestibular folds ("false vocal cords") are superior to the vocal folds. They contain the vestibular ligament, the free inferior end of the quadrangular membrane. The fissure between the vestibular folds is the rima vestibuli, which is broader than the rima glottidis. *Note:* The loose connective tissue of the laryngeal inlet may become markedly swollen (e.g., insect bite, inflammatory process), obstructing the rima vestibuli. This laryngeal edema (often incorrectly called "glottic edema") presents clinically with dyspnea and poses an asphyxiation risk.

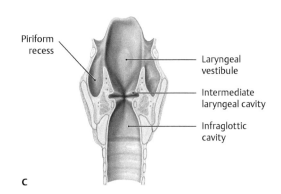

C

Table 13.2 Divisions of the laryngeal cavity

Laryngeal level	Boundaries
I: Laryngeal vestibule (supraglottic space)	Laryngeal inlet (aditus laryngis) to vestibular folds
II: Intermediate laryngeal cavity (transglottic space)	Vestibular folds across the laryngeal ventricle (lateral evagination of mucosa) to vocal folds
III: Infraglottic cavity (subglottic space)	Vocal folds to inferior border of cricoid cartilage

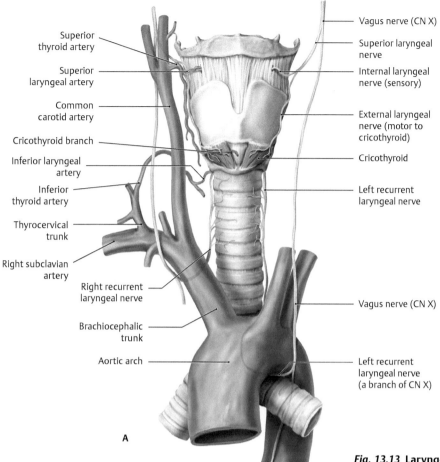

Superior thyroid artery

Superior laryngeal artery

Common carotid artery

Cricothyroid branch

Inferior laryngeal artery

Inferior thyroid artery

Thyrocervical trunk

Right subclavian artery

Right recurrent laryngeal nerve

Brachiocephalic trunk

Aortic arch

Vagus nerve (CN X)

Superior laryngeal nerve

Internal laryngeal nerve (sensory)

External laryngeal nerve (motor to cricothyroid)

Cricothyroid

Left recurrent laryngeal nerve

Vagus nerve (CN X)

Left recurrent laryngeal nerve (a branch of CN X)

A

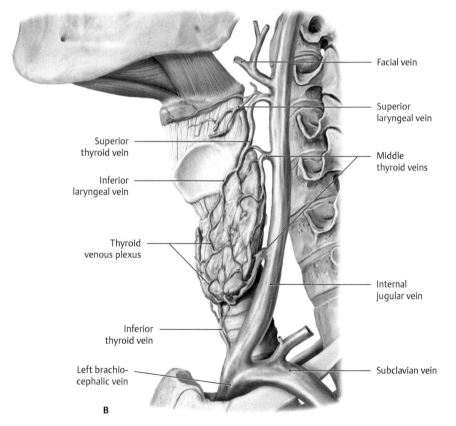

Superior thyroid vein

Inferior laryngeal vein

Thyroid venous plexus

Inferior thyroid vein

Left brachio-cephalic vein

Facial vein

Superior laryngeal vein

Middle thyroid veins

Internal jugular vein

Subclavian vein

B

Fig. 13.13 Laryngeal blood vessels and nerves

A Arteries and nerves, anterior view. **B** Veins, left lateral view.

Arteries: The larynx derives its blood supply primarily from the superior and inferior laryngeal arteries. The superior laryngeal artery arises from the superior thyroid artery (a branch of the external carotid artery). The inferior laryngeal artery arises from the inferior thyroid artery (a branch of the thyrocervical trunk).

Nerves: The larynx is innervated by the superior laryngeal nerve and the recurrent laryngeal nerve (of the vagus nerve). The superior laryngeal nerve splits into an internal (sensory) and an external (motor) laryngeal nerve. The external laryngeal nerve innervates the cricothyroid. The remaining intrinsic laryngeal muscles receive motor innervation from the recurrent laryngeal nerve, which branches from the vagus nerve below the larynx and ascends. *Note:* The left recurrent laryngeal nerve wraps around the aortic arch, and the right recurrent laryngeal nerve wraps around the subclavian artery. A left-sided aortic aneurysm may cause left recurrent laryngeal nerve palsy, resulting in hoarseness (see p. 353).

Veins: The larynx is drained by a superior and an inferior laryngeal vein. The superior laryngeal vein drains to the internal jugular vein (via the superior thyroid vein); the inferior laryngeal vein drains to the left brachiocephalic vein (via the thyroid venous plexus to the inferior thyroid vein).

363

Larynx: Topography

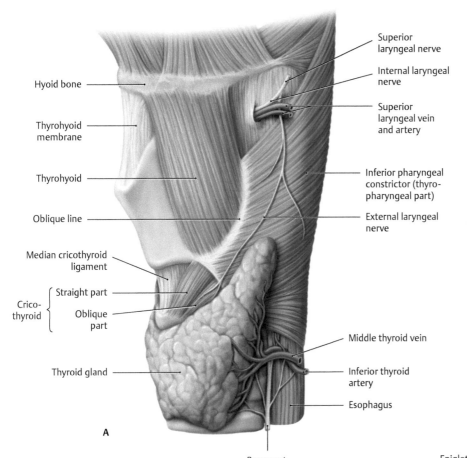

Superior laryngeal nerve

Internal laryngeal nerve

Superior laryngeal vein and artery

Hyoid bone

Thyrohyoid membrane

Thyrohyoid

Inferior pharyngeal constrictor (thyropharyngeal part)

Oblique line

External laryngeal nerve

Median cricothyroid ligament

Cricothyroid — Straight part / Oblique part

Middle thyroid vein

Thyroid gland

Inferior thyroid artery

Esophagus

A

Recurrent laryngeal nerve

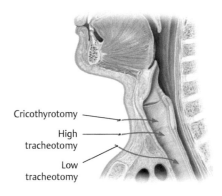

Cricothyrotomy

High tracheotomy

Low tracheotomy

Fig. 13.15 Approaches to the larynx and trachea
Midsagittal section, left lateral view. When an acute edematous obstruction of the larynx (e. g., due to an allergic reaction) poses an acute risk of asphyxiation, the following surgical approaches are available for creating an emergency airway:

- Division of the median cricothyroid ligament (cricothyrotomy)
- Incision of the trachea (tracheotomy) at a level just below the cricoid cartilage (high tracheotomy) or just superior to the jugular notch (low tracheotomy).

Fig. 13.14 Topography of the larynx
Left lateral view. **A** Superficial dissection. **B** Deep dissection (cricothyroid and left thyroid lamina removed with pharyngeal mucosa retracted).
Neurovascular structures enter the larynx posteriorly. The larynx receives sensory and motor innervation from branches of the vagus nerve (CN X).
Sensory innervation: The upper larynx (above the vocal folds) receives sensory innervation from the internal laryngeal nerve, and the infraglottic cavity receives sensory innervation from the recurrent laryngeal nerve.
Motor innervation: The cricothyroid receives motor innervation from the external laryngeal nerve, and the rest of the intrinsic muscles of the larynx receive motor innervation from the recurrent laryngeal nerve.

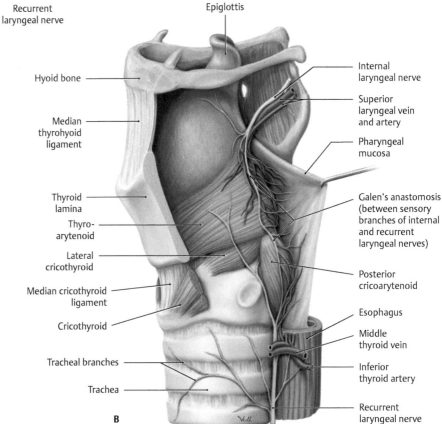

Epiglottis

Internal laryngeal nerve

Superior laryngeal vein and artery

Pharyngeal mucosa

Hyoid bone

Median thyrohyoid ligament

Thyroid lamina

Thyroarytenoid

Lateral cricothyroid

Median cricothyroid ligament

Cricothyroid

Galen's anastomosis (between sensory branches of internal and recurrent laryngeal nerves)

Posterior cricoarytenoid

Esophagus

Middle thyroid vein

Inferior thyroid artery

Tracheal branches

Trachea

B

Recurrent laryngeal nerve

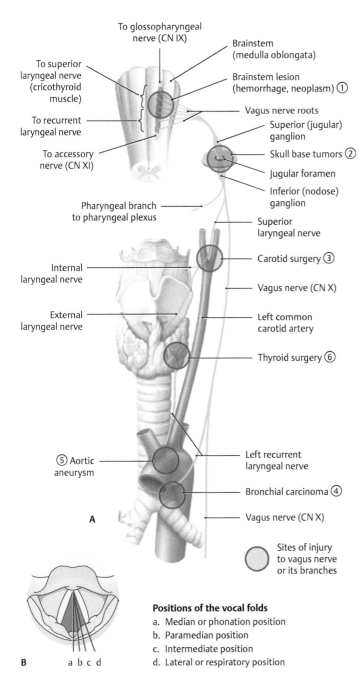

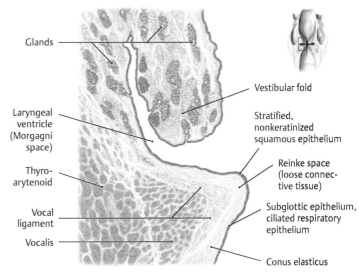

Fig. 13.16 Vagus nerve lesions
The vagus nerve (CN X) provides branchiomotor innervation to the pharyngeal and laryngeal muscles and somatic sensory innervation to the larynx. *Note:* The vagus nerve also conveys parasympathetic motor fibers and visceral sensory fibers to and from the thoracic and abdominal viscera.
Branchiomotor innervation: The nucleus ambiguus contains the cell bodies of lower motor neurons whose branchiomotor fibers travel in CN IX, X, and XI. The nuclei of the vagus nerve are located in the middle region of the nucleus ambiguus in the brainstem (the cranial portions of the nucleus send axons via the glossopharyngeal nerve, and the caudal portions send axons via the accessory nerve). Fibers emerge from the middle portion of the nucleus ambiguus as roots and combine into CN X, which passes through the jugular foramen. Branchiomotor fibers are distributed to the pharyngeal plexus via the pharyngeal branch and the cricothyroid muscle via the external laryngeal nerve (a branch of the superior laryngeal nerve). The remaining branchiomotor fibers leave the vagus nerve as the recurrent laryngeal nerves, which ascend along the trachea to reach the larynx.
Sensory innervation: General somatic sensory fibers travel from the laryngeal mucosa to the spinal nucleus of the trigeminal nerve via the vagus nerve. The cell bodies of these primary sensory neurons are located in the inferior (nodose) ganglion. *Note:* The superior (jugular) ganglion contains the cell bodies of viscerosensory neurons.

Fig. 13.17 Vocal folds
Schematic coronal histologic section, posterior view. The vocal fold, which is exposed to severe mechanical stresses, is covered by nonkeratinized squamous epithelium, unlike the adjacent subglottic space, which is covered by ciliated respiratory epithelium. The mucosa of the vocal folds and subglottic space overlies loose connective tissue. Chronic irritation of the subglottic mucosa (e.g., from cigarette smoke) may cause chronic edema in the subglottic space, resulting in a harsh voice. Degenerative changes in the vocal fold mucosa may lead to thickening, loss of elasticity, and squamous cell carcinoma.

Table 13.3 Vagus nerve lesions

Lesions of the laryngeal nerves (**Fig. 13.16A**) may cause sensory loss or motor paralysis, which disrupts the position of the vocal folds (**Fig. 13.16B**).

Level of nerve lesion and effects on vocal fold position		Sensory loss
① Central lesion (brainstem or higher)*		
E.g., due to tumor or hemorrhage. Spastic paralysis (if nucleus ambiguus is disrupted), flaccid paralysis, and muscle atrophy (if motor neurons or axons are destroyed).	b,c	None
② Skull base lesion*		
E.g., due to nasopharyngeal tumors. Flaccid paralysis of all intrinsic and extrinsic laryngeal muscles on affected side. Glottis cannot be closed, causing severe hoarseness.	b,c	Entire affected (ipsilateral) side
③ Superior laryngeal nerve lesions		
E.g., due to carotid surgery. Hypotonicity of the cricothyroid, resulting in mild hoarseness with a weak voice, especially at high frequencies.	d	Above vocal fold
④, ⑤, ⑥ Recurrent laryngeal nerve lesions**		
E.g., due to bronchial carcinoma ④, aortic aneurysm ⑤, or thyroid surgery ⑥. Paralysis of all intrinsic laryngeal muscles on affected side. This results in mild hoarseness, poor tonal control, rapid voice fatigue, but not dyspnea.	a,b	Below vocal fold

*Other motor deficits include drooping of the soft palate and deviation of the uvula toward the affected side, diminished gag and cough reflexes, difficulty swallowing (dysphagia), and hypernasal speech due to deficient closure of the pharyngeal isthmus. Sensory defects include the sensation of a foreign body in the throat.

**Transection of both recurrent laryngeal nerves can cause significant dyspnea and inspiratory stridor (high-pitched noise indicating obstruction), necessitating tracheotomy in acute cases.

Endotracheal Intubation

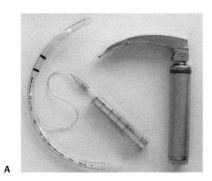

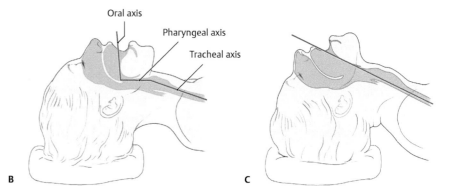

Fig. 13.18 Equipment and positioning of the head for endotracheal intubation

A Endotracheal (ET) tube with an inflatable cuff (left) and laryngoscope with handle and curved spatula (right).

B, C Unfavorable and optimal positioning of the head for endotracheal intubation.

Endotracheal intubation, inserting a tube into the trachea of a patient, is the safest way to keep the airways clear to allow for effective ventilation. Depending on access there are four ways to achieve endotracheal intubation:

- orotracheal = via the mouth (gold standard),
- nasotracheal = via the nose (performed if orotracheal intubation is not possible), and
- pertracheal = intubation through tracheostomy (used for longterm ventilation), and
- cricothyrotomy (used only in an emergencies when there is the threat of impending suffocation).

Endotracheal intubation requires the use of a laryngoscope and an ET tube **(A)**. The tubes are available in different sizes (10–22 cm) and diameters (2.5–8 mm). They have a circular cross piece that has a proximal connector for a ventilation hose and a beveled distal end. An inflatable cuff on the ET ensures that the trachea is hermetically sealed (see **Fig. 13.20**). With orotracheal intubation, the oral, pharyngeal, and tracheal axes should lie on a straight line (the so-called "sniffing position", see **C**).This facilitates direct visualization of the laryngeal inlet (see **Fig. 13.19**) and shortens the distance between the teeth and glottis in young adults (13–16 cm).

Note: In patients with suspected cervical spine injury, manipulation of the head position without maintaining the stability of the cervical spine is contraindicated.

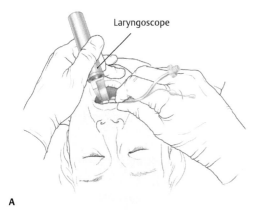

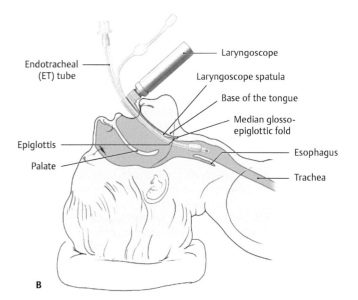

Fig. 13.19 Placement of the laryngoscope and the endotracheal tube (ET)

A Handling and placement of the laryngoscope from the perspective of the physician. **B** Placement of the ET tube.

To place the ET tube, the physician stands at the head of the patient and introduces the spatula of the laryngoscope into the patient's mouth. The spatula is then used to push the patient's tongue to the left to get a clear view of the larynx.

Under direct visualization, the spatula tip is then advanced until its lies in the vallecula. Note: If the spatula is introduced too deep, its tip reaches behind the epiglottis, and orientation is difficult.

The physician then pulls the spatula in the direction of floor of mouth without using the upper teeth as a fulcrum. This elevates the epiglottis and the base of the tongue such that the physician now has an unobstructed view of the laryngeal inlet (see **Fig. 13.20A**). The physician

then pushes the ET tube through the rima glottidis into the trachea (see **Fig. 13.20B**). Placement under laryngoscopic control ensures that the ET tube is placed in the trachea and does not accidentally enter the esophagus.

Note: The ET tube has markings in centimeter increments that serve as an orientation aid to the physician. The distance from the upper teeth to the center of the trachea in the adult is about 22 cm and in newborns is about 11 cm. Distances greater than these might indicate that the tube is inserted too deeply and is in the right main bronchus.

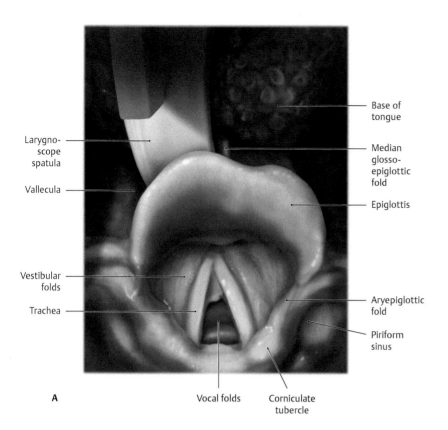

Laryngoscope spatula

Vallecula

Vestibular folds

Trachea

Base of tongue

Median glosso-epiglottic fold

Epiglottis

Aryepiglottic fold

Piriform sinus

A

Vocal folds

Corniculate tubercle

Fig. 13.20 View of the laryngeal inlet and location of the endotracheal tube after intubation

A Laryngoscopic view of larynx, epiglottis, and median glossoepiglottic fold. **B** Median sagittal section viewed from the right of an ET tube in situ with its cuff inflated.

The inflatable cuff seals the trachea in all directions and eliminates leakage during ventilation and prevents aspiration of foreign bodies, mucus, or gastric juice.

To check if the ET tube has been placed correctly, the physician looks at the patient's chest to evaluate if chest movement is symmetrical, he auscultates for equal breath sounds over both lung fields and the absence of breath sounds over the stomach. Further indicators that the ET tube is placed correctly include vapor condensation on the inside of the ET tube with exhalation and measurement of endtidal carbon dioxide. If there is any doubt as to the positioning of the tube, it should be removed.

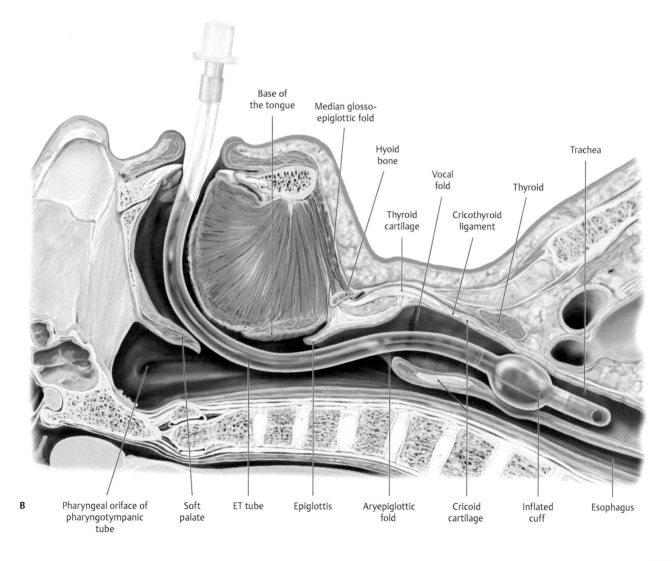

Base of the tongue

Median glosso-epiglottic fold

Hyoid bone

Vocal fold

Trachea

Thyroid

Thyroid cartilage

Cricothyroid ligament

B

Pharyngeal oriface of pharyngotympanic tube

Soft palate

ET tube

Epiglottis

Aryepiglottic fold

Cricoid cartilage

Inflated cuff

Esophagus

Thyroid & Parathyroid Glands

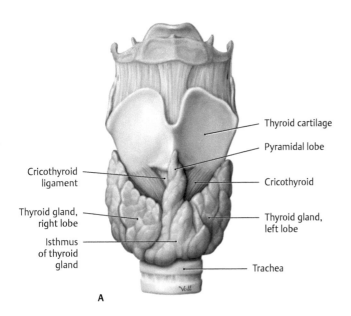

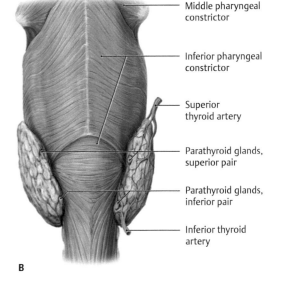

Fig. 13.21 Thyroid and parathyroid glands
A Anterior view. **B** Posterior view.
The thyroid gland consists of two laterally situated lobes and a central narrowing (isthmus). A pyramidal lobe may be found in place of the isthmus; the apex points to the embryonic origin of the thyroid at the base of the tongue (on occasion, a persistent thyroglossal duct may be present, connecting the pyramidal lobe with the foramen cecum of the tongue). The parathyroid glands (generally four in number) show considerable variation in number and location. *Note:* Because the parathyroid glands are usually contained within the thyroid capsule, there is considerable risk of inadvertently removing them during thyroid surgery. This causes decreased plasma calcium (Ca^{2+}) levels, resulting in tetany (muscle twitching and cramps). Tetany involving the laryngeal and respiratory muscles may cause dyspnea (shortness of breath), which could be fatal if untreated.

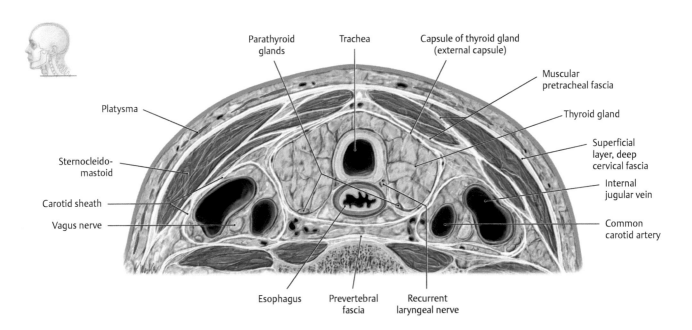

Fig. 13.22 Topography of the thyroid gland
Transverse section through the neck at the T1 level, superior view. The thyroid gland partially surrounds the trachea and is bordered posterolaterally by the carotid sheath. When the thyroid gland is pathologically enlarged (e. g., due to iodine-deficiency goiter), it may gradually compress and narrow the tracheal lumen, causing respiratory distress. The thyroid gland is surrounded by a fibrous capsule composed of an internal and external layer. The delicate internal layer (*internal capsule*, not shown here) directly invests the thyroid gland and is fused with its glandular parenchyma. Vascularized fibrous slips extend from the internal capsule into the substance of the gland, subdividing it into lobules. The internal capsule is covered by the tough *external capsule*, which is part of the pretracheal layer of the deep cervical fascia. This capsule invests the thyroid gland and parathyroid glands and is also called the "surgical capsule" because it must be opened to gain surgical access to the thyroid gland. Between the external and internal capsules is a potential space that is traversed by vascular branches and is occupied by the parathyroid glands.

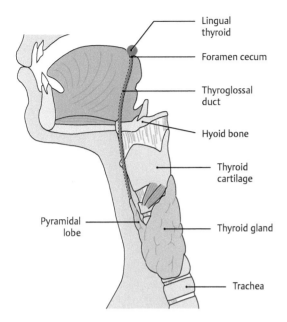

Lingual thyroid

Foramen cecum

Thyroglossal duct

Hyoid bone

Thyroid cartilage

Thyroid gland

Pyramidal lobe

Trachea

Fig. 13.23 Ectopic Thyroid Gland
Left lateral view. Ectopic thyroid is a rare condition in which the entire thyroid gland or thyroid tissues are found outwith their normal position in the neck inferolateral to the thyroid cartilage. Dentists may encounter this as a firm midline mass on the dorsal tongue, just posterior to the foramen cecum (the embryonic origin on the thyroid gland). This mass may appear as light pink to bright red, and may be regular or irregular. This is known as a lingual thyroid and represents approximately 90% of ectopic thyroid cases. Symptoms of lingual thyroid may include cough, pain, dysphagia (difficulty swallowing), dysphonia (difficulty speaking), and dyspnea (shortness of breath). Treatment involves administration of thyroxine to suppress thyroid stimulating hormone (TSH) production and therefore reduce the size of the mass. Surgical excision may be necessary if symptoms are severe, especially if they threaten the airway.

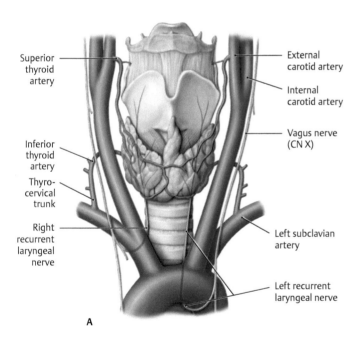

Superior thyroid artery

External carotid artery

Internal carotid artery

Vagus nerve (CN X)

Inferior thyroid artery

Thyro-cervical trunk

Right recurrent laryngeal nerve

Left subclavian artery

Left recurrent laryngeal nerve

A

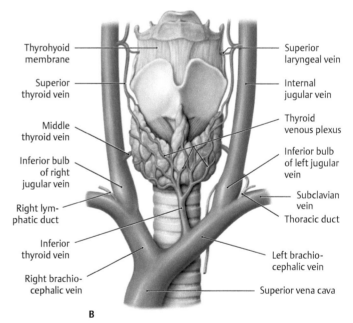

Thyrohyoid membrane

Superior thyroid vein

Middle thyroid vein

Inferior bulb of right jugular vein

Right lymphatic duct

Inferior thyroid vein

Right brachio-cephalic vein

Superior laryngeal vein

Internal jugular vein

Thyroid venous plexus

Inferior bulb of left jugular vein

Subclavian vein

Thoracic duct

Left brachio-cephalic vein

Superior vena cava

B

Fig. 13.24 Blood supply and innervation of the thyroid gland
Anterior view.

A Arterial supply: The thyroid gland derives most of its arterial blood supply from the superior and inferior thyroid arteries. The superior thyroid artery, a branch of the external carotid artery, runs forward and downward to supply the gland. It is supplied from below by the inferior thyroid artery, which branches from the thyrocervical trunk. All of these arteries, which course on the right and left sides of the organ, must be ligated during surgical removal of the thyroid gland. In addition, a rare branch, the thyroid ima, may arise from the brachiocephalic trunk or right common carotid artery to supply the gland from below. It is a potential source of bleeding when performing midline procedures on the neck, for example, a tracheostomy.

Note: Operations on the thyroid gland carry a risk of injury to the recurrent laryngeal nerve, which is closely related to the posterior surface of the gland. Because it supplies important laryngeal muscles, unilateral injury to the nerve will cause postoperative hoarseness; bilateral injury may additionally result in dyspnea (difficulty in breathing). Prior to thyroid surgery, therefore, an otolaryngologist should confirm the integrity of the nerve supply to the laryngeal muscles and exclude any preexisting nerve lesion.

B Venous drainage: The thyroid gland is drained anteroinferiorly by a well-developed *thyroid venous plexus*, which usually drains through the inferior thyroid vein to the left brachiocephalic vein. Blood from the thyroid gland also drains to the internal jugular vein via the superior and middle thyroid veins.

Radiographs of the Larynx

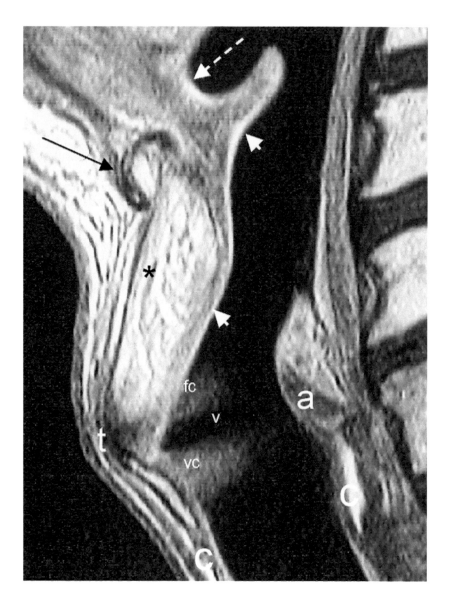

***Fig. 13.25* Normal anatomy of the preepiglottic space.**
Parasagittal, contrast-enhanced T1W MR image obtained in a healthy volunteer. Asterisk = preepiglottic space; short arrows = epiglottis; long thin arrow = hyoid bone; t = thyroid cartilage; c = cricoid cartilage; a = arytenoid cartilage; thm = thyrohyoid membrane; hepl = hyoepiglottic ligament; v = laryngeal ventricle; fc = false cord; vc = true vocal cord; dashed arrow = vallecula. (Source: Becker M. Normal Anatomy. In: Valvassori G, Mafee M, Becker M, ed. Imaging of the Head and Neck. 2nd edition. Stuttgart: Thieme; 2004.)

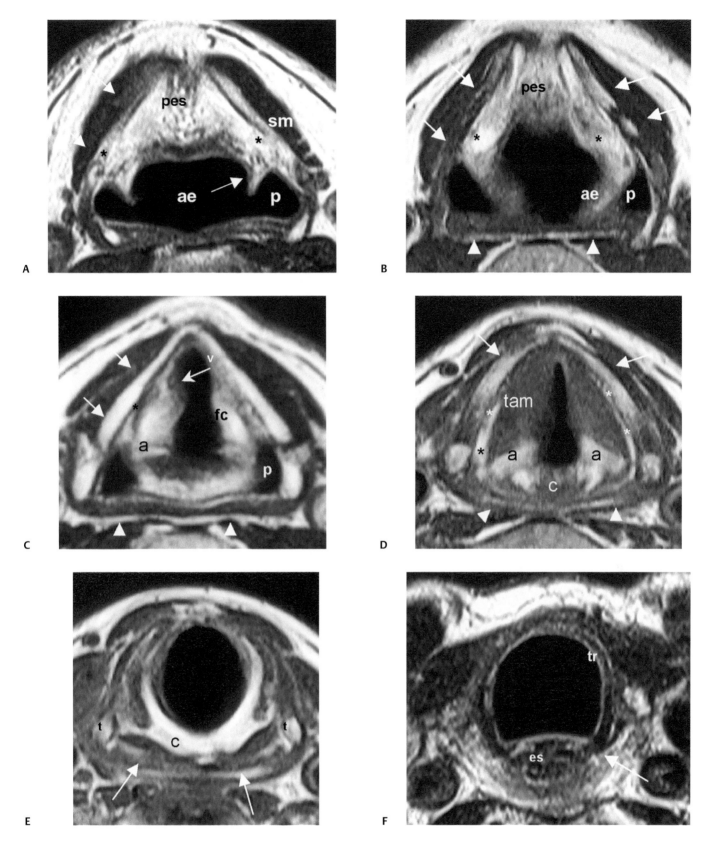

Fig. 13.26
Normal laryngeal and hypopharyngeal anatomy as seen on axial unenhanced T1W MR images.

A–C Supraglottic level. pes = preepiglottic space; asterisks = paraglottic space; ae = aryepiglottic folds; fc = false cords; v = ventricle; p = piriform sinus; arrows = thyroid cartilage; a = arytenoid cartilage; arrowheads = pharyngeal constrictor muscles; sm = strap muscles.

D Glottic level. Asterisks = paraglottic space; tam = thyroarytenoid muscle; arrows = thyroid cartilage; a = arytenoid cartilages; c = cricoid cartilage; arrowheads = pharyngeal constrictor muscles.

E Subglottic level. c = cricoid cartilage; arrows = esophageal verge; t = inferior cornu of the thyroid cartilage.
F Level of the cervical trachea (tr). es = cervical esophagus; arrow = tracheo-esophageal groove.

(Source: Becker M. Normal Anatomy. In: Valvassori G, Mafee M, Becker M, ed. Imaging of the Head and Neck. 2nd edition. Stuttgart: Thieme; 2004.)

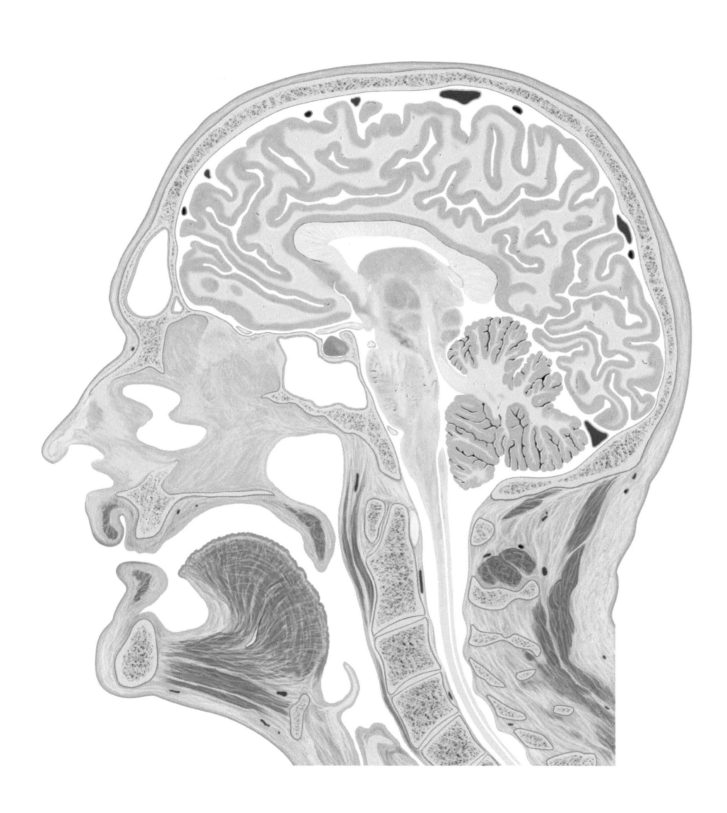

Sectional Anatomy

Coronal Sections of the Head (I): Anterior

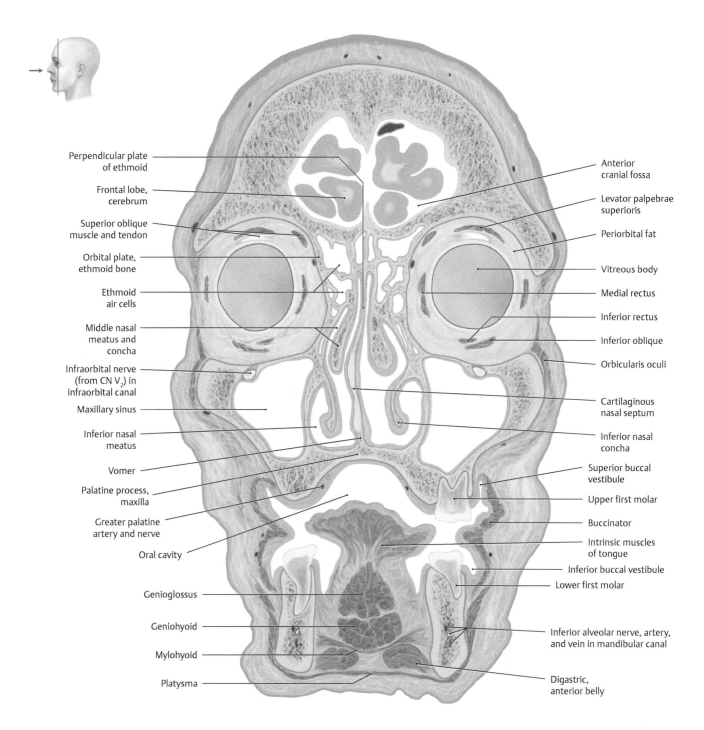

Perpendicular plate of ethmoid

Frontal lobe, cerebrum

Superior oblique muscle and tendon

Orbital plate, ethmoid bone

Ethmoid air cells

Middle nasal meatus and concha

Infraorbital nerve (from CN V₂) in infraorbital canal

Maxillary sinus

Inferior nasal meatus

Vomer

Palatine process, maxilla

Greater palatine artery and nerve

Oral cavity

Genioglossus

Geniohyoid

Mylohyoid

Platysma

Anterior cranial fossa

Levator palpebrae superioris

Periorbital fat

Vitreous body

Medial rectus

Inferior rectus

Inferior oblique

Orbicularis oculi

Cartilaginous nasal septum

Inferior nasal concha

Superior buccal vestibule

Upper first molar

Buccinator

Intrinsic muscles of tongue

Inferior buccal vestibule

Lower first molar

Inferior alveolar nerve, artery, and vein in mandibular canal

Digastric, anterior belly

Fig. 14.1 Coronal section through the anterior orbital margin
Anterior view. This section of the skull can be roughly subdivided into four regions: the oral cavity, the nasal cavity and paranasal sinuses, the orbit, and the anterior cranial fossa. Inspecting the region in and around the **oral cavity**, we observe the muscles of the oral floor, the apex of the tongue, the neurovascular structures in the mandibular canal, and the first molar. The hard palate separates the oral cavity from the **nasal cavity**, which is divided into left and right halves by the nasal septum. The inferior and middle nasal conchae can be identified along with the laterally situated maxillary sinus. Notice in **Figs. 14.2** and **14.3**, as the coronal sections progress backward through the eye, the middle concha no longer is associated with the ethmoidal air cells but instead with the maxillary sinus. The structure bulging down into the

roof of the sinus is the infraorbital canal, which transmits the infraorbital nerve (branch of the maxillary division of the trigeminal nerve, CN V₂). The plane of section is so far anterior that it does not cut the lateral bony walls of the **orbits** because of the lateral curvature of the skull. The section passes through the transparent vitreous body and four of the six extraocular muscles, which can be identified in the periorbital fat. Two additional muscles can be seen in the next deeper plane of section (**Fig. 14.2**). The space between the two orbits is occupied by the ethmoid air cells. *Note:* The bony orbital plate is very thin (lamina papyracea) and may be penetrated by infection, trauma, and neoplasms.
In the **anterior cranial fossa**, the section passes through both frontal lobes of the brain in the most anterior portions of the cerebral gray matter. Very little white matter is visible at this level.

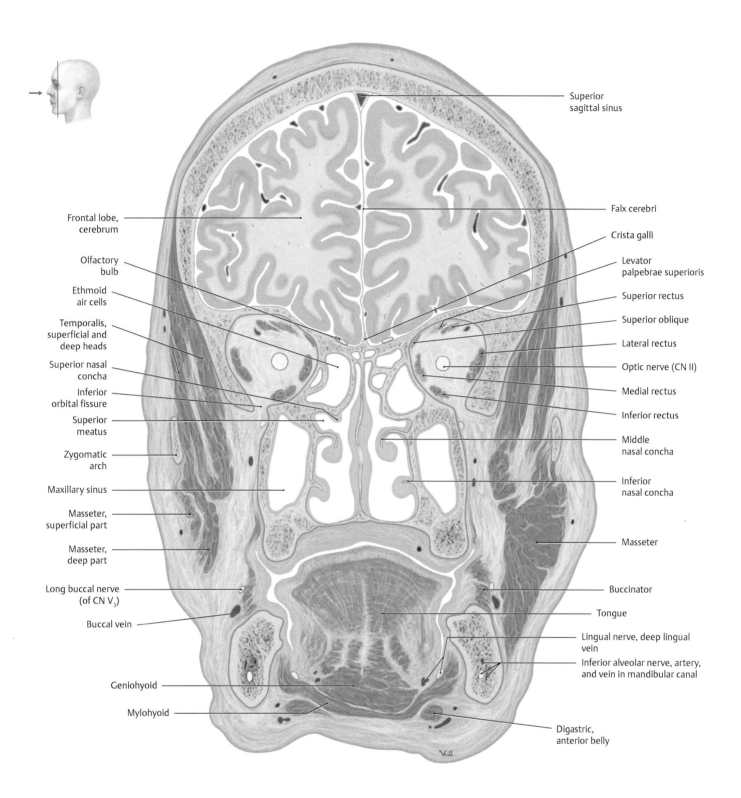

Superior
sagittal sinus

Falx cerebri

Frontal lobe,
cerebrum

Crista galli

Olfactory
bulb

Levator
palpebrae superioris

Ethmoid
air cells

Superior rectus

Temporalis,
superficial and
deep heads

Superior oblique

Lateral rectus

Superior nasal
concha

Optic nerve (CN II)

Inferior
orbital fissure

Medial rectus

Superior
meatus

Inferior rectus

Zygomatic
arch

Middle
nasal concha

Maxillary sinus

Inferior
nasal concha

Masseter,
superficial part

Masseter,
deep part

Masseter

Long buccal nerve
(of CN V₃)

Buccinator

Buccal vein

Tongue

Lingual nerve, deep lingual
vein

Inferior alveolar nerve, artery,
and vein in mandibular canal

Geniohyoid

Mylohyoid

Digastric,
anterior belly

Fig. 14.2 Coronal section through the retrobulbar space
Anterior view. Here, the tongue is cut at a more posterior level than in
Fig. 14.1 and therefore appears broader. In addition to the oral floor
muscles, we see the muscles of mastication on the sides of the skull. In
the orbital region we can identify the retrobulbar space with its fatty
tissue, the extraocular muscles, and the optic nerve. The orbit communicates laterally with the infratemporal fossa through the inferior
orbital fissure. This section cuts through both olfactory bulbs in the anterior cranial fossa, and the superior sagittal sinus can be recognized
in the midline.

375

Coronal Sections of the Head (II): Posterior

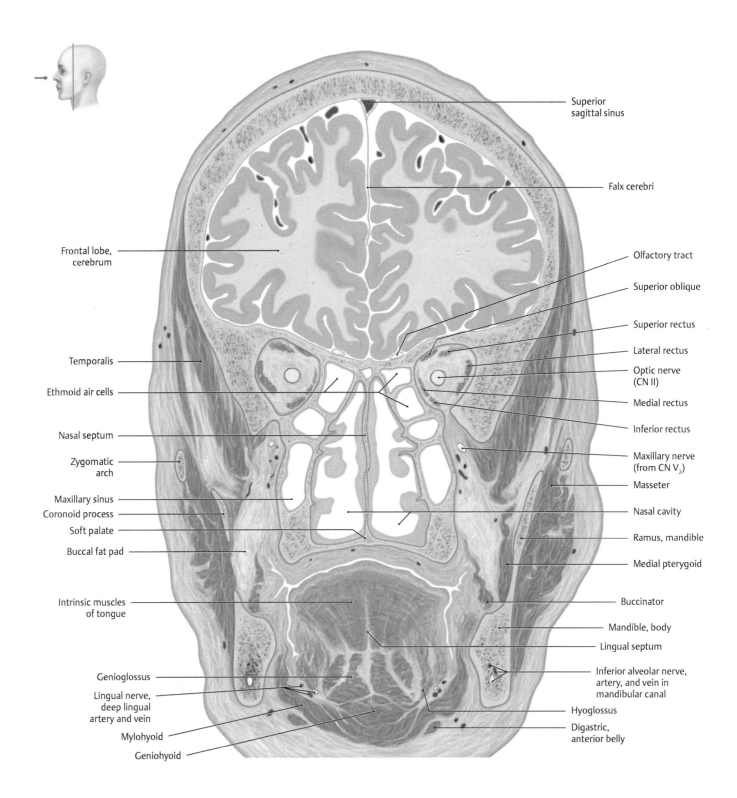

Superior sagittal sinus

Falx cerebri

Frontal lobe, cerebrum

Olfactory tract

Superior oblique

Superior rectus

Temporalis

Lateral rectus

Ethmoid air cells

Optic nerve (CN II)

Medial rectus

Nasal septum

Inferior rectus

Zygomatic arch

Maxillary nerve (from CN V₂)

Masseter

Maxillary sinus

Coronoid process

Nasal cavity

Soft palate

Buccal fat pad

Ramus, mandible

Medial pterygoid

Intrinsic muscles of tongue

Buccinator

Mandible, body

Lingual septum

Genioglossus

Inferior alveolar nerve, artery, and vein in mandibular canal

Lingual nerve, deep lingual artery and vein

Hyoglossus

Digastric, anterior belly

Mylohyoid

Geniohyoid

Fig. 14.3 Coronal section through the orbital apex
Anterior view. The soft palate replaces the hard palate in this plane of section, and the nasal septum becomes osseous at this level. The buccal fat pad is also visible in this plane. The buccal pad fat is reduced in wasting diseases; this is why the cheeks are sunken in patients with end-stage cancer. This coronal section is slightly angled, producing an apparent discontinuity in the mandibular ramus on the left side of the figure (compare with the continuous ramus on the right side).

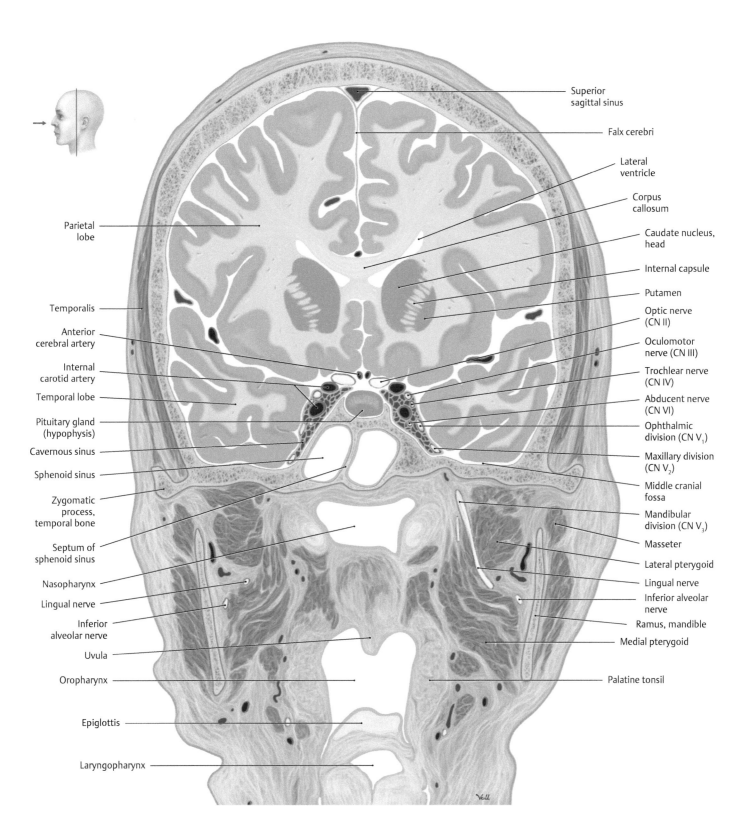

Parietal lobe
Temporalis
Anterior cerebral artery
Internal carotid artery
Temporal lobe
Pituitary gland (hypophysis)
Cavernous sinus
Sphenoid sinus
Zygomatic process, temporal bone
Septum of sphenoid sinus
Nasopharynx
Lingual nerve
Inferior alveolar nerve
Uvula
Oropharynx
Epiglottis
Laryngopharynx

Superior sagittal sinus
Falx cerebri
Lateral ventricle
Corpus callosum
Caudate nucleus, head
Internal capsule
Putamen
Optic nerve (CN II)
Oculomotor nerve (CN III)
Trochlear nerve (CN IV)
Abducent nerve (CN VI)
Ophthalmic division (CN V$_1$)
Maxillary division (CN V$_2$)
Middle cranial fossa
Mandibular division (CN V$_3$)
Masseter
Lateral pterygoid
Lingual nerve
Inferior alveolar nerve
Ramus, mandible
Medial pterygoid
Palatine tonsil

Fig. 14.4 Coronal section through the pituitary

Anterior view. The nasopharynx, oropharynx, and laryngopharynx can now be identified. This section cuts the epiglottis, below which is the supraglottic space. The plane cuts the ramus of the mandible on both sides, and a relatively long segment of the mandibular division of the trigeminal nerve (CN V$_3$) can be identified on the left side. Above the roof of the sphenoid sinuses is the pituitary gland (hypophysis), which lies in the hypophyseal fossa. In the cranial cavity, the plane of section passes through the middle cranial fossa. Due to the presence of the carotid siphon (a 180-degree bend in the cavernous part of the internal carotid artery), the section cuts the internal carotid artery twice on each side. Cranial nerves can be seen passing through the cavernous sinus on their way from the middle cranial fossa to the orbit. The superior sagittal sinus appears in cross section at the attachment of the falx cerebri. At the level of the cerebrum, the plane of section passes through the parietal and temporal lobes.

377

Coronal MRIs of the Head

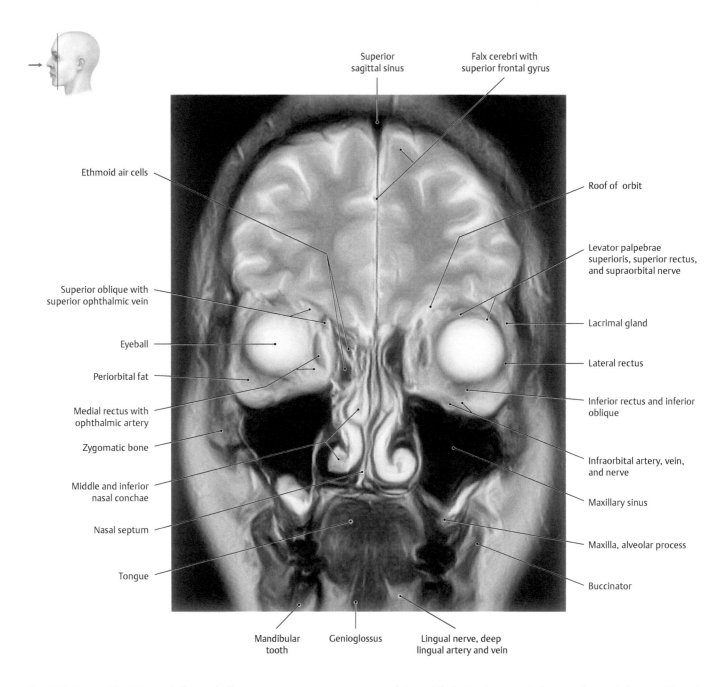

Superior sagittal sinus

Falx cerebri with superior frontal gyrus

Ethmoid air cells

Roof of orbit

Levator palpebrae superioris, superior rectus, and supraorbital nerve

Superior oblique with superior ophthalmic vein

Lacrimal gland

Eyeball

Lateral rectus

Periorbital fat

Inferior rectus and inferior oblique

Medial rectus with ophthalmic artery

Zygomatic bone

Infraorbital artery, vein, and nerve

Middle and inferior nasal conchae

Maxillary sinus

Nasal septum

Maxilla, alveolar process

Tongue

Buccinator

Mandibular tooth

Genioglossus

Lingual nerve, deep lingual artery and vein

Fig. 14.5 Coronal MRI through the eyeball
Anterior view. In this plane of section, the falx cerebri completely divides the cerebral hemispheres. The extraocular muscles can be used to find the orbital neurovasculature: the supraorbital nerve runs superior to the levator palpebrae superioris and superior rectus, the superior ophthalmic vein runs medial and superior to the superior oblique, and the ophthalmic artery runs inferior to the medial rectus. The infraorbital canal (containing the infraorbital artery, vein, and nerve) runs inferior to the inferior rectus and oblique. The region medial to the mandibular tooth and lateral to the genioglossus contains the sublingual gland as well as the lingual nerve, deep lingual artery and vein, hypoglossal nerve (CN XII), and submandibular duct.

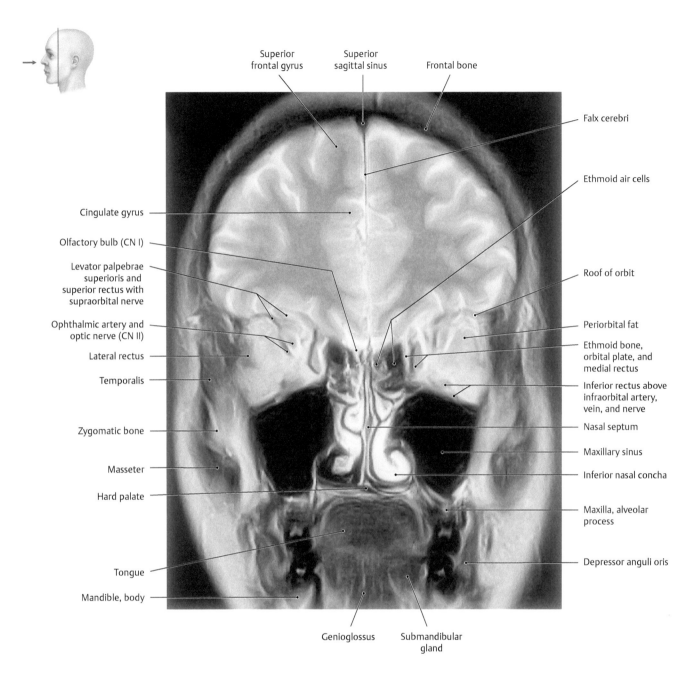

Superior frontal gyrus
Superior sagittal sinus
Frontal bone
Falx cerebri
Ethmoid air cells
Cingulate gyrus
Olfactory bulb (CN I)
Levator palpebrae superioris and superior rectus with supraorbital nerve
Roof of orbit
Ophthalmic artery and optic nerve (CN II)
Periorbital fat
Ethmoid bone, orbital plate, and medial rectus
Lateral rectus
Temporalis
Inferior rectus above infraorbital artery, vein, and nerve
Zygomatic bone
Nasal septum
Maxillary sinus
Masseter
Inferior nasal concha
Hard palate
Maxilla, alveolar process
Depressor anguli oris
Tongue
Mandible, body
Genioglossus
Submandibular gland

Fig. 14.6 Coronal MRI through the posterior orbit
Anterior view. The inferior margin of the falx cerebri is now superior to the cingulate gyrus. In the orbit, the supraorbital nerve runs with the levator palpebrae superioris and superior rectus, and the oculomotor nerve (CN III) runs lateral to the inferior rectus, which in turn runs supe-rior to the infraorbital canal. The ophthalmic artery can be used to find the more medially located optic nerve (CN II), both of which emerge from the optic canal. Note the asymmetrical nature of the nasal cavi-ties. The submandibular gland is more prominent in this section be-tween the genioglossus and the body of the mandible.

379

Coronal MRIs of the Neck (I): Anterior

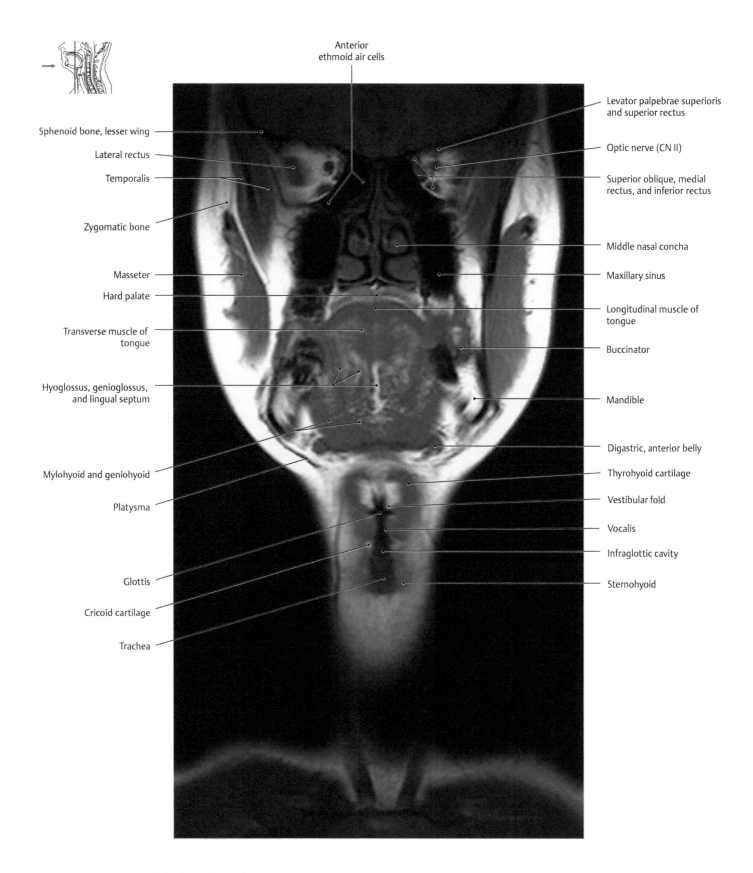

Anterior ethmoid air cells

Sphenoid bone, lesser wing

Lateral rectus

Temporalis

Zygomatic bone

Masseter

Hard palate

Transverse muscle of tongue

Hyoglossus, genioglossus, and lingual septum

Mylohyoid and geniohyoid

Platysma

Glottis

Cricoid cartilage

Trachea

Levator palpebrae superioris and superior rectus

Optic nerve (CN II)

Superior oblique, medial rectus, and inferior rectus

Middle nasal concha

Maxillary sinus

Longitudinal muscle of tongue

Buccinator

Mandible

Digastric, anterior belly

Thyrohyoid cartilage

Vestibular fold

Vocalis

Infraglottic cavity

Sternohyoid

Fig. 14.7 Coronal MRI of the lingual muscles
Anterior view. This plane of section lies just posterior to the previous one and transects the extrinsic (genioglossus and hyoglossus) and intrinsic (longitudinal and transverse) lingual muscles. The muscles of mastication (temporalis and masseter) are visible, as are the buccinator, mylohyoid, and geniohyoid. This section cuts the larynx and trachea, revealing the vestibular fold, vocalis muscle, and cricoid cartilage.

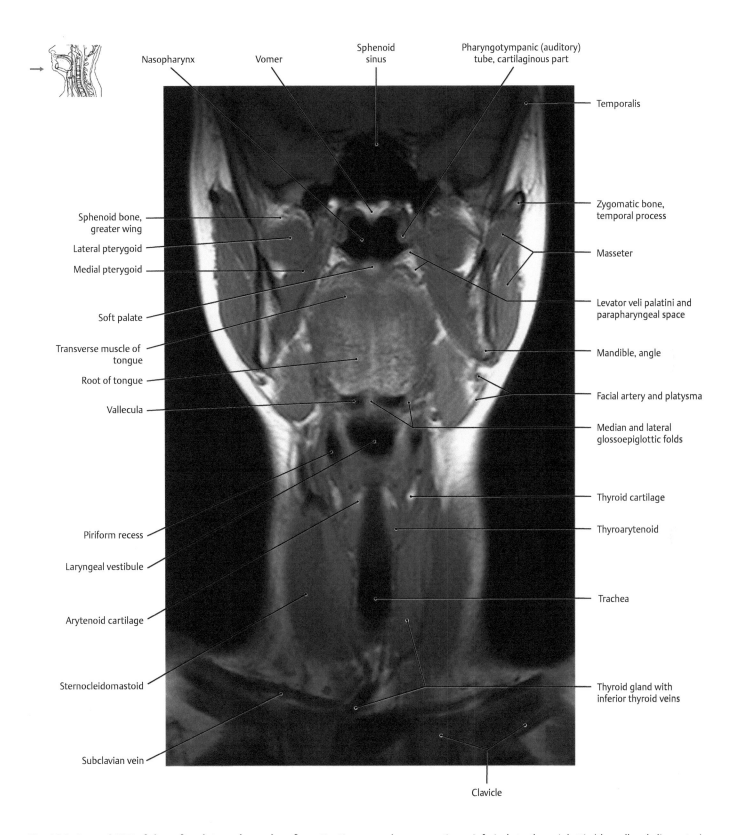

Fig. 14.8 **Coronal MRI of the soft palate and muscles of mastication**
Anterior view. This section illustrates the convergence of the air- and foodways in the pharynx. The nasopharynx lies inferior to the sphenoid sinus and superior to the soft palate. It converges with the foodway in the oropharynx, located posterior to the uvula (not shown). The oro- pharynx continues inferiorly to the epiglottis (the vallecula lies anterior to this). The air- and foodways then diverge into the larynx and laryn- gopharynx, respectively. The laryngeal vestibule is the superior portion of the larynx, above the vocal folds. This section reveals the thyroid and arytenoid cartilage of the larynx. Compare this image to **Fig. 14.9.**

381

Coronal MRIs of the Neck (II): Middle

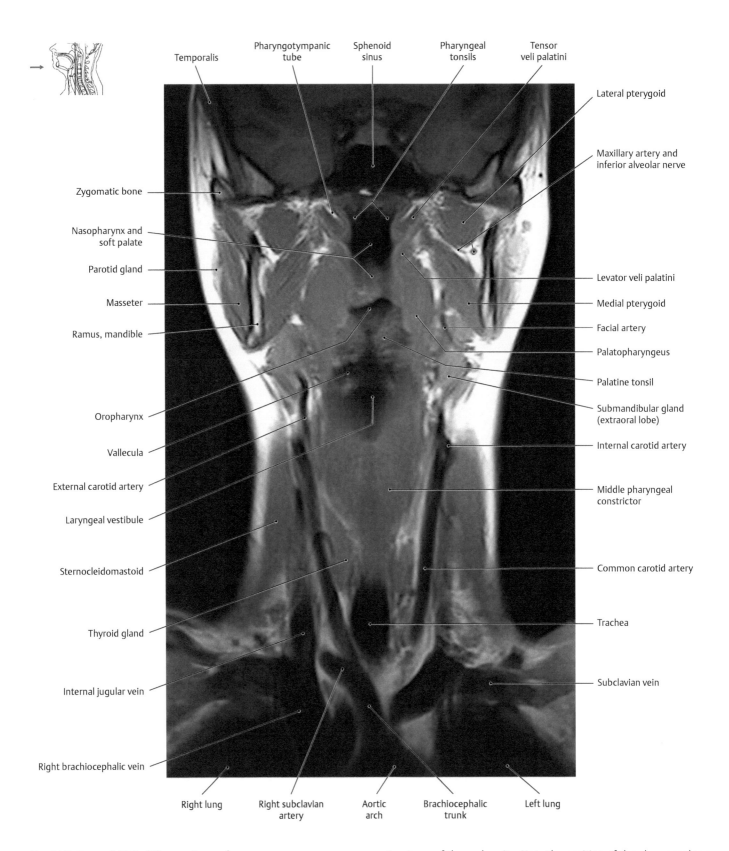

Fig. 14.9 Coronal MRI of the great vessels

Anterior view. This image clearly demonstrates the course of the great vessels in the neck. This image is also an excellent demonstration of the structures of the oral cavity. Note the position of the pharyngeal tonsils on the roof of the nasopharynx and the extent of the palatine tonsils in the oropharynx.

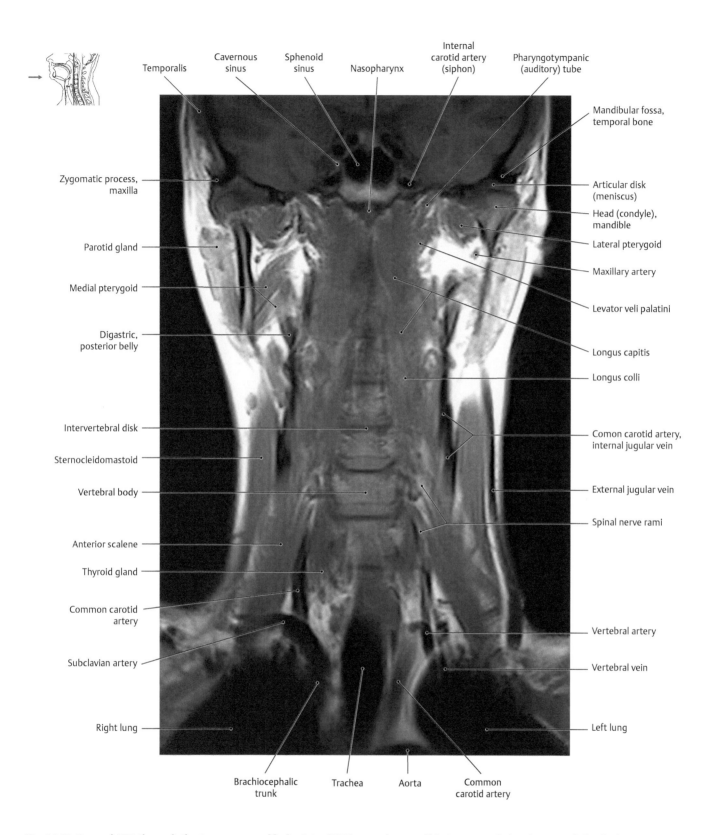

Fig. 14.10 Coronal MRI through the temporomandibular joint (TMJ)
Anterior view. This image clearly demonstrates the structures of the TMJ, in particular the articular disk and mandibular head. The ramus of the mandible is seen medial to the parotid gland. This image shows the cervical vertebrae with intervertebral disks.

Coronal MRIs of the Neck (III): Posterior

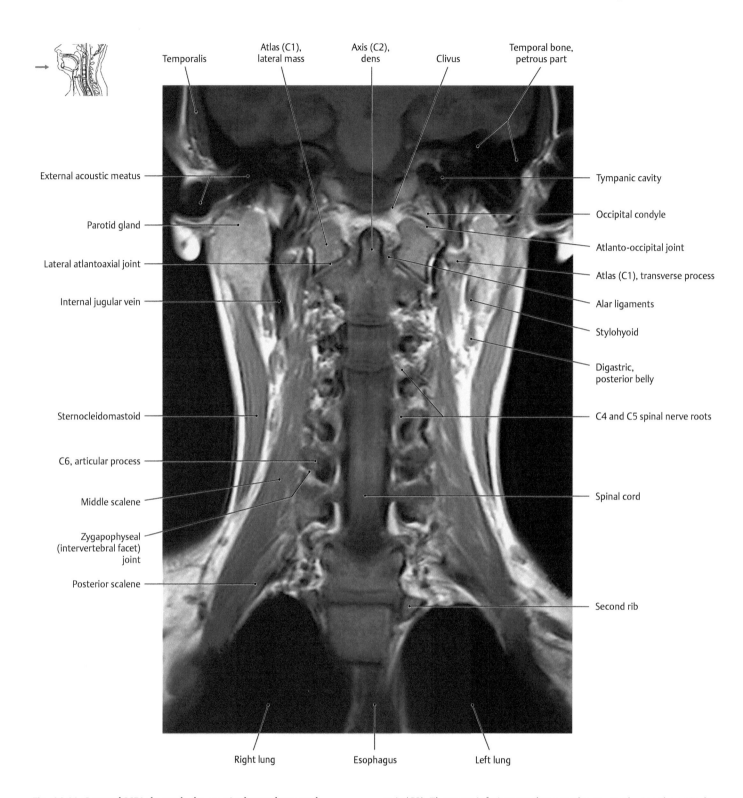

Temporalis

Atlas (C1), lateral mass

Axis (C2), dens

Clivus

Temporal bone, petrous part

External acoustic meatus

Parotid gland

Lateral atlantoaxial joint

Internal jugular vein

Sternocleidomastoid

C6, articular process

Middle scalene

Zygapophyseal (intervertebral facet) joint

Posterior scalene

Tympanic cavity

Occipital condyle

Atlanto-occipital joint

Atlas (C1), transverse process

Alar ligaments

Stylohyoid

Digastric, posterior belly

C4 and C5 spinal nerve roots

Spinal cord

Second rib

Right lung

Esophagus

Left lung

***Fig. 14.11* Coronal MRI through the cervical vertebrae and spinal nerves**
Anterior view. This image clearly shows the C1 through T2 vertebrae. The lateral masses of the atlas (C1) can be seen flanking the dens of the axis (C2). The more inferior vertebrae can be counted using the articular processes of the cervical vertebrae. The spinal nerve roots emerge between the articular processes (note for counting purposes: the C3 root emerges inferior to C2 and superior to the articular processes of C3).

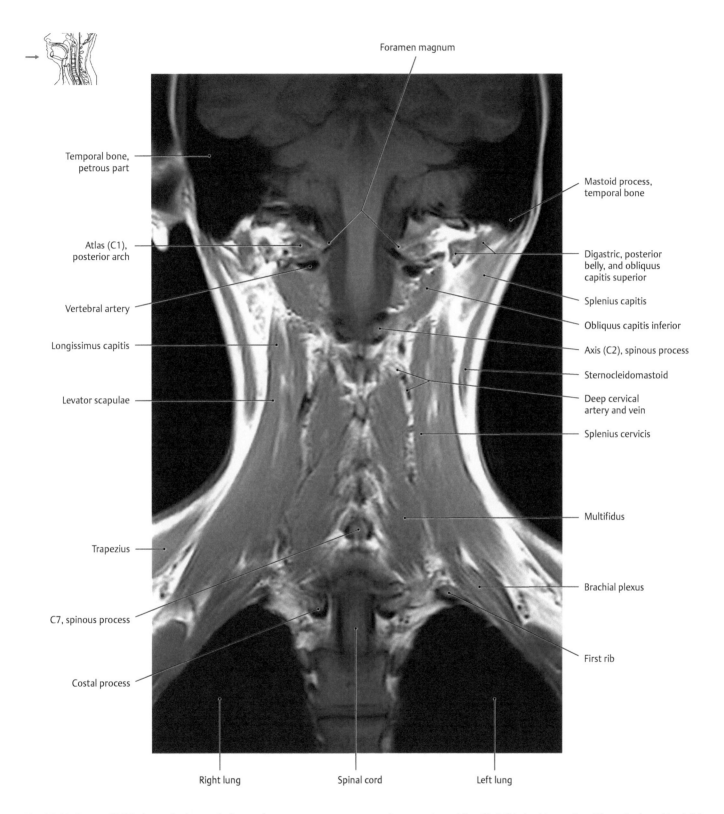

Foramen magnum

Temporal bone, petrous part

Atlas (C1), posterior arch

Vertebral artery

Longissimus capitis

Levator scapulae

Trapezius

C7, spinous process

Costal process

Mastoid process, temporal bone

Digastric, posterior belly, and obliquus capitis superior

Splenius capitis

Obliquus capitis inferior

Axis (C2), spinous process

Sternocleidomastoid

Deep cervical artery and vein

Splenius cervicis

Multifidus

Brachial plexus

First rib

Right lung

Spinal cord

Left lung

Fig. 14.12 Coronal MRI through the nuchal muscles
Anterior view. This image clearly shows the relations of the muscles in the neck. *Note:* The elongated spinous process of the C7 vertebra (ver- tebra prominens) is still visible in this section. The spinal cord is visible both during its passage through the foramen magnum and more cau- dally, posterior to the T1 vertebral body.

Transverse Sections of the Head (I): Cranial

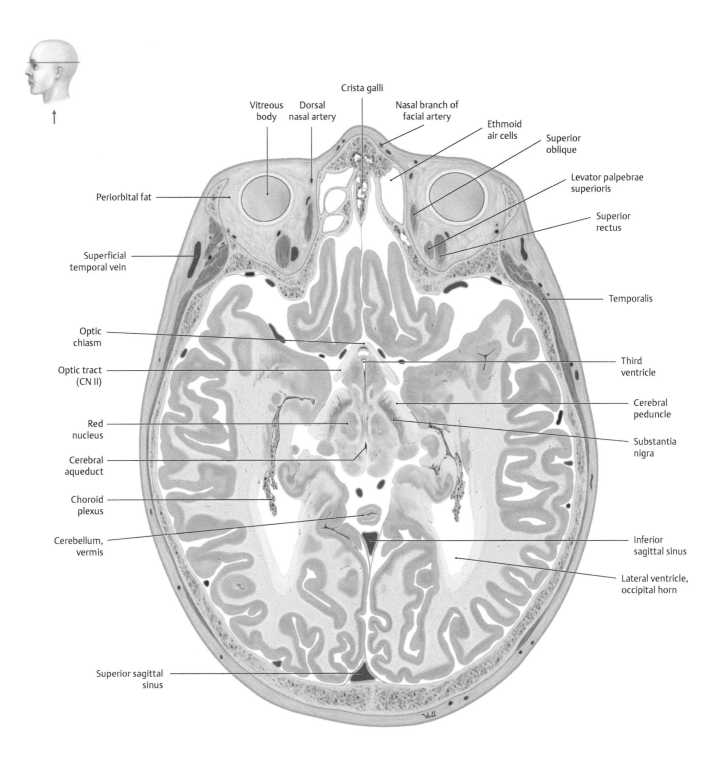

Fig. 14.13 Transverse section through the upper level of the orbits
Inferior view. The highest section in this series displays the muscles in the upper level of the orbit (the orbital levels are described on p. 250). The section cuts the bony crista galli in the anterior cranial fossa, flanked on each side by cells of the ethmoid sinus. The sections of the optic chiasm and adjacent optic tract are parts of the diencephalon, which surrounds the third ventricle at the center of the section. The red nucleus and substantia nigra are visible in the mesencephalon. The pyramidal tract descends in the cerebral peduncles. The section passes through the posterior (occipital) horns of the lateral ventricles and barely cuts the vermis of the cerebellum in the midline.

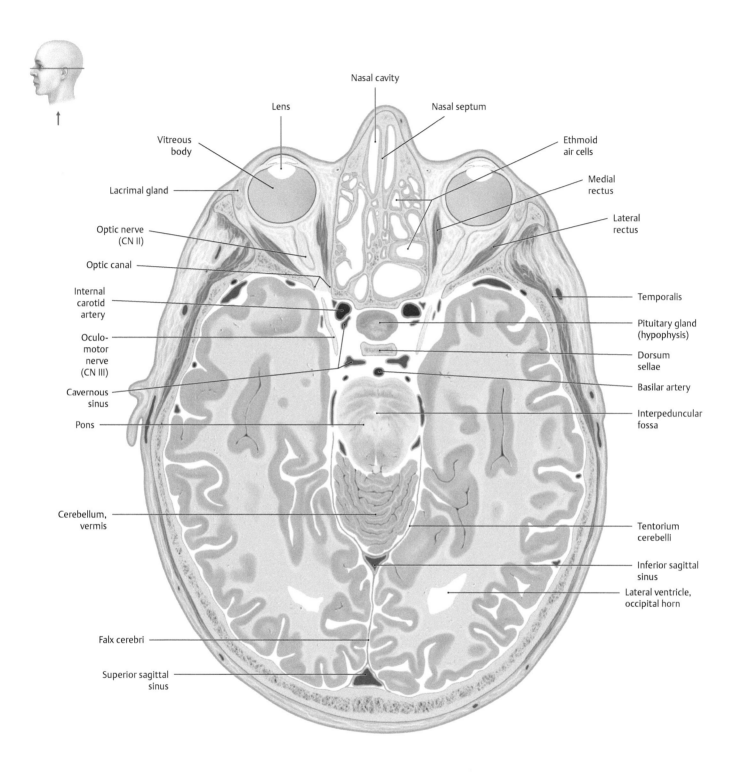

Nasal cavity

Lens

Nasal septum

Vitreous body

Ethmoid air cells

Lacrimal gland

Medial rectus

Optic nerve (CN II)

Lateral rectus

Optic canal

Internal carotid artery

Temporalis

Oculo-motor nerve (CN III)

Pituitary gland (hypophysis)

Dorsum sellae

Cavernous sinus

Basilar artery

Pons

Interpeduncular fossa

Cerebellum, vermis

Tentorium cerebelli

Inferior sagittal sinus

Lateral ventricle, occipital horn

Falx cerebri

Superior sagittal sinus

Fig. 14.14 Transverse section through the optic nerve and pituitary Inferior view. The optic nerve is seen just before its entry into the optic canal, indicating that the plane of section passes through the middle level of the orbit. Because the nerve completely fills the canal, growth disturbances of the bone at this level may cause pressure injury to the nerve. This plane cuts the ocular lenses and the cells of the ethmoid labyrinth. The internal carotid artery can be identified in the middle cranial fossa, embedded in the cavernous sinus. The section cuts the oculomotor nerve on either side, which courses in the lateral wall of the cavernous sinus. The pons and cerebellar vermis are also seen. The falx cerebri and tentorium cerebelli appear as thin lines that come together at the straight sinus.

Transverse Sections of the Head (II)

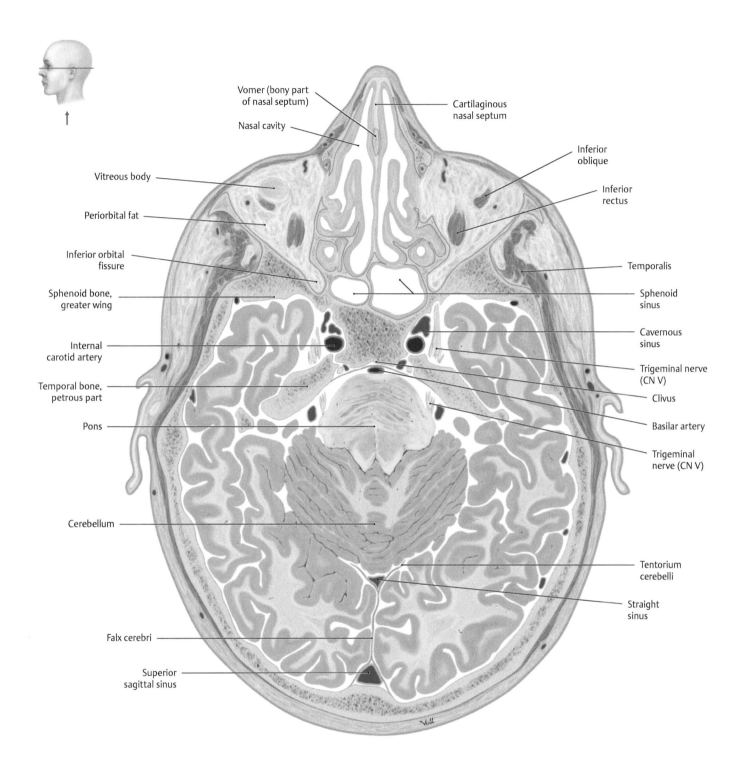

Vomer (bony part of nasal septum)

Cartilaginous nasal septum

Nasal cavity

Inferior oblique

Inferior rectus

Vitreous body

Periorbital fat

Temporalis

Inferior orbital fissure

Sphenoid sinus

Sphenoid bone, greater wing

Cavernous sinus

Internal carotid artery

Trigeminal nerve (CN V)

Temporal bone, petrous part

Clivus

Pons

Basilar artery

Trigeminal nerve (CN V)

Cerebellum

Tentorium cerebelli

Straight sinus

Falx cerebri

Superior sagittal sinus

Fig. 14.15 Transverse section through the sphenoid sinus
Inferior view. This section cuts the infratemporal fossa on the lateral aspect of the skull and the temporalis muscle that lies within it. The plane passes through the lower level of the orbit, which is continuous posteriorly with the inferior orbital fissure. This section displays the anterior extension of the two greater wings of the sphenoid bone and the posterior extension of the two petrous parts of the temporal bones, which mark the boundary between the middle and posterior cranial fossae. The clivus is part of the posterior cranial fossa and lies in contact with the basilar artery. The pontine origin of the trigeminal nerve is visible. *Note:* The trigeminal nerve passes superior to the petrous portion of the temporal bone to enter the middle cranial fossa.

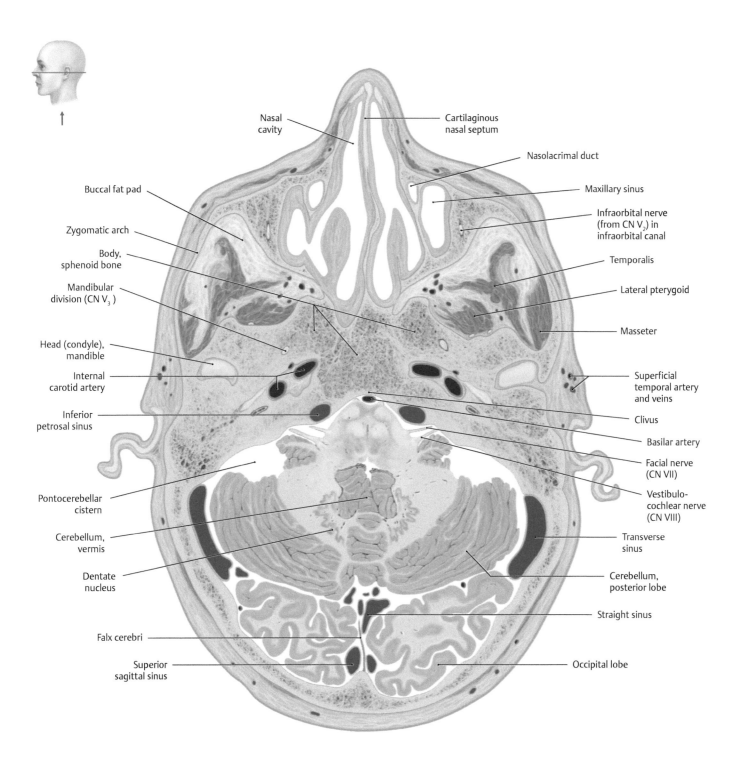

Fig. 14.16 Transverse section through the middle nasal concha
Inferior view. This section below the orbit passes through the infraorbital nerve and canal. Medial to the infraorbital nerve is the roof of the maxillary sinus. The zygomatic arch is visible in its entirety, with portions of the muscles of mastication (masseter, temporalis, and lateral pterygoid) and the upper part of the head of the mandible. The mandibular division of the trigeminal nerve (CN V₃) appears in cross section in its bony canal, the foramen ovale. The body of the sphenoid bone forms the bony center of the base of the skull. The facial and vestibulocochlear nerves (CNs VII and VIII) emerge from the brainstem and enter the internal acoustic meatus. The dentate nucleus lies within the white matter of the cerebellum. The space around the anterior part of the cerebellum, the pontocerebellar cistern, is filled with cerebrospinal fluid in the living individual. The transverse sinus is prominent among the dural sinuses of the brain.

389

Transverse Sections of the Head (III): Caudal

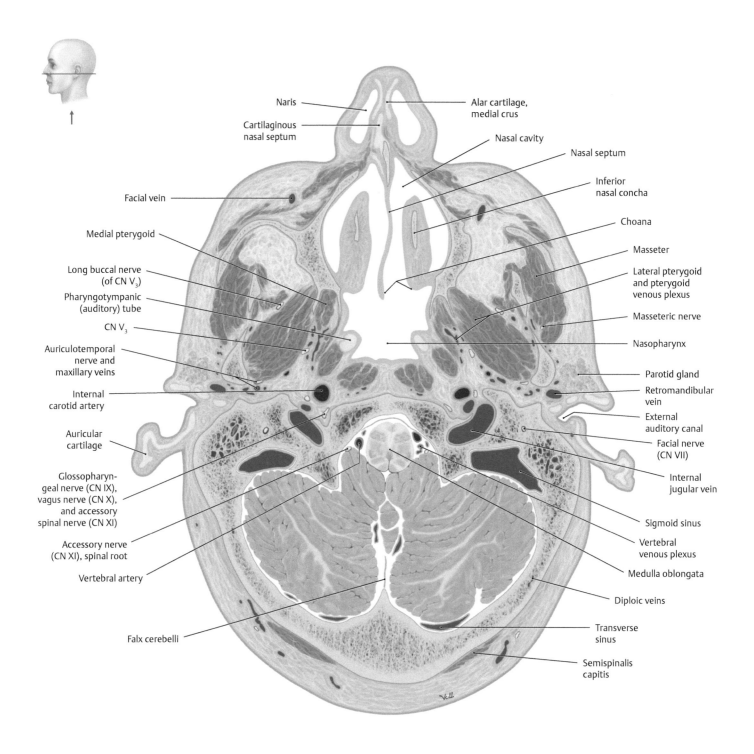

Fig. 14.17 Transverse section through the nasopharynx

Inferior view. This section passes through the external nose and portions of the cartilaginous nasal skeleton. The nasal cavities communicate with the nasopharynx through the choanae. Cartilaginous portions of the pharyngotympanic tube project into the nasopharynx. The internal jugular vein travels with the vagus nerve (CN X) and common carotid artery as a neurovascular bundle within the carotid sheath, a fascial covering that extends from the base of the skull to the arch of the aorta. The glossopharyngeal, accessory spinal, and hypoglossal nerves (CN IX, XI, and XII) also pierce the upper portion of the carotid sheath. However, these neurovascular structures do not all enter and exit the skull base together. The jugular foramen consists of a neural and a venous portion. The neural portion conducts the glossopharyngeal (CN IX), vagus (CN X), and accessory spinal (CN XI) nerves, and the venous portion contains the jugular bulb, which receives blood from the sigmoid sinus. (*Note:* The internal jugular vein begins at the inferior portion of the jugular foramen.) The internal carotid artery enters the carotid canal, and the hypoglossal (CN XII) nerve enters the hypoglossal canal.

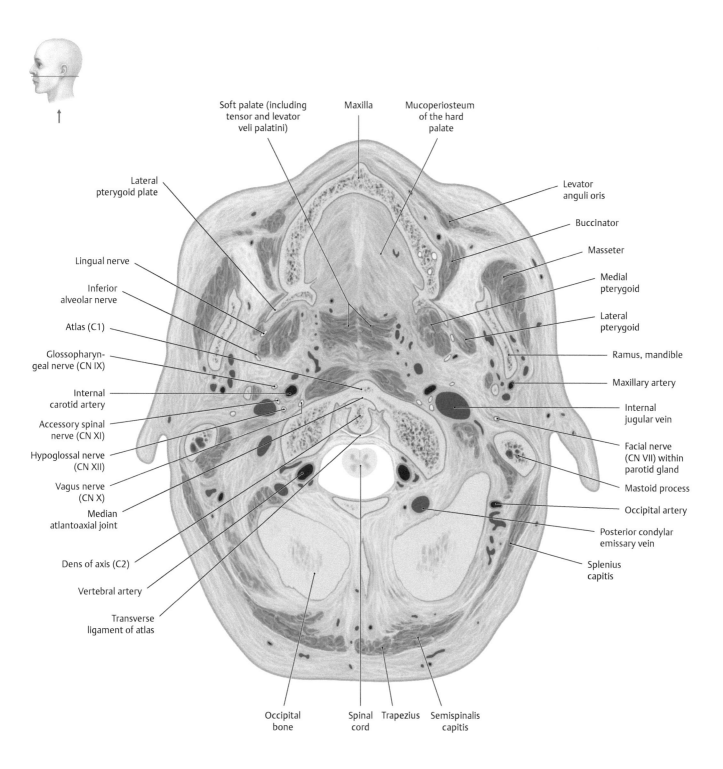

Soft palate (including tensor and levator veli palatini)

Maxilla

Mucoperiosteum of the hard palate

Lateral pterygoid plate

Levator anguli oris

Buccinator

Masseter

Lingual nerve

Medial pterygoid

Inferior alveolar nerve

Lateral pterygoid

Atlas (C1)

Ramus, mandible

Glossopharyn-geal nerve (CN IX)

Maxillary artery

Internal carotid artery

Internal jugular vein

Accessory spinal nerve (CN XI)

Facial nerve (CN VII) within parotid gland

Hypoglossal nerve (CN XII)

Mastoid process

Vagus nerve (CN X)

Occipital artery

Median atlantoaxial joint

Posterior condylar emissary vein

Dens of axis (C2)

Splenius capitis

Vertebral artery

Transverse ligament of atlas

Occipital bone

Spinal cord

Trapezius

Semispinalis capitis

Fig. 14.18 Transverse section through the median atlantoaxial joint
Inferior view. The section at this level passes through the connective tissue sheet that stretches over the bone of the hard palate. Portions of the upper pharyngeal muscles are sectioned close to their origin. The neurovascular structures in the carotid sheath are also well displayed. The dens of the axis articulates in the median atlantoaxial joint with the facet for the dens on the posterior surface of the anterior arch of the atlas. The transverse ligament of the atlas that helps to stabilize this joint can also be identified. The vertebral artery and its accompanying veins are displayed in cross section, as is the spinal cord. In the occipital region, the section passes through the upper portion of the posterior neck muscles.

Transverse Sections of the Neck (I): Cranial

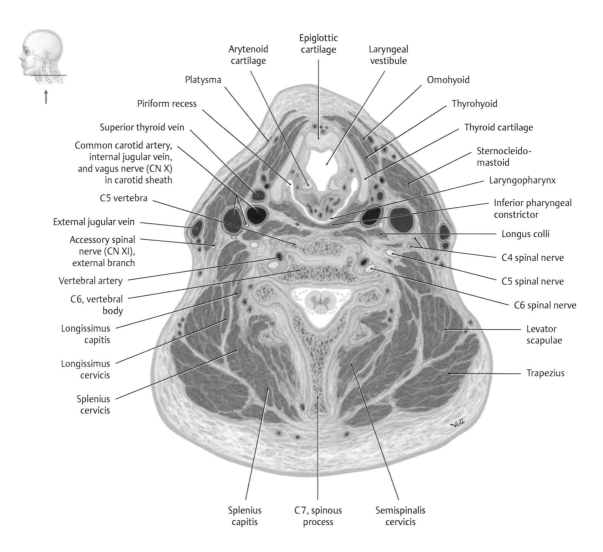

Arytenoid cartilage

Epiglottic cartilage

Laryngeal vestibule

Platysma

Omohyoid

Piriform recess

Thyrohyoid

Superior thyroid vein

Thyroid cartilage

Common carotid artery, internal jugular vein, and vagus nerve (CN X) in carotid sheath

Sternocleido-mastoid

C5 vertebra

Laryngopharynx

External jugular vein

Inferior pharyngeal constrictor

Accessory spinal nerve (CN XI), external branch

Longus colli

Vertebral artery

C4 spinal nerve

C6, vertebral body

C5 spinal nerve

Longissimus capitis

C6 spinal nerve

Longissimus cervicis

Levator scapulae

Splenius cervicis

Trapezius

Splenius capitis

C7, spinous process

Semispinalis cervicis

Fig. 14.19 Transverse section at the level of the C5 vertebral body Inferior view. The internal jugular vein travels with the common carotid artery and vagus nerve in the carotid sheath. The accessory spinal nerve (CN XI) is medial to the sternocleidomastoid; more proximal to the skull base it will pierce the carotid sheath to enter the jugular foramen with the internal jugular vein, as well as CN IX and X. The elongated spinous process of the C7 vertebra (vertebra prominens) is visible at this level, owing to the lordotic curvature of the neck. Note that the triangular shape of the arytenoid cartilage is clearly demonstrated in the laryngeal cross section.

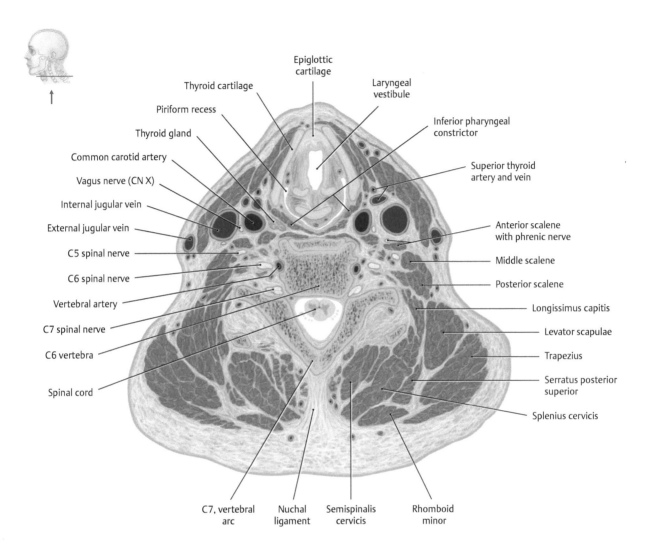

Epiglottic
cartilage

Thyroid cartilage

Laryngeal
vestibule

Piriform recess

Inferior pharyngeal
constrictor

Thyroid gland

Common carotid artery

Superior thyroid
artery and vein

Vagus nerve (CN X)

Internal jugular vein

External jugular vein

Anterior scalene
with phrenic nerve

C5 spinal nerve

Middle scalene

C6 spinal nerve

Posterior scalene

Vertebral artery

Longissimus capitis

C7 spinal nerve

Levator scapulae

C6 vertebra

Trapezius

Spinal cord

Serratus posterior
superior

Splenius cervicis

C7, vertebral
arc

Nuchal
ligament

Semispinalis
cervicis

Rhomboid
minor

Fig. 14.20 Transverse section through the C6 vertebral body
Inferior view. The piriform recess can be identified at this level, and
the vertebral artery is visible in its course along the vertebral body.
The vagus nerve (CN X) lies in a posterior angle between the common
carotid artery and internal jugular vein within the carotid sheath. The
phrenic nerve, which arises from the anterior rami of cervical spinal
nerves C3–C5, lies on the anterior scalene muscle on the left side.

Transverse Sections of the Neck (II): Caudal

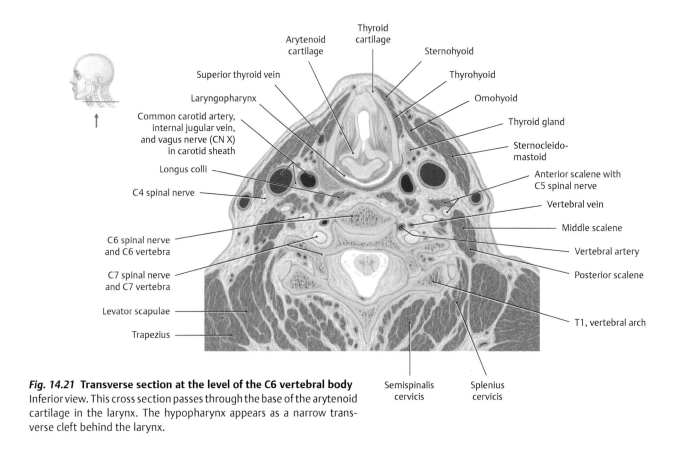

Fig. 14.21 Transverse section at the level of the C6 vertebral body
Inferior view. This cross section passes through the base of the arytenoid cartilage in the larynx. The hypopharynx appears as a narrow transverse cleft behind the larynx.

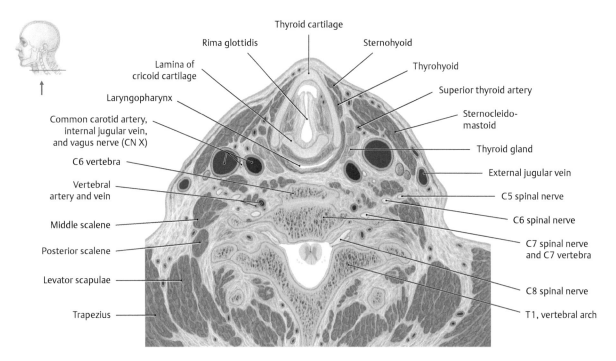

Fig. 14.22 Transverse section at the level of the C6/C7 vertebral junction
Inferior view. This cross section passes through the larynx at the level of the vocal folds. The thyroid gland appears considerably smaller at this level than in subsequent views.

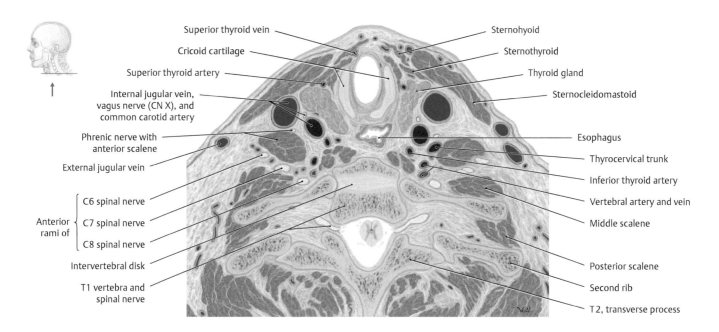

Fig. 14.23 Transverse section at the level of the C7/T1 vertebral junction

Inferior view. This cross section clearly displays the anterior and middle scalenes and the interval between them, which is traversed by the C6–C8 roots of the brachial plexus. Note the neurovascular structures (common carotid artery, internal jugular vein, vagus nerve) that lie within the carotid sheath between the sternocleidomastoid, anterior scalene, and thyroid gland.

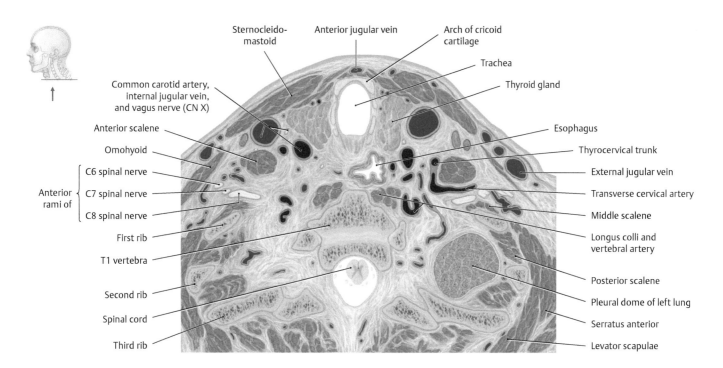

Fig. 14.24 Transverse section at the level of the T1/T2 vertebral junction

Inferior view. Due to the curvature of the neck in this specimen, the section also cuts the intervertebral disk between T1 and T2. This section includes the C6–C8 nerve roots of the brachial plexus and a small section of the left pleural dome. The proximity of the pulmonary apex to the brachial plexus shows why the growth of an apical lung tumor may damage the brachial plexus roots. Note also the thyroid gland and its proximity to the trachea and neurovascular bundle in the carotid sheath.

Transverse MRIs of the Head

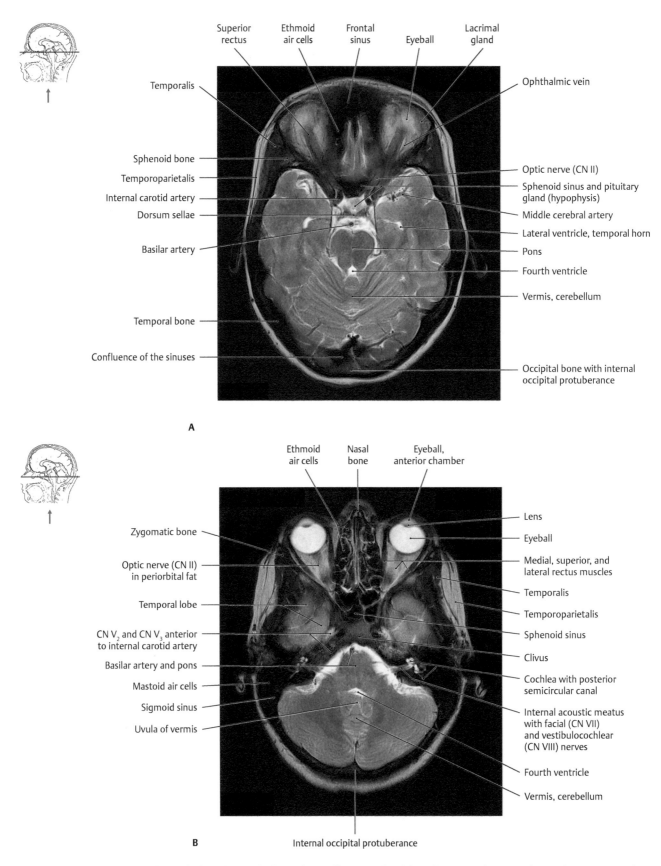

A

B

Fig. 14.25 **Transverse MRIs through the orbit and ethmoid air cells** Inferior view. **A** Superior orbit. This section demonstrates the relationship of the frontal and sphenoid sinuses to the orbit and nasal cavity. **B** Section through optic nerve (CN II). The divisions of the eye can be clearly seen along with the extraocular muscles located in the peri-orbital fat. The sigmoid sinus is located posterior to the mastoid air cells and lateral to the cerebellum. This section clearly displays the internal acoustic meatus, which conducts the facial (CN VII) and vestibulocochlear (CN VIII) nerves.

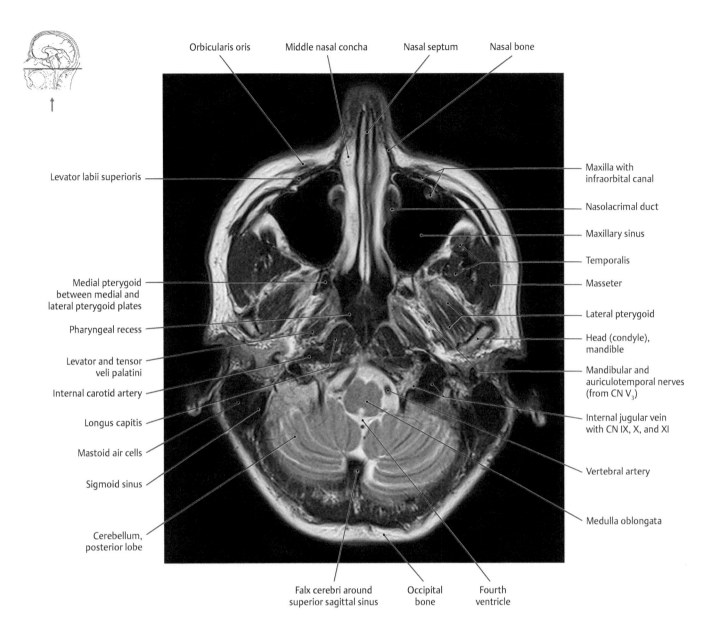

Orbicularis oris — Middle nasal concha — Nasal septum — Nasal bone

Levator labii superioris

Maxilla with infraorbital canal

Nasolacrimal duct

Maxillary sinus

Temporalis

Masseter

Medial pterygoid between medial and lateral pterygoid plates

Lateral pterygoid

Pharyngeal recess

Head (condyle), mandible

Levator and tensor veli palatini

Mandibular and auriculotemporal nerves (from CN V₃)

Internal carotid artery

Internal jugular vein with CN IX, X, and XI

Longus capitis

Mastoid air cells

Vertebral artery

Sigmoid sinus

Medulla oblongata

Cerebellum, posterior lobe

Falx cerebri around superior sagittal sinus — Occipital bone — Fourth ventricle

Fig. 14.26 Transverse MRI through the orbit and nasolacrimal duct
Inferior view. This section clearly demonstrates the relationships of the infraorbital canal and nasolacrimal duct to the maxillary sinus. The medial and lateral pterygoid plates can be seen flanking the medial pterygoid. The pharyngeal recess is visible, anterior to the lon-gus capitis. The mandibular division of the trigeminal nerve (CN V₃) is lateral to the levator and tensor veli palatini and medial to the lateral pterygoid. The glossopharyngeal, vagus, and accessory spinal nerves (CN IX, X, and XI) run just anteromedial to the internal jugular vein.

Transverse MRIs of the Oral Cavity

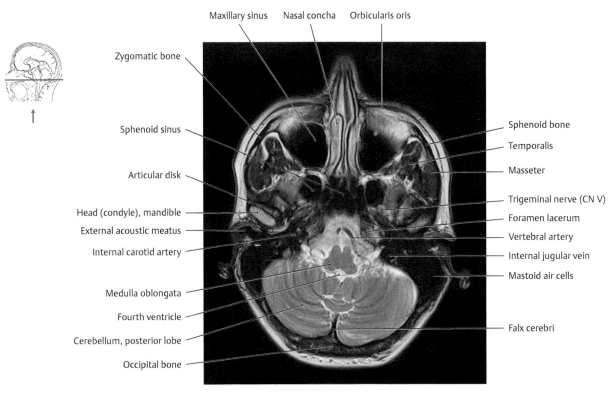

Fig. 14.27 Transverse MRI through the temporomandibular joint (TMJ)
Inferior view. *Note:* The plane of this section is slightly higher than **Fig. 14.26**. It has been included here in order to show the articular disk of the TMJ and the full extent of the mandible.

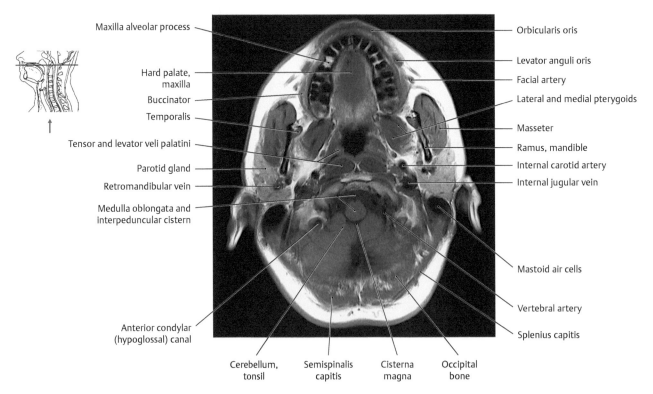

Fig. 14.28 Transverse MRI through the hard and soft palates
Inferior view. This section demonstrates the relation of the ramus of the mandible to the muscles of mastication in the infratemporal fossa.

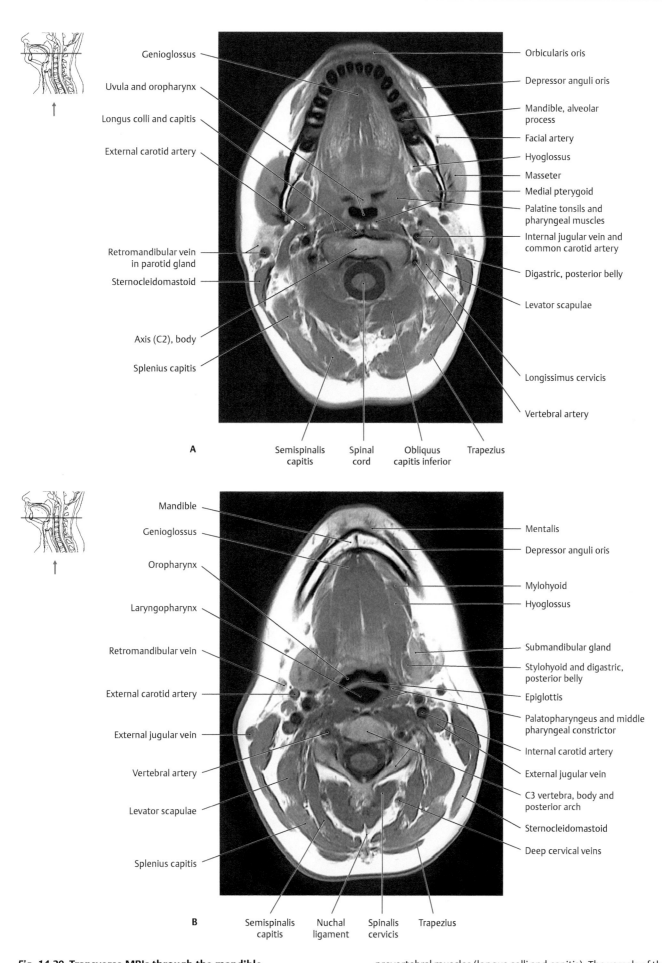

A

Genioglossus
Uvula and oropharynx
Longus colli and capitis
External carotid artery
Retromandibular vein in parotid gland
Sternocleidomastoid
Axis (C2), body
Splenius capitis

Semispinalis capitis
Spinal cord
Obliquus capitis inferior
Trapezius

Orbicularis oris
Depressor anguli oris
Mandible, alveolar process
Facial artery
Hyoglossus
Masseter
Medial pterygoid
Palatine tonsils and pharyngeal muscles
Internal jugular vein and common carotid artery
Digastric, posterior belly
Levator scapulae
Longissimus cervicis
Vertebral artery

B

Mandible
Genioglossus
Oropharynx
Laryngopharynx
Retromandibular vein
External carotid artery
External jugular vein
Vertebral artery
Levator scapulae
Splenius capitis

Semispinalis capitis
Nuchal ligament
Spinalis cervicis
Trapezius

Mentalis
Depressor anguli oris
Mylohyoid
Hyoglossus
Submandibular gland
Stylohyoid and digastric, posterior belly
Epiglottis
Palatopharyngeus and middle pharyngeal constrictor
Internal carotid artery
External jugular vein
C3 vertebra, body and posterior arch
Sternocleidomastoid
Deep cervical veins

Fig. 14.29 Transverse MRIs through the mandible

Inferior view. **A** Section through mandibular arch. This section demonstrates the relationship of the oropharynx to the soft palate (uvula) and prevertebral muscles (longus colli and capitis). The vessels of the carotid sheath are clearly visible, along with the retromandibular vein in the parotid gland. **B** Section through body of mandible and laryngopharynx.

399

Transverse MRIs of the Neck

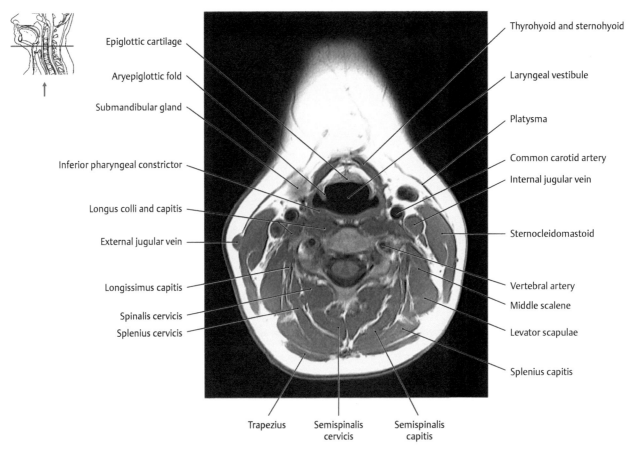

Epiglottic cartilage

Aryepiglottic fold

Submandibular gland

Inferior pharyngeal constrictor

Longus colli and capitis

External jugular vein

Longissimus capitis

Spinalis cervicis

Splenius cervicis

Thyrohyoid and sternohyoid

Laryngeal vestibule

Platysma

Common carotid artery

Internal jugular vein

Sternocleidomastoid

Vertebral artery

Middle scalene

Levator scapulae

Splenius capitis

Trapezius   Semispinalis   Semispinalis
             cervicis   capitis

Fig. 14.30 Transverse MRI through the C4 vertebral body
Inferior view. This section demonstrates the aryepiglottic fold in the laryngeal vestibule. Note the proximity of the prevertebral muscles to the pharyngeal constrictors.

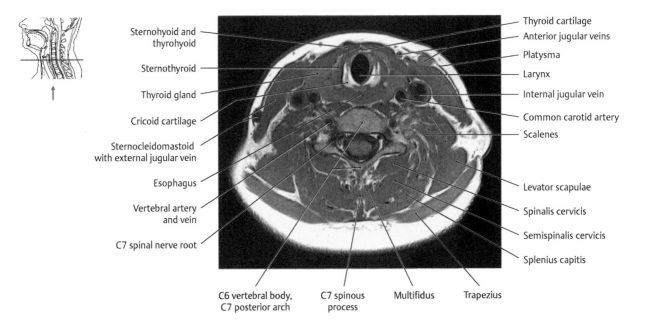

Sternohyoid and
thyrohyoid

Sternothyroid

Thyroid gland

Cricoid cartilage

Sternocleidomastoid
with external jugular vein

Esophagus

Vertebral artery
and vein

C7 spinal nerve root

Thyroid cartilage

Anterior jugular veins

Platysma

Larynx

Internal jugular vein

Common carotid artery

Scalenes

Levator scapulae

Spinalis cervicis

Semispinalis cervicis

Splenius capitis

C6 vertebral body,   C7 spinous   Multifidus   Trapezius
C7 posterior arch   process

Fig. 14.31 Transverse MRI through the C6 vertebral body
Inferior view. This section demonstrates the cricoid and thyroid cartilage of the larynx (note the change in shape of the larynx). Due to lordosis of the cervical spine, this section includes the C6 vertebral body and the C7 spinous process with posterior arch.

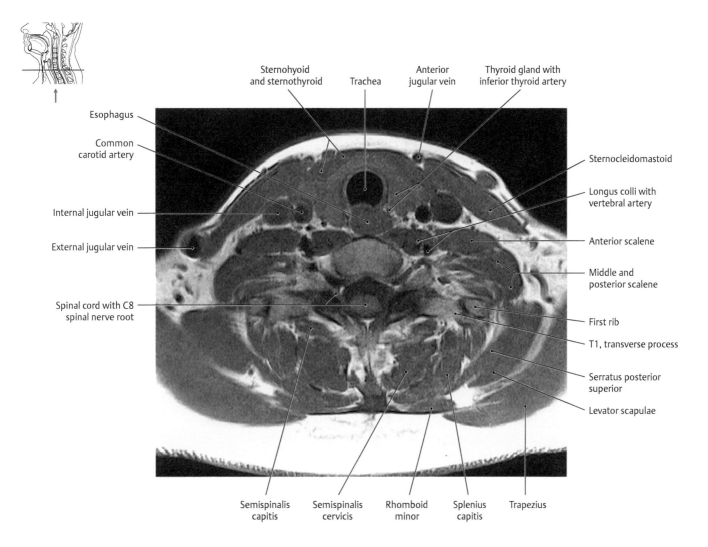

Esophagus

Common carotid artery

Internal jugular vein

External jugular vein

Spinal cord with C8 spinal nerve root

Sternohyoid and sternothyroid

Trachea

Anterior jugular vein

Thyroid gland with inferior thyroid artery

Sternocleidomastoid

Longus colli with vertebral artery

Anterior scalene

Middle and posterior scalene

First rib

T1, transverse process

Serratus posterior superior

Levator scapulae

Semispinalis capitis

Semispinalis cervicis

Rhomboid minor

Splenius capitis

Trapezius

Fig. 14.32 Transverse MRI through the C7 vertebra
Inferior view. This section demonstrates the relationship of the trachea to the esophagus. Note the position of the carotid sheath (containing the common carotid artery, internal jugular vein, and vagus nerve [CN X]) with respect to the thyroid gland. The C8 spinal nerve root can be seen emerging from the spinal cord. Note the first rib and transverse process of the thoracic vertebra.

Sagittal Sections of the Head (I): Medial

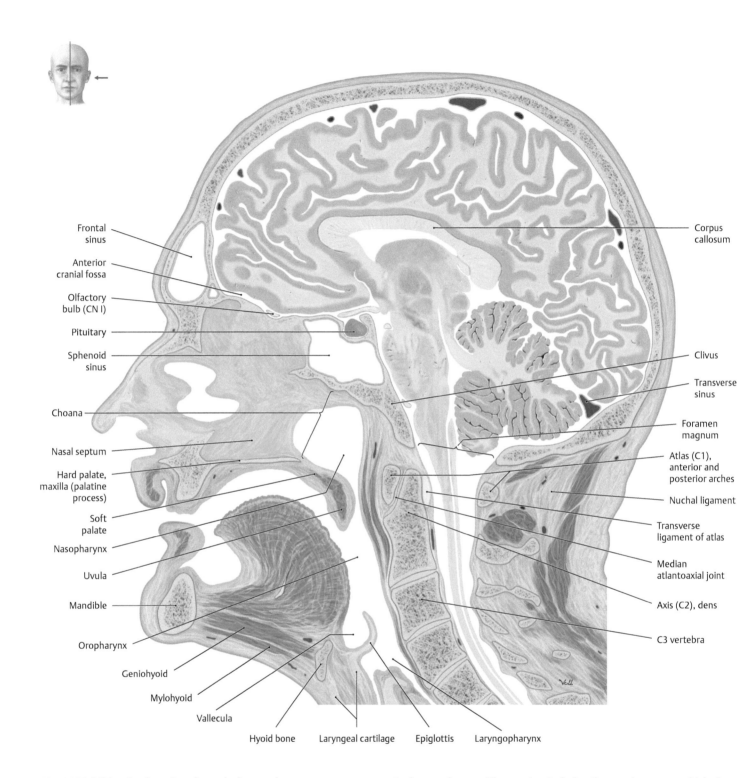

Frontal sinus

Anterior cranial fossa

Olfactory bulb (CN I)

Pituitary

Sphenoid sinus

Choana

Nasal septum

Hard palate, maxilla (palatine process)

Soft palate

Nasopharynx

Uvula

Mandible

Oropharynx

Geniohyoid

Mylohyoid

Vallecula

Hyoid bone   Laryngeal cartilage   Epiglottis   Laryngopharynx

Corpus callosum

Clivus

Transverse sinus

Foramen magnum

Atlas (C1), anterior and posterior arches

Nuchal ligament

Transverse ligament of atlas

Median atlantoaxial joint

Axis (C2), dens

C3 vertebra

Fig. 14.33 Midsagittal section through the nasal septum
Left lateral view. The anatomical structures at this level can be roughly assigned to the face or neurocranium (cranial vault). This section also passes through the epiglottis and the larynx below it, which are considered part of the cervical viscera. *Note:* The vallecula, located in the oropharynx, is bounded by the root of the tongue and the epiglottis. The hard and soft palate with the uvula define the boundary between the oral and nasal cavities. Posterior to the uvula is the oropharynx. The section includes the nasal septum, which divides the nasal cavity into two cavities that communicate with the nasopharynx through the choanae. Posterior to the frontal sinus is the anterior cranial fossa, which is part of the neurocranium. This section passes through the medial surface of the brain (the falx cerebri has been removed). The cut edge of the corpus callosum, the olfactory bulb, and the pituitary gland are also shown.

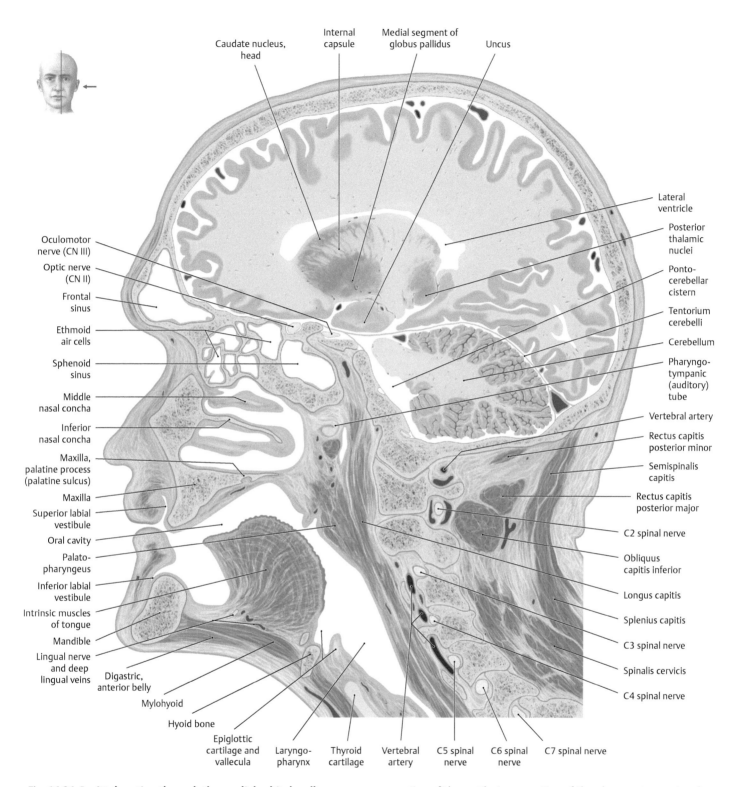

Caudate nucleus, head

Internal capsule

Medial segment of globus pallidus

Uncus

Oculomotor nerve (CN III)

Optic nerve (CN II)

Frontal sinus

Ethmoid air cells

Sphenoid sinus

Middle nasal concha

Inferior nasal concha

Maxilla, palatine process (palatine sulcus)

Maxilla

Superior labial vestibule

Oral cavity

Palato-pharyngeus

Inferior labial vestibule

Intrinsic muscles of tongue

Mandible

Lingual nerve and deep lingual veins

Digastric, anterior belly

Mylohyoid

Hyoid bone

Epiglottic cartilage and vallecula

Laryngo-pharynx

Thyroid cartilage

Vertebral artery

C5 spinal nerve

C6 spinal nerve

C7 spinal nerve

Lateral ventricle

Posterior thalamic nuclei

Ponto-cerebellar cistern

Tentorium cerebelli

Cerebellum

Pharyngo-tympanic (auditory) tube

Vertebral artery

Rectus capitis posterior minor

Semispinalis capitis

Rectus capitis posterior major

C2 spinal nerve

Obliquus capitis inferior

Longus capitis

Splenius capitis

C3 spinal nerve

Spinalis cervicis

C4 spinal nerve

Fig. 14.34 Sagittal section through the medial orbital wall
Left lateral view. This section passes through the inferior and middle nasal conchae within the nasal cavity. Above the middle nasal concha are the ethmoid air cells. The only parts of the nasopharynx visible in this section are a small luminal area and the lateral wall, which bears a section of the cartilaginous portion of the pharyngotympanic tube. The sphenoid sinus is also displayed. In the region of the cervical spine, the section cuts the vertebral artery at multiple levels. The lateral sites where the spinal nerves emerge from the intervertebral foramina are clearly displayed. *Note:* This section is lateral to the geniohyoid.

403

Sagittal Sections of the Head (II): Lateral

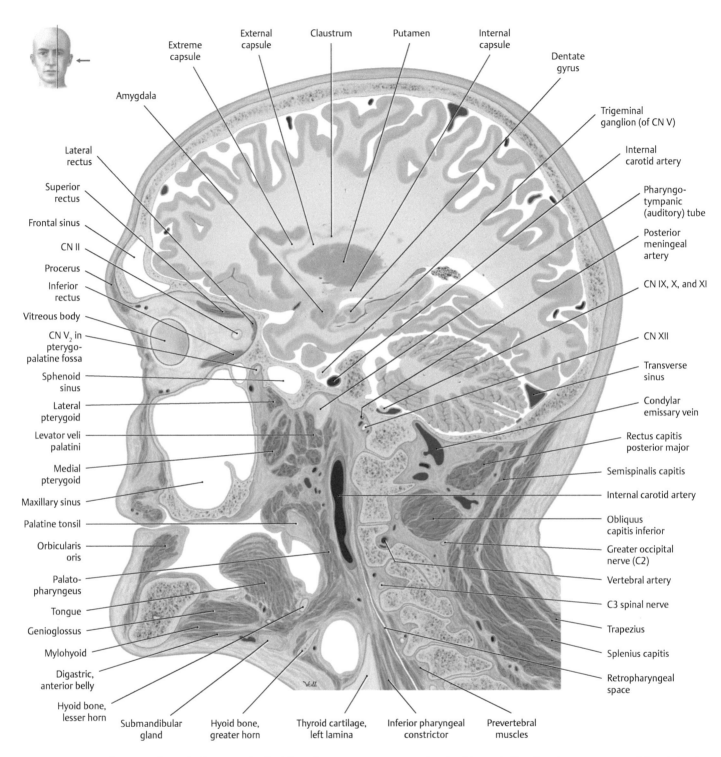

Fig. 14.35 Sagittal section through the inner third of the orbit
Left lateral view. This section passes through the maxillary and frontal sinuses while displaying one ethmoid air cell and the peripheral part of the sphenoid sinus. It passes through the medial portion of the internal carotid artery and submandibular gland. The pharyngeal and masticatory muscles are grouped about the cartilaginous part of the pharyn-

gotympanic tube. The eyeball and optic nerve are cut obliquely by the section, which displays relatively long segments of the superior and inferior rectus muscles. Sectioned brain structures include the external and internal capsules and the intervening putamen. The amygdala can be identified near the base of the brain. A section of the trigeminal ganglion appears below the cerebrum.

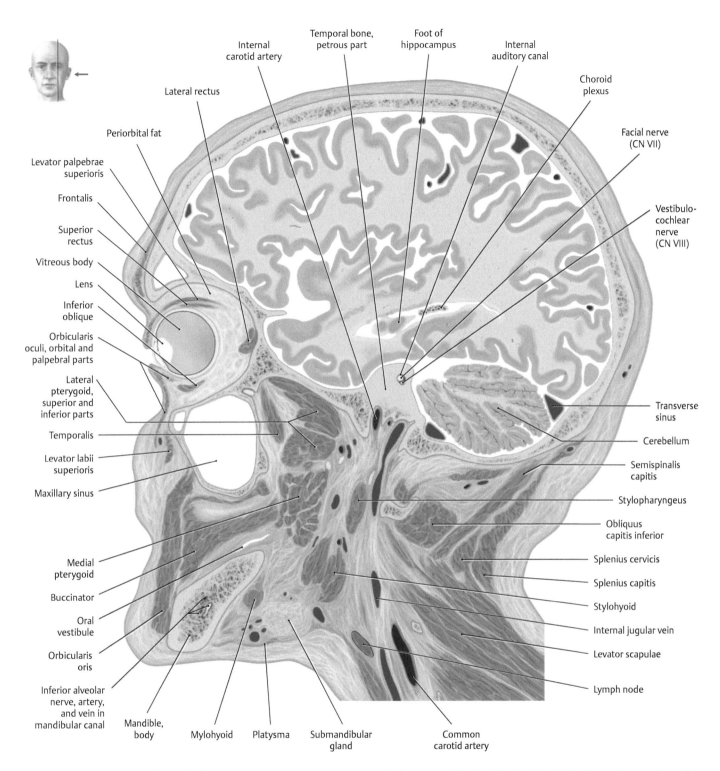

Fig. 14.36 Sagittal section through the approximate center of the orbit

Left lateral view. Due to the obliquity of this section, the dominant structure in the oral floor region is the mandible, whereas the oral vestibule appears as a narrow slit. The buccal and masticatory muscles are prominently displayed. Much of the orbit is occupied by the eyeball, which appears in longitudinal section. Aside from a few sections of the extraocular muscles, the orbit in this plane is filled with periorbital fat. Both the internal carotid artery and the internal jugular vein are demonstrated. Except for the foot of the hippocampus, the only visible cerebral structures are the white matter and cortex. The facial nerve and vestibulocochlear nerve can be identified in the internal auditory canal.

405

Sagittal MRIs of the Head

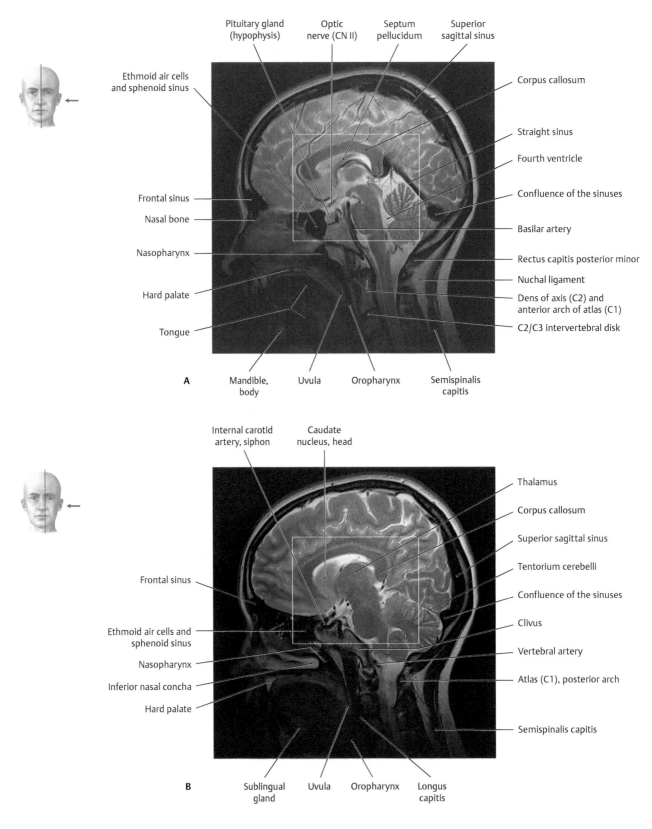

Fig. 14.37 Sagittal sections through the nasal cavity
Left lateral view. **A** Midsagittal section through nasal septum. **B** Para-sagittal section through inferior and middle nasal conchae. These sections demonstrate the relationship of the nasopharynx to the oro-pharynx. The optic nerve (CN II) is visible as the optic chiasm in **A**. The pituitary gland (hypophysis) can be seen inferior to it, just posterior to the sphenoid sinus. The siphon of the internal carotid artery is beautifully displayed in **B**.

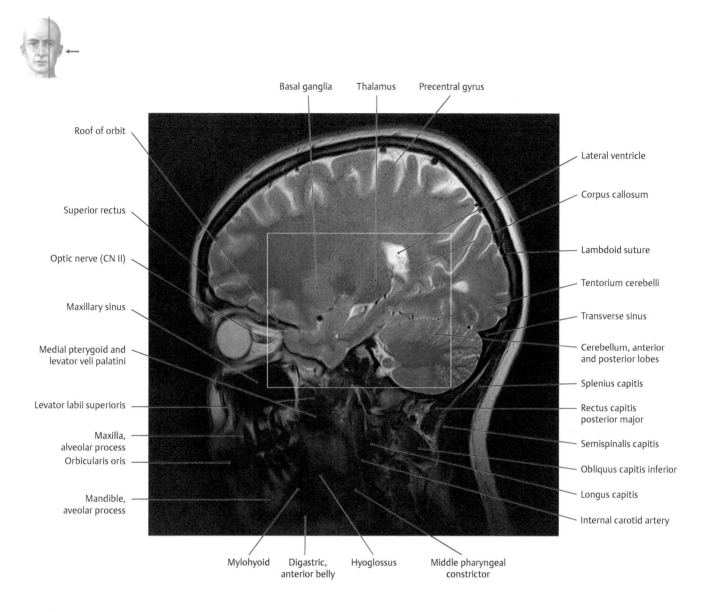

Basal ganglia   **Thalamus**   **Precentral gyrus**

Roof of orbit

Superior rectus

Optic nerve (CN II)

Maxillary sinus

Medial pterygoid and
levator veli palatini

Levator labii superioris

Maxilla,
alveolar process

Orbicularis oris

Mandible,
aveolar process

Lateral ventricle

Corpus callosum

Lambdoid suture

Tentorium cerebelli

Transverse sinus

Cerebellum, anterior
and posterior lobes

Splenius capitis

Rectus capitis
posterior major

Semispinalis capitis

Obliquus capitis inferior

Longus capitis

Internal carotid artery

Mylohyoid   Digastric,   Hyoglossus   Middle pharyngeal
anterior belly   constrictor

Fig. 14.38 **Parasagittal section through the orbit**
Left lateral view. This view exposes the superior and inferior rectus
muscles within the periorbital fat. The course of the optic nerve (CN II)
within the orbit can be seen. Note the proximity of the maxillary teeth
to the maxillary sinus. Roots of the maxillary teeth may erupt into the
maxillary sinus.

Sagittal MRIs of the Neck

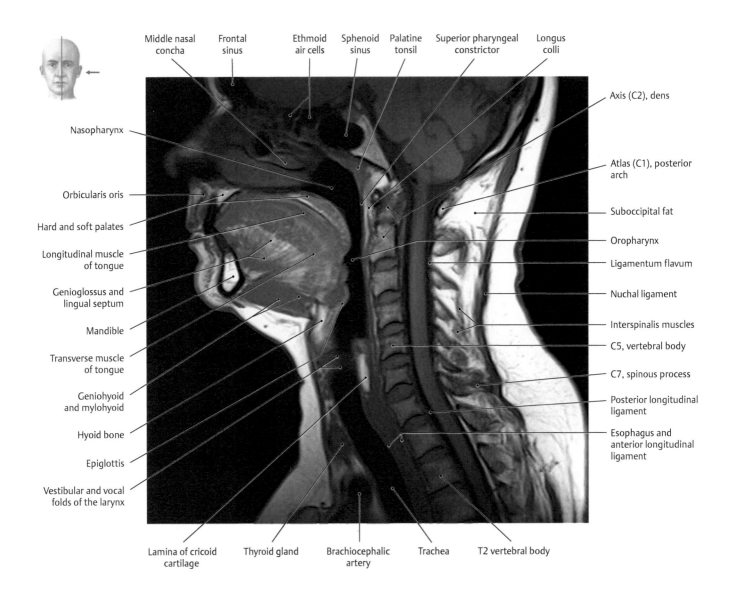

Middle nasal concha · Frontal sinus · Ethmoid air cells · Sphenoid sinus · Palatine tonsil · Superior pharyngeal constrictor · Longus colli

Nasopharynx

Orbicularis oris

Hard and soft palates

Longitudinal muscle of tongue

Genioglossus and lingual septum

Mandible

Transverse muscle of tongue

Geniohyoid and mylohyoid

Hyoid bone

Epiglottis

Vestibular and vocal folds of the larynx

Axis (C2), dens

Atlas (C1), posterior arch

Suboccipital fat

Oropharynx

Ligamentum flavum

Nuchal ligament

Interspinalis muscles

C5, vertebral body

C7, spinous process

Posterior longitudinal ligament

Esophagus and anterior longitudinal ligament

Lamina of cricoid cartilage · Thyroid gland · Brachiocephalic artery · Trachea · T2 vertebral body

Fig. 14.39 Midsagittal section
Left lateral view. This section illustrates the relations between the nasal cavity and ethmoid air cells. The nasal cavity communicates posteriorly (via the choanae) with the nasopharynx, which is separated from the oral cavity by the soft palate and uvula. Inferior to the uvula, the naso-pharynx and oral cavity converge in the oropharynx. Air goes anteriorly into the larynx. Food goes into the laryngopharynx, then the esophagus. Note how closely opposed the esophagus is to the anterior surface of the vertebral bodies. This section also reveals the cervical vertebrae and ligaments.

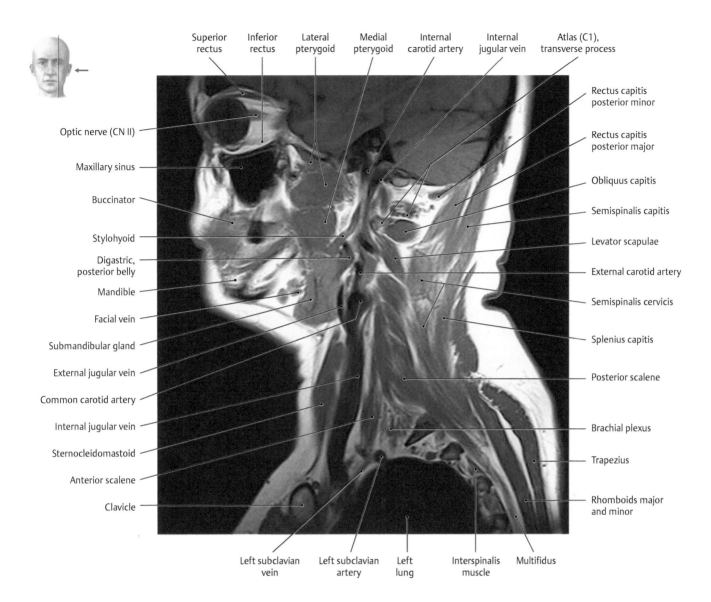

Superior rectus · Inferior rectus · Lateral pterygoid · Medial pterygoid · Internal carotid artery · Internal jugular vein · Atlas (C1), transverse process

Optic nerve (CN II)

Maxillary sinus

Buccinator

Stylohyoid

Digastric, posterior belly

Mandible

Facial vein

Submandibular gland

External jugular vein

Common carotid artery

Internal jugular vein

Sternocleidomastoid

Anterior scalene

Clavicle

Rectus capitis posterior minor

Rectus capitis posterior major

Obliquus capitis

Semispinalis capitis

Levator scapulae

External carotid artery

Semispinalis cervicis

Splenius capitis

Posterior scalene

Brachial plexus

Trapezius

Rhomboids major and minor

Left subclavian vein · Left subclavian artery · Left lung · Interspinalis muscle · Multifidus

Fig. 14.40 Sagittal section through carotid bifurcation
Left lateral view. This section shows the common and external carotid arteries, as well as the internal and external jugular veins. The cranio-vertebral joint muscles are visible along with the nuchal muscles. Note the position of the brachial plexus between the medial and posterior scalenes. The extent of the submandibular gland can be appreciated in this view.

409

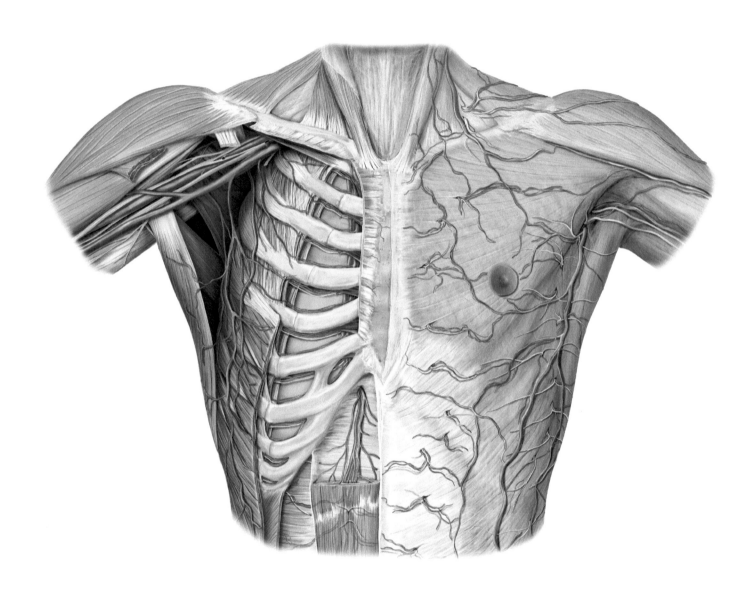

Rest of Body Anatomy

Clavicle & Scapula

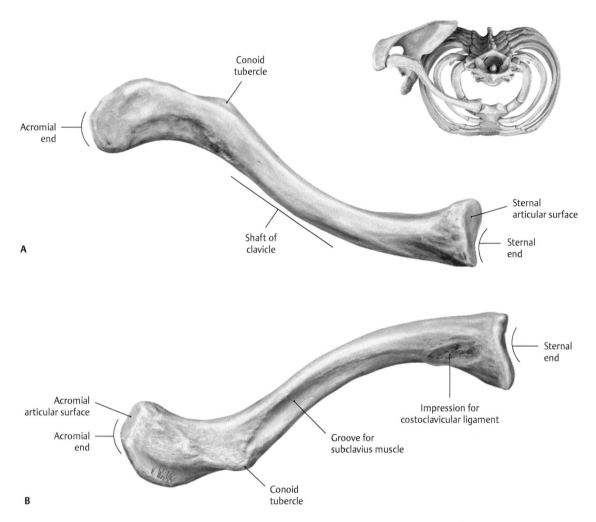

Fig. 15.1 Clavicle
Right clavicle. **A** Superior view. **B** Inferior view. The S-shaped clavicle is visible and palpable along its entire length. Its medial end articulates with the sternum at the sternoclavicular joint. Its lateral end articulates with the scapula at the acromioclavicular joint. The clavicle and scapula connect the bones of the upper limb to the thoracic cage.

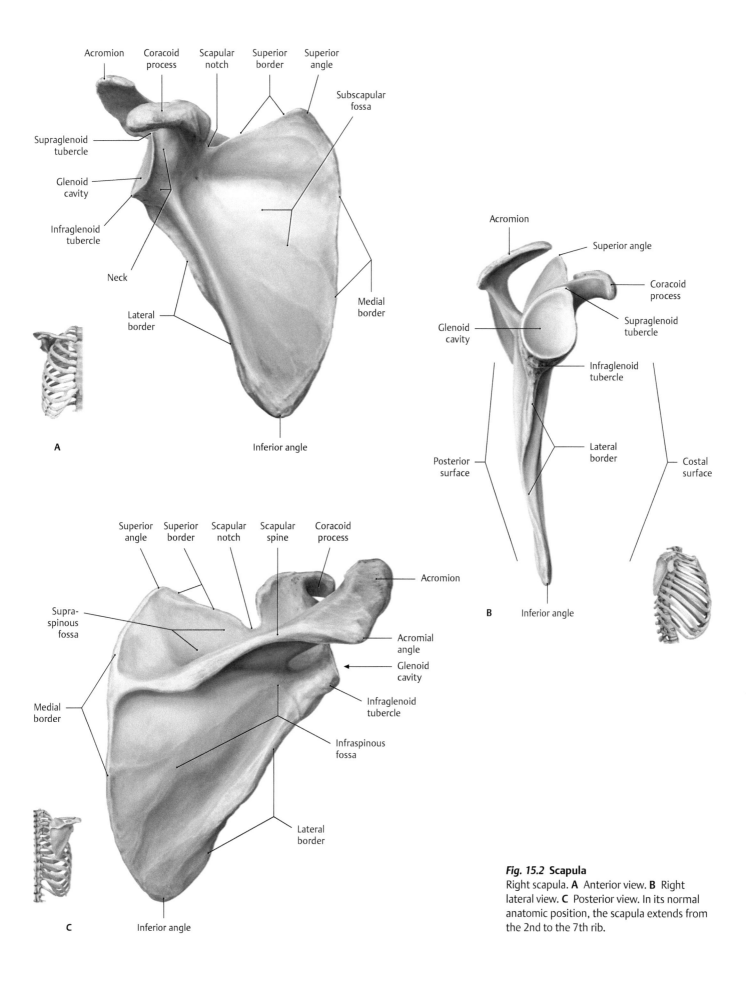

Acromion Coracoid process Scapular notch Superior border Superior angle

Subscapular fossa

Supraglenoid tubercle

Glenoid cavity

Infraglenoid tubercle

Neck

Lateral border

Medial border

A

Inferior angle

Acromion

Superior angle

Coracoid process

Glenoid cavity

Supraglenoid tubercle

Infraglenoid tubercle

Lateral border

Posterior surface

Costal surface

B Inferior angle

Superior angle Superior border Scapular notch Scapular spine Coracoid process

Acromion

Supra-spinous fossa

Acromial angle

Glenoid cavity

Medial border

Infraglenoid tubercle

Infraspinous fossa

Lateral border

C Inferior angle

***Fig. 15.2* Scapula**
Right scapula. **A** Anterior view. **B** Right lateral view. **C** Posterior view. In its normal anatomic position, the scapula extends from the 2nd to the 7th rib.

413

Humerus & Glenohumeral Joint

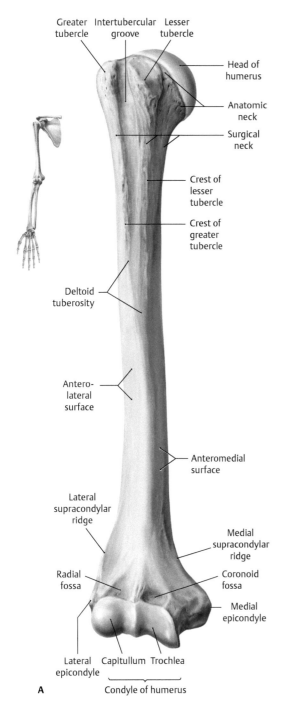

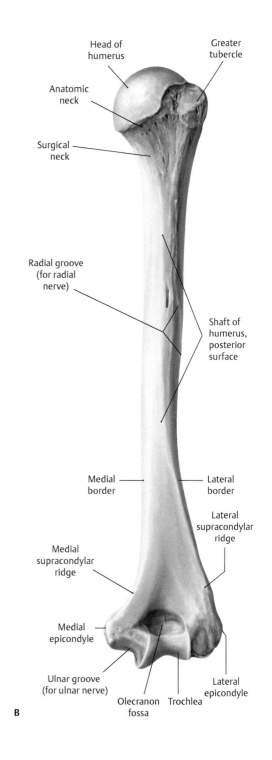

A

Greater tubercle
Intertubercular groove
Lesser tubercle
Head of humerus
Anatomic neck
Surgical neck
Crest of lesser tubercle
Crest of greater tubercle
Deltoid tuberosity
Antero-lateral surface
Anteromedial surface
Lateral supracondylar ridge
Medial supracondylar ridge
Radial fossa
Coronoid fossa
Medial epicondyle
Lateral epicondyle
Capitullum
Trochlea
Condyle of humerus

B

Head of humerus
Greater tubercle
Anatomic neck
Surgical neck
Radial groove (for radial nerve)
Shaft of humerus, posterior surface
Medial border
Lateral border
Lateral supracondylar ridge
Medial supracondylar ridge
Medial epicondyle
Ulnar groove (for ulnar nerve)
Olecranon fossa
Trochlea
Lateral epicondyle

Fig. 15.3 **Humerus**
Right humerus. **A** Anterior view. **B** Posterior view.
The head of the humerus articulates with the scapula at the gleno-humeral joint. The capitullum and trochlea of the humerus articulate with the radius and ulna, respectively, at the elbow (cubital) joint.

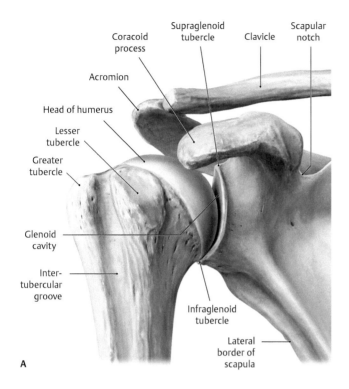

A

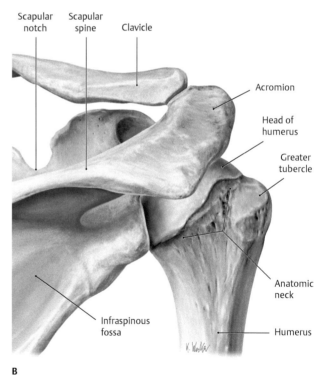

B

***Fig. 15.4* Glenohumeral joint: Bony elements**
Right shoulder. **A** Anterior view. **B** Posterior view.

Bones of Forearm, Wrist, & Hand

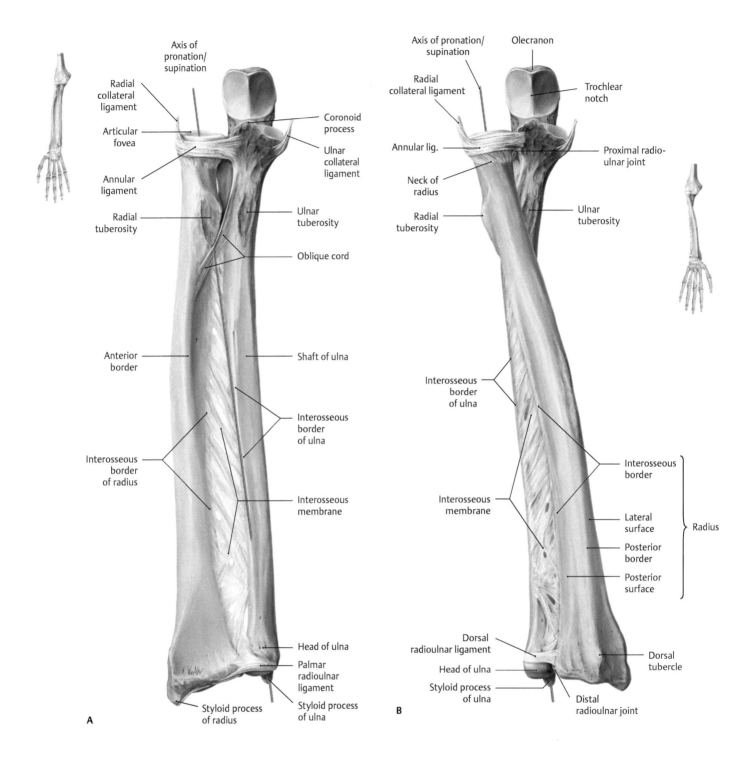

Fig. 15.5 Radius and Ulna
Right forearm, anterior view. **A** Supination. **B** Pronation.

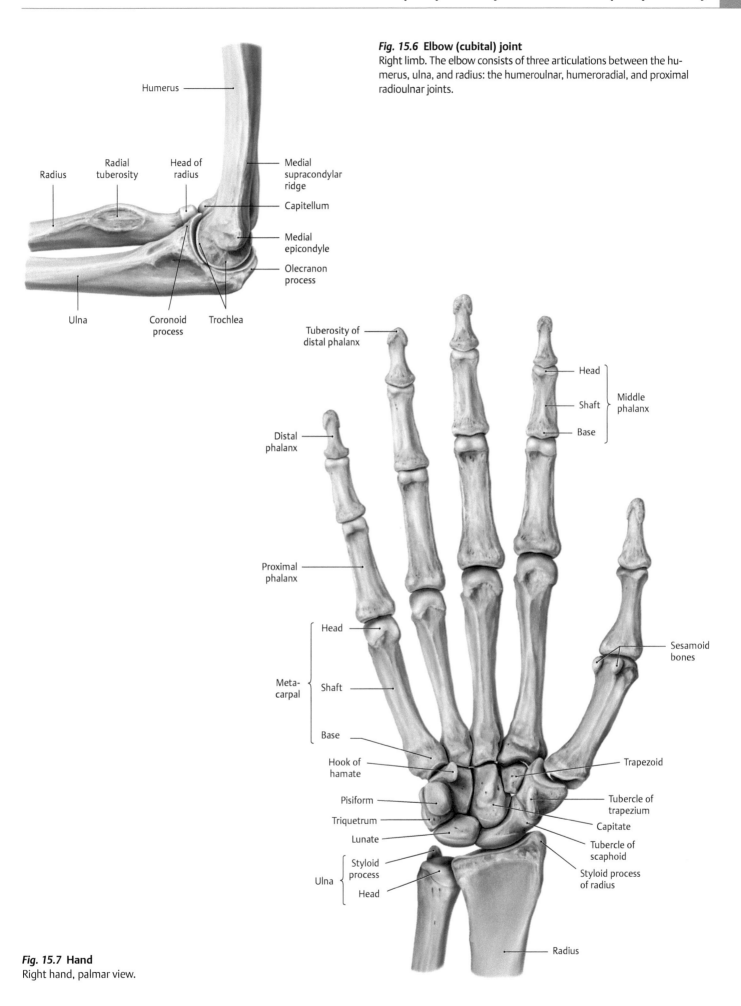

Humerus

Radius

Radial tuberosity

Head of radius

Medial supracondylar ridge

Capitellum

Medial epicondyle

Olecranon process

Ulna

Coronoid process

Trochlea

Fig. 15.6 Elbow (cubital) joint
Right limb. The elbow consists of three articulations between the humerus, ulna, and radius: the humeroulnar, humeroradial, and proximal radioulnar joints.

Tuberosity of distal phalanx

Head
Middle phalanx
Shaft
Base

Distal phalanx

Proximal phalanx

Head
Meta-carpal
Shaft
Base

Sesamoid bones

Hook of hamate

Trapezoid

Pisiform

Triquetrum

Lunate

Tubercle of trapezium

Capitate

Tubercle of scaphoid

Ulna
Styloid process
Head

Styloid process of radius

Radius

Fig. 15.7 Hand
Right hand, palmar view.

417

Muscles of the Shoulder (I)

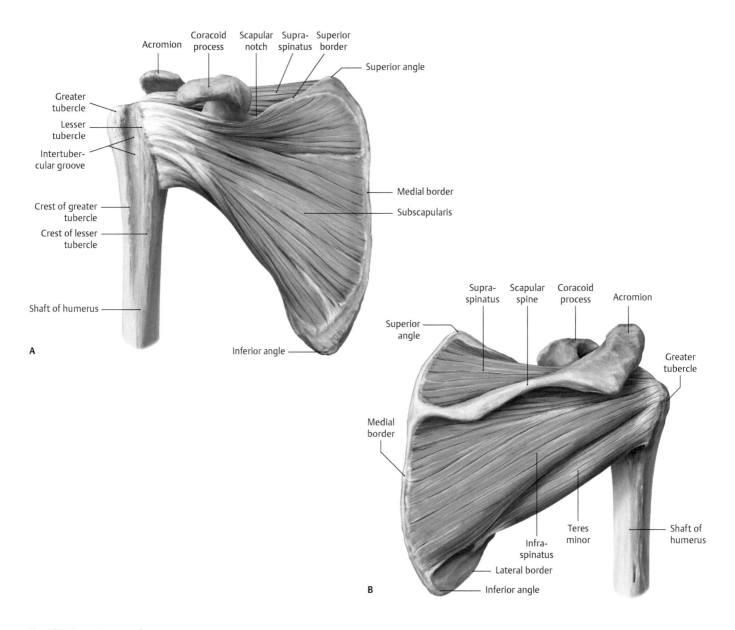

***Fig. 15.8* Serratus anterior**
Right shoulder. **A** Anterior view. **B** Posterior view.
The rotator cuff consists of four muscles: supraspinatus, infraspinatus,
teres minor, and subscapularis.

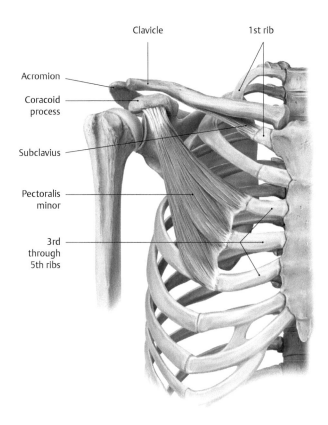

Fig. 15.9 **Subclavius and pectoralis minor**
Right side, anterior view.

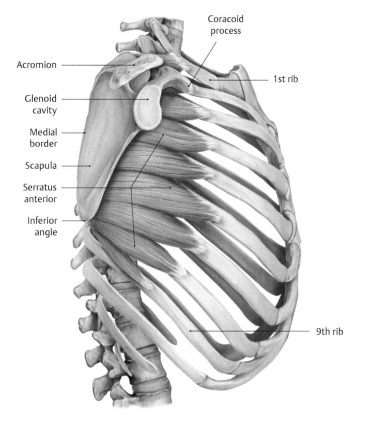

Fig. 15.10 **Serratus anterior**
Right lateral view.

Muscles of the Shoulder (II) & Arm

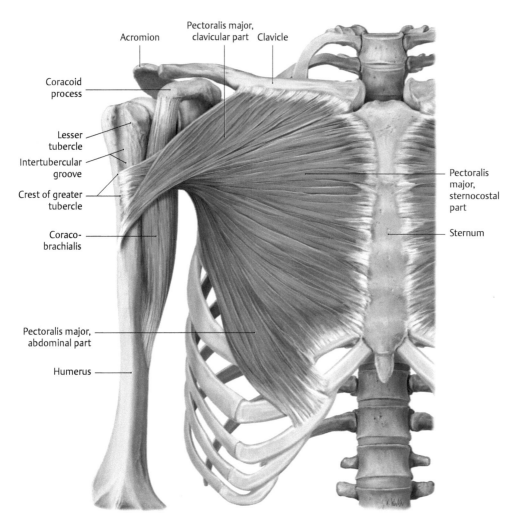

Fig. 15.11 Pectoralis major and coracobrachialis
Anterior view.

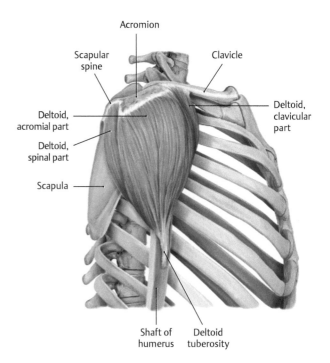

Fig. 15.12 Deltoid
Right shoulder, right lateral view.

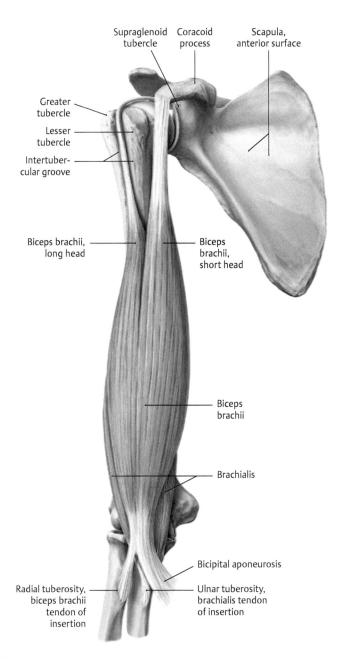

Supraglenoid tubercle

Coracoid process

Scapula, anterior surface

Greater tubercle

Lesser tubercle

Intertuber-cular groove

Biceps brachii, long head

Biceps brachii, short head

Biceps brachii

Brachialis

Bicipital aponeurosis

Radial tuberosity, biceps brachii tendon of insertion

Ulnar tuberosity, brachialis tendon of insertion

Fig. 15.13 Right shoulder, right lateral view
Right arm, anterior view.

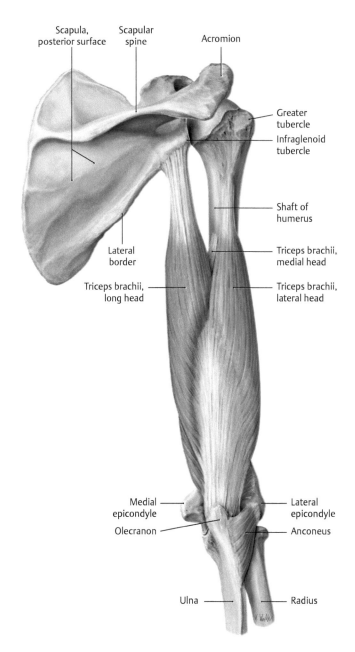

Scapula, posterior surface

Scapular spine

Acromion

Greater tubercle

Infraglenoid tubercle

Shaft of humerus

Lateral border

Triceps brachii, medial head

Triceps brachii, long head

Triceps brachii, lateral head

Medial epicondyle

Lateral epicondyle

Olecranon

Anconeus

Ulna

Radius

Fig. 15.14 Triceps brachii and anconeus
Right arm, posterior view.

421

Muscles of the Forearm

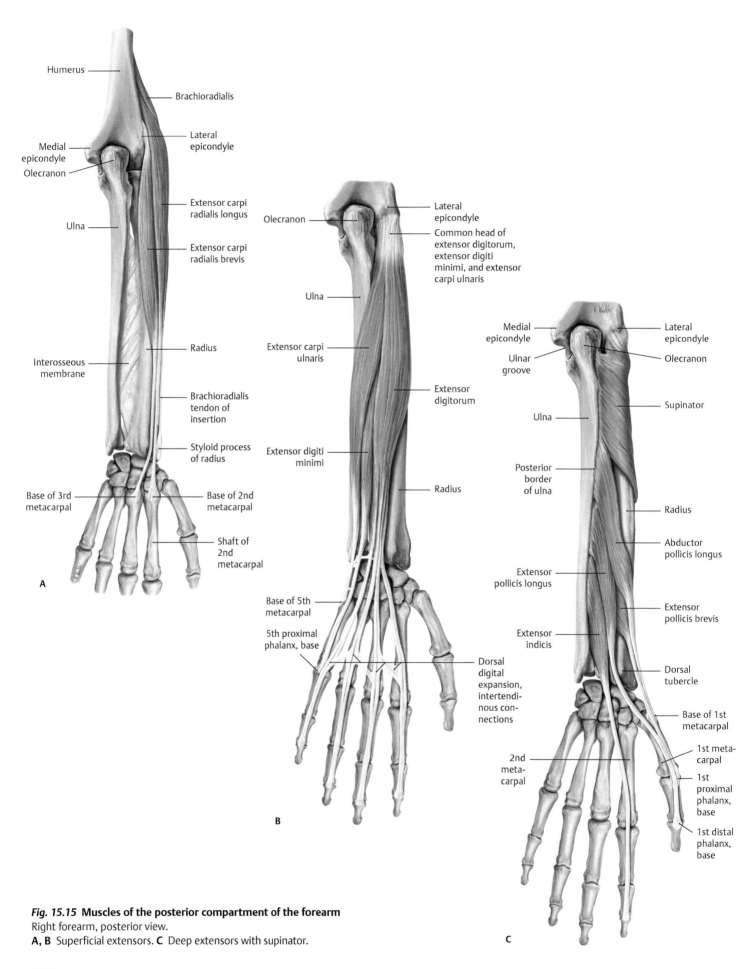

Fig. 15.15 **Muscles of the posterior compartment of the forearm**
Right forearm, posterior view.
A, B Superficial extensors. **C** Deep extensors with supinator.

422

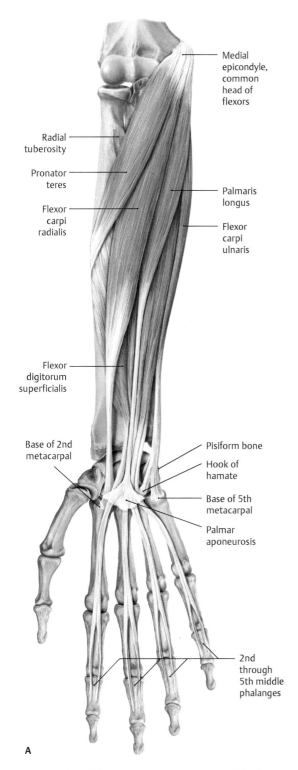

A

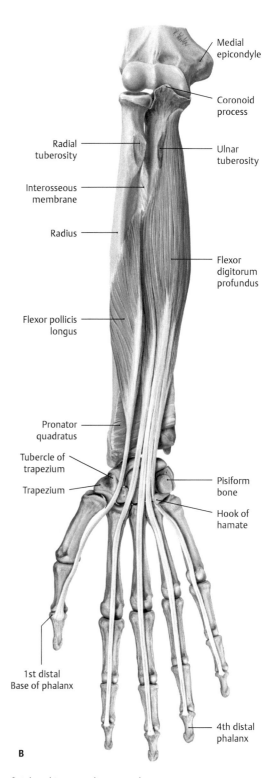

B

Fig. 15.16 **Muscles of the anterior compartment of the forearm**
Right forearm, anterior view.

A Superficial and intermediate muscles.
B Deep muscles.

Muscles of the Wrist & Hand

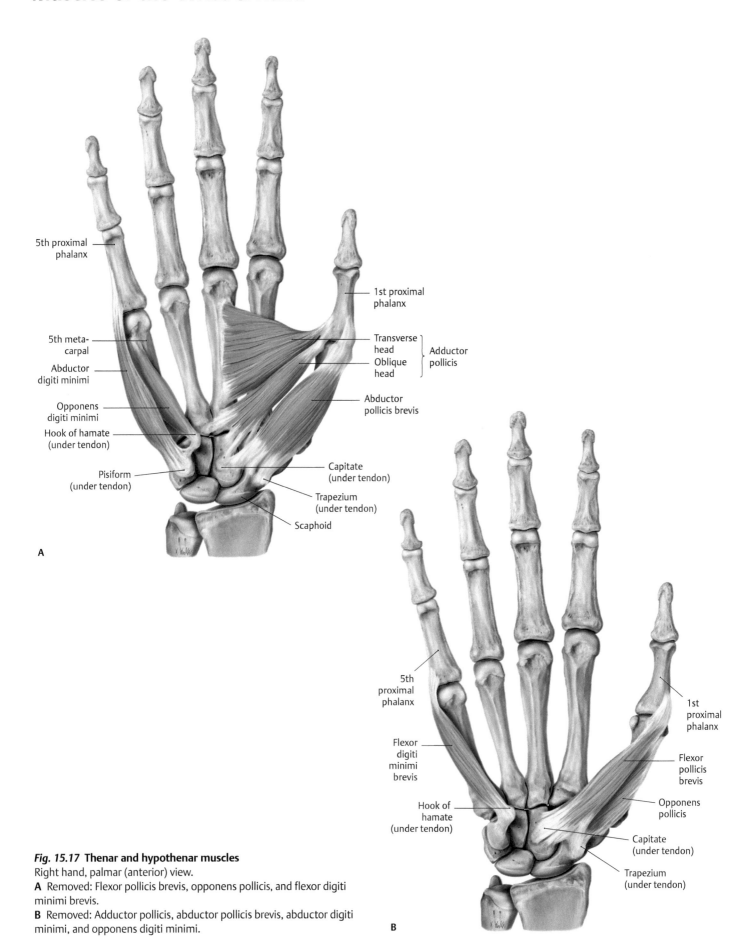

5th proximal phalanx

5th meta-carpal

Abductor digiti minimi

Opponens digiti minimi

Hook of hamate (under tendon)

Pisiform (under tendon)

1st proximal phalanx

Transverse head

Oblique head

Adductor pollicis

Abductor pollicis brevis

Capitate (under tendon)

Trapezium (under tendon)

Scaphoid

A

5th proximal phalanx

Flexor digiti minimi brevis

Hook of hamate (under tendon)

1st proximal phalanx

Flexor pollicis brevis

Opponens pollicis

Capitate (under tendon)

Trapezium (under tendon)

B

Fig. 15.17 Thenar and hypothenar muscles
Right hand, palmar (anterior) view.
A Removed: Flexor pollicis brevis, opponens pollicis, and flexor digiti minimi brevis.
B Removed: Adductor pollicis, abductor pollicis brevis, abductor digiti minimi, and opponens digiti minimi.

424

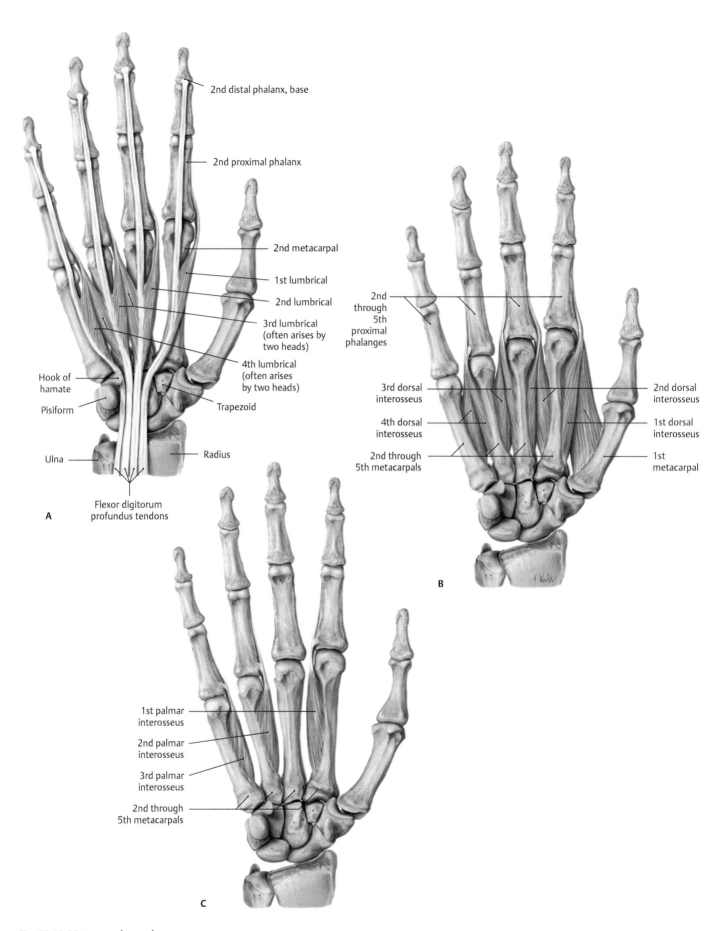

2nd distal phalanx, base

2nd proximal phalanx

2nd metacarpal

1st lumbrical

2nd lumbrical

3rd lumbrical
(often arises by
two heads)

4th lumbrical
(often arises
by two heads)

Hook of
hamate

Pisiform

Trapezoid

Ulna

Radius

Flexor digitorum
profundus tendons

A

2nd
through
5th
proximal
phalanges

3rd dorsal
interosseus

4th dorsal
interosseus

2nd through
5th metacarpals

2nd dorsal
interosseus

1st dorsal
interosseus

1st
metacarpal

B

1st palmar
interosseus

2nd palmar
interosseus

3rd palmar
interosseus

2nd through
5th metacarpals

C

Fig. 15.18 **Metacarpal muscles**
Right hand, palmar (anterior) view.
A Lumbrical muscles.
B Dorsal interosseus muscles.
C Palmar interosseus muscles.

425

Arteries & Veins of the Upper Limb

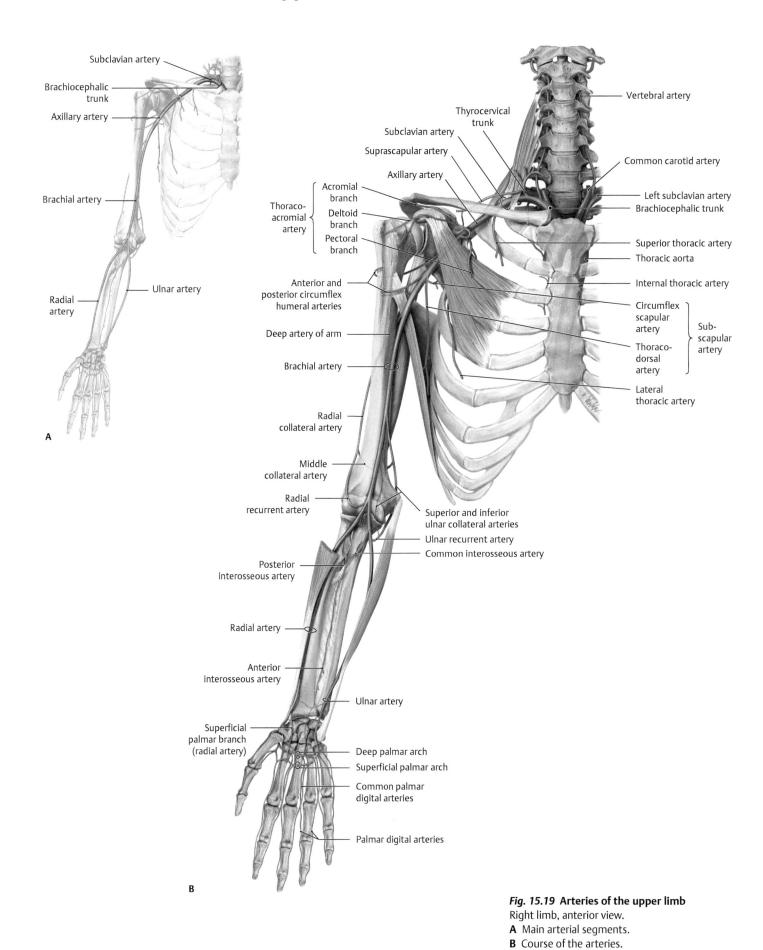

Subclavian artery
Brachiocephalic trunk
Axillary artery
Brachial artery
Ulnar artery
Radial artery

A

Thyrocervical trunk
Subclavian artery
Suprascapular artery
Axillary artery
Acromial branch
Thoraco-acromial artery — Deltoid branch
Pectoral branch
Anterior and posterior circumflex humeral arteries
Deep artery of arm
Brachial artery
Radial collateral artery
Middle collateral artery
Radial recurrent artery
Posterior interosseous artery
Radial artery
Anterior interosseous artery
Ulnar artery
Superficial palmar branch (radial artery)

Vertebral artery
Common carotid artery
Left subclavian artery
Brachiocephalic trunk
Superior thoracic artery
Thoracic aorta
Internal thoracic artery
Circumflex scapular artery
Thoraco-dorsal artery } Sub-scapular artery
Lateral thoracic artery
Superior and inferior ulnar collateral arteries
Ulnar recurrent artery
Common interosseous artery

Deep palmar arch
Superficial palmar arch
Common palmar digital arteries
Palmar digital arteries

B

Fig. 15.19 **Arteries of the upper limb**
Right limb, anterior view.
A Main arterial segments.
B Course of the arteries.

426

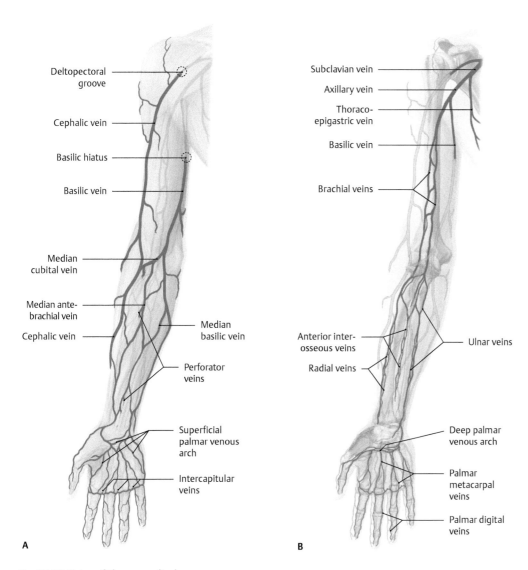

Deltopectoral groove

Cephalic vein

Basilic hiatus

Basilic vein

Median cubital vein

Median ante-brachial vein

Cephalic vein

Median basilic vein

Perforator veins

Superficial palmar venous arch

Intercapitular veins

A

Subclavian vein

Axillary vein

Thoraco-epigastric vein

Basilic vein

Brachial veins

Anterior inter-osseous veins

Radial veins

Ulnar veins

Deep palmar venous arch

Palmar metacarpal veins

Palmar digital veins

B

Fig. 15.20 Veins of the upper limb
Right limb, anterior view.
A Superficial veins.
B Deep veins.

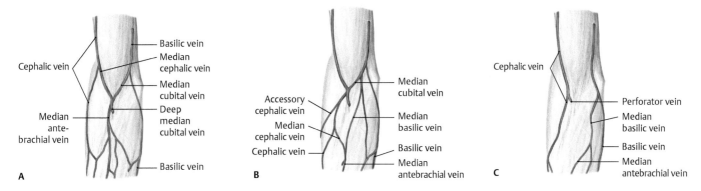

Cephalic vein

Basilic vein

Median cephalic vein

Median cubital vein

Deep median cubital vein

Median ante-brachial vein

Basilic vein

A

Accessory cephalic vein

Median cephalic vein

Cephalic vein

Median cubital vein

Median basilic vein

Basilic vein

Median antebrachial vein

B

Cephalic vein

Perforator vein

Median basilic vein

Basilic vein

Median antebrachial vein

C

Fig. 15.21 Veins of the cubital fossa
Right limb, anterior view. The subcutaneous veins of the cubital fossa
have a highly variable course.
A M-shaped.
B With accessory cephalic vein.
C Without median cubital vein.

Brachial Plexus

Almost all muscles in the upper limb are innervated by the brachial plexus, which arises from spinal cord segments C5 to T1. The anterior rami of the spinal nerves give off direct branches (supraclavicular part of the brachial plexus) and merge to form three trunks, six divisions (three anterior and three posterior), and three cords. The infraclavicular part of the brachial plexus consists of short branches that arise directly from the cords and long (terminal) branches that traverse the limb.

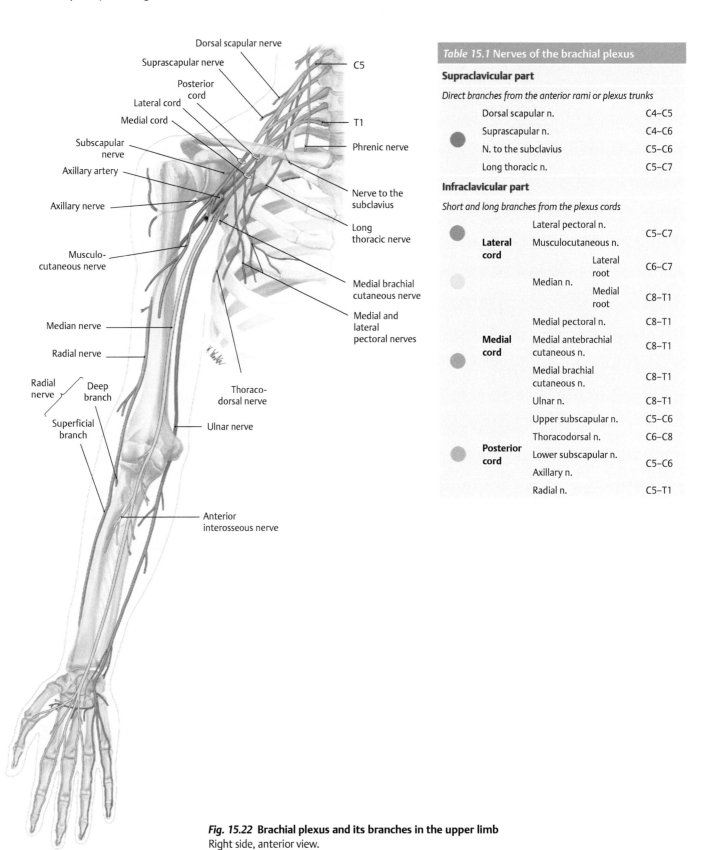

Fig. 15.22 Brachial plexus and its branches in the upper limb
Right side, anterior view.

Table 15.1 Nerves of the brachial plexus

Supraclavicular part

Direct branches from the anterior rami or plexus trunks

	Dorsal scapular n.	C4–C5
	Suprascapular n.	C4–C6
	N. to the subclavius	C5–C6
	Long thoracic n.	C5–C7

Infraclavicular part

Short and long branches from the plexus cords

Lateral cord	Lateral pectoral n.		C5–C7
	Musculocutaneous n.		
	Median n.	Lateral root	C6–C7
		Medial root	C8–T1
Medial cord	Medial pectoral n.		C8–T1
	Medial antebrachial cutaneous n.		C8–T1
	Medial brachial cutaneous n.		C8–T1
	Ulnar n.		C8–T1
Posterior cord	Upper subscapular n.		C5–C6
	Thoracodorsal n.		C6–C8
	Lower subscapular n.		C5–C6
	Axillary n.		
	Radial n.		C5–T1

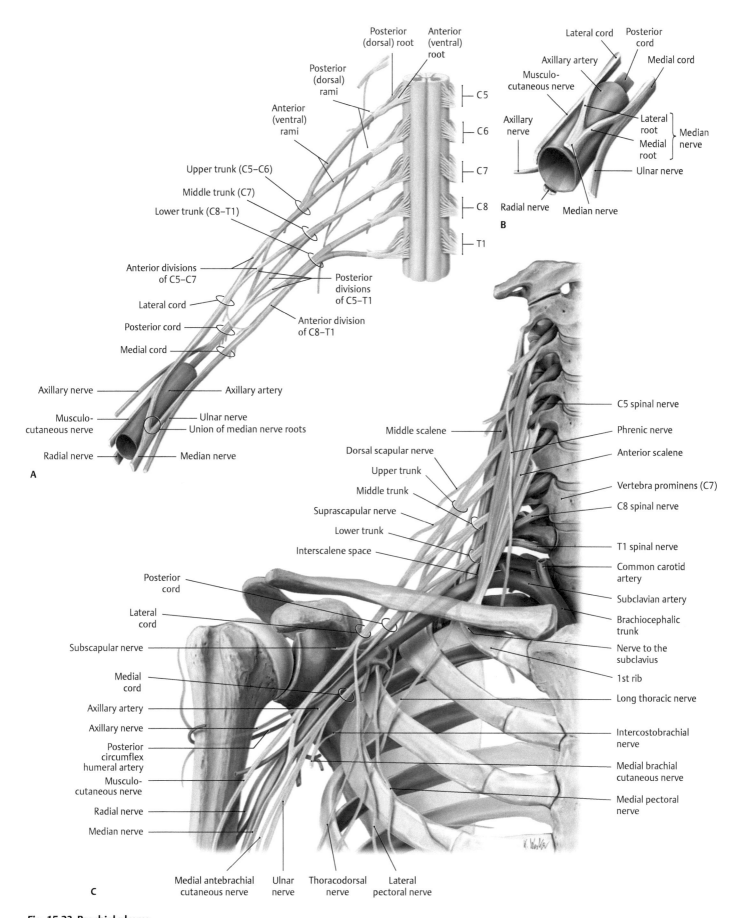

Posterior (dorsal) root

Anterior (ventral) root

Posterior (dorsal) rami

Anterior (ventral) rami

Upper trunk (C5–C6)

Middle trunk (C7)

Lower trunk (C8–T1)

Anterior divisions of C5–C7

Lateral cord

Posterior cord

Medial cord

Posterior divisions of C5–T1

Anterior division of C8–T1

C5

C6

C7

C8

T1

Axillary nerve

Musculo-cutaneous nerve

Radial nerve

Axillary artery

Ulnar nerve

Union of median nerve roots

Median nerve

A

Lateral cord

Posterior cord

Axillary artery

Musculo-cutaneous nerve

Axillary nerve

Radial nerve

Medial cord

Lateral root

Medial root

Median nerve

Ulnar nerve

Median nerve

B

Middle scalene

Dorsal scapular nerve

Upper trunk

Middle trunk

Suprascapular nerve

Lower trunk

Interscalene space

C5 spinal nerve

Phrenic nerve

Anterior scalene

Vertebra prominens (C7)

C8 spinal nerve

T1 spinal nerve

Common carotid artery

Subclavian artery

Brachiocephalic trunk

Nerve to the subclavius

1st rib

Long thoracic nerve

Intercostobrachial nerve

Medial brachial cutaneous nerve

Medial pectoral nerve

Posterior cord

Lateral cord

Subscapular nerve

Medial cord

Axillary artery

Axillary nerve

Posterior circumflex humeral artery

Musculo-cutaneous nerve

Radial nerve

Median nerve

Medial antebrachial cutaneous nerve

Ulnar nerve

Thoracodorsal nerve

Lateral pectoral nerve

C

Fig. 15.23 **Brachial plexus**

Right side, anterior view.

A Structure of the brachial plexus.

B Division of the cords into terminal branches.

C Course of the brachial plexus, stretched for clarity.

429

Thoracic Skeleton

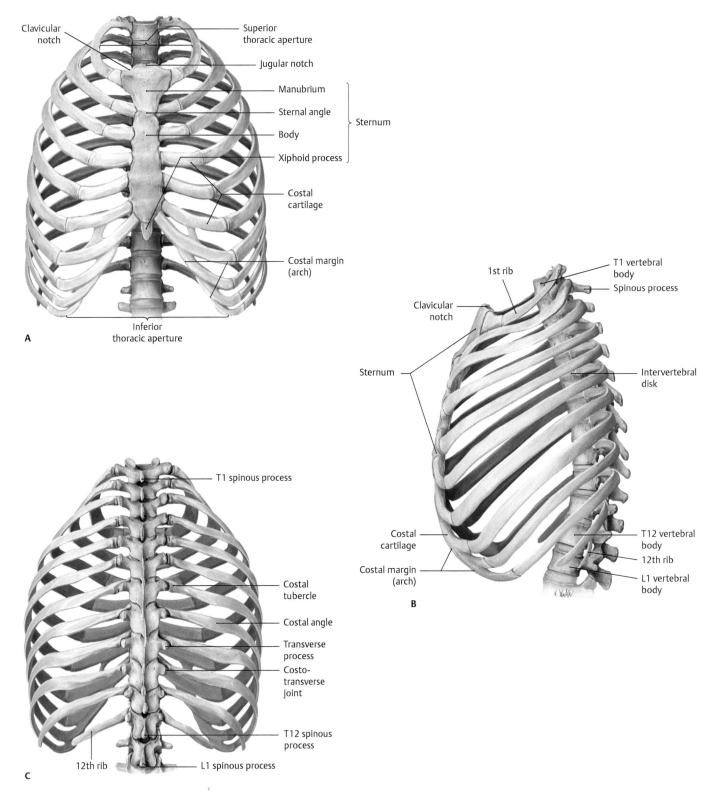

Clavicular notch
Superior thoracic aperture
Jugular notch
Manubrium
Sternal angle
Body
Xiphoid process
Sternum
Costal cartilage
Costal margin (arch)
Inferior thoracic aperture

A

1st rib
Clavicular notch
Sternum
Costal cartilage
Costal margin (arch)
T1 vertebral body
Spinous process
Intervertebral disk
T12 vertebral body
12th rib
L1 vertebral body

B

T1 spinous process
Costal tubercle
Costal angle
Transverse process
Costo-transverse joint
T12 spinous process
12th rib
L1 spinous process

C

***Fig. 15.24* Thoracic skeleton**
A Anterior view. **B** Left lateral view.
C Posterior view.

430

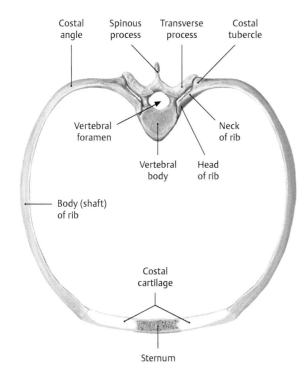

Fig. 15.25 Structure of a thoracic segment
Superior view of 6th rib pair.

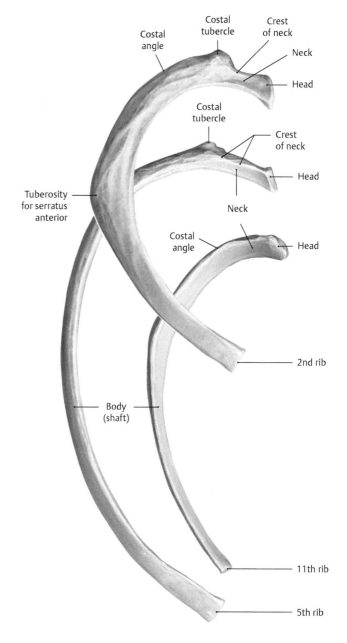

Fig. 15.26 Ribs
Right ribs, superior view.

Muscles & Neurovascular Topography of the Thoracic Wall

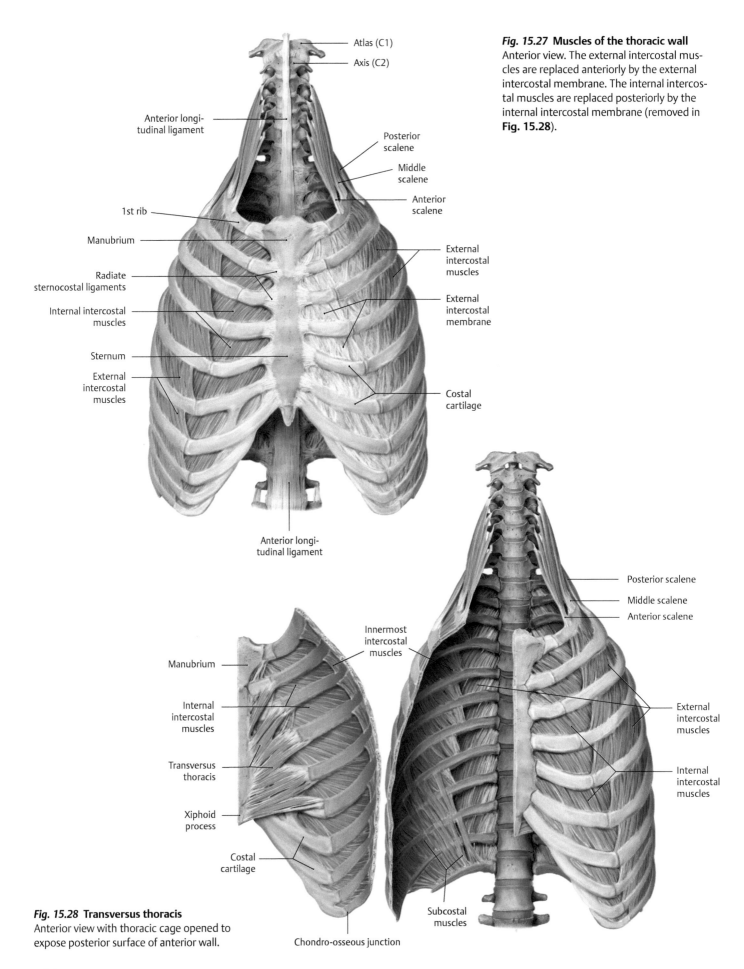

Atlas (C1)

Axis (C2)

Anterior longi-
tudinal ligament

Posterior
scalene

Middle
scalene

Anterior
scalene

1st rib

Manubrium

External
intercostal
muscles

Radiate
sternocostal ligaments

External
intercostal
membrane

Internal intercostal
muscles

Sternum

External
intercostal
muscles

Costal
cartilage

Anterior longi-
tudinal ligament

Fig. 15.27 Muscles of the thoracic wall
Anterior view. The external intercostal muscles are replaced anteriorly by the external intercostal membrane. The internal intercostal muscles are replaced posteriorly by the internal intercostal membrane (removed in **Fig. 15.28**).

Innermost
intercostal
muscles

Manubrium

Internal
intercostal
muscles

Transversus
thoracis

Xiphoid
process

Costal
cartilage

Posterior scalene

Middle scalene

Anterior scalene

External
intercostal
muscles

Internal
intercostal
muscles

Subcostal
muscles

Chondro-osseous junction

Fig. 15.28 Transversus thoracis
Anterior view with thoracic cage opened to expose posterior surface of anterior wall.

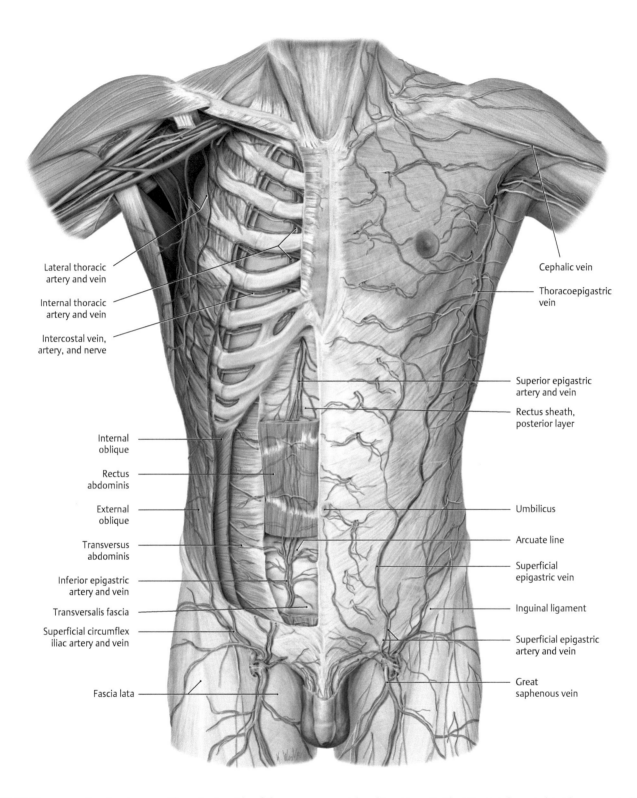

Lateral thoracic
artery and vein

Internal thoracic
artery and vein

Intercostal vein,
artery, and nerve

Internal
oblique

Rectus
abdominis

External
oblique

Transversus
abdominis

Inferior epigastric
artery and vein

Transversalis fascia

Superficial circumflex
iliac artery and vein

Fascia lata

Cephalic vein

Thoracoepigastric
vein

Superior epigastric
artery and vein

Rectus sheath,
posterior layer

Umbilicus

Arcuate line

Superficial
epigastric vein

Inguinal ligament

Superficial epigastric
artery and vein

Great
saphenous vein

Fig. 15.29 Neurovascular structures on the anterior side of the anterior trunk wall

Anterior view. The superficial (subcutaneous) neurovascular structures are demonstrated on the left side of the trunk and the deep neurovascular structures on the right side.

Removed on right side: pectoralis major and minor, external and internal obliques (partially removed), rectus abdominus (partially removed or rendered transparent). The intercostal spaces have been exposed to display the course of the intercostal vessels and nerves.

Note: The intercostal vessels run in the costal groove. From superior to inferior they are vein, artery, and nerve.

433

Female Breast

The female breast, a modified sweat gland in the subcutaneous tissue layer, consists of glandular tissue, fibrous stroma, and fat. The breast extends from the 2nd to the 6th rib and is loosely attached to the pectoral, axillary, and superficial abdominal fascia by connective tissue. The breast is additionally supported by suspensory ligaments. An extension of the breast tissue into the axilla, the axillary tail, is often present.

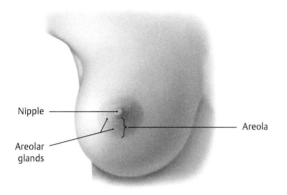

Fig. 15.30 Female breast
Right breast, anterior view.

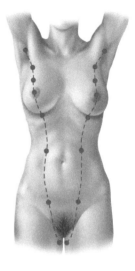

Fig. 15.31 Mammary ridges
Rudimentary mammary glands form in both sexes along the mammary ridges. Occasionally, these may persist in humans to form accessory nipples (*polythelia*), although only the thoracic pair normally remains.

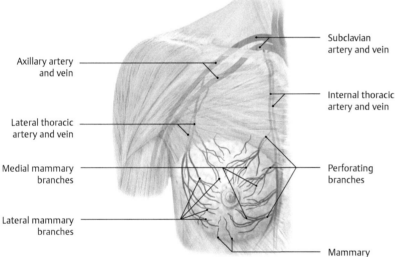

Fig. 15.32 Blood supply to the breast

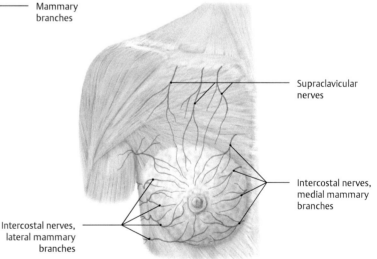

Fig. 15.33 Sensory innervation of the breast

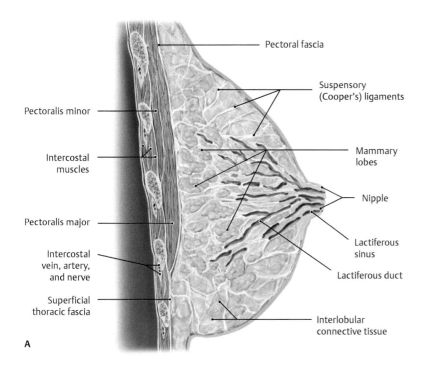

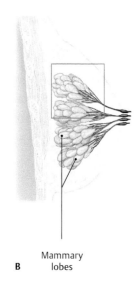

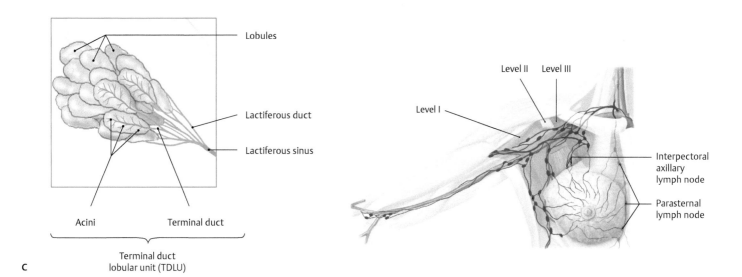

Fig. 15.34 Structures of the breast
A Sagittal section along midclavicular line. **B** Duct system and portions of a lobe, sagittal section. In the nonlactating breast (shown here), the lobules contain clusters of rudimentary acini. **C** Terminal duct lobular unit (TDLU). The clustered acini composing the lobule empty into a terminal ductule; these structures are collectively known as the TDLU.

The glandular tissue is composed of 10 to 20 individual lobes, each with its own lactiferous duct. The gland ducts open on the elevated nipple at the center of the pigmented areola. Just proximal to the duct opening is a dilated portion called the lactiferous sinus. Areolar elevations are the openings of the areolar glands (sebaceous). The glands and lactiferous ducts are surrounded by firm, fibrofatty tissue with a rich blood supply.

The most common type of breast cancer, invasive ductal carcinoma, arises from the lining of the lactiferous ducts. Typically it metastasizes through lymphatic channels, most abundantly to axillary nodes, but it may also travel to supraclavicular nodes, the contralateral breast and the abdomen. Obstruction of the lymphatic drainage and fibrosis (shortening) of the suspensory ligaments can cause a leathery (peau d' orange) and dimpled appearance of the skin. Because the intercostal veins that drain the breast communicate with the azygos system, and through that, the vertebral venous plexus, breast cancer can spread to the vertebrae, cranium and brain. Elevation of the breast with contraction of the pectoralis major muscle suggests invasion of the retromammary space.

Fig. 15.35 Lymphatic drainage of the breast
The lymphatic vessels of the breast (not shown) are divided into three systems: superficial, subcutaneous, and deep. These drain primarily into the axillary lymph nodes, which are classified based on their relationship to the pectoralis muscle as Levels I, II, and III. Level I is lateral to pectoralis major; Level II is along this muscle; Level III is medial to it. The medial portion of the breast is drained by the parasternal lymph nodes, which are associated with the internal thoracic vessels.

435

Diaphragm

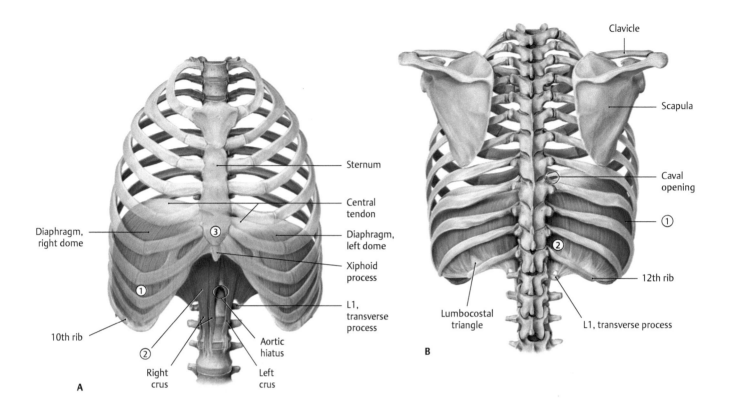

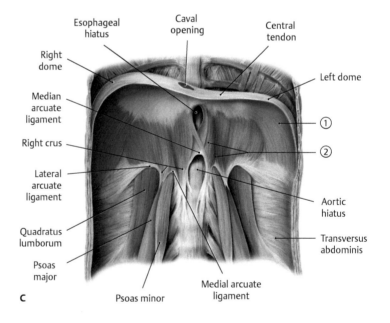

Fig. 15.36 Diaphragm
A Anterior view.
B Posterior view.
C Coronal section with diaphragm in intermediate position.
The diaphragm, which separates the thorax from the abdomen, has two asymmetric domes and three apertures (for the aorta, vena cava, and esophagus; see **C**).

Table 15.2 Diaphragm					
Muscle		**Origin**	**Insertion**	**Innervation**	**Action**
Diaphragm	① Costal part	7th to 12th ribs (inner surface; lower margin of costal arch)	Central tendon	Phrenic n. (C3–C5, cervical plexus)	Principal muscle of respiration (diaphragmatic and thoracic breathing); aids in compressing abdominal viscera (abdominal press)
	② Lumbar part	Medial part: L1–L3 vertebral bodies, intervertebral disks, and anterior longitudinal ligament as right and left crura			
		Lateral parts: lateral and medial arcuate ligaments			
	③ Sternal part	Xiphoid process (posterior surface)			

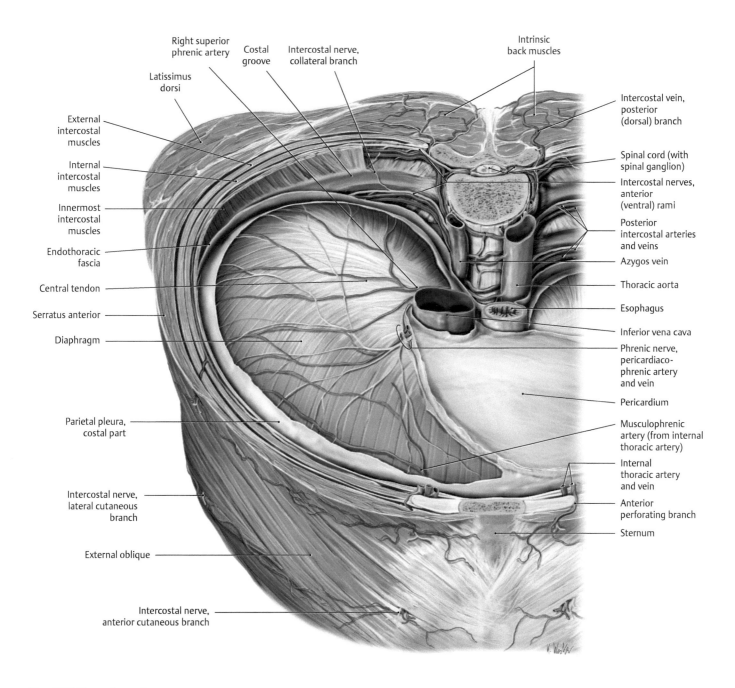

Right superior phrenic artery

Costal groove

Intercostal nerve, collateral branch

Intrinsic back muscles

Latissimus dorsi

External intercostal muscles

Internal intercostal muscles

Innermost intercostal muscles

Endothoracic fascia

Central tendon

Serratus anterior

Diaphragm

Parietal pleura, costal part

Intercostal nerve, lateral cutaneous branch

External oblique

Intercostal nerve, anterior cutaneous branch

Intercostal vein, posterior (dorsal) branch

Spinal cord (with spinal ganglion)

Intercostal nerves, anterior (ventral) rami

Posterior intercostal arteries and veins

Azygos vein

Thoracic aorta

Esophagus

Inferior vena cava

Phrenic nerve, pericardiaco-phrenic artery and vein

Pericardium

Musculophrenic artery (from internal thoracic artery)

Internal thoracic artery and vein

Anterior perforating branch

Sternum

Fig. 15.37 **Thoracic section**
Transverse section, anterosuperior view.

437

Neurovasculature of the Diaphragm

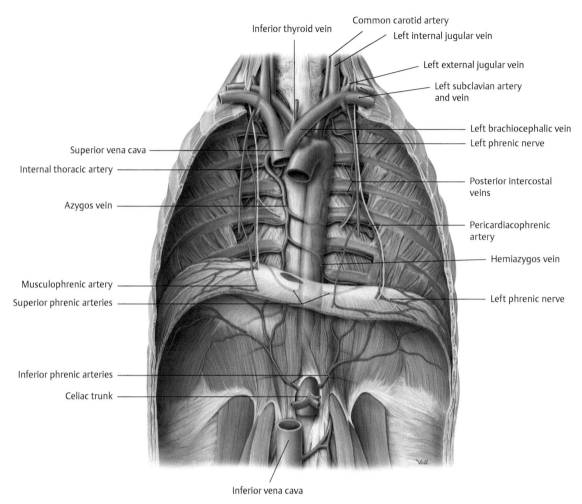

Fig. 15.38 Neurovasculature of the diaphragm
Anterior view of opened thoracic cage.

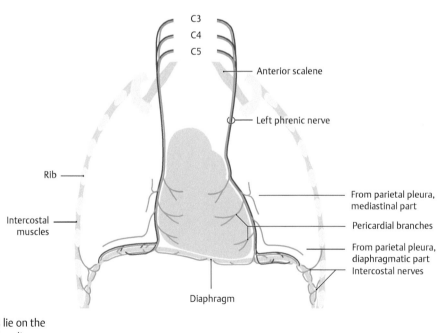

Fig. 15.39 Innervation of the diaphragm
Anterior view. The phrenic nerves lie on the lateral surfaces of the fibrous pericardium together with the pericardiacophrenic arteries and veins. Note: The phrenic nerves also innervate the pericardium.

438

Artery	Origin	Vein	Drainage
Inferior phrenic aa. (chief blood supply)	Abdominal aorta; occasionally from celiac trunk	Inferior phrenic vv.	Inferior vena cava
Superior phrenic aa.	Thoracic aorta	Superior phrenic vv.	Azygos v. (right side), hemiazygos v. (left side)
Pericardiacophrenic aa.	Internal thoracic aa.	Pericardiacophrenic vv.	Internal thoracic vv. or brachiocephalic vv.
Musculophrenic aa.		Musculophrenic vv.	Internal thoracic vv.

Table 15.3 Blood vessels of the diaphragm

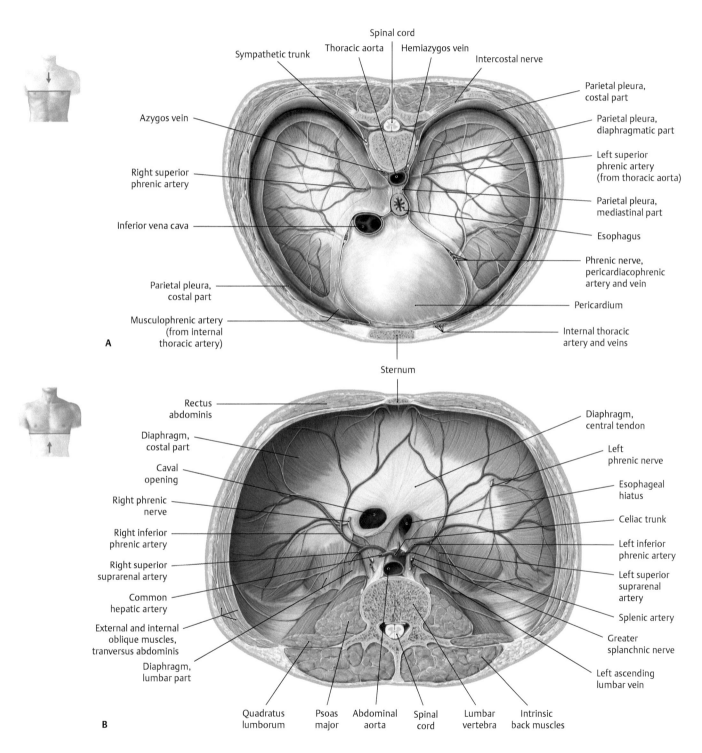

Fig. 15.40 Arteries and nerves of the diaphragm
A Superior view.
B Inferior view. *Removed:* Parietal peritoneum.
Note: The margins of the diaphragm receive sensory innervation from
the lowest intercostal nerves.

439

Divisions of the Thoracic Cavity & Lymphatics

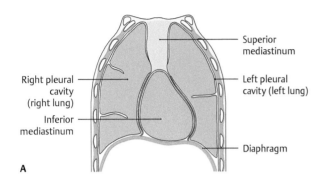

Right pleural cavity (right lung)

Superior mediastinum

Left pleural cavity (left lung)

Inferior mediastinum

Diaphragm

A

Table 15.4 Major structures of the thoracic cavity			
Mediastinum	Superior mediastinum		Thymus, great vessels, trachea, esophagus, and thoracic duct
	Inferior mediastinum	Anterior	Thymus (especially in children)
		Middle	Heart, pericardium, and roots of great vessels
		Posterior	Thoracic aorta, thoracic duct, esophagus, and azygos venous system
Pleural cavities	Right pleural cavity		Right lung
	Left pleural cavity		Left lung

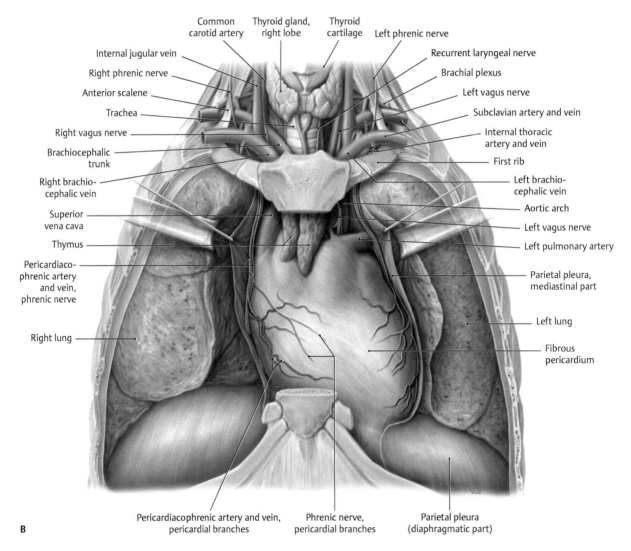

Common carotid artery

Thyroid gland, right lobe

Thyroid cartilage

Left phrenic nerve

Internal jugular vein

Right phrenic nerve

Anterior scalene

Trachea

Right vagus nerve

Brachiocephalic trunk

Right brachio-cephalic vein

Superior vena cava

Thymus

Pericardiaco-phrenic artery and vein, phrenic nerve

Right lung

Recurrent laryngeal nerve

Brachial plexus

Left vagus nerve

Subclavian artery and vein

Internal thoracic artery and vein

First rib

Left brachio-cephalic vein

Aortic arch

Left vagus nerve

Left pulmonary artery

Parietal pleura, mediastinal part

Left lung

Fibrous pericardium

B

Pericardiacophrenic artery and vein, pericardial branches

Phrenic nerve, pericardial branches

Parietal pleura (diaphragmatic part)

Fig. 15.41 Thoracic cavity

Coronal section, anterior view.

A Divisions of the thoracic cavity. The thoracic cavity is divided into three large spaces, the mediastinum (p. 446) and the two pleural cavities (p. 460).

B Opened thoracic cavity. *Removed:* Thoracic wall; connective tissue of anterior mediastinum

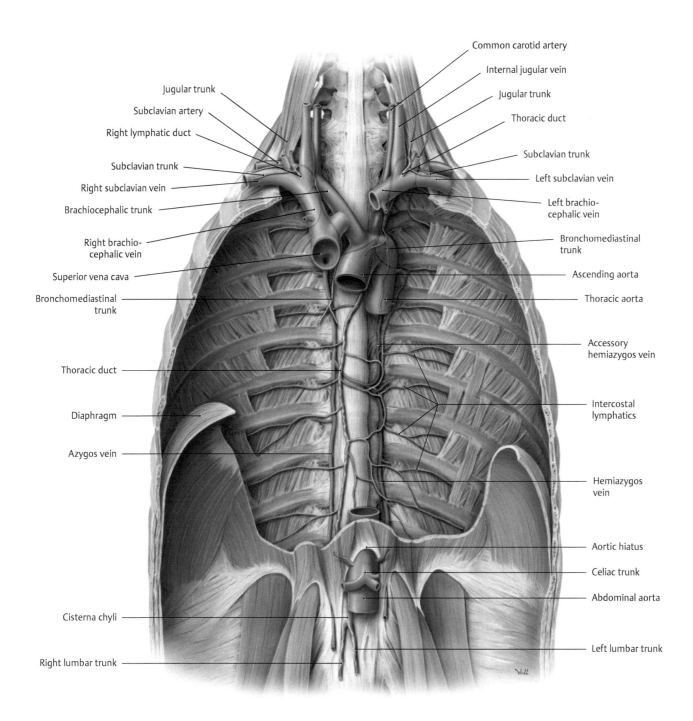

Common carotid artery

Internal jugular vein

Jugular trunk

Thoracic duct

Subclavian trunk

Left subclavian vein

Left brachio-cephalic vein

Bronchomediastinal trunk

Ascending aorta

Thoracic aorta

Accessory hemiazygos vein

Intercostal lymphatics

Hemiazygos vein

Aortic hiatus

Celiac trunk

Abdominal aorta

Left lumbar trunk

Jugular trunk

Subclavian artery

Right lymphatic duct

Subclavian trunk

Right subclavian vein

Brachiocephalic trunk

Right brachio-cephalic vein

Superior vena cava

Bronchomediastinal trunk

Thoracic duct

Diaphragm

Azygos vein

Cisterna chyli

Right lumbar trunk

Fig. 15.42 **Lymphatic trunks in the thorax**
Anterior view of opened thorax.
The body's chief lymph vessel is the thoracic duct. Beginning in the abdomen at the level of L1 as the *cisterna chyli*, the thoracic duct empties into the junction of the left internal jugular and subclavian veins. The right lymphatic duct drains to the right junction of the internal jugular and subclavian veins.

441

Thoracic Vasculature

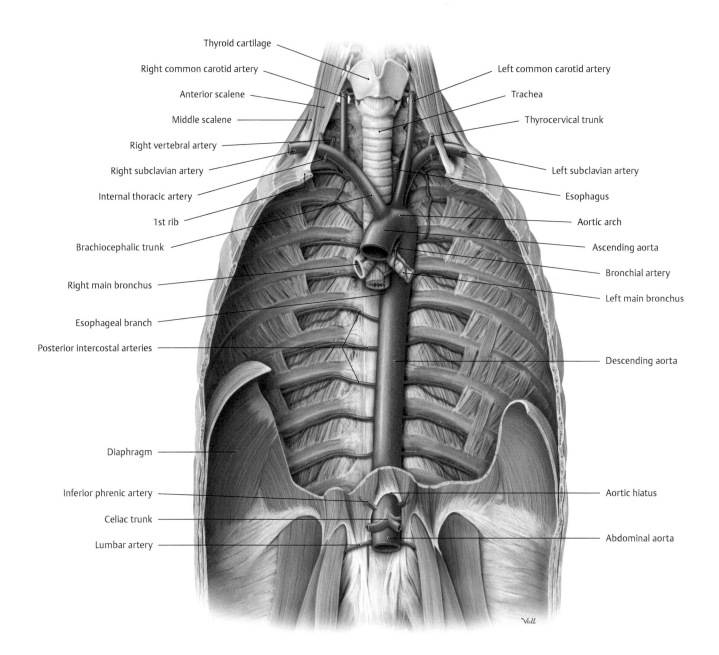

Thyroid cartilage

Right common carotid artery

Anterior scalene

Middle scalene

Right vertebral artery

Right subclavian artery

Internal thoracic artery

1st rib

Brachiocephalic trunk

Right main bronchus

Esophageal branch

Posterior intercostal arteries

Diaphragm

Inferior phrenic artery

Celiac trunk

Lumbar artery

Left common carotid artery

Trachea

Thyrocervical trunk

Left subclavian artery

Esophagus

Aortic arch

Ascending aorta

Bronchial artery

Left main bronchus

Descending aorta

Aortic hiatus

Abdominal aorta

Fig. 15.43 **Thoracic aorta in situ**
Anterior view. Removed: Heart, lungs, and portions of the diaphragm.

Table 15.5 Thoracic tributaries of the superior vena cava			
Major vein	**Tributaries**		**Region drained**
Brachiocephalic vv.	Inferior thyroid v.		Esophagus, trachea, thyroid gland
	Internal jugular vv.		
	External jugular vv.		
	Subclavian vv.		Head, neck, upper limb
	Supreme intercostal vv.		
	Pericardial vv.		
	Left superior intercostal v.		
Azygos system (left side: accessory hemiazygos v.; right side: azygos v.)	Visceral branches		Trachea, bronchi, esophagus
	Parietal branches	Posterior intercostal vv.	Inner chest wall and diaphragm
		Superior phrenic vv.	
		Right superior intercostal v.	
Internal thoracic v.	Thymic vv.		Thymus
	Mediastinal tributaries		Posterior mediastinum
	Anterior intercostal vv.		Anterior chest wall
	Pericardiacophrenic v.		Pericardium
	Musculophrenic v.		Diaphragm

Note: Structures of the superior mediastinum may also drain directly to the brachiocephalic veins via the tracheal, esophageal, and mediastinal veins.

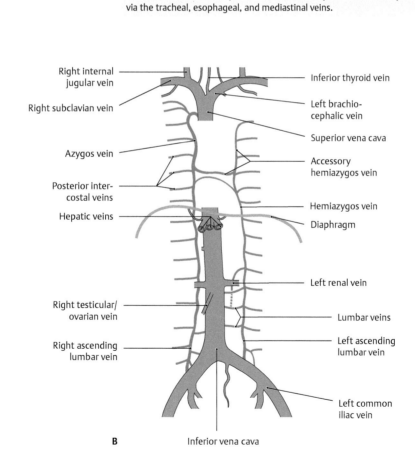

Fig. 15.44 Superior vena cava
Anterior view. **A** Projection of venae cavae onto chest. **B** Veins of the thoracic cavity.

Nerves of the Thoracic Cavity

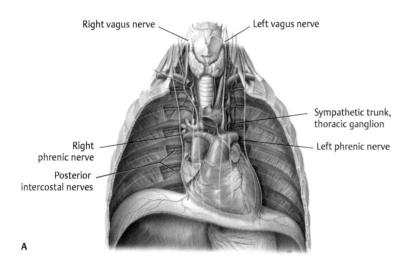

A

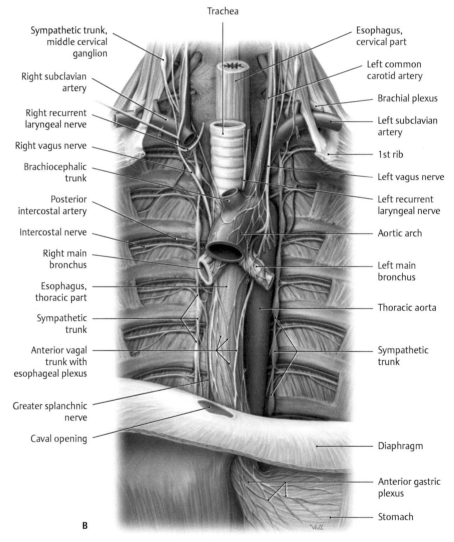

B

Fig. 15.45 Nerves in the thorax
Anterior view of opened thorax.
Thoracic innervation is mostly autonomic, arising from the paravertebral sympathetic trunks and parasympathetic vagus nerves. There are two exceptions: the phrenic nerves innervate the pericardium and diaphragm and the intercostal nerves innervate the thoracic wall.

A Thoracic innervation.
B Nerves of the thorax in situ. *Note:* The recurrent laryngeal nerves have been slightly anteriorly retracted; normally, they occupy the groove between the trachea and the esophagus, making them vulnerable during thyroid gland surgery.

444

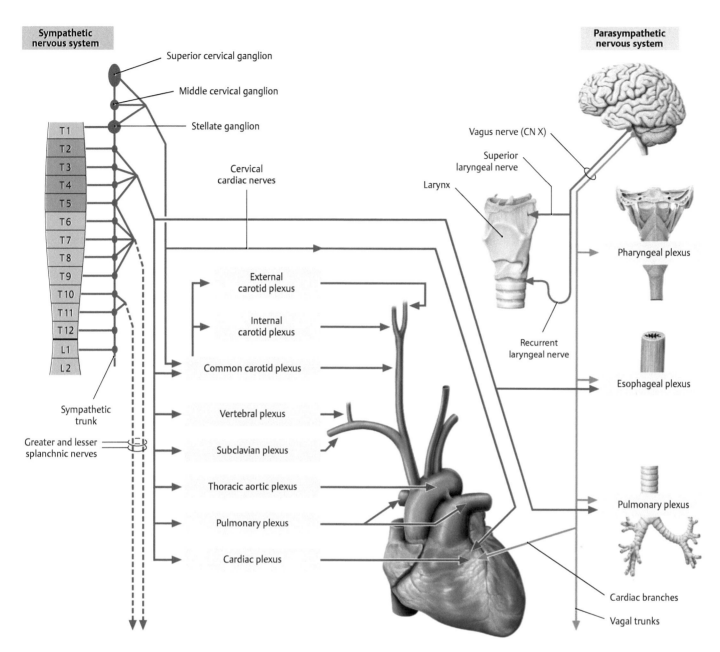

Fig. 15.46 Sympathetic and parasympathetic nervous systems in the thorax
The autonomic nervous system innervates smooth muscle, cardiac muscle, and glands. It is
subdivided into the sympathetic (red) and parasympathetic (blue) nervous systems, which
together regulate blood flow, secretions, and organ function.

Table 15.6 Peripheral sympathetic nervous system

Origin of pre-ganglionic fibers*	Ganglion cells	Course of post-ganglionic fibers	Target
Spinal cord	Sympathetic trunk	Follow intercostal nn.	Blood vessels and glands in chest wall
		Accompany intrathoracic aa.	Visceral targets

*The axons of preganglionic neurons exit the spinal cord via the anterior roots
 and synapse with *post*ganglionic neurons in the sympathetic ganglia.

Table 15.7 Peripheral parasympathetic nervous system

Origin of pre-ganglionic fibers	Course of preganglionic motor axons*		Target
Brainstem	Vagus n. (CN X)	Cardiac branches	Cardiac plexus
		Esophageal branches	Esophageal plexus
		Tracheal branches	Trachea
		Bronchial branches	Pulmonary plexus (bronchi, pulmonary vessels)

*The ganglion cells of the parasympathetic nervous system are scattered in
 microscopic groups in their target organs. The vagus nerve thus carries the
 *pre*ganglionic motor axons to these targets.
CN, cranial nerve.

445

Mediastinum: Overview

The mediastinum is the space in the thorax between the pleural sacs of the lungs. It is divided into two parts: superior and inferior. The inferior mediastinum is further divided into anterior, middle, and posterior portions. The sternal angle (the articulation between the manubrium and body of the sternum) can be used as a landmark for multiple thoracic structures. It marks the level of the division between the superior and inferior mediastinum, which passes through the level of the T4/T5 intervertebral disc. Anteriorly, the second rib attaches at this location. In addition, this is the plane at which: the arch of the aorta begins and ends, the trachea divides into primary bronchi, the pulmonary trunk divides into pulmonary arteries, the azygos vein drains into the superior vena cava, and the thoracic duct crosses the midline from right to left.

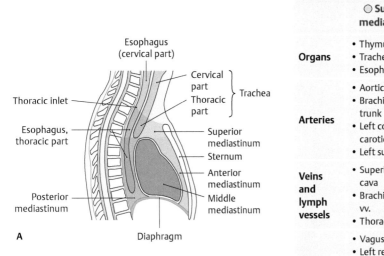

A

Table 15.8 Contents of the mediastinum

	○ **Superior mediastinum**	**Inferior mediastinum**		
		○ *Anterior*	◉ *Middle*	○ *Posterior*
Organs	• Thymus • Trachea • Esophagus	• Thymus	• Heart • Pericardium	• Esophagus
Arteries	• Aortic arch • Brachiocephalic trunk • Left common carotid a. • Left subclavian a.	• Smaller vessels	• Ascending aorta • Pulmonary trunk and branches • Pericardiacophrenic aa.	• Thoracic aorta and branches
Veins and lymph vessels	• Superior vena cava • Brachiocephalic vv. • Thoracic duct	• Smaller vessels, lymphatics, and lymph nodes	• Superior vena cava • Azygos v. • Pulmonary vv. • Pericardiacophrenic vv.	• Azygos v. • Hemiazygos v. • Thoracic duct
Nerves	• Vagus nn. • Left recurrent laryngeal n. • Cardiac nn. • Phrenic nn.	• None	• Phrenic nn.	• Vagus nn.

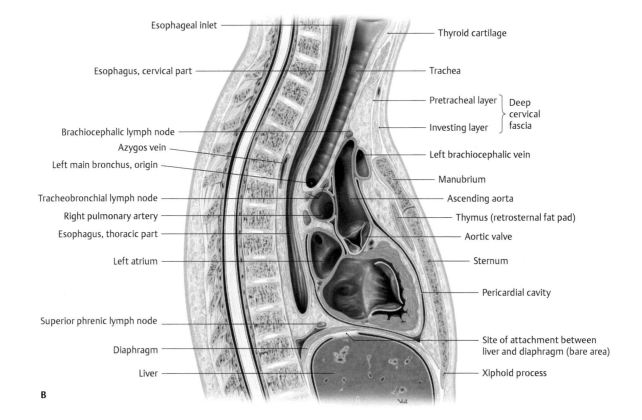

B

Fig. 15.47 Divisions of the mediastinum
A Schematic. **B** Midsagittal section, right lateral view.

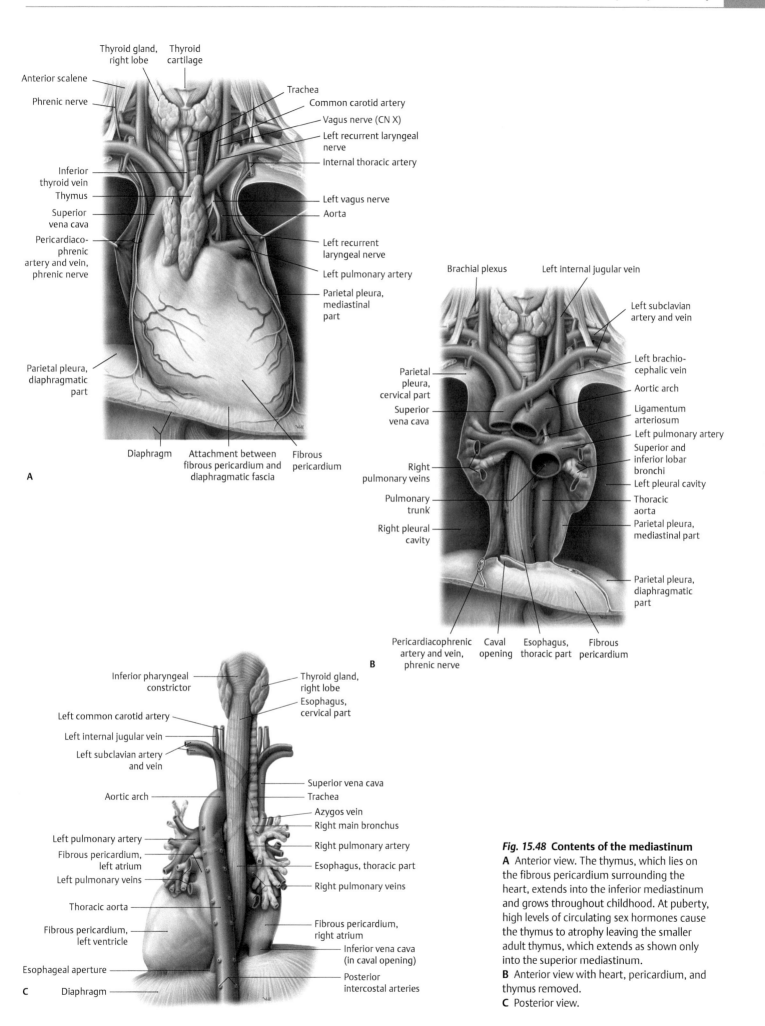

A

Thyroid gland, right lobe
Thyroid cartilage
Anterior scalene
Phrenic nerve
Trachea
Common carotid artery
Vagus nerve (CN X)
Left recurrent laryngeal nerve
Internal thoracic artery
Inferior thyroid vein
Thymus
Superior vena cava
Left vagus nerve
Aorta
Pericardiaco-phrenic artery and vein, phrenic nerve
Left recurrent laryngeal nerve
Left pulmonary artery
Parietal pleura, mediastinal part
Parietal pleura, diaphragmatic part
Diaphragm
Attachment between fibrous pericardium and diaphragmatic fascia
Fibrous pericardium

B

Brachial plexus
Left internal jugular vein
Left subclavian artery and vein
Left brachio-cephalic vein
Aortic arch
Ligamentum arteriosum
Left pulmonary artery
Superior and inferior lobar bronchi
Left pleural cavity
Thoracic aorta
Parietal pleura, mediastinal part
Parietal pleura, diaphragmatic part
Parietal pleura, cervical part
Superior vena cava
Right pulmonary veins
Pulmonary trunk
Right pleural cavity
Pericardiacophrenic artery and vein, phrenic nerve
Caval opening
Esophagus, thoracic part
Fibrous pericardium

C

Inferior pharyngeal constrictor
Thyroid gland, right lobe
Esophagus, cervical part
Left common carotid artery
Left internal jugular vein
Left subclavian artery and vein
Aortic arch
Left pulmonary artery
Fibrous pericardium, left atrium
Left pulmonary veins
Thoracic aorta
Fibrous pericardium, left ventricle
Esophageal aperture
Diaphragm
Superior vena cava
Trachea
Azygos vein
Right main bronchus
Right pulmonary artery
Esophagus, thoracic part
Right pulmonary veins
Fibrous pericardium, right atrium
Inferior vena cava (in caval opening)
Posterior intercostal arteries

Fig. 15.48 Contents of the mediastinum
A Anterior view. The thymus, which lies on the fibrous pericardium surrounding the heart, extends into the inferior mediastinum and grows throughout childhood. At puberty, high levels of circulating sex hormones cause the thymus to atrophy leaving the smaller adult thymus, which extends as shown only into the superior mediastinum.
B Anterior view with heart, pericardium, and thymus removed.
C Posterior view.

447

Mediastinum: Structures

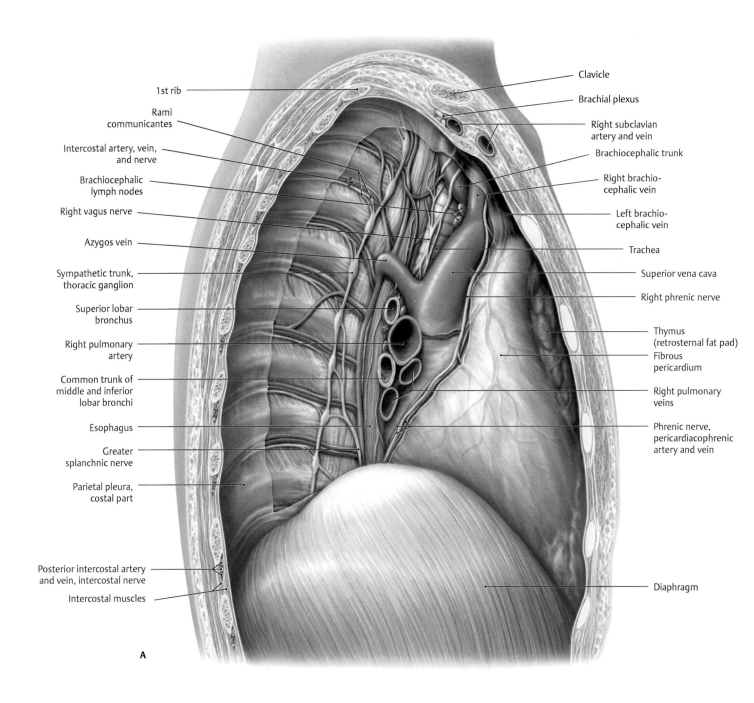

1st rib

Rami communicantes

Intercostal artery, vein, and nerve

Brachiocephalic lymph nodes

Right vagus nerve

Azygos vein

Sympathetic trunk, thoracic ganglion

Superior lobar bronchus

Right pulmonary artery

Common trunk of middle and inferior lobar bronchi

Esophagus

Greater splanchnic nerve

Parietal pleura, costal part

Posterior intercostal artery and vein, intercostal nerve

Intercostal muscles

Clavicle

Brachial plexus

Right subclavian artery and vein

Brachiocephalic trunk

Right brachiocephalic vein

Left brachiocephalic vein

Trachea

Superior vena cava

Right phrenic nerve

Thymus (retrosternal fat pad)

Fibrous pericardium

Right pulmonary veins

Phrenic nerve, pericardiacophrenic artery and vein

Diaphragm

A

Fig. 15.49 **Mediastinum**
A Right lateral view, parasagittal section. Note the many structures passing between the superior and inferior (middle and posterior) mediastinum.

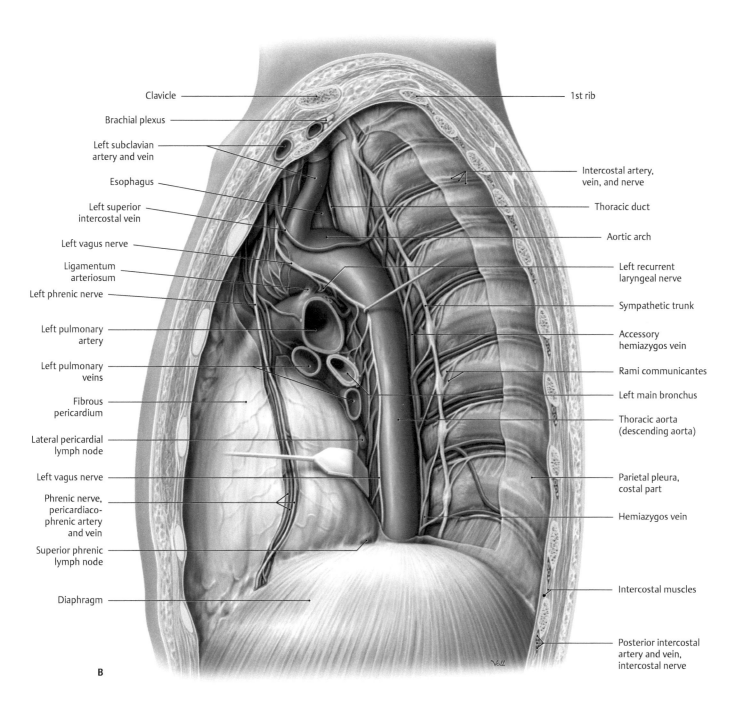

Clavicle

Brachial plexus

Left subclavian
artery and vein

Esophagus

Left superior
intercostal vein

Left vagus nerve

Ligamentum
arteriosum

Left phrenic nerve

Left pulmonary
artery

Left pulmonary
veins

Fibrous
pericardium

Lateral pericardial
lymph node

Left vagus nerve

Phrenic nerve,
pericardiaco-
phrenic artery
and vein

Superior phrenic
lymph node

Diaphragm

1st rib

Intercostal artery,
vein, and nerve

Thoracic duct

Aortic arch

Left recurrent
laryngeal nerve

Sympathetic trunk

Accessory
hemiazygos vein

Rami communicantes

Left main bronchus

Thoracic aorta
(descending aorta)

Parietal pleura,
costal part

Hemiazygos vein

Intercostal muscles

Posterior intercostal
artery and vein,
intercostal nerve

B

B Left lateral view, parasagittal section. Removed: Left lung and parietal
pleura. *Revealed:* Posterior mediastinal structures.

Heart: Surfaces & Chambers

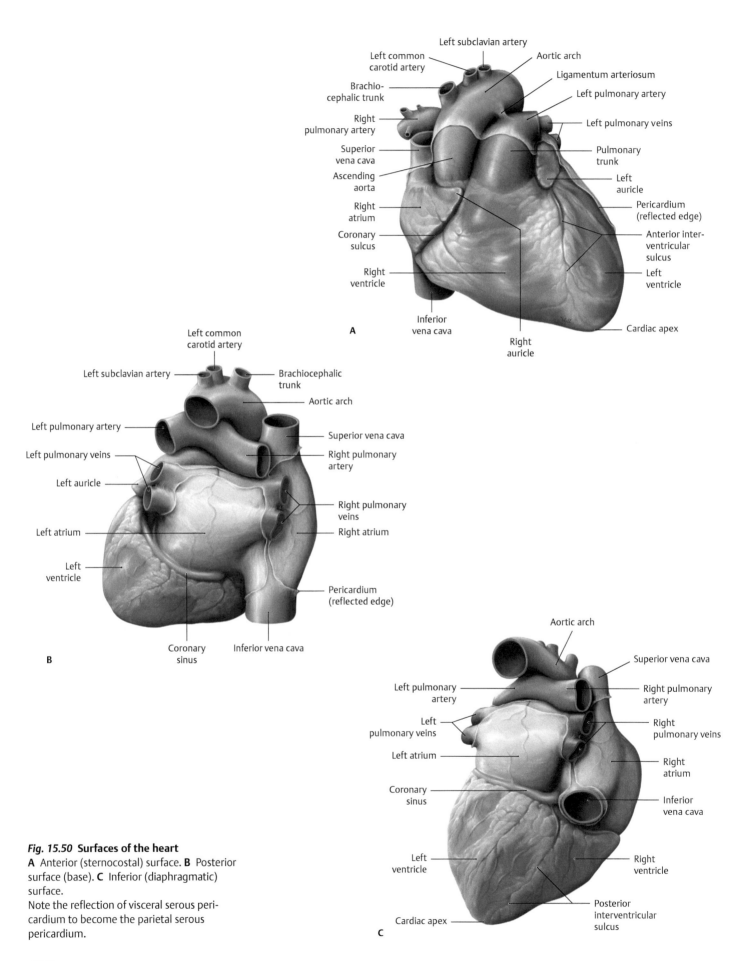

Fig. 15.50 Surfaces of the heart
A Anterior (sternocostal) surface. **B** Posterior surface (base). **C** Inferior (diaphragmatic) surface.
Note the reflection of visceral serous pericardium to become the parietal serous pericardium.

450

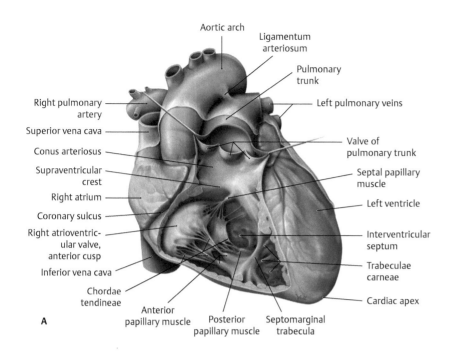

Aortic arch

Ligamentum arteriosum

Pulmonary trunk

Right pulmonary artery

Left pulmonary veins

Superior vena cava

Conus arteriosus

Valve of pulmonary trunk

Supraventricular crest

Septal papillary muscle

Right atrium

Left ventricle

Coronary sulcus

Right atrioventricular valve, anterior cusp

Interventricular septum

Inferior vena cava

Trabeculae carneae

Chordae tendineae

Cardiac apex

Anterior papillary muscle

Posterior papillary muscle

Septomarginal trabecula

A

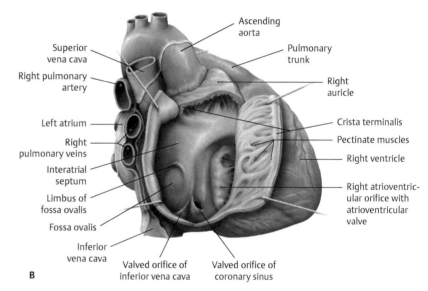

Ascending aorta

Superior vena cava

Pulmonary trunk

Right pulmonary artery

Right auricle

Left atrium

Crista terminalis

Right pulmonary veins

Pectinate muscles

Interatrial septum

Right ventricle

Limbus of fossa ovalis

Right atrioventricular orifice with atrioventricular valve

Fossa ovalis

Inferior vena cava

Valved orifice of inferior vena cava

Valved orifice of coronary sinus

B

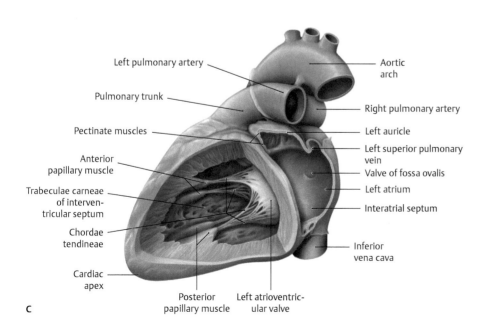

Left pulmonary artery

Aortic arch

Pulmonary trunk

Right pulmonary artery

Pectinate muscles

Left auricle

Anterior papillary muscle

Left superior pulmonary vein

Trabeculae carneae of interventricular septum

Valve of fossa ovalis

Left atrium

Chordae tendineae

Interatrial septum

Cardiac apex

Inferior vena cava

Posterior papillary muscle

Left atrioventricular valve

C

Fig. 15.51 **Chambers of the heart**
A Right ventricle, anterior view. Note the supraventricular crest, which marks the adult boundary between the embryonic ventricle and the bulbus cordis (now the conus arteriosus).
B Right atrium, right lateral view.
C Left atrium and ventricle, left lateral view. Note the irregular trabeculae carneae characteristic of the ventricular wall.

451

Heart: Valves, Arteries, & Veins

The cardiac valves are divided into two groups: semilunar and atrio-ventricular. The two semilunar valves (aortic and pulmonary), located at the base of the two great arteries of the heart, regulate passage of blood from the ventricles to the aorta and pulmonary trunk. The two atrioventricular valves (left and right) lie at the interface between the atria and ventricles.

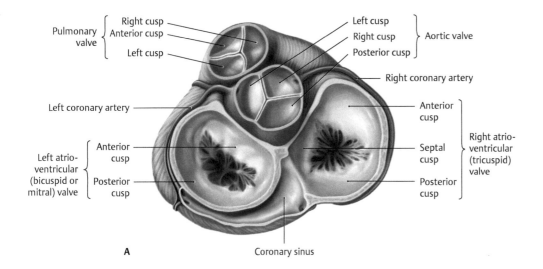

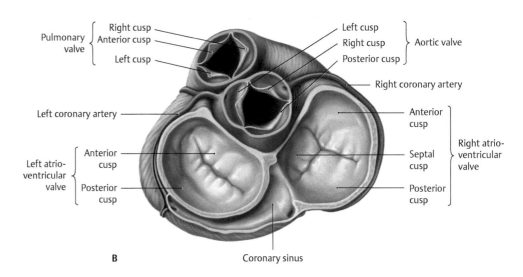

Fig. 15.52 Cardiac valves
Plane of cardiac valves, superior view. *Removed:* Atria and great arteries.
A Ventricular diastole (relaxation of the ventricles). *Closed:* Semilunar valves. *Open:* Atrioventricular valves.

B Ventricular systole (contraction of the ventricles). *Closed:* Atrioventricular valves. *Open:* Semilunar valves.

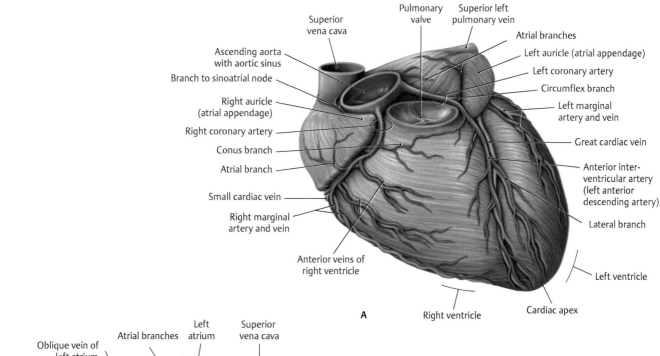

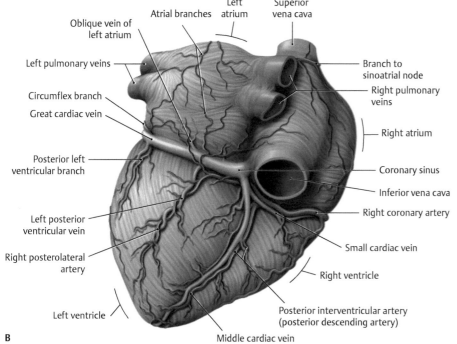

Fig. 15.53 Coronary arteries and cardiac veins

A Anterior view.

B Posteroinferior view. *Note:* The right and left coronary arteries typically anastomose posteriorly at the left atrium and ventricle.

Table 15.9 Branches of the coronary arteries	
Left coronary artery	**Right coronary artery**
Circumflex branch • Atrial branch • Left marginal a. • Posterior left ventricular branch	Branch to SA node
	Conus branch
	Atrial branch
	Right marginal a.
Anterior interventricular branch (left anterior descending) • Conus branch • Lateral branch • Interventricular septal branches	Posterior interventricular branch (posterior descending) • Interventricular septal branches
	Branch to AV node
	Right posterolateral a.

Abbreviations: AV, atrioventricular; SA, sinoatrial.

Table 15.10 Divisions of the cardiac veins		
Vein	**Tributaries**	**Drainage to**
Anterior cardiac vv. (not shown)		Right atrium
Great cardiac v.	Anterior interventricular v.	Coronary sinus
	Left marginal v.	
	Oblique v. of left atrium	
Left posterior ventricular v.		
Middle cardiac v. (posterior interventricular v.)		
Small cardiac v.	Anterior vv. of right ventricle	
	Right marginal v.	

453

Heart: Conduction & Innervation

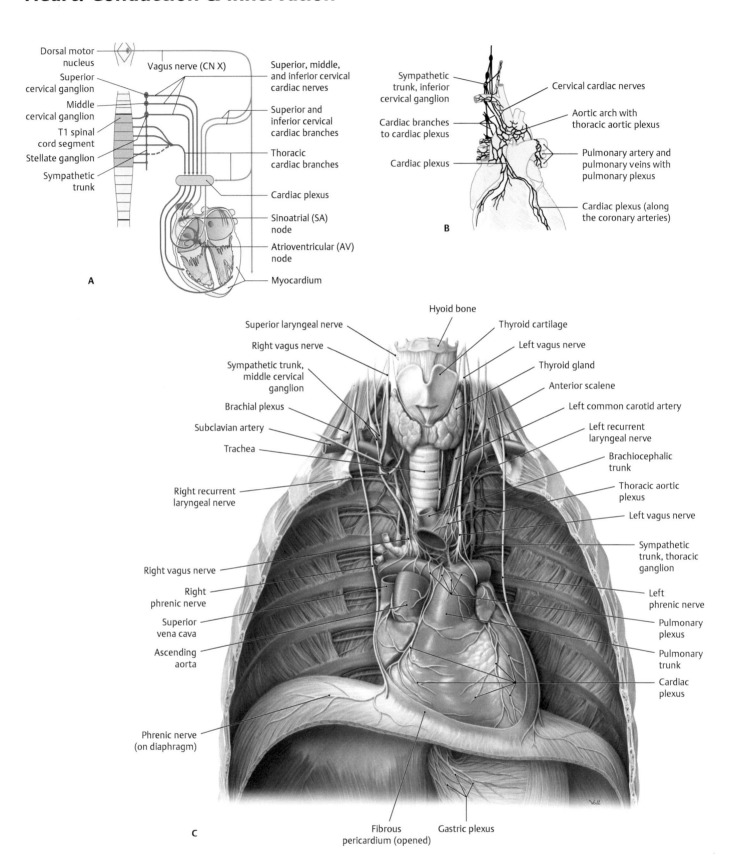

Fig. 15.54 Autonomic innervation of the heart

A Schematic. **Sympathetic innervation:** Preganglionic neurons from T1 to T6 spinal cord segments send fibers to synapse on postganglionic neurons in the cervical and upper thoracic sympathetic ganglia. The three cervical cardiac nerves and their thoracic cardiac branches contribute to the cardiac plexus. **Parasympathetic innervation:** Pregan-

glionic neurons and fibers reach the heart via cardiac branches, some of which also arise in the cervical region. They synapse on postganglionic neurons near the SA node and along the coronary arteries.
B Autonomic plexuses of the heart, right lateral view. Note the continuity between the cardiac, aortic, and pulmonary plexuses.
C Autonomic nerves of the heart. Anterior view of opened thorax.

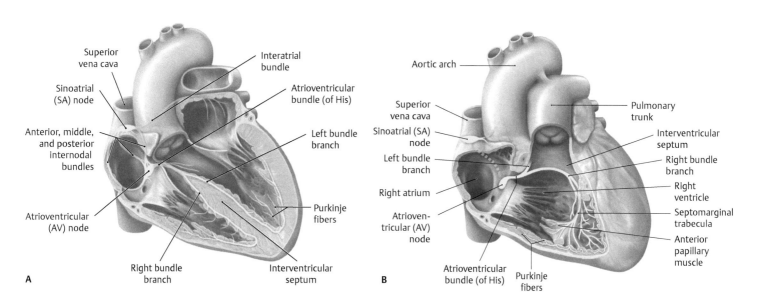

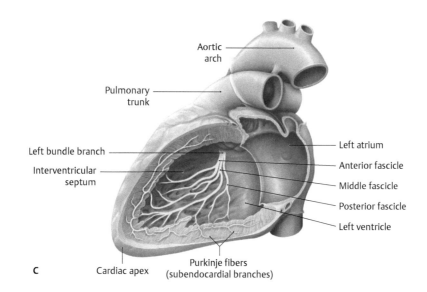

Fig. 15.55 Cardiac conduction system
A Anterior view. *Opened:* All four chambers.
B Right lateral view. *Opened:* Right atrium and ventricle.
C Left lateral view. *Opened:* Left atrium and ventricle.

Contraction of cardiac muscle is modulated by the cardiac conduction system. This system of specialized myocardial cells (Purkinje fibers) generates and conducts excitatory impulses in the heart. The conduction system contains two nodes, both located in the atria: the sinoatrial (SA) node, known as the pacemaker, and the atrioventricular (AV) node.

Pre- & Postnatal Circulation

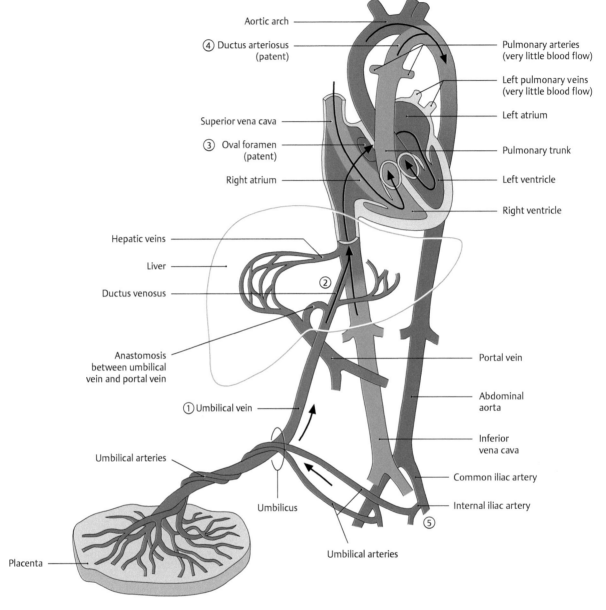

Fig. 15.56 Prenatal circulation (after Fritsch and Kühnel)

① Oxygenated and nutrient-rich fetal blood from the placenta passes to the fetus via the umbilical *vein*.

② Approximately half of this blood bypasses the liver (via the ductus venosus) and enters the inferior vena cava. The remainder enters the portal vein to supply the liver with nutrients and oxygen.

③ Blood entering the right atrium from the inferior vena cava bypasses the right ventricle (as the lungs are not yet functioning) to enter the left atrium via the oval foramen, a right-to-left shunt.

④ Blood from the superior vena cava enters the right atrium, passes to the right ventricle, and moves into the pulmonary trunk. Most of this blood enters the aorta via the ductus arteriosus, a right-to-left shunt.

⑤ The partially oxygenated blood in the aorta returns to the placenta via the paired umbilical arteries that arise from the internal iliac arteries.

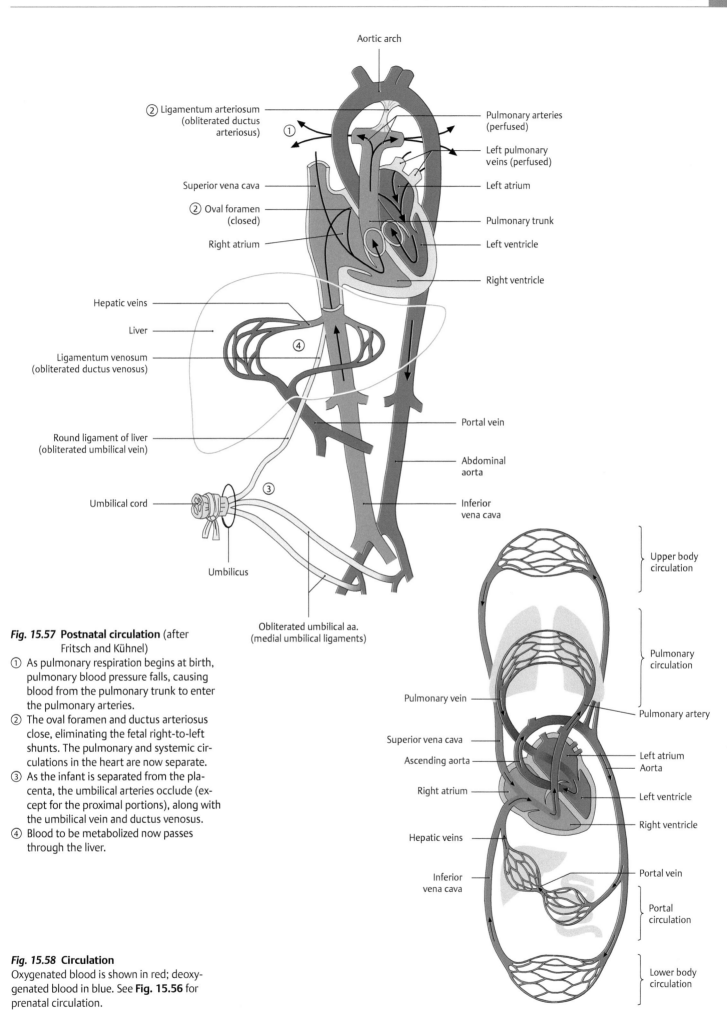

Aortic arch

② Ligamentum arteriosum
(obliterated ductus
arteriosus)

①

Pulmonary arteries
(perfused)

Left pulmonary
veins (perfused)

Superior vena cava

Left atrium

② Oval foramen
(closed)

Pulmonary trunk

Right atrium

Left ventricle

Right ventricle

Hepatic veins

Liver

④

Ligamentum venosum
(obliterated ductus venosus)

Round ligament of liver
(obliterated umbilical vein)

Portal vein

Abdominal
aorta

Umbilical cord

③

Inferior
vena cava

Umbilicus

Obliterated umbilical aa.
(medial umbilical ligaments)

***Fig. 15.57* Postnatal circulation** (after
Fritsch and Kühnel)
① As pulmonary respiration begins at birth,
pulmonary blood pressure falls, causing
blood from the pulmonary trunk to enter
the pulmonary arteries.
② The oval foramen and ductus arteriosus
close, eliminating the fetal right-to-left
shunts. The pulmonary and systemic cir-
culations in the heart are now separate.
③ As the infant is separated from the placenta, the umbilical arteries occlude (except for the proximal portions), along with
the umbilical vein and ductus venosus.
④ Blood to be metabolized now passes
through the liver.

Pulmonary vein

Upper body
circulation

Pulmonary
circulation

Pulmonary artery

Superior vena cava

Ascending aorta

Left atrium
Aorta

Right atrium

Left ventricle

Right ventricle

Hepatic veins

Portal vein

Inferior
vena cava

Portal
circulation

***Fig. 15.58* Circulation**
Oxygenated blood is shown in red; deoxy-
genated blood in blue. See **Fig. 15.56** for
prenatal circulation.

Lower body
circulation

Esophagus

The esophagus is divided into three parts: cervical (C6–T1), thoracic (T1 to the esophageal hiatus of the diaphragm), and abdominal (the diaphragm to the cardiac orifice of the stomach). It descends slightly to the right of the thoracic aorta and pierces the diaphragm slightly to the left, just below the xiphoid process of the sternum.

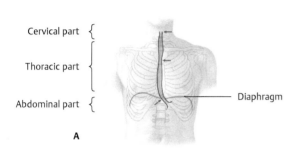

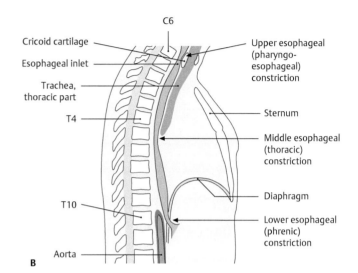

Fig. 15.59 Esophagus: Location and constrictions
A Projection of esophagus onto chest wall. Esophageal constrictions are indicated with arrows.
B Esophageal constrictions, right lateral view.

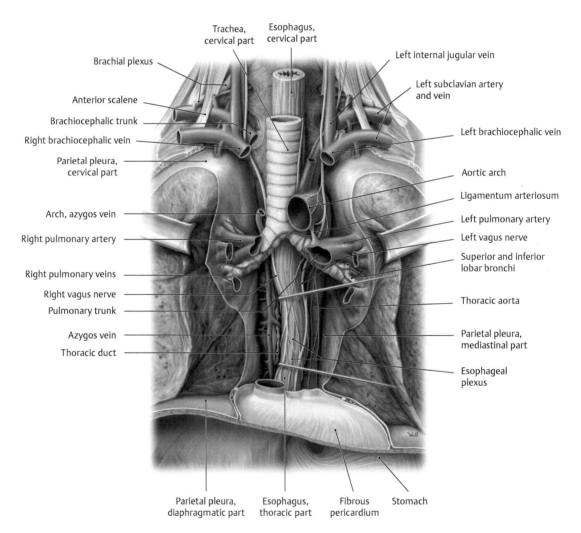

Fig. 15.60 Esophagus in situ
Anterior view.

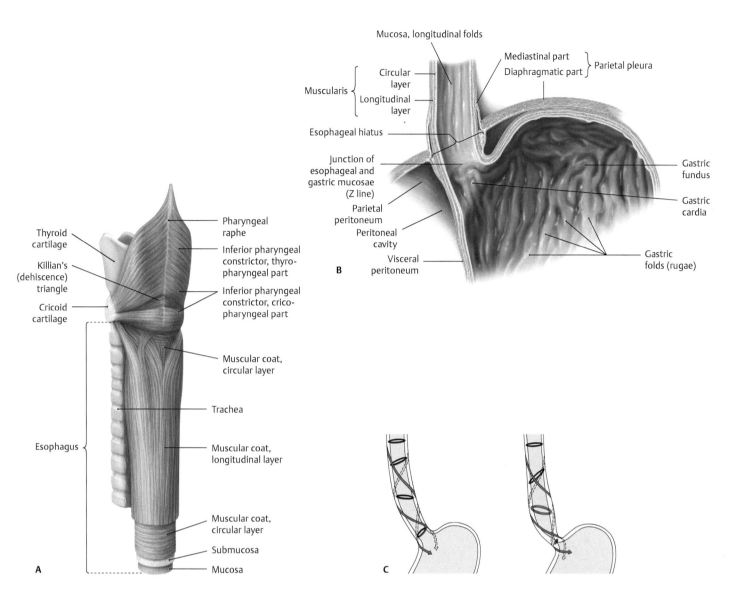

Fig. 15.61 Structure of the esophagus
A Esophageal wall, oblique left posterior view.
B Esophagogastric junction, anterior view. A true sphincter is not identifiable at this junction; instead, the diaphragmatic muscle of the esophageal hiatus functions as a sphincter. It is often referred to as the "Z line" because of its zigzag form.
C Functional architecture of esophageal muscle.

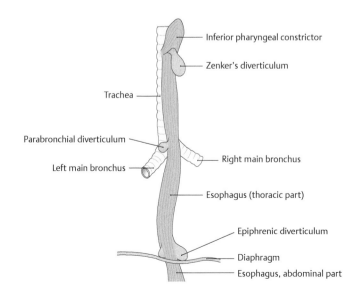

Fig. 15.62 Esophageal diverticula
Diverticula (abnormal outpouchings or sacs) generally develop at weak spots in the esophageal wall. There are three main types of esophageal diverticula:
— **Hypopharyngeal (pharyngo-esophageal) diverticula:** outpouchings occurring at the junction of the pharynx and the esophagus. These include Zenker's diverticula (70% of cases).
— **"True" traction diverticula:** protrusion of all wall layers, not typically occurring at characteristic weak spots. However, they generally result from an inflammatory process (e.g., lymphangitis) and are thus common at sites where the esophagus closely approaches the bronchi and bronchial lymph nodes (thoracic or parabronchial diverticula).
— **"False" pulsion diverticula:** herniations of the mucosa and submucosa through weak spots in the muscular coat due to a rise in esophageal pressure (e.g., during normal swallowing). These include parahiatal and epiphrenic diverticula occurring above the esophageal aperture of the diaphragm (10% of cases).

459

Pleura

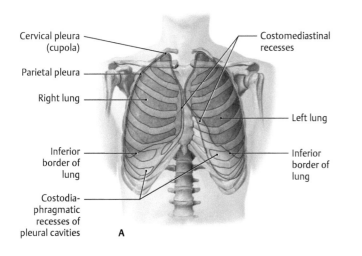

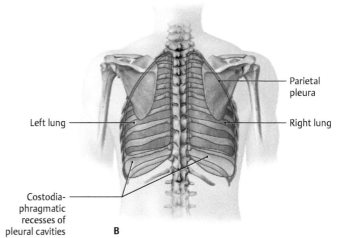

Fig. 15.63 Vertical reference lines of the thorax
A Anterior view. **B** Right lateral view.

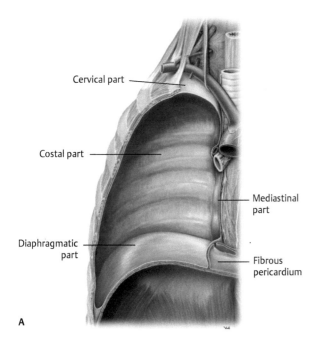

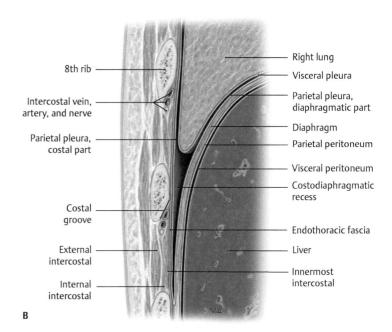

Fig. 15.64 Parietal pleura
A Parts of the parietal pleura. *Opened:* Right pleural cavity, anterior view.
B Costodiaphragmatic recess, coronal section, anterior view. Reflection
of the diaphragmatic pleura onto the inner thoracic wall (becoming the
costal pleura) forms the costodiaphragmatic recess.
The pleural cavity is bounded by two serous layers. The visceral (pulmonary) pleura covers the lungs, and the parietal pleura lines the inner surface of the thoracic cavity. The four parts of the parietal pleura (costal,
diaphragmatic, mediastinal, and cervical) are continuous.

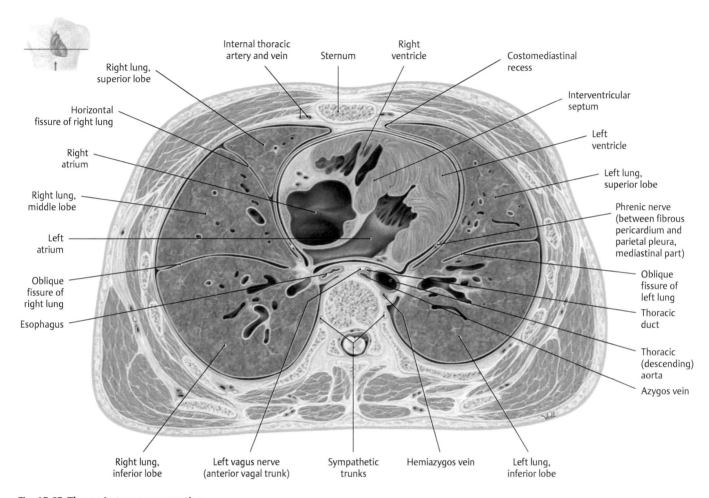

Internal thoracic
artery and vein

Sternum

Right
ventricle

Costomediastinal
recess

Right lung,
superior lobe

Horizontal
fissure of right lung

Interventricular
septum

Right
atrium

Left
ventricle

Right lung,
middle lobe

Left lung,
superior lobe

Left
atrium

Phrenic nerve
(between fibrous
pericardium and
parietal pleura,
mediastinal part)

Oblique
fissure of
right lung

Oblique
fissure of
left lung

Esophagus

Thoracic
duct

Thoracic
(descending)
aorta

Azygos vein

Right lung,
inferior lobe

Left vagus nerve
(anterior vagal trunk)

Sympathetic
trunks

Hemiazygos vein

Left lung,
inferior lobe

Fig. 15.65 **Thorax in transverse section**
Transverse section through T8, inferior view.

Lungs in situ

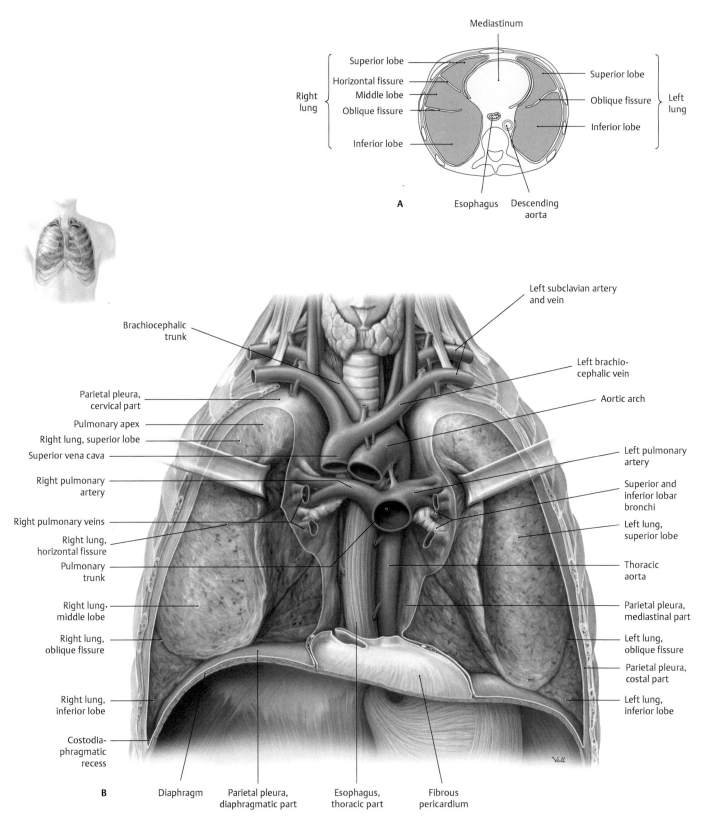

Mediastinum

Right lung
- Superior lobe
- Horizontal fissure
- Middle lobe
- Oblique fissure
- Inferior lobe

Left lung
- Superior lobe
- Oblique fissure
- Inferior lobe

A Esophagus Descending aorta

Brachiocephalic trunk

Parietal pleura, cervical part

Pulmonary apex

Right lung, superior lobe

Superior vena cava

Right pulmonary artery

Right pulmonary veins

Right lung, horizontal fissure

Pulmonary trunk

Right lung, middle lobe

Right lung, oblique fissure

Right lung, inferior lobe

Costodiaphragmatic recess

Left subclavian artery and vein

Left brachiocephalic vein

Aortic arch

Left pulmonary artery

Superior and inferior lobar bronchi

Left lung, superior lobe

Thoracic aorta

Parietal pleura, mediastinal part

Left lung, oblique fissure

Parietal pleura, costal part

Left lung, inferior lobe

B Diaphragm Parietal pleura, diaphragmatic part Esophagus, thoracic part Fibrous pericardium

***Fig. 15.66* Lungs in situ**
The left and right lungs occupy the full volume of the pleural cavity. Note that the left lung is slightly smaller than the right due to the asymmetrical position of the heart.

A Topographical relations of the lungs, transverse section, inferior view.
B Anterior view with lungs retracted.

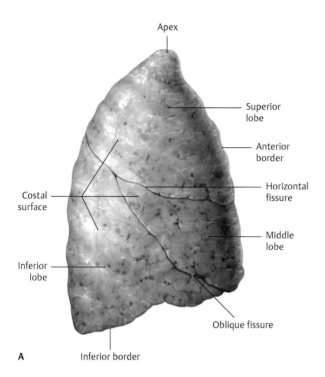

Apex

Superior
lobe

Anterior
border

Horizontal
fissure

Costal
surface

Middle
lobe

Inferior
lobe

Oblique fissure

A   Inferior border

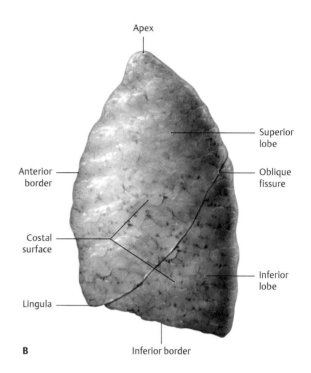

Apex

Superior
lobe

Oblique
fissure

Anterior
border

Costal
surface

Inferior
lobe

Lingula

B   Inferior border

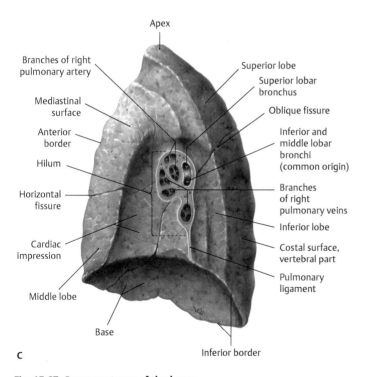

Apex

Branches of right
pulmonary artery

Superior lobe

Superior lobar
bronchus

Mediastinal
surface

Oblique fissure

Anterior
border

Inferior and
middle lobar
bronchi
(common origin)

Hilum

Branches
of right
pulmonary veins

Horizontal
fissure

Inferior lobe

Cardiac
impression

Costal surface,
vertebral part

Middle lobe

Pulmonary
ligament

Base

C   Inferior border

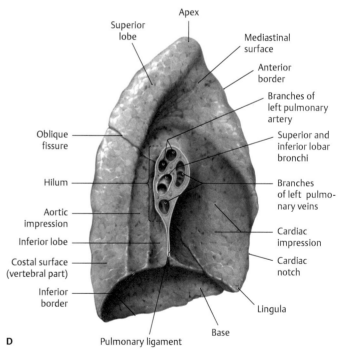

Apex

Superior
lobe

Mediastinal
surface

Anterior
border

Branches of
left pulmonary
artery

Oblique
fissure

Superior and
inferior lobar
bronchi

Hilum

Branches
of left pulmo-
nary veins

Aortic
impression

Inferior lobe

Cardiac
impression

Costal surface
(vertebral part)

Cardiac
notch

Inferior
border

Lingula

Base

D   Pulmonary ligament

Fig. 15.67 Gross anatomy of the lungs
A Right lung, lateral view. **B** Left lung, lateral view.
C Right lung, medial view. **D** Left lung, medial view.
The oblique and horizontal fissures divide the right lung into three lobes: superior, middle, and inferior. The oblique fissure divides the left lung into two lobes: superior and inferior. The apex of each lung extends into the root of the neck. The hilum is the location at which the bronchi and neurovascular structures connect to the lung.

463

Pulmonary Arteries & Veins

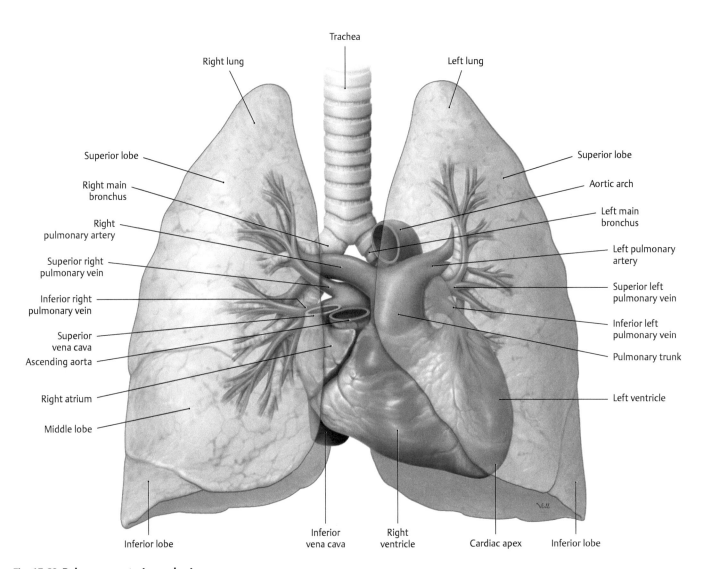

Trachea

Right lung

Left lung

Superior lobe

Right main
bronchus

Right
pulmonary artery

Superior right
pulmonary vein

Inferior right
pulmonary vein

Superior
vena cava

Ascending aorta

Right atrium

Middle lobe

Superior lobe

Aortic arch

Left main
bronchus

Left pulmonary
artery

Superior left
pulmonary vein

Inferior left
pulmonary vein

Pulmonary trunk

Left ventricle

Inferior lobe

Inferior
vena cava

Right
ventricle

Cardiac apex

Inferior lobe

Fig. 15.68 **Pulmonary arteries and veins**
Anterior view. The pulmonary trunk arises from the right ventricle and
divides into a left and right pulmonary artery for each lung. The paired
pulmonary veins open into the left atrium on each side. The pulmonary
arteries accompany and follow the branching of the bronchial tree,
whereas the pulmonary veins do not, being located at the margins of
the pulmonary lobules.

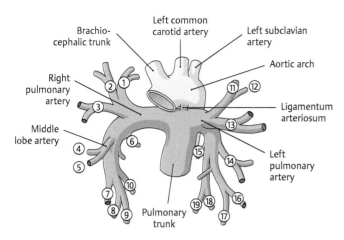

Fig. 15.69 Pulmonary arteries
Schematic.

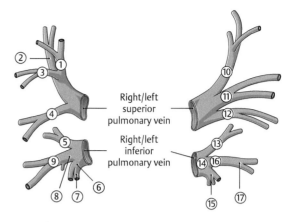

Fig. 15.70 Pulmonary veins
Schematic.

Table 15.11 Pulmonary arteries and their branches		
Right pulmonary artery	**Left pulmonary artery**	
Superior lobe arteries		
① Apical segmental a.		⑪
② Posterior segmental a.		⑫
③ Anterior segmental a.		⑬
Middle lobe arteries		
④ Lateral segmental a.	Lingular a.	⑭
⑤ Medial segmental a.		
Inferior lobe arteries		
⑥ Superior segmental a.		⑮
⑦ Anterior basal segmental a.		⑯
⑧ Lateral basal segmental a.		⑰
⑨ Posterior basal segmental a.		⑱
⑩ Medial basal segmental a.		⑲

Table 15.12 Pulmonary veins and their tributaries		
Right pulmonary vein	**Left pulmonary vein**	
Superior pulmonary veins		
① Apical v.	Apicoposterior v.	⑩
② Posterior v.		
③ Anterior v.	Anterior v.	⑪
④ Middle lobe v.	Lingular v.	⑫
Inferior pulmonary veins		
⑤ Superior v.		⑬
⑥ Common basal v.		⑭
⑦ Inferior basal v.		⑮
⑧ Superior basal v.		⑯
⑨ Anterior basal v.		⑰

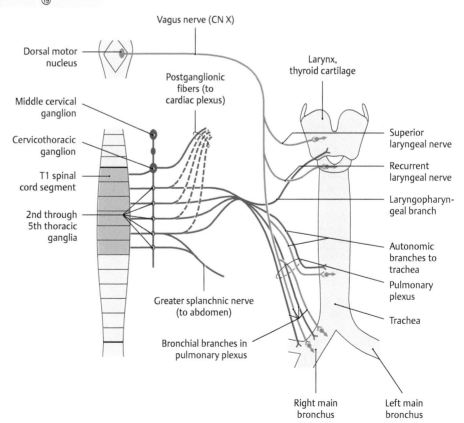

Fig. 15.71 Autonomic innervation of the tracheobronchial tree
Sympathetic innervation (red); parasympathetic innervation (blue).

465

Surface Anatomy & Muscles of the Abdominal Wall

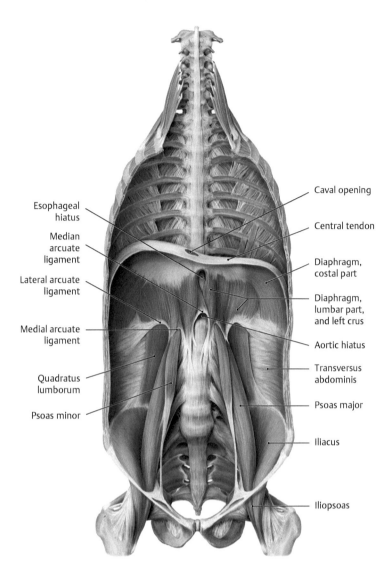

Esophageal
hiatus

Median
arcuate
ligament

Lateral arcuate
ligament

Medial arcuate
ligament

Quadratus
lumborum

Psoas minor

Caval opening

Central tendon

Diaphragm,
costal part

Diaphragm,
lumbar part,
and left crus

Aortic hiatus

Transversus
abdominis

Psoas major

Iliacus

Iliopsoas

Fig. 15.72 **Muscles of the posterior abdominal wall**
Coronal section with diaphragm in intermediate position.

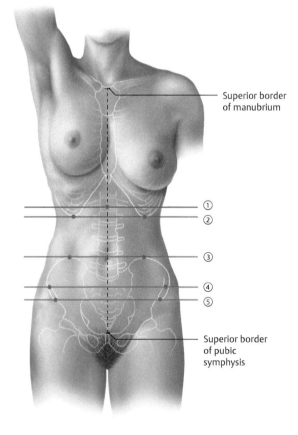

Superior border
of manubrium

① ② ③ ④ ⑤

Superior border
of pubic
symphysis

Fig. 15.73 **Transverse planes through the abdomen**
Anterior view. See **Table 15.13**.

Table 15.13 Transverse planes through the abdomen	
① Transpyloric plane	Transverse plane midway between the superior borders of the pubic symphysis and the manubrium
② Subcostal plane	Plane at the lowest level of the costal margin (the inferior margin of the tenth costal cartilage)
③ Supracrestal plane	Plane passing through the summits of the iliac crests
④ Transtubercular plane	Plane at the level of the iliac tubercles (the iliac tubercle lies ~5 cm posterolateral to the anterior superior iliac spine)
⑤ Interspinous plane	Plane at the level of the anterior superior iliac spine

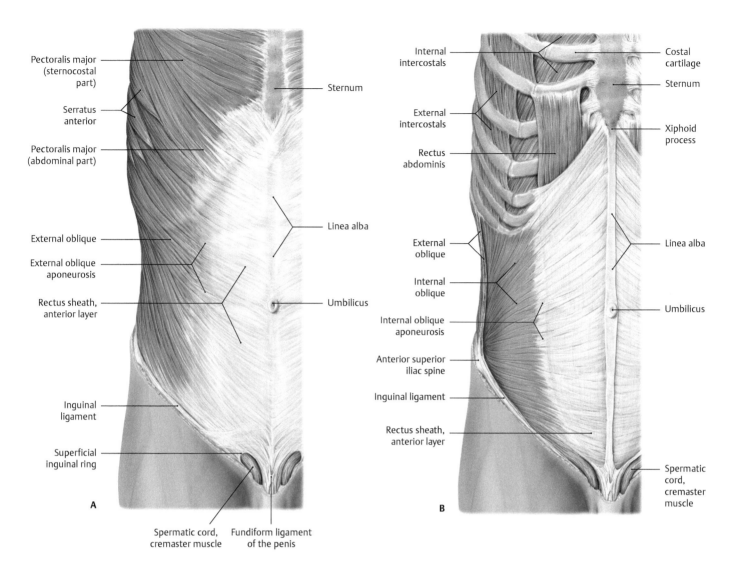

Fig. 15.74 Muscles of the abdominal wall
Right side, anterior view.
A Superficial abdominal wall muscles.
B *Removed:* External oblique, pectoralis major, and serratus anterior.

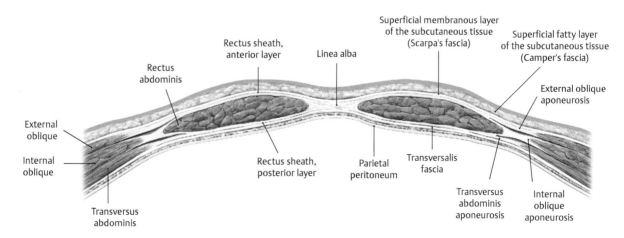

Fig. 15.75 Anterior abdominal wall and rectus sheath
Transverse section, superior to the arcuate line.
The rectus sheath is created by fusion of the aponeuroses of the transversus abdominis and abdominal oblique muscles. The inferior edge of the posterior layer of the rectus sheath is called the arcuate line.

Arteries of the Abdominal Wall & Abdomen

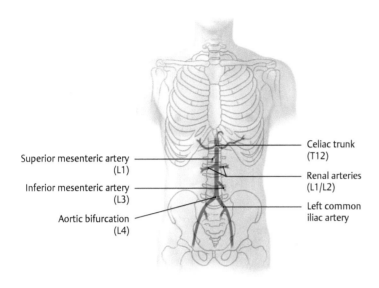

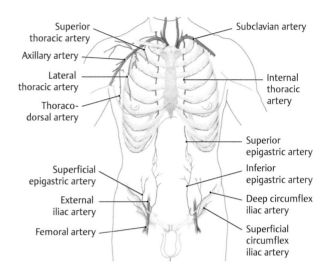

Fig. 15.76 Abdominal aorta and major branches

Anterior view. The abdominal aorta enters the abdomen at the T12 level through the aortic hiatus of the diaphragm. Before bifurcating at L4 into its terminal branches, the common iliac arteries, the abdominal aorta gives off the renal arteries and three major trunks that supply the organs of the alimentary canal:

Celiac trunk: supplies the structures of the foregut, the anterior portion of the alimentary canal. The foregut consists of the esophagus (abdominal 1.25 cm), stomach, duodenum (proximal half), liver, gallbladder, and pancreas (superior portion).

Superior mesenteric artery: supplies the structures of the midgut: the duodenum (distal half), jejunum and ileum, cecum and appendix,

Fig. 15.77 Arteries of the abdominal wall

The superior and inferior epigastric arteries form a potential anastomosis, or bypass for blood, from the subclavian and femoral arteries. This effectively allows blood to bypass the abdominal aorta.

ascending colon, right colic flexure, and the proximal one half of the transverse colon.

Inferior mesenteric artery: supplies the structures of the hindgut: the transverse colon (distal half), left colic flexure, descending and sigmoid colons, rectum, and anal canal (upper part).

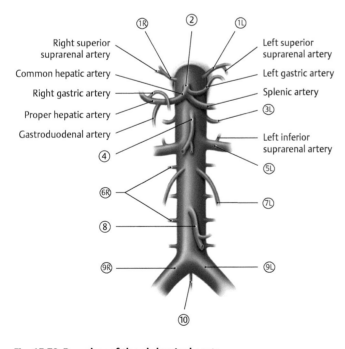

Fig. 15.78 Branches of the abdominal aorta

Anterior view. See **Table 15.14**.

Table 15.14 Branches of the abdominal aorta

The abdominal aorta gives rise to three major unpaired trunks (bold) and the unpaired median sacral artery, as well as six paired branches.

Branch from abdominal aorta			Branches	
①R	①L	Inferior phrenic aa. (paired)	Superior suprarenal aa.	
②		**Celiac trunk**	Left gastric a.	
			Splenic a.	
			Common hepatic a.	Proper hepatic a.
				Right gastric a.
				Gastroduodenal a.
③R	③L	Middle suprarenal aa. (paired)		
④		**Superior mesenteric a.**		
⑤R	⑤L	Renal aa. (paired)	Inferior suprarenal aa.	
⑥R	⑥L	Lumbar aa. (1st through 4th, paired)		
⑦R	⑦L	Testicular/ovarian aa. (paired)		
⑧		**Inferior mesenteric a.**		
⑨R	⑨L	Common iliac aa. (paired)	External iliac a.	
			Internal iliac a.	
	⑩	Median sacral a.		

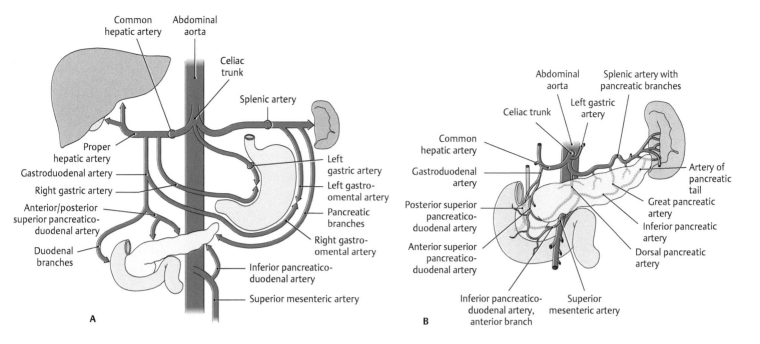

Fig. 15.79 Celiac trunk
A Celiac trunk distribution. **B** Arterial supply to the pancreas.

Fig. 15.80 Abdominal arterial anastomoses
The three major anastomoses provide overlap in the arterial supply to abdominal areas to ensure adequate blood flow. These are between
① the celiac trunk and the superior mesenteric artery via the pancreaticoduodenal arteries,
② the superior and inferior mesenteric arteries via the middle and left colic arteries, and
③ the inferior mesenteric and the internal iliac arteries via the superior and middle or inferior rectal arteries.

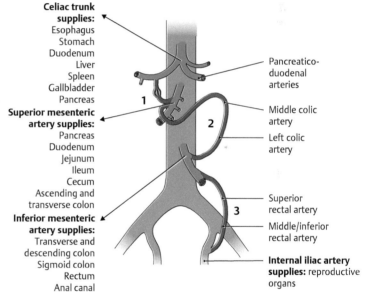

Celiac trunk supplies:
Esophagus
Stomach
Duodenum
Liver
Spleen
Gallbladder
Pancreas

Superior mesenteric artery supplies:
Pancreas
Duodenum
Jejunum
Ileum
Cecum
Ascending and transverse colon

Inferior mesenteric artery supplies:
Transverse and descending colon
Sigmoid colon
Rectum
Anal canal

Internal iliac artery supplies: reproductive organs

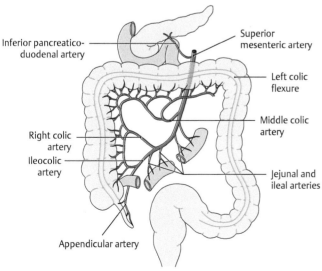

Fig. 15.81 Superior mesenteric artery

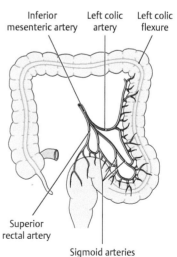

Fig. 15.82 Inferior mesenteric artery

469

Divisions of the Abdominopelvic Cavity

Organs in the abdominopelvic cavity are classified by the presence of surrounding peritoneum (the serous membrane lining the cavity) and a mesentery (a double layer of peritoneum that connects the organ to the abdominal wall) (see **Table 15.15**).

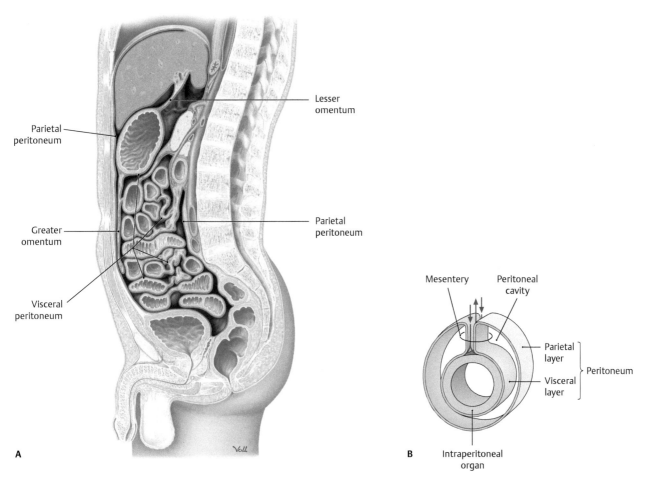

Fig. 15.83 Peritoneal cavity
A Midsagittal section through the male abdominopelvic cavity, viewed from the left. The peritoneum is shown in red.
B An intraperitoneal organ, showing the mesentery and surrounding peritoneum. Arrows indicate location of blood vessels in the mesentery.

Table 15.15 Organs of the abdominopelvic cavity classified by their relationship to the peritoneum		
Location	**Organs**	
Intraperitoneal organs: These organs have a mesentery and are completely covered by the peritoneum.		
Abdominal peritoneal	• Stomach • Small intestine (jejunum, ileum, some of the superior part of the duodenum) • Spleen • Liver	• Gallbladder • Cecum with vermiform appendix • Large intestine (transverse and sigmoid colons)
Pelvic peritoneal	• Uterus (fundus and body)　　• Ovaries	• Uterine tubes
Extraperitoneal organs: These organs either have no mesentery or lost it during development.		
Retroperitoneal — Primarily	• Kidneys and ureters　　• Suprarenal glands	• Uterine cervix
Retroperitoneal — Secondarily	• Duodenum (descending, horizontal, and ascending) • Pancreas	• Ascending and descending colon • Rectum (upper 2/3)
Infraperitoneal/subperitoneal	• Urinary bladder　　• Seminal vesicle • Distal ureters　　• Uterine cervix • Prostate	• Vagina • Rectum (lower 1/3)

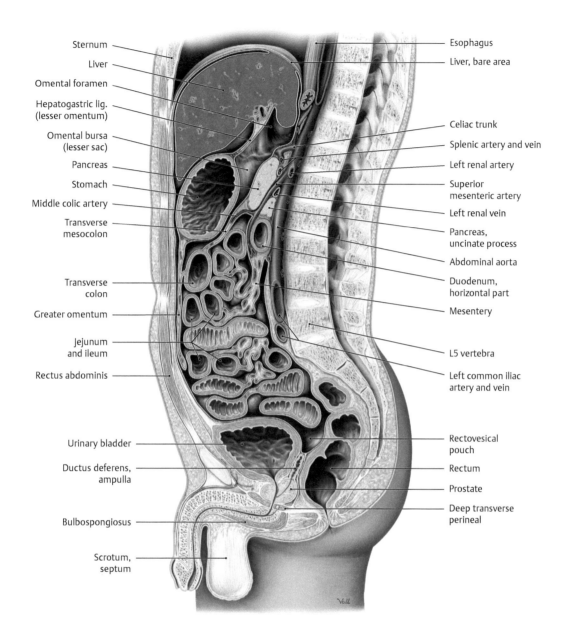

Sternum

Liver

Omental foramen

Hepatogastric lig.
(lesser omentum)

Omental bursa
(lesser sac)

Pancreas

Stomach

Middle colic artery

Transverse
mesocolon

Transverse
colon

Greater omentum

Jejunum
and ileum

Rectus abdominis

Urinary bladder

Ductus deferens,
ampulla

Bulbospongiosus

Scrotum,
septum

Esophagus

Liver, bare area

Celiac trunk

Splenic artery and vein

Left renal artery

Superior
mesenteric artery

Left renal vein

Pancreas,
uncinate process

Abdominal aorta

Duodenum,
horizontal part

Mesentery

L5 vertebra

Left common iliac
artery and vein

Rectovesical
pouch

Rectum

Prostate

Deep transverse
perineal

**Fig. 15.84 Peritoneal relationships of the
abdominopelvic organs**
Midsagittal section through the male abdominopelvic cavity, viewed from the left.

Peritoneal Cavity, Greater Sac, & Mesenteries (I)

The peritoneal cavity is divided into the large greater sac and small omental bursa (lesser sac). The greater omentum is an apron-like fold of peritoneum suspended from the greater curvature of the stomach and covering the anterior surface of the transverse colon. The attachment of the transverse mesocolon on the anterior surface of the descending part of the duodenum and the pancreas divides the peritoneal cavity into a supracolic compartment (liver, gallbladder, and stomach) and an infracolic compartment (intestines).

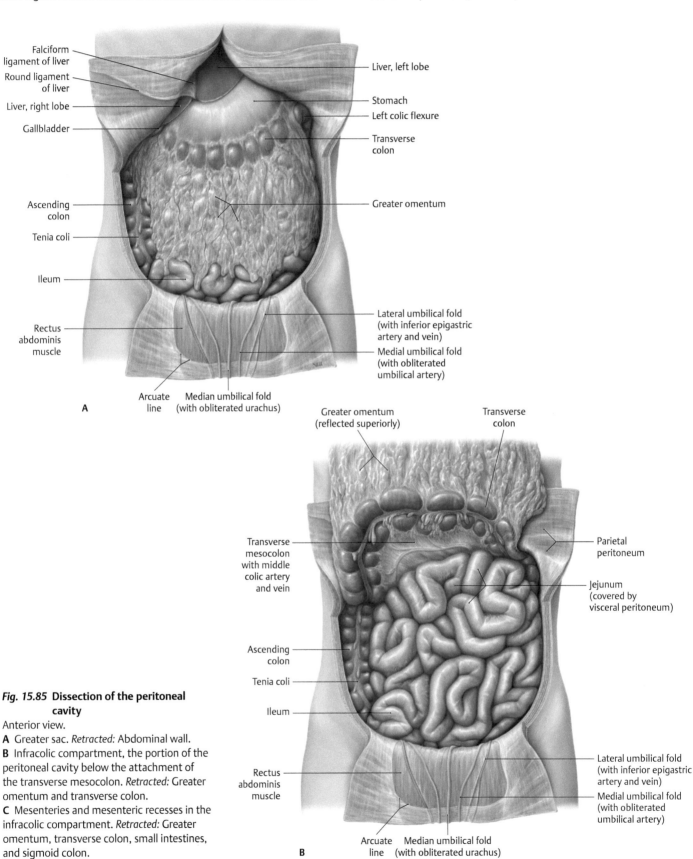

Fig. 15.85 Dissection of the peritoneal cavity

Anterior view.
A Greater sac. *Retracted:* Abdominal wall.
B Infracolic compartment, the portion of the peritoneal cavity below the attachment of the transverse mesocolon. *Retracted:* Greater omentum and transverse colon.
C Mesenteries and mesenteric recesses in the infracolic compartment. *Retracted:* Greater omentum, transverse colon, small intestines, and sigmoid colon.

472

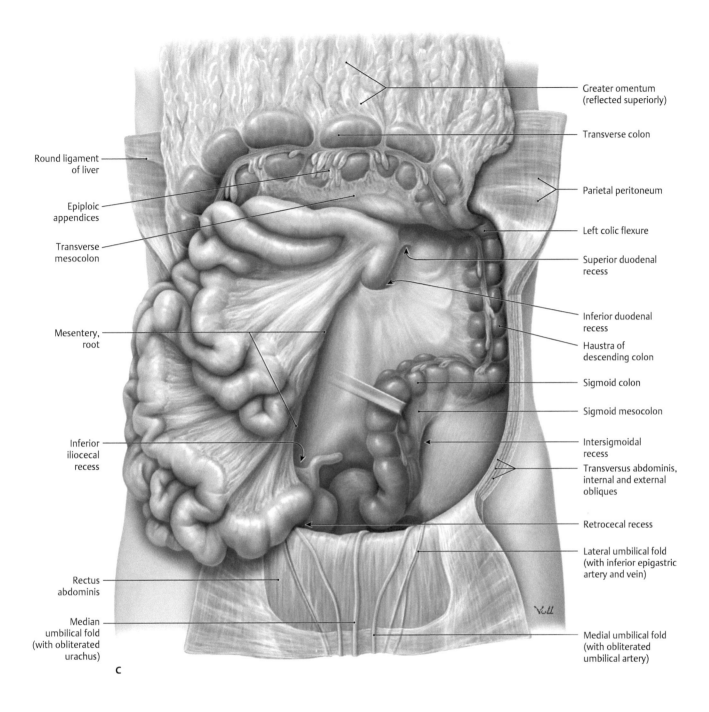

Round ligament of liver

Epiploic appendices

Transverse mesocolon

Mesentery, root

Inferior iliocecal recess

Rectus abdominis

Median umbilical fold (with obliterated urachus)

Greater omentum (reflected superiorly)

Transverse colon

Parietal peritoneum

Left colic flexure

Superior duodenal recess

Inferior duodenal recess

Haustra of descending colon

Sigmoid colon

Sigmoid mesocolon

Intersigmoidal recess

Transversus abdominis, internal and external obliques

Retrocecal recess

Lateral umbilical fold (with inferior epigastric artery and vein)

Medial umbilical fold (with obliterated umbilical artery)

C

Stomach & Omental Bursa

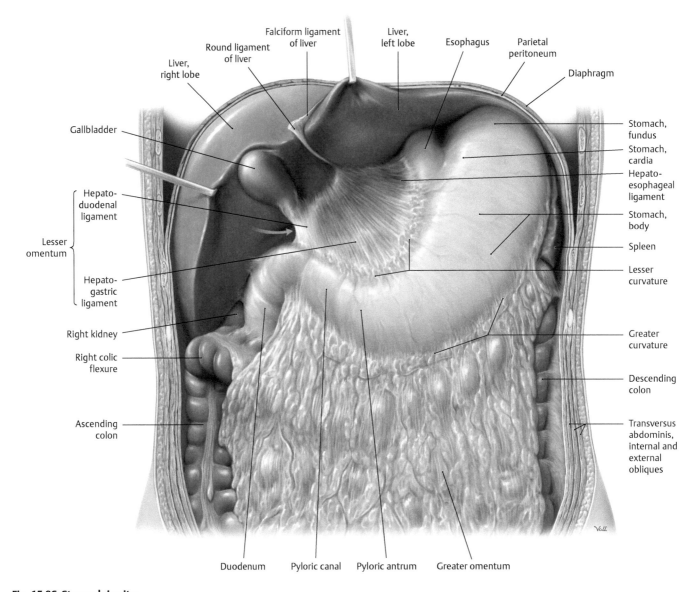

Fig. 15.86 Stomach in situ
Anterior view of the opened upper abdomen. Arrow indicates the omental foramen.

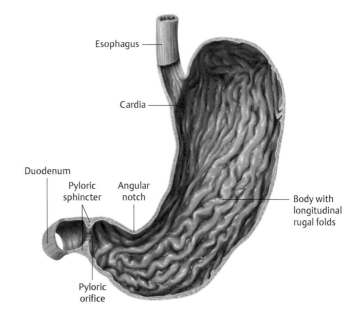

Fig. 15.87 Stomach
Anterior view. *Removed:* Anterior wall.

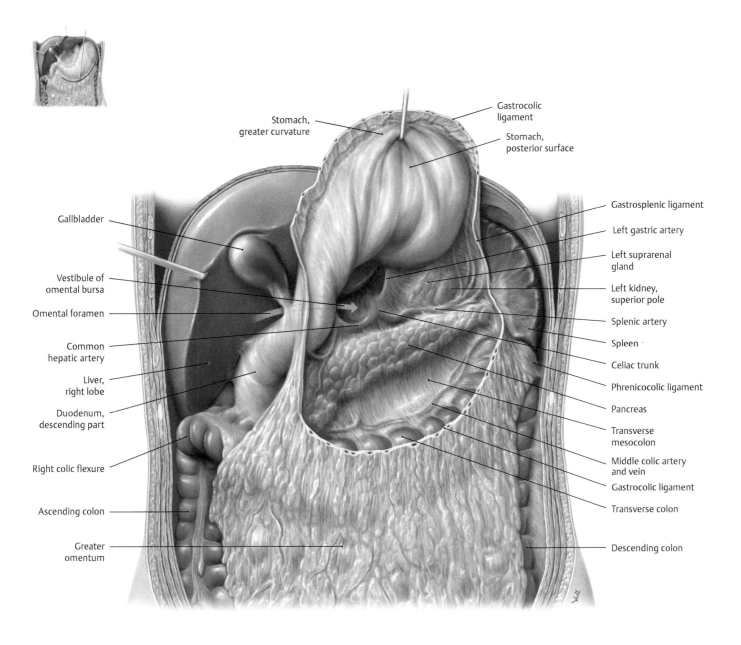

Stomach,
greater curvature

Gastrocolic
ligament

Stomach,
posterior surface

Gallbladder

Vestibule of
omental bursa

Omental foramen

Common
hepatic artery

Liver,
right lobe

Duodenum,
descending part

Right colic flexure

Ascending colon

Greater
omentum

Gastrosplenic ligament

Left gastric artery

Left suprarenal
gland

Left kidney,
superior pole

Splenic artery

Spleen

Celiac trunk

Phrenicocolic ligament

Pancreas

Transverse
mesocolon

Middle colic artery
and vein

Gastrocolic ligament

Transverse colon

Descending colon

Fig. 15.88 **Omental bursa**
Anterior view. *Divided:* Gastrocolic ligament.
Retracted: Liver. *Reflected:* Stomach.

475

Mesenteries (II) & Bowel

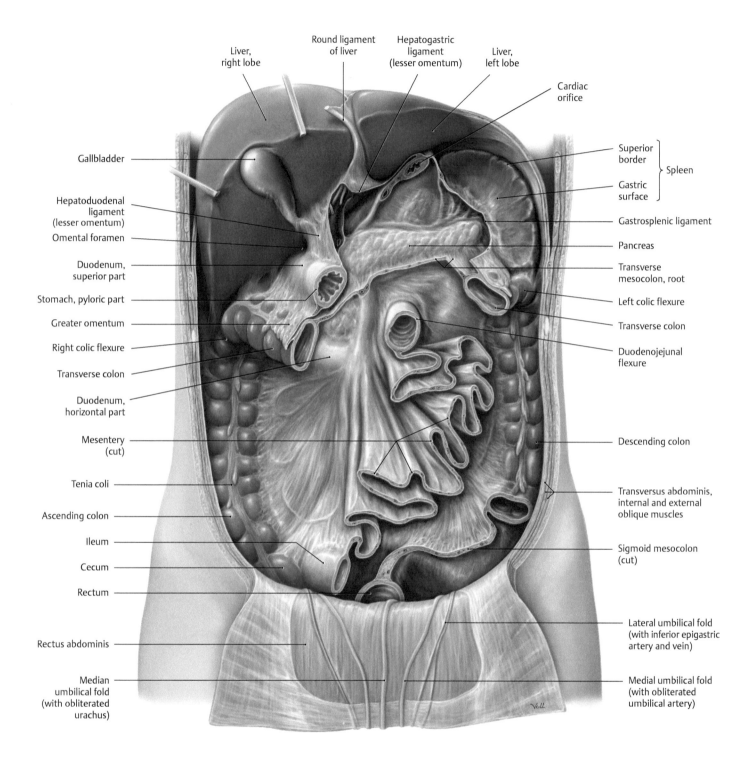

Fig. 15.89 Mesenteries and organs of the peritoneal cavity
Anterior view. *Removed:* Stomach, transerse colon, jejunum, ileum, and sigmoid colon. *Retracted:* Liver.

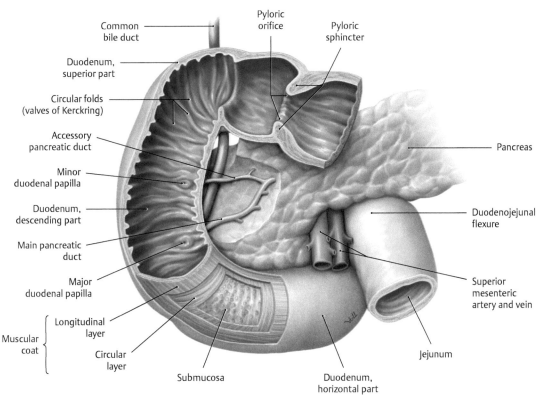

Fig. 15.90 Duodenum
Anterior view with the anterior wall opened. The small intestine consists of the duodenum, jejunum, and ileum. The duodenum is primarily retroperitoneal and is divided into four parts: superior, descending, horizontal, and ascending.

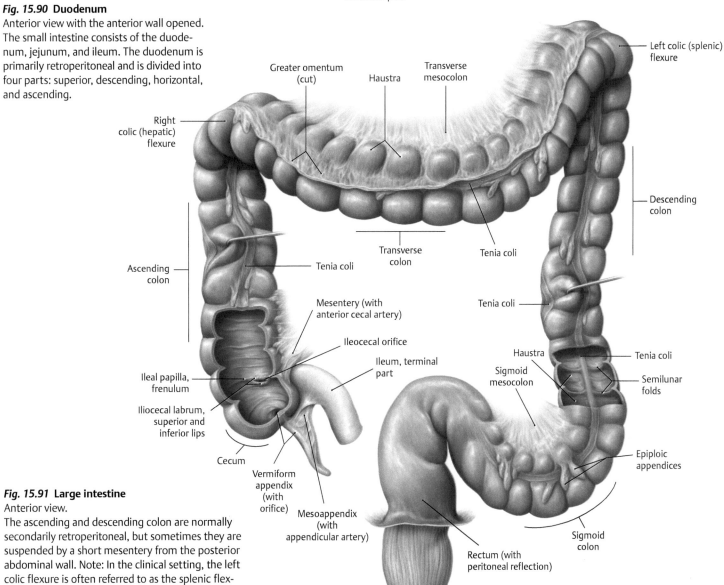

Fig. 15.91 Large intestine
Anterior view.
The ascending and descending colon are normally secondarily retroperitoneal, but sometimes they are suspended by a short mesentery from the posterior abdominal wall. Note: In the clinical setting, the left colic flexure is often referred to as the splenic flexure and the right colic flexure, as the hepatic flexure.

Liver, Gallbladder, & Biliary Tract

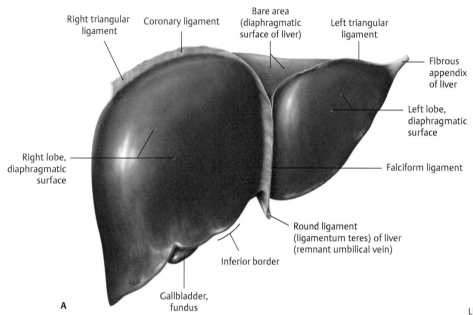

Right triangular ligament
Coronary ligament
Bare area (diaphragmatic surface of liver)
Left triangular ligament
Fibrous appendix of liver
Left lobe, diaphragmatic surface
Right lobe, diaphragmatic surface
Falciform ligament
Round ligament (ligamentum teres) of liver (remnant umbilical vein)
Inferior border
Gallbladder, fundus
A

Fig. 15.92 Surfaces of the liver
A Anterior view. **B** Inferior view.
The liver is divided into four lobes by its ligaments: right, left, caudate, and quadrate. The falciform ligament, a double layer of parietal peritoneum that reflects off the anterior abdominal wall and extends to the liver, spreading out over its surface as visceral peritoneum, divides the liver into right and left anatomic lobes. The round ligament of the liver is found in the free edge of the falciform ligament and contains the obliterated umbilical vein, which once extended from the umbilicus to the liver.

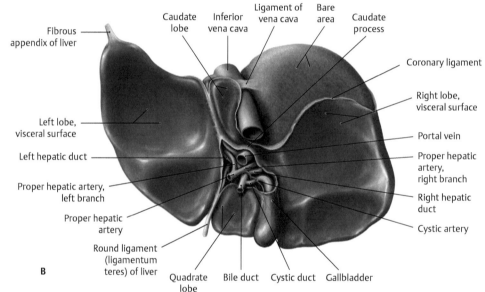

Caudate lobe
Inferior vena cava
Ligament of vena cava
Bare area
Caudate process
Coronary ligament
Fibrous appendix of liver
Right lobe, visceral surface
Left lobe, visceral surface
Portal vein
Left hepatic duct
Proper hepatic artery, right branch
Proper hepatic artery, left branch
Right hepatic duct
Proper hepatic artery
Cystic artery
Round ligament (ligamentum teres) of liver
Quadrate lobe
Bile duct
Cystic duct
Gallbladder
B

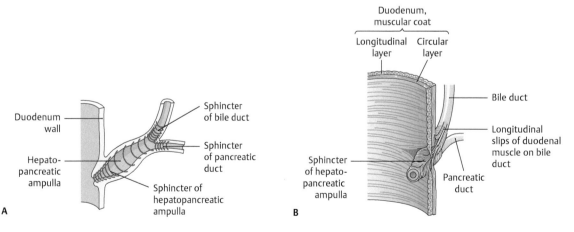

Duodenum wall
Sphincter of bile duct
Sphincter of pancreatic duct
Hepato-pancreatic ampulla
Sphincter of hepatopancreatic ampulla
A

Duodenum, muscular coat
Longitudinal layer
Circular layer
Bile duct
Longitudinal slips of duodenal muscle on bile duct
Sphincter of hepato-pancreatic ampulla
Pancreatic duct
B

Fig. 15.93 Biliary sphincter system
A Sphincters of the pancreatic and bile ducts. **B** Sphincter system in the duodenal wall.

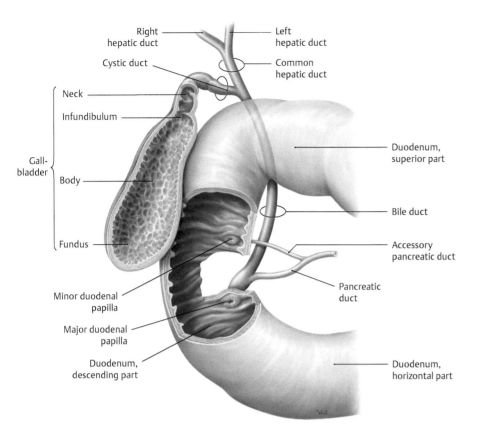

Fig. 15.94 Extrahepatic bile ducts
Anterior view. *Opened:* Gallbladder and duodenum.

Fig. 15.95 Biliary tract in situ
Anterior view. *Removed:* Stomach, small intestine, transverse colon, and large portions of the liver. The gallbladder is intraperitoneal and covered by visceral peritoneum where it is not attached to the liver.

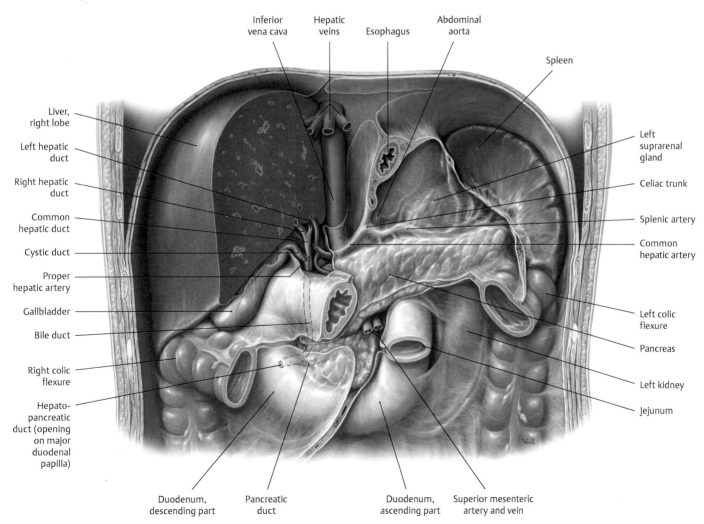

479

Abdominal Aorta & Celiac Trunk

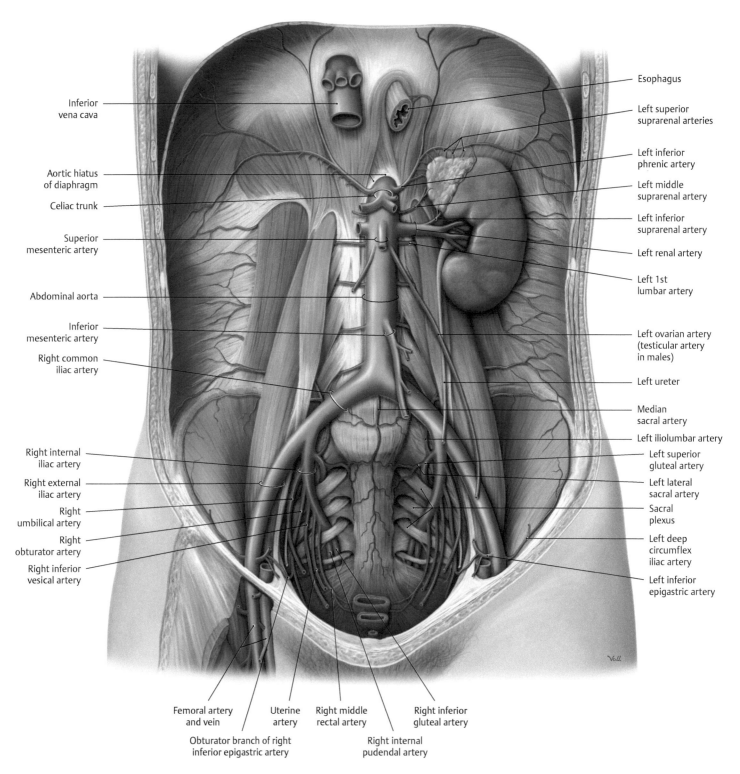

Inferior vena cava

Aortic hiatus of diaphragm

Celiac trunk

Superior mesenteric artery

Abdominal aorta

Inferior mesenteric artery

Right common iliac artery

Right internal iliac artery

Right external iliac artery

Right umbilical artery

Right obturator artery

Right inferior vesical artery

Esophagus

Left superior suprarenal arteries

Left inferior phrenic artery

Left middle suprarenal artery

Left inferior suprarenal artery

Left renal artery

Left 1st lumbar artery

Left ovarian artery (testicular artery in males)

Left ureter

Median sacral artery

Left iliolumbar artery

Left superior gluteal artery

Left lateral sacral artery

Sacral plexus

Left deep circumflex iliac artery

Left inferior epigastric artery

Femoral artery and vein

Uterine artery

Right middle rectal artery

Right inferior gluteal artery

Obturator branch of right inferior epigastric artery

Right internal pudendal artery

Fig. 15.96 Abdominal aorta
Anterior view of the female abdomen. *Removed:* All organs except the left kidney band suprarenal gland. The abdominal aorta is the distal continuation of the thoracic aorta (see **Fig. 15.43**, p. 442). It enters the abdomen at the T12 level and bifurcates into the common iliac arteries at L4.

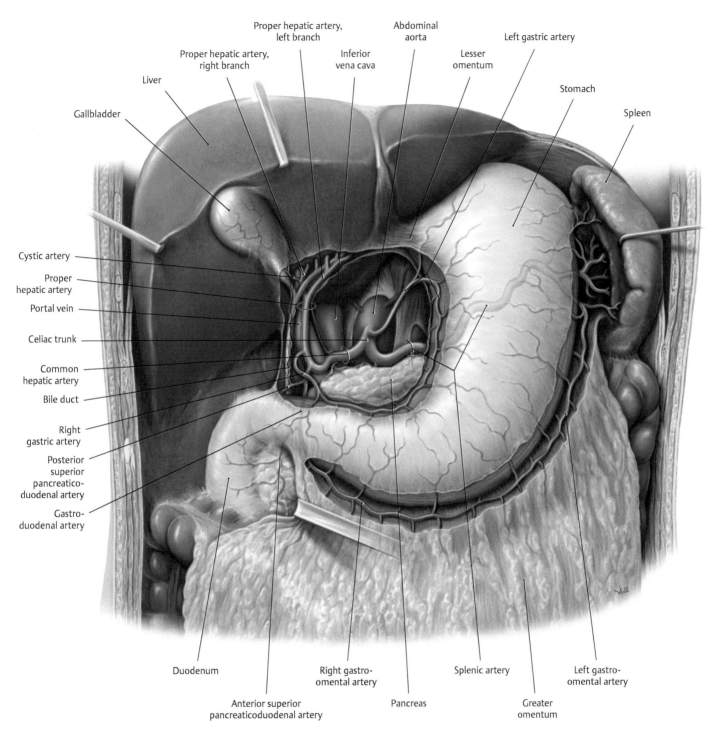

Proper hepatic artery,
left branch

Proper hepatic artery,
right branch

Liver

Gallbladder

Abdominal
aorta

Inferior
vena cava

Lesser
omentum

Left gastric artery

Stomach

Spleen

Cystic artery

Proper
hepatic artery

Portal vein

Celiac trunk

Common
hepatic artery

Bile duct

Right
gastric artery

Posterior
superior
pancreatico-
duodenal artery

Gastro-
duodenal artery

Duodenum

Right gastro-
omental artery

Splenic artery

Left gastro-
omental artery

Anterior superior
pancreaticoduodenal artery

Pancreas

Greater
omentum

Fig. 15.97 Celiac trunk: Stomach, liver, and gallbladder
Anterior view. *Opened:* Lesser omentum. *Incised:* Greater omentum. The
celiac trunk arises from the abdominal aorta at about the level of T12.

481

Superior & Inferior Mesenteric Arteries

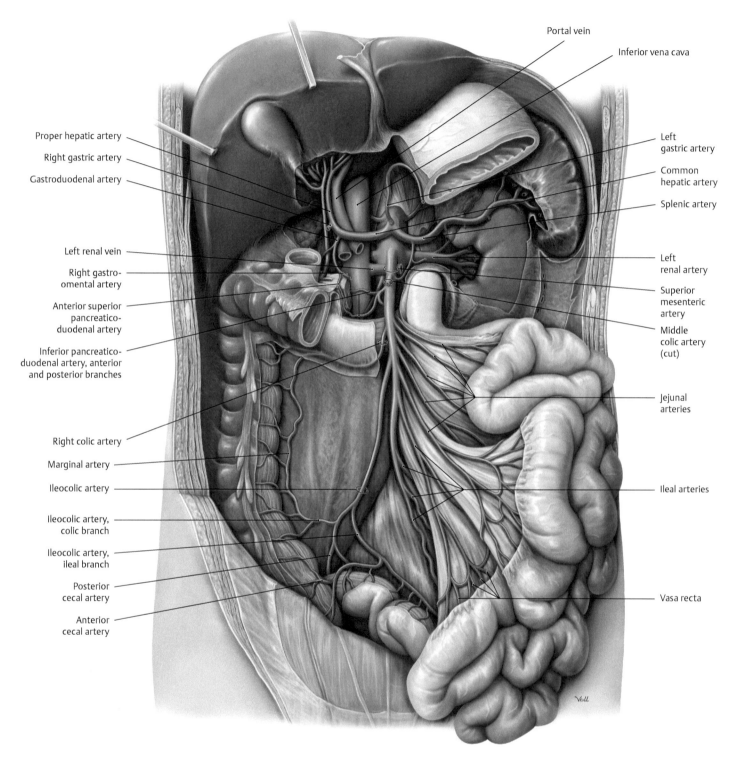

Portal vein

Inferior vena cava

Proper hepatic artery

Right gastric artery

Gastroduodenal artery

Left gastric artery

Common hepatic artery

Splenic artery

Left renal vein

Right gastro-omental artery

Anterior superior pancreatico-duodenal artery

Inferior pancreatico-duodenal artery, anterior and posterior branches

Left renal artery

Superior mesenteric artery

Middle colic artery (cut)

Jejunal arteries

Right colic artery

Marginal artery

Ileocolic artery

Ileocolic artery, colic branch

Ileocolic artery, ileal branch

Posterior cecal artery

Anterior cecal artery

Ileal arteries

Vasa recta

Fig. 15.98 **Superior mesenteric artery**
Anterior view. *Partially removed:* Stomach, duodenum, and peritoneum.
Reflected: Liver and gallbladder. *Note:* The middle colic artery has been
truncated (see **Fig. 15.99**). The superior and inferior mesenteric arteries
arise from the aorta opposite L2 and L3, respectively.

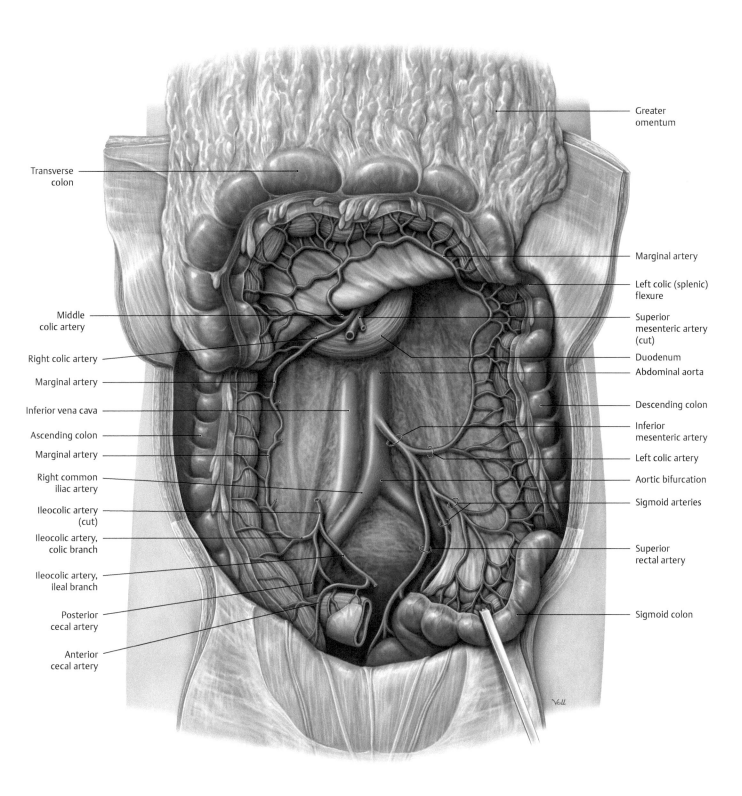

Greater omentum

Transverse colon

Marginal artery

Left colic (splenic) flexure

Middle colic artery

Superior mesenteric artery (cut)

Right colic artery

Duodenum

Abdominal aorta

Marginal artery

Inferior vena cava

Descending colon

Ascending colon

Inferior mesenteric artery

Marginal artery

Left colic artery

Right common iliac artery

Aortic bifurcation

Ileocolic artery (cut)

Sigmoid arteries

Ileocolic artery, colic branch

Superior rectal artery

Ileocolic artery, ileal branch

Posterior cecal artery

Sigmoid colon

Anterior cecal artery

Fig. 15.99 **Inferior mesenteric artery**
Anterior view. *Removed:* Jejunum and ileum. *Reflected:* Transverse colon.

Veins of the Abdomen

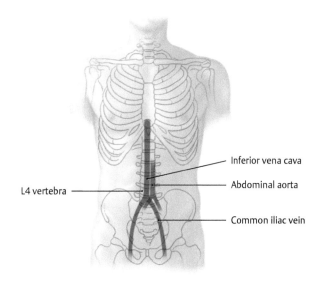

Fig. 15.100 Location of the inferior vena cava
Anterior view.

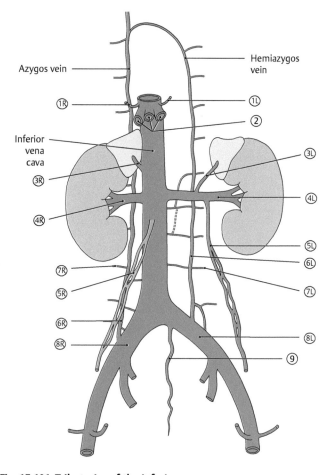

Fig. 15.101 Tributaries of the inferior vena cava
Schematic. See **Table 15.16**.

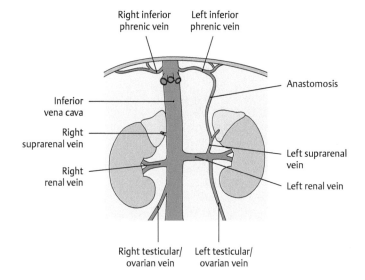

Fig. 15.102 Tributaries of the renal veins
Anterior view.

Table 15.16	Tributaries of the inferior vena cava	
①R	①L	Inferior phrenic vv. (paired)
	②	Hepatic vv. (3)
③R	③L	Suprarenal vv. (the right vein is a direct tributary)
④R	④L	Renal vv. (paired)
⑤R	⑤L	Testicular/ovarian vv. (the right vein is a direct tributary)
⑥R	⑥L	Ascending lumbar vv. (paired), not direct tributaries
⑦R	⑦L	Lumbar vv.
⑧R	⑧L	Common iliac vv. (paired)
	⑨	Median sacral v.

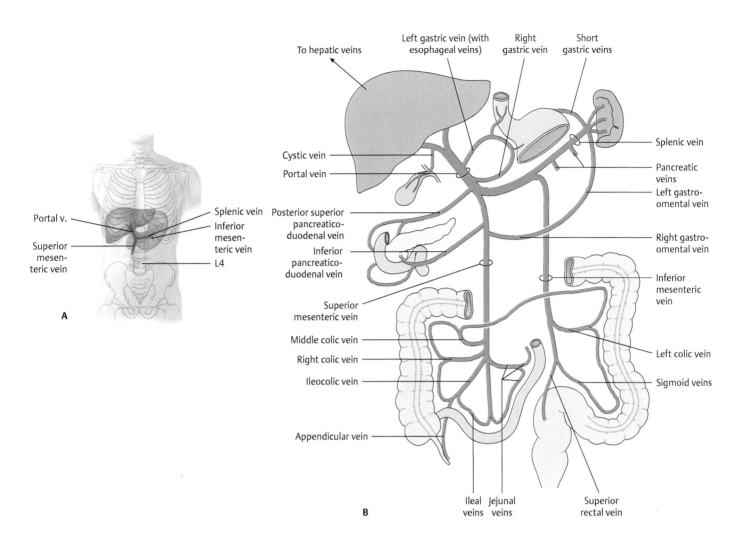

A — labels: To hepatic veins; Left gastric vein (with esophageal veins); Right gastric vein; Short gastric veins; Portal v.; Splenic vein; Inferior mesenteric vein; Superior mesenteric vein; L4

B — labels: Left gastric vein (with esophageal veins); Right gastric vein; Short gastric veins; Cystic vein; Portal vein; Splenic vein; Pancreatic veins; Left gastro-omental vein; Posterior superior pancreatico-duodenal vein; Inferior pancreatico-duodenal vein; Right gastro-omental vein; Inferior mesenteric vein; Superior mesenteric vein; Middle colic vein; Right colic vein; Ileocolic vein; Left colic vein; Sigmoid veins; Appendicular vein; Ileal veins; Jejunal veins; Superior rectal vein

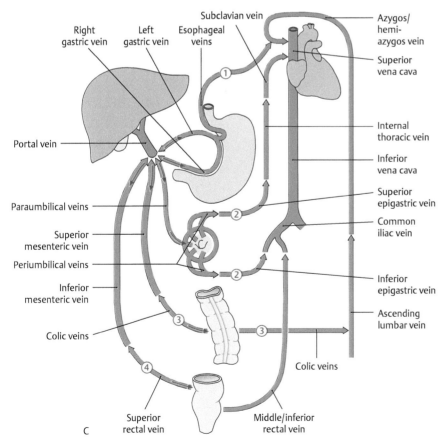

C — labels: Right gastric vein; Left gastric vein; Esophageal veins; Subclavian vein; Azygos/hemi-azygos vein; Superior vena cava; Portal vein; Internal thoracic vein; Inferior vena cava; Paraumbilical veins; Superior epigastric vein; Superior mesenteric vein; Common iliac vein; Periumbilical veins; Inferior mesenteric vein; Inferior epigastric vein; Colic veins; Ascending lumbar vein; Colic veins; Superior rectal vein; Middle/inferior rectal vein

Fig. 15.103 Portal vein
The portal vein drains venous blood from the abdominopelvic organs supplied by the celiac trunk and superior and inferior mesenteric arteries.
A Location, anterior view.
B Portal vein distribution.
C Collateral pathways between the portal system and the heart. When the portal system is compromised, the portal vein can divert blood away from the liver back to its supplying veins, which return this nutrient-rich blood to the heart via the venae cavae. The red arrows indicate the flow reversal in the (1) esophageal veins, (2) paraumbilical veins, (3) colic veins, and (4) middle and inferior rectal veins.

485

Inferior Vena Cava & Inferior Mesenteric Veins

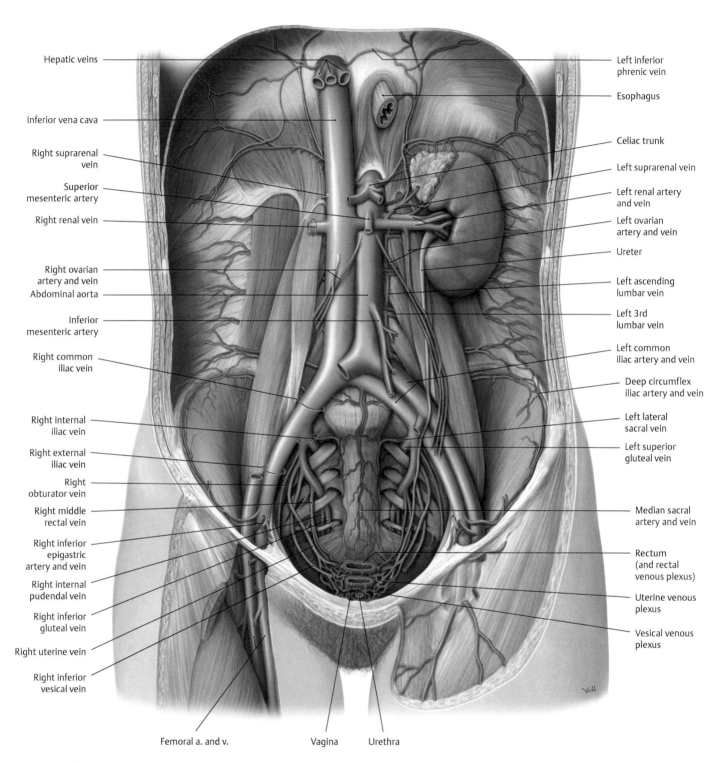

Hepatic veins

Inferior vena cava

Right suprarenal vein

Superior mesenteric artery

Right renal vein

Right ovarian artery and vein

Abdominal aorta

Inferior mesenteric artery

Right common iliac vein

Right internal iliac vein

Right external iliac vein

Right obturator vein

Right middle rectal vein

Right inferior epigastric artery and vein

Right internal pudendal vein

Right inferior gluteal vein

Right uterine vein

Right inferior vesical vein

Left inferior phrenic vein

Esophagus

Celiac trunk

Left suprarenal vein

Left renal artery and vein

Left ovarian artery and vein

Ureter

Left ascending lumbar vein

Left 3rd lumbar vein

Left common iliac artery and vein

Deep circumflex iliac artery and vein

Left lateral sacral vein

Left superior gluteal vein

Median sacral artery and vein

Rectum (and rectal venous plexus)

Uterine venous plexus

Vesical venous plexus

Femoral a. and v.   Vagina   Urethra

Fig. 15.104 Inferior vena cava
Anterior view of the female abdomen. *Removed:* All organs except the left kidney and suprarenal gland.

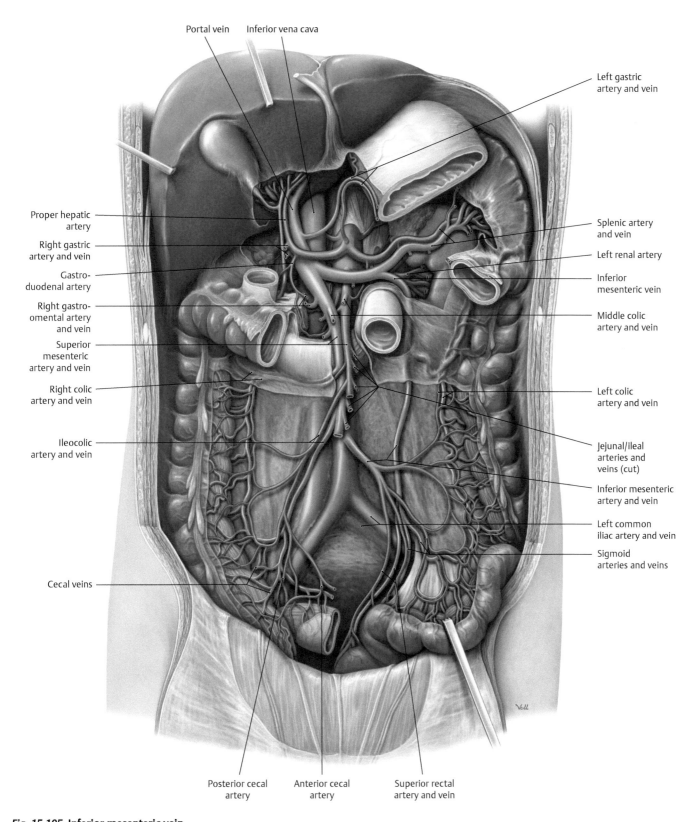

Portal vein   Inferior vena cava

Left gastric
artery and vein

Proper hepatic
artery

Right gastric
artery and vein

Gastro-
duodenal artery

Right gastro-
omental artery
and vein

Superior
mesenteric
artery and vein

Right colic
artery and vein

Ileocolic
artery and vein

Cecal veins

Splenic artery
and vein

Left renal artery

Inferior
mesenteric vein

Middle colic
artery and vein

Left colic
artery and vein

Jejunal/ileal
arteries and
veins (cut)

Inferior mesenteric
artery and vein

Left common
iliac artery and vein

Sigmoid
arteries and veins

Posterior cecal
artery

Anterior cecal
artery

Superior rectal
artery and vein

Fig. 15.105 Inferior mesenteric vein
Anterior view. *Partially removed:* Stomach, duodenum, and peritoneum.
Removed: Pancreas, greater omentum, transverse colon, and small intes-
tine. *Reflected:* Liver and gallbladder.
The inferior mesenteric vein is part of the portal system.

487

Autonomic Plexuses & Sectional Anatomy of the Abdomen

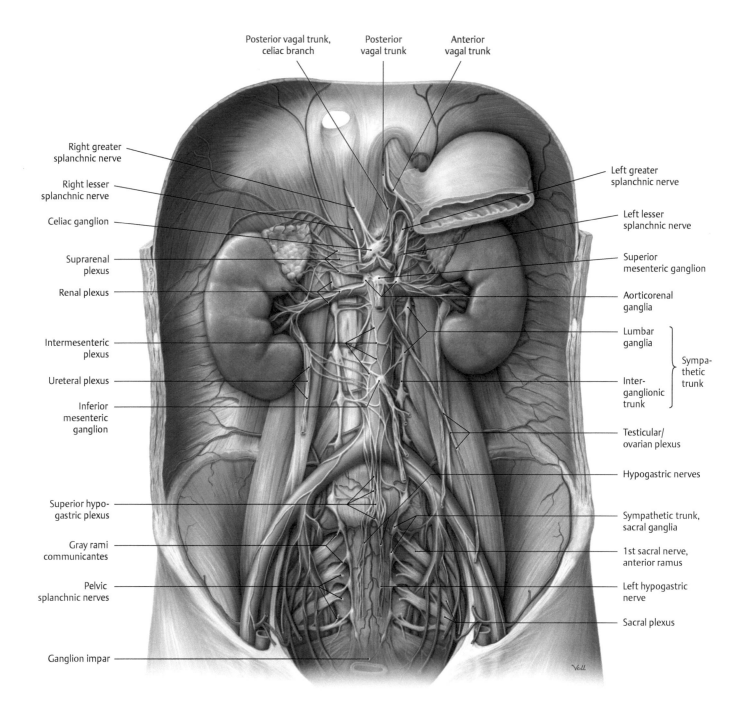

Fig. 15.106 Autonomic plexuses in the abdomen and pelvis
Anterior view of the male abdomen and pelvis. *Removed:* Peritoneum,
majority of the stomach, and all other abdominal organs except kidneys
and suprarenal glands.

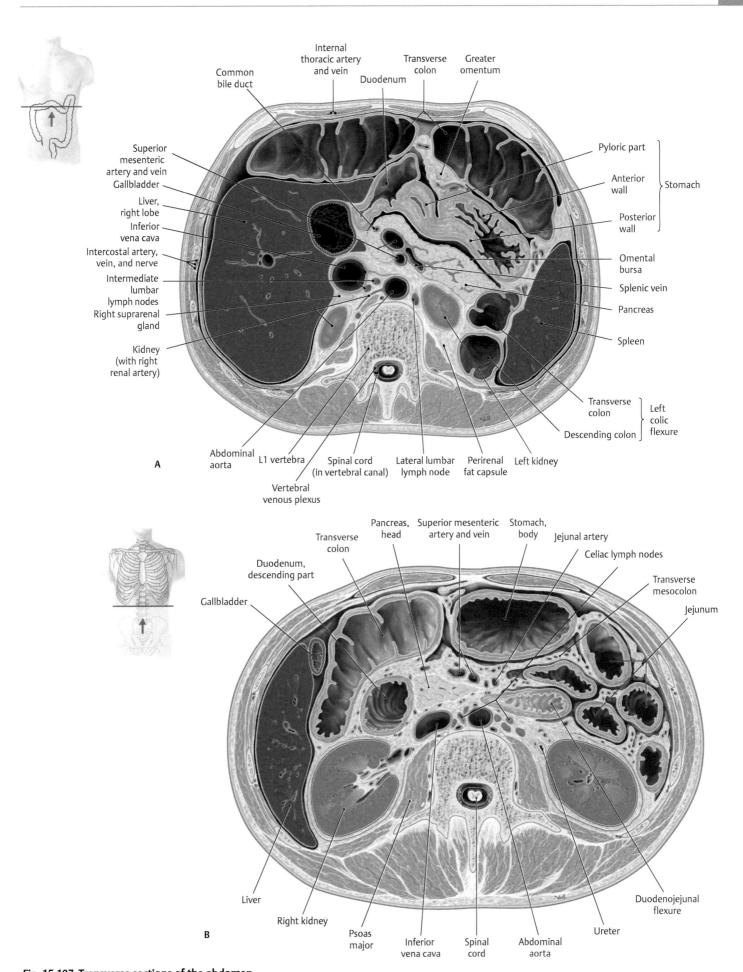

Fig. 15.107 Transverse sections of the abdomen
Inferior view. **A** Section through L1 vertebra. **B** Section through L2 vertebra.

Pelvic Girdle & Ligaments of the Pelvis

Fig. 15.108 Pelvic girdle

Anterosuperior view. The pelvic girdle surrounds the pelvis, the region of the body inferior to the abdomen. It consists of the two hip bones and the sacrum that together connect the vertebral column to the femur. The stability of the pelvic girdle is necessary for the transfer of trunk loads to the lower limb, which occurs in normal gait.

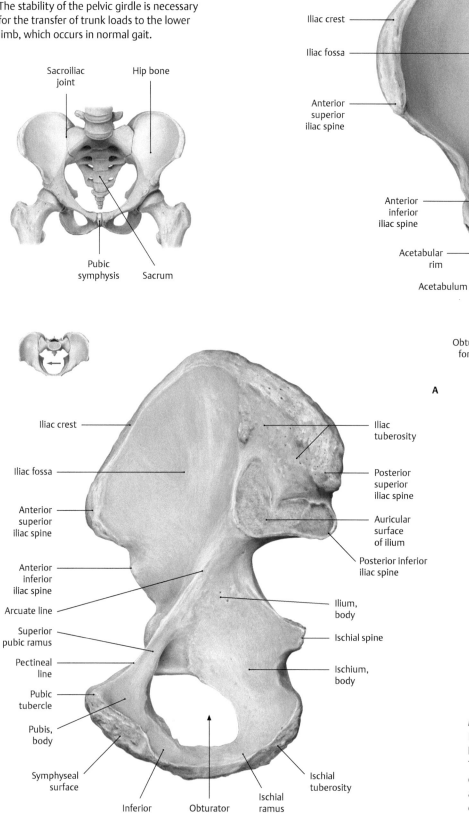

Sacroiliac joint
Hip bone
Pubic symphysis
Sacrum

Iliac crest
Iliac fossa
Anterior superior iliac spine
Anterior inferior iliac spine
Acetabular rim
Acetabulum
Obturator foramen
Ischial tuberosity

Iliac tuberosity
Auricular surface of ilium
Arcuate line
Ischial spine
Pectineal line
Symphyseal surface

A

Iliac crest
Iliac fossa
Anterior superior iliac spine
Anterior inferior iliac spine
Arcuate line
Superior pubic ramus
Pectineal line
Pubic tubercle
Pubis, body
Symphyseal surface
Inferior pubic ramus
Obturator foramen
Ischial ramus
Ischial tuberosity

Iliac tuberosity
Posterior superior iliac spine
Auricular surface of ilium
Posterior inferior iliac spine
Ilium, body
Ischial spine
Ischium, body

B

Fig. 15.109 Hip bone

Right hip bone (male). **A** Anterior view. **B** Medial view.

The two hip bones are connected to each other at the cartilaginous pubic symphysis and to the sacrum via the sacroiliac joints, creating the pelvic brim (seen in red in **Fig. 15.108**).

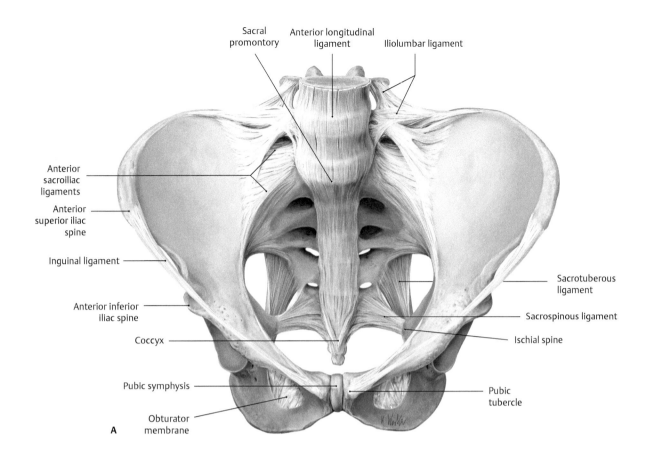

Sacral promontory

Anterior longitudinal ligament

Iliolumbar ligament

Anterior sacroiliac ligaments

Anterior superior iliac spine

Inguinal ligament

Anterior inferior iliac spine

Coccyx

Pubic symphysis

Obturator membrane

Sacrotuberous ligament

Sacrospinous ligament

Ischial spine

Pubic tubercle

A

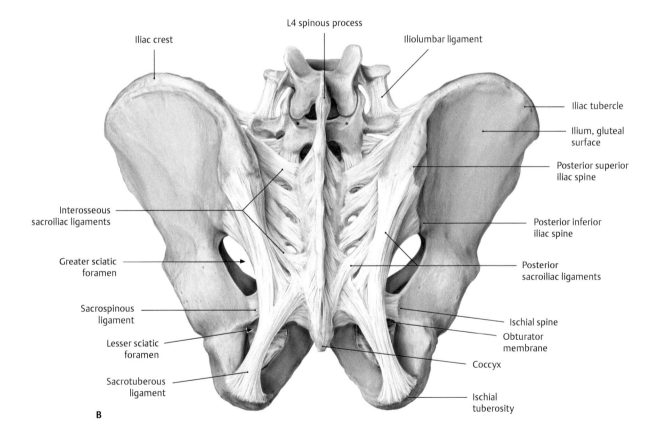

Iliac crest

L4 spinous process

Iliolumbar ligament

Iliac tubercle

Ilium, gluteal surface

Posterior superior iliac spine

Interosseous sacroiliac ligaments

Greater sciatic foramen

Sacrospinous ligament

Lesser sciatic foramen

Sacrotuberous ligament

Posterior inferior iliac spine

Posterior sacroiliac ligaments

Ischial spine

Obturator membrane

Coccyx

Ischial tuberosity

B

Fig. 15.110 **Ligaments of the pelvis**
Male pelvis. **A** Anterosuperior view. **B** Posterior view. *Removed on the right side:* some of the posterior sacroiliac ligaments to reveal the interosseous sacroiliac ligaments.

Contents of the Pelvis

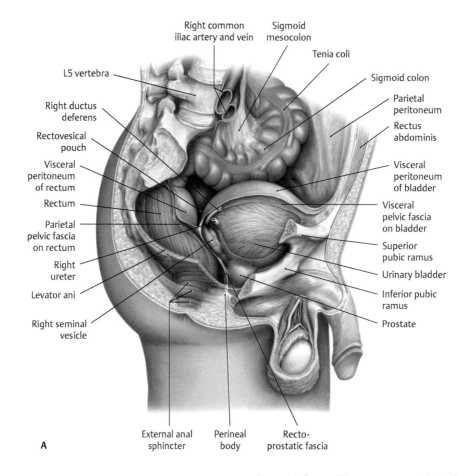

A

Right common iliac artery and vein
Sigmoid mesocolon
Tenia coli
L5 vertebra
Sigmoid colon
Right ductus deferens
Parietal peritoneum
Rectovesical pouch
Rectus abdominis
Visceral peritoneum of rectum
Visceral peritoneum of bladder
Rectum
Visceral pelvic fascia on bladder
Parietal pelvic fascia on rectum
Superior pubic ramus
Right ureter
Urinary bladder
Levator ani
Inferior pubic ramus
Right seminal vesicle
Prostate
External anal sphincter
Perineal body
Recto-prostatic fascia

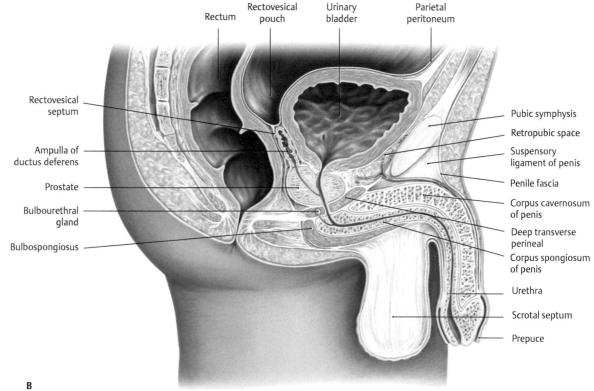

B

Rectum
Rectovesical pouch
Urinary bladder
Parietal peritoneum
Rectovesical septum
Pubic symphysis
Retropubic space
Ampulla of ductus deferens
Suspensory ligament of penis
Prostate
Penile fascia
Bulbourethral gland
Corpus cavernosum of penis
Bulbospongiosus
Deep transverse perineal
Corpus spongiosum of penis
Urethra
Scrotal septum
Prepuce

Fig. 15.111 **Male pelvis**
A Parasagittal section, viewed from the right side. **B** Midsagittal section, viewed from the right side.

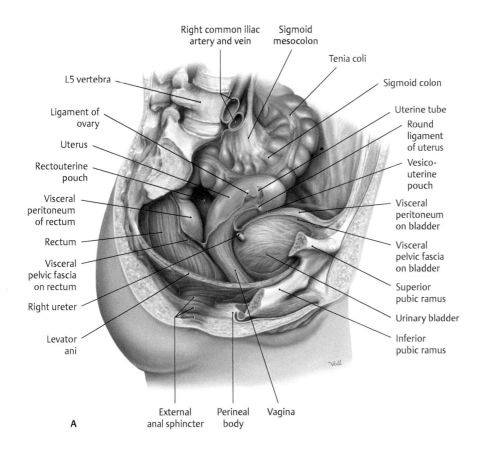

Right common iliac artery and vein

Sigmoid mesocolon

Tenia coli

Sigmoid colon

Uterine tube

Round ligament of uterus

Vesico-uterine pouch

Visceral peritoneum on bladder

Visceral pelvic fascia on bladder

Superior pubic ramus

Urinary bladder

Inferior pubic ramus

L5 vertebra

Ligament of ovary

Uterus

Rectouterine pouch

Visceral peritoneum of rectum

Rectum

Visceral pelvic fascia on rectum

Right ureter

Levator ani

External anal sphincter

Perineal body

Vagina

A

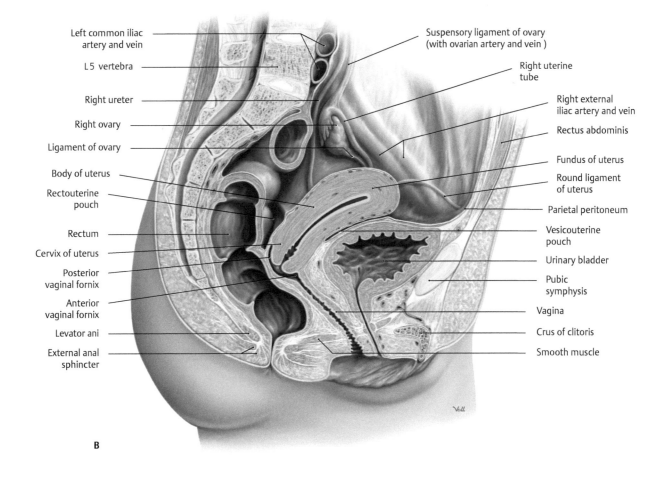

Left common iliac artery and vein

L5 vertebra

Right ureter

Right ovary

Ligament of ovary

Body of uterus

Rectouterine pouch

Rectum

Cervix of uterus

Posterior vaginal fornix

Anterior vaginal fornix

Levator ani

External anal sphincter

Suspensory ligament of ovary (with ovarian artery and vein)

Right uterine tube

Right external iliac artery and vein

Rectus abdominis

Fundus of uterus

Round ligament of uterus

Parietal peritoneum

Vesicouterine pouch

Urinary bladder

Pubic symphysis

Vagina

Crus of clitoris

Smooth muscle

B

Fig. 15.112 **Female pelvis**
A Parasagittal section, viewed from the right side. **B** Midsagittal section, viewed from the right side.

Arteries & Veins of the Pelvis

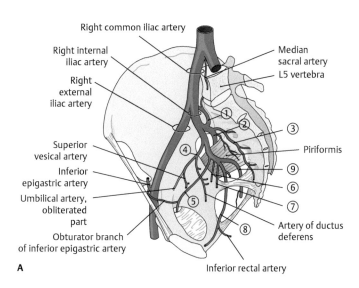

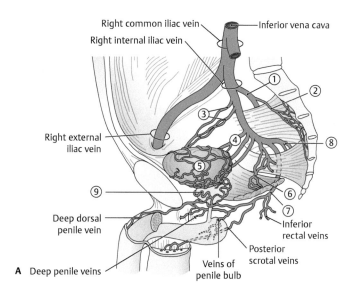

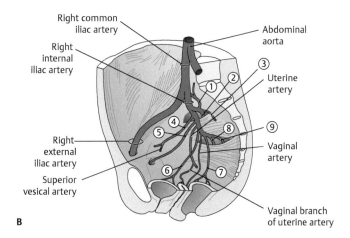

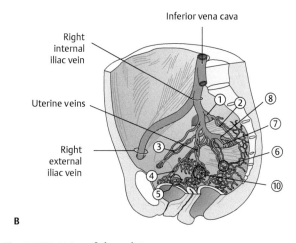

Fig. 15.113 Arteries of the pelvis
A Male pelvis. **B** Female pelvis. See **Table 15.17**.

Fig. 15.114 Veins of the pelvis
A Male pelvis. **B** Female pelvis. See **Table 15.18**.

Table 15.17 Branches of the internal iliac artery

The internal iliac artery gives off five parietal (pelvic wall) and four visceral (pelvic organs) branches.* Parietal branches are shown in italics.

Branches

①	*Iliolumbar a.*	
②	*Superior gluteal a.*	
③	*Lateral sacral a.*	
④	Umbilical a.	A. of ductus deferens Superior vesical a.
⑤	*Obturator a.*	
⑥	Inferior vesical a.	
⑦	Middle rectal a.	
⑧	Internal pudendal a.	Inferior rectal a.
⑨	*Inferior gluteal a.*	

* In the female pelvis, the uterine and vaginal arteries arise directly from the anterior division of the internal iliac artery.

Table 15.18 Venous drainage of the pelvis

Tributaries

①	Superior gluteal v.
②	Lateral sacral v.
③	Obturator vv.
④	Vesical vv.
⑤	Vesical venous plexus
⑥	Middle rectal vv. (rectal venous plexus) (also superior and inferior rectal vv., not shown)
⑦	Internal pudendal v.
⑧	Inferior gluteal vv.
⑨	Prostatic venous plexus
⑩	Uterine and vaginal venous plexus

The male pelvis also contains veins draining the penis and scrotum.

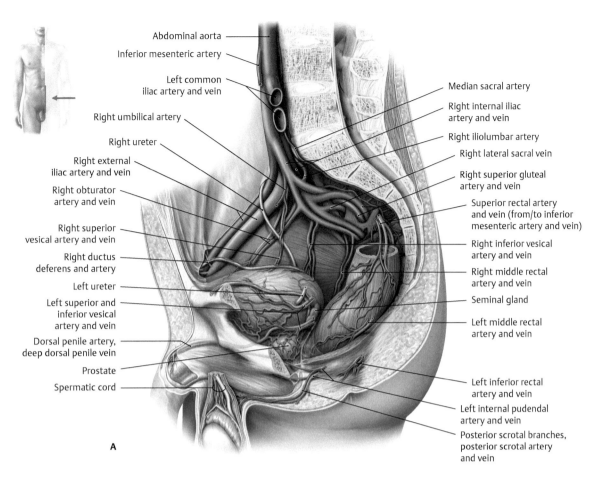

Abdominal aorta

Inferior mesenteric artery

Left common iliac artery and vein

Right umbilical artery

Right ureter

Right external iliac artery and vein

Right obturator artery and vein

Right superior vesical artery and vein

Right ductus deferens and artery

Left ureter

Left superior and inferior vesical artery and vein

Dorsal penile artery, deep dorsal penile vein

Prostate

Spermatic cord

Median sacral artery

Right internal iliac artery and vein

Right iliolumbar artery

Right lateral sacral vein

Right superior gluteal artery and vein

Superior rectal artery and vein (from/to inferior mesenteric artery and vein)

Right inferior vesical artery and vein

Right middle rectal artery and vein

Seminal gland

Left middle rectal artery and vein

Left inferior rectal artery and vein

Left internal pudendal artery and vein

Posterior scrotal branches, posterior scrotal artery and vein

A

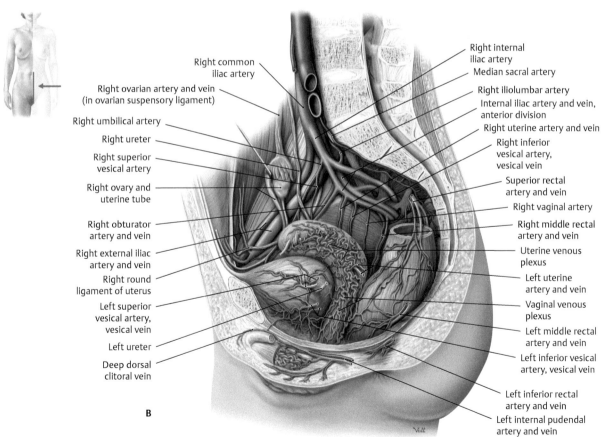

Right common iliac artery

Right ovarian artery and vein (in ovarian suspensory ligament)

Right umbilical artery

Right ureter

Right superior vesical artery

Right ovary and uterine tube

Right obturator artery and vein

Right external iliac artery and vein

Right round ligament of uterus

Left superior vesical artery, vesical vein

Left ureter

Deep dorsal clitoral vein

Right internal iliac artery

Median sacral artery

Right iliolumbar artery

Internal iliac artery and vein, anterior division

Right uterine artery and vein

Right inferior vesical artery, vesical vein

Superior rectal artery and vein

Right vaginal artery

Right middle rectal artery and vein

Uterine venous plexus

Left uterine artery and vein

Vaginal venous plexus

Left middle rectal artery and vein

Left inferior vesical artery, vesical vein

Left inferior rectal artery and vein

Left internal pudendal artery and vein

B

Fig. 15.115 Blood vessels of the pelvis
Idealized right hemipelvis, left lateral view. **A** Male pelvis.
B Female pelvis.

Appendices

General Principles of Local Anesthesia

Physiology of Peripheral Nerve Depolarization

When a nerve is inactive (not generating action potentials), there is a potential difference across its membrane, which is known as the resting membrane potential (RMP) and is measured in millivolts (mV). Nerve cells have an RMP of −70 mV, which is established by differences in potassium and sodium ion concentrations across the resting cell membrane — high potassium concentration intercellularly and high sodium ion concentration extracellularly. At rest, the nerve cell is relatively resistant to ion passage, but on excitation, voltage-gated sodium channels open, and there is a slow influx of sodium ions into the cell. When a threshold potential is reached, depolarization occurs, and there is a fast influx of sodium ions into the cell, causing the potential across the membrane to become positive (+40mV). The sodium channels quickly close again, preventing further sodium influx. At the same time, potassium channels open, and there is potassium efflux from the cell. This causes repolarization of the cell membrane back to the RMP.

The depolarization of a nerve cell initiates a sequential series of depolarizations along the nerve fiber, thus propagating the impulse (action potential) along the fiber. In myelinated nerve fibers, the depolarizations "jump" from one node of Ranvier to the next (saltatory conduction). In unmyelinated fibers (which do not have nodes of Ranvier), the depolarization spreads to adjacent cells.

Mechanism of Action of Local Anesthetics

Local anesthetics block the inner (cytoplasmic) gate of sodium channels in nerve cells, preventing sodium influx and action potential initiation and propagation. Termination of action of the anesthetic at the site of injection is by diffusion of the active drug into the systemic circulation, followed by metabolism and elimination

Duration of Anesthesia

Duration of dental local anesthesia can be defined in terms of duration of pulpal anesthesia versus the duration of soft tissue anesthesia. Usually, dentists try to maximize the duration of pulpal anesthesia and minimize the undesirable persistence of soft tissue anesthesia. The duration of pulpal anesthesia and the duration of soft tissue anesthesia of some of the main local anesthetic agents following maxillary infiltration and an inferior alveolar nerve block are listed in **Table A.1**.

General Injection Technique

The fingers of the supporting hand retract the soft tissue around the injection site, enabling the dentist to visualize the target area. These fingers may also be used to provide stability for the syringe and can act as reference points for some injections.

When ready to inject, the needle is inserted gently and directly in one continuous movement to the target area. The dentist should then aspirate to ensure that the tip of the needle does not lie within a blood vessel. Most dental syringes are "self-aspirating," meaning that if the plunger of the syringe is slightly deployed, it bounces back, aspirating (sucking) as it does so. If the syringe is not self-aspirating, aspiration is performed by drawing back slightly on the plunger. The absence of blood in the local anesthetic cartridge suggests that no vessel has been breached. If there is blood in the cartridge, the needle tip should be repositioned slightly and aspiration repeated. Following a negative aspiration result, the local anesthetic is injected slowly, exerting as little pressure as possible. Injection into the hard palate and interdental papillae are exceptions because the mucosa is tightly adherent to the supporting periosteum in these areas, necessitating that some pressure is used.

Classification of Injection Techniques

Infiltration

Local anesthetic solution is deposited at the level of the tooth apices and through alveolar bone to bathe the periapical nerves.

Nerve Blocks

Local anesthetic solution is deposited around the main nerve trunk and therefore anesthetizes all of the branches distal to this.

Table A.1	Duration of anesthesia with some local anesthetic agents				
Local anesthetic agent	Maxillary infiltration		Inferior alveolar nerve block	
	Duration of pulpal anesthesia (min)	Duration of soft tissue anesthesia (min)	Duration of pulpal anesthesia (min)	Duration of soft tissue anesthesia (min)
Lidocaine 2% with 1:100,000 epinephrine*	45–60	170	85	190
Articaine 4% with 1:100,000 epinephrine*	45–60	190	90	230
Bupivacaine 0.5% with 1:200,000 epinephrine*	90	340	240	440
Prilocaine 4% plain	20	105	55	190
Mepivacaine 3% plain	25	90	40	165
* The duration of action is prolonged when combined with epinephrine, a vasoconstrictor. A "plain" solution contains no vasoconstrictive agent.					

Overview of Nerves Anesthetized

Injections given within the oral cavity anesthetize a branch or branches of either the maxillary or mandibular division of the trigeminal nerve (CN V_2 or CN V_3, respectively) on the same side as the injection (**Figs. A.1** and **A.2**).

Failure of Anesthesia

Patient Variation

A typical dose of local anesthetic profoundly anesthetizes some patients and may not sufficiently anesthetize others. The dentist must try to ascertain whether failure is due to patient variation or improper injection technique. If due to the former, then more local anesthetic may be given to achieve adequate anesthesia. Likewise, differences occur between patients in the duration of action of anesthetics. The best way to mitigate these differences is to begin treatment as soon as anesthesia is achieved: ~2 minutes after injection for an infiltration and ~5 minutes after injection for a block.

Acute Pulpitis or Apical Abscess

Acute pulpitis (pulpal inflammation) results in a hyperemic tooth (a tooth in which the pulpal blood vessels dilate causing a painful increase in pressure) that is difficult to adequately anesthetize. The pus of an apical abscess can prevent proper diffusion of the local anesthetic solution to the periapical nerves and vessels.

Intravascular Injection

If all or part of an injection of local anesthetic is deposited intravascularly, then there may be little or no anesthesia achieved.

Injection into Muscles or Their Fascia

If the local anesthetic is deposited in a muscle or its fascia instead of into the bone near the teeth apices, then the distance the anesthetic has to diffuse to reach the apical nerves and vessels is increased, resulting in reduced anesthesia. Injection into a muscle can also produce trismus (restricted mouth opening).

Complications and Their Treatment

Fainting

This is the most common systemic complication and is likely attributed to anxiety over the procedure. It can be minimized by administering local anesthetic with the patient supine. If fainting does occur, place the patient in a supine position, and recovery will occur rapidly.

Allergic Reactions

Allergy to local anesthetic is uncommon but possible. It may be due to allergy to the drug, allergy to the additives for compounding the drug, or latex allergy to the rubber bung located at one end of a local anesthetic cartridge. Allergy manifests as facial flushing, swelling, rash, itching, and wheezing. The patient should be sent for allergy testing to determine the precise cause. For minor allergic reactions, provide reassurance, and antihistamines if necessary. For severe (anaphylactic) reactions, urgently call for an ambulance, place the patient in a supine position, and give emergency medication as needed (e.g., intramuscular epinephrine, intravenous hydrocortisone, and oxygen by mask).

Cardiovascular Collapse

Cardiovascular collapse may be precipitated by, or exacerbated by stress, excessive amounts of local anesthetic, and improper aspiration, leading to deposition of local anesthetic in a blood vessel. Epinephrine in the local anesthetic can act directly on the heart, which, if previously diseased, can cause arrhythmias.

If this occurs, urgently call for an ambulance, place the patient in a supine position, and maintain airway and circulation.

Hematomas

Small hematomas are of little consequence. Larger hematomas can compromise the airway.

No treatment is needed for small hematomas; large hematomas due to arterial bleeding, if they are not self-limiting, may require ligation of the vessel.

Trismus

Trismus is the inability to open the mouth normally. It usually occurs after an inferior alveolar nerve block that is given too low, resulting in hematoma formation in the medial pterygoid. This may be accompanied by infection.

Treatment includes reassurance, antibiotics, and encouragement to progressively try to open the mouth.

Facial Paralysis

Facial paralysis (or palsy) may occur following an improperly placed inferior alveolar nerve block. If the needle is directed too far posteriorly, the tip may enter the superficial layer of deep cervical fascia that surrounds the parotid gland. Local anesthetic is therefore able to penetrate the gland and anesthetize the five branches of the facial nerve that are embedded within it. This is manifested by the patient's inability to frown or blink and drooping of the mouth on the affected side. The facial paralysis is transient, normally lasting for ~1 hour.

Treatment includes reassurance and a protective eye covering until the blink reflex returns.

499

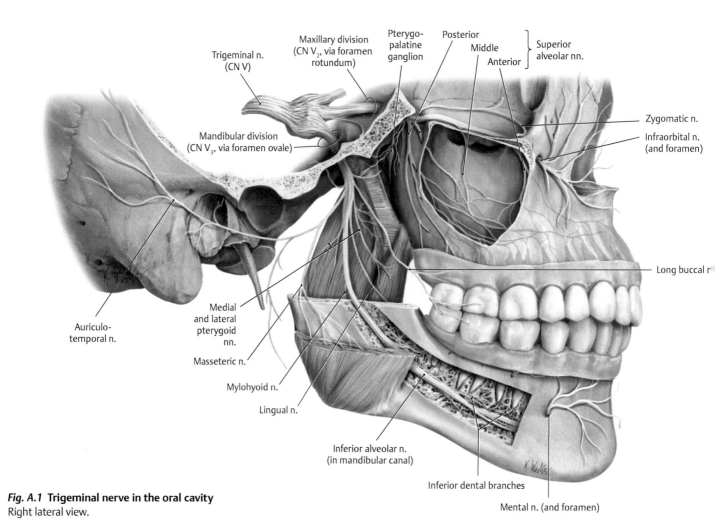

Fig. A.1 Trigeminal nerve in the oral cavity
Right lateral view.

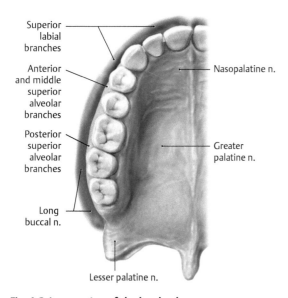

Fig. A.2 Innervation of the hard palate
Inferior view.

Maxillary Anesthesia

Maxillary Incisors and Canines

Anatomy

The incisors and canines and their associated periodontal ligaments, buccal gingiva, mucosa, and supporting bone are innervated by the anterior superior alveolar nerves, which branch off the infraorbital nerve just before it emerges from the infraorbital foramen (**Table A.2**). These nerves anastomose over the midline. The palatal gingiva, mucosa, and supporting bone are innervated by the nasopalatine nerve, which emerges through the incisive foramen.

The medial spread of local anesthetic may be hindered by the labial frenulum that anchors the lip to the attached gingiva in the midline.

The maxillary bone has a thin, porous lamina (layer) easily penetrated by an infiltration of local anesthetic solution.

Injection Technique

- Insert the needle in the mucobuccal fold immediately superior to the crown of the tooth being anesthetized and pass it axially toward the apex of the tooth (**Fig. A.3A** and **B**). The needle should be in close proximity to the bone to ensure that the local anesthetic solution has minimal diffusion distance before it bathes the periapical nerves and vessels.

- Following a negative aspiration result, slowly inject 1.0 to 1.8 mL of local anesthetic.

- For central incisors, the injection is best placed distally due to the close proximity of the anterior nasal spine.

Clinical Considerations

- A mucobuccal fold infiltration is sufficient for cavity preparation and pulpal procedures.

- Extractions will require supplementary anesthesia of the palatal gingiva, mucosa, and supporting bone, either by local infiltration of the palate (p. 508) or by a nasopalatine block (p. 507).

- Painful injection

Table A.2	Anesthesia of maxillary incisors and canine
Areas anesthetized* (see Fig. A.3C and D)	**Nerve (Fig. A.3B)**
Maxillary central, lateral incisor** and canine*** and their associated periodontal ligaments, buccal gingiva, mucosa, and supporting bone	Anterior superior alveolar nerve
Lateral aspect of the nose	External nasal branch fibers of the infraorbital nerve
Upper lip	Superior labial branch fibers of the infraorbital nerve

* On the same side as the injection.
** This applies when the injection is placed superior to the maxillary lateral incisor.
*** The root of the canine is longer, and the apical part of the root is often distally oriented; therefore, the maxillary right canine may not be sufficiently anesthetized for cavity preparation from this injection alone.

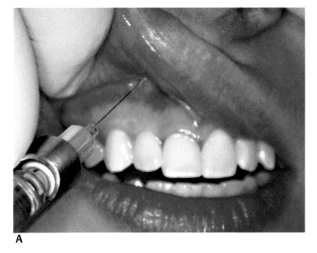

A

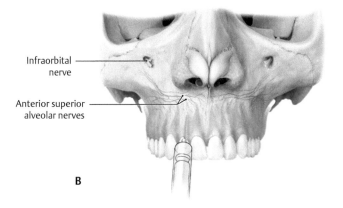

B

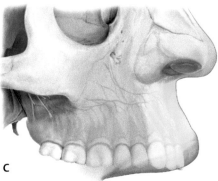

C

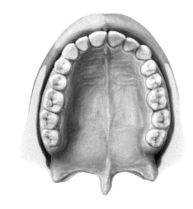

D

Fig. A.3 **Infiltration of the maxillary lateral incisor**
A Injection technique.
B Nerves anesthetized, anterior view.
C Areas anesthetized, right lateral view.

D Areas anesthetized, inferior view. Note the lips roughly extend to the first premolar region on each side; the cheeks are colored gray.

Infraorbital Nerve Block

Anatomy

The infraorbital nerve is a continuation of the maxillary nerve as it enters the infraorbital canal. The anterior superior alveolar nerve and middle superior alveolar nerve (when present) branch from this nerve just before it exits the infraorbital canal and are therefore also anesthetized by diffusion of local anesthetic from the injection site (**Table A.3**).

Injection Technique

- Palpate the center of the inferior margin of the orbit with the index finger of the supporting hand. At a point ~1 cm below the orbital margin, the infraorbital foramen can be palpated. Hold the index finger at that point, while retracting the upper lip with the thumb of the supporting hand. Insert the needle at the mucobuccal fold immediately superior to the 1st maxillary premolar, parallel to the long axis of the tooth, toward the tip of the index finger (**Fig. A.4A** and **B**).

- Following a negative aspiration result, slowly inject ~1 mL of local anesthetic.

Clinical Considerations

- To avoid having to give more than one injection, an infraorbital block may be used to anesthetize multiple teeth for cavity preparation or pulpal procedures. It may also be used when infiltration has failed to achieve pulpal anesthesia or is contraindicated (e.g., infiltration would require an injection into an infected area).

- Extractions of any of the teeth anesthetized by an infraorbital block will require supplementary anesthesia of the palatal gingiva by a nasopalatine or greater palatine block or by local infiltration of the palate.

- Hematoma is rare with this injection, but there is potential for iatrogenic (accidental, clinician-induced) damage to the patient's eye.

- To obtain complete anesthesia of the central incisor on the same side as the injection, it may be necessary to block anastomosing fibers from the anterior superior alveolar nerve on the contralateral side of the midline. This is achieved by placing a supplemental 0.5 mL of local anesthetic in the contralateral buccal fold, just distal to the central incisor.

Table A.3	Anesthesia following an infraorbital nerve block
Areas anesthetized (Fig. A.4C and D)	**Nerve (Fig. A.4B)**
Incisors and canine and their associated periodontal ligament, buccal gingival, mucosa, and supporting bone	Anterior superior alveolar nerve
Premolars and possibly the mesiobuccal cusp of the 1st molar and their associated periodontal ligament, buccal gingival, mucosa, and supporting bone	Middle superior alveolar nerve or fibers from the superior dental plexus
Lateral aspect of the nose	External nasal branches of the infraorbital nerve
Lower eyelid	Inferior palpebral branches of the infraorbital nerve
Upper lip and mucosa	Superior labial branches of the infraorbital nerve

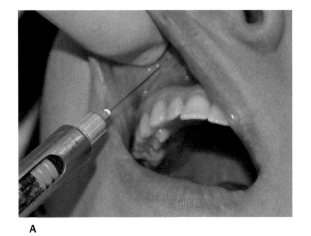

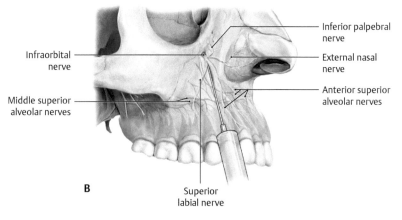

B

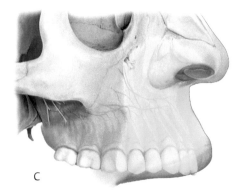

C

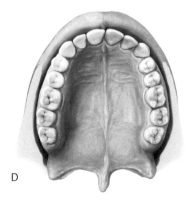

D

Fig. A.4 Infraorbital nerve block
A Injection technique.
B Nerves anesthetized, right lateral view.
C Areas anesthetized, right lateral view.
D Areas anesthetized, inferior view.

Maxillary Premolars

Anatomy

The premolar area is innervated by the superior dental plexus, which is formed by convergent branches from the posterior superior alveolar nerve and the anterior superior alveolar nerve. Sometimes there is a middle superior alveolar nerve that, when present, innervates the premolars, their periodontal ligaments, buccal gingiva, and supporting bone, and often the mesiobuccal root of the first molar (**Table A.4**). The palatal gingiva, mucosa, and supporting bone adjacent to the premolars is mainly innervated by the greater palatine nerve, but the area of the first premolar may also be innervated by fibers of the nasopalatine nerve.

Diffusion of local anesthetic deposited in the mucobuccal fold is especially good in this area because the bone lamina is thin, and the apices of the premolars lie very close to the lamina. Consequently, small volumes of local anesthetic are required, and the palatal roots of the premolars are almost always anesthetized by this one injection.

Injection Technique

The same infiltration technique is used as for the incisors and canines. Deposit 1.0 to 1.5 mL of local anesthetic solution around the apex of the premolars (**Fig. A.5A** and **B**).

Clinical Considerations

- A mucobuccal fold infiltration is sufficient for cavity preparation and pulpal procedures.

- Extractions will require supplementary anesthesia of the palatal gingiva, mucosa, and supporting bone, usually by one local infiltration injection of the palate between the premolars.

Table A.4	**Anesthesia of maxillary premolars**
Area anesthetized* (Figs. A.5C and D)	**Nerve (Fig. A.5B)**
Both maxillary premolars* and their associated periodontal ligaments, buccal gingival, mucosa, and supporting bone	Middle superior alveolar nerve or branches of the superior dental plexus
Canine and the mesiobuccal cusp of the 1st molar** and their associated periodontal ligaments, buccal gingival, mucosa, and supporting bone	
* This applies when the injection is placed between the premolars. ** These teeth, soft tissues, and bone may also be anesthetized to a lesser extent.	

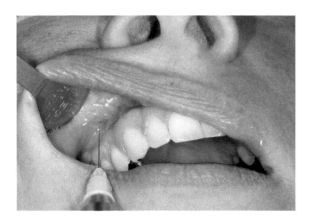

A

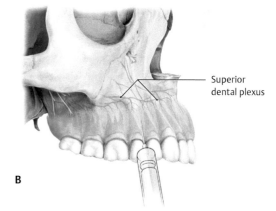

B

Superior dental plexus

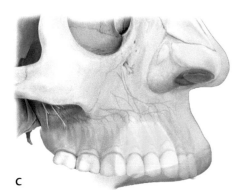

C

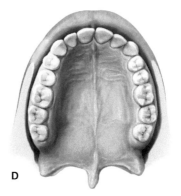

D

***Fig. A.5* Infiltration of the maxillary premolars**
A Injection technique.
B Nerves anesthetized, right lateral view.
C Areas anesthetized, right lateral view.
D Areas anesthetized, inferior view.

Maxillary Molars

Anatomy

The molar region of the maxilla is innervated by the posterior superior alveolar nerve, which branches from the infraorbital nerve before it enters the infraorbital canal. These branches enter foramina on the infratemporal surface of the maxilla, where they enter to innervate the maxillary molars and their associated periodontal ligaments, buccal gingiva, mucosa, and supporting bone (**Table A.5**). The distance between the mucobuccal fold and the apices of the maxillary molars varies from patient to patient. This distance may be increased by the lower margin of the zygomatic arch or when the maxillary sinus extends down between the buccal and palatal roots. This can lead to failure of a buccal infiltration injection.

Injection Technique

- The same infiltration technique as for incisors and canines is used. Introduce the needle to the mucobuccal fold slightly mesially to the maxillary first molar (**Fig. A.6A** and **B**). A second injection may be given in the mucobuccal fold at the distal aspect of the maxillary first molar to ensure the tooth is adequately anesthetized.

- Following a negative aspiration result, slowly inject 1.0 to 1.8 mL of local anesthetic.

Clinical Considerations

- A mucobuccal fold infiltration injected is usually sufficient for cavity preparation and pulpal procedures. Rarely, it may be necessary to perform a palatal injection to achieve complete anesthesia of the palatal root.

- Extractions will require supplementary anesthesia of the palatal gingiva, mucosa, and supporting bone by greater palatine block or by local infiltration.

- For infiltration injections of the maxillary third molars, the patient should not be asked to open too widely; otherwise, the coronoid process of the mandible is moved anteriorly and can cover the injection site.

Table A.5	Anesthesia of maxillary molars
Area anesthetized* (Fig. A.6C and D)	**Nerve (Fig. A.6B)**
Mesiobuccal cusp of the 1st molar	Middle superior alveolar nerve (if present)
1st and 2nd molar* and their associated periodontal ligaments, buccal gingival, mucosa, and supporting bone	Posterior superior alveolar nerve
Lateral aspect of the lip (may be very slight or absent)	Superior labial branches of the infraorbital nerve
* This applies when injection is placed mesially and distally to the 1st molar.	

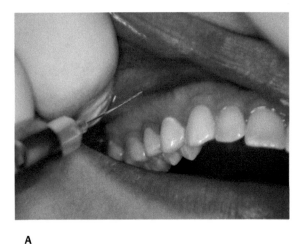

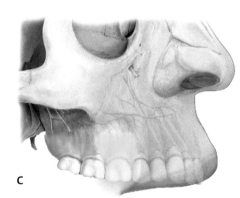

A

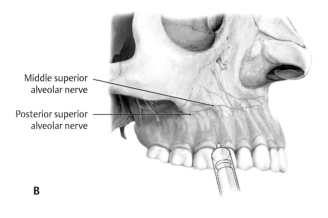

Middle superior alveolar nerve

Posterior superior alveolar nerve

B

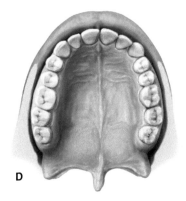

C

D

Fig. A.6 Infiltration of the maxillary molars
A Injection technique.
B Nerves anesthetized, right lateral view.
C Areas anesthetized, right lateral view.
D Areas anesthetized, inferior view.

Posterior Superior Alveolar Nerve Block

Anatomy

The posterior superior alveolar nerve is located in the infratemporal fossa and lies in close proximity to the pterygoid plexus of veins (**Table A.6**).

Injection Technique

- Instruct the patient to open his or her mouth and swing the mandible toward the same side to allow better visualization of the injection site and more room to maneuver.

- Insert the needle into the mucobuccal fold just superior to the maxillary second molar, between the medial border of the ramus of the mandible and the maxillary tuberosity. Then advance the needle inward, backward, and upward 1.5 to 2.0 cm (**Fig. A.7A** and **B**).

- Following a negative aspiration result, slowly deposit 1.0 to 1.8 mL of local anesthetic.

Clinical Considerations

- This injection is sufficient for cavity preparation and pulpal procedures on all of the maxillary molars.

- Extractions will require supplementary anesthesia of the palatal gingiva, mucosa, and supporting bone by a greater palatine nerve block or by local infiltration.

Notes

There is a significant risk of hematoma by introduction of the needle into the pterygoid plexus. Short needles and careful aspiration reduce this risk.

Table A.6	Anesthesia following a posterior superior alveolar nerve block	
Areas anesthetized* (Fig. A.7C and D)	**Nerve (Fig. A.7B)**	
Maxillary 1st,* 2nd, and 3rd molars and their associated periodontal ligaments, buccal gingival, mucosa, and supporting bone	Posterior superior alveolar nerve	
* The mesiobuccal root of the 1st molar may not be anesthetized and may therefore require supplemental buccal infiltration anesthesia mesial to the 1st molar (to anesthetize the middle superior alveolar nerve).		

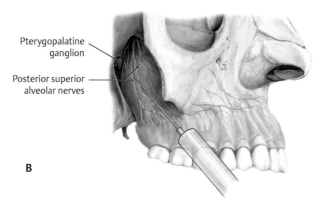

Pterygopalatine ganglion

Posterior superior alveolar nerves

B

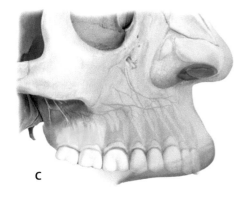

A

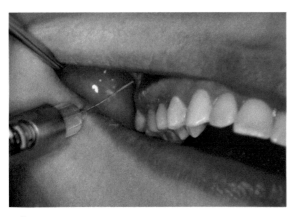

C

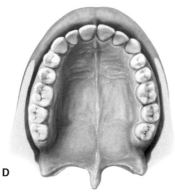

D

Fig. A.7 Posterior superior alveolar nerve block
A Injection technique.
B Nerves anesthetized, right lateral view.

C Areas anesthetized, right lateral view.
D Areas anesthetized, inferior view.

Maxillary Division Block

Anatomy

The maxillary division block is an advanced local anesthetic technique. It uses the greater palatine canal to reach the pterygopalatine fossa and therefore enables the dentist to anesthetize all branches of the maxillary nerve (**Table A.7**). The canal is usually vertical, thus aiding this procedure.

Injection Technique

- Locate the greater palatine foramen with a cotton swab applicator, which can be felt to sink slightly into the foramen. Inject a small amount of anesthetic. This lessens patient's discomfort for the next part of the procedure.

- Insert the needle into the greater palatine foramen ~28 to 30 mm. The needle tip should now be located in the pterygopalatine fossa (**Fig. A.8A** and **B**).

- Following a negative aspiration result, slowly inject 1 to 2 mL of local anesthetic.

Clinical Considerations

- This injection is useful when extensive restorative dentistry and surgical procedures are needed.

- The needle should never be forced into the greater palatine foramen to avoid fracture of the wall of the greater palatine canal.

- If the needle is placed too far superiorly, the anesthetic can be deposited in the eye, affecting vision.

- Hematoma formation may occur due to rupture of the vessels that also run in the greater palatine canal.

Table A.7 Anesthesia following a maxillary division block	
Areas anesthetized (Fig. A.8C and D)	**Nerve (Fig. A.8B)**
All maxillary teeth and their associated periodontal ligaments, buccal gingiva, mucosa, and supporting bone	Anterior, middle (if present), and posterior superior alveolar nerves
All palatal gingival, mucosa, and supporting bone	Nasopalatine nerve (anterior one-third) and greater palatine nerve (posterior two-thirds)
Lateral aspect of the nose	External nasal branches of the infraorbital nerve
Lower eyelid	Inferior palpebral branches of the infraorbital nerve
Upper lip	Superior labial branches of the infraorbital nerve

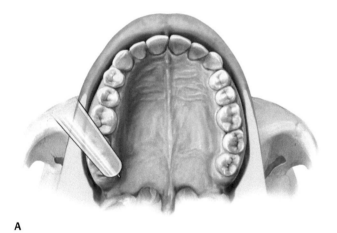

A

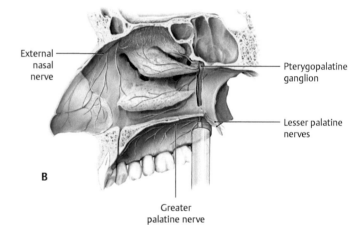

External nasal nerve

Pterygopalatine ganglion

Lesser palatine nerves

B

Greater palatine nerve

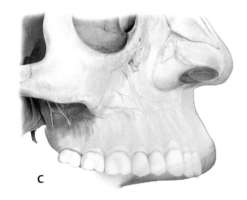

C

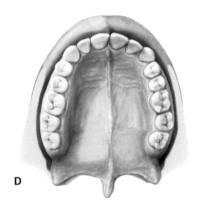

D

***Fig. A.8* Maxillary division block**
A Injection technique, inferior view.
B Nerves anesthetized, left lateral view of the right lateral nasal wall with the pterygopalatine ganglion exposed. .

C Areas anesthetized, right lateral view.
D Areas anesthetized, inferior view.

Nasopalatine Nerve Block

Anatomy

The nasopalatine nerve is a branch of the maxillary nerve that passes through the pterygopalatine ganglion (**Table A.8**). It enters the nasal cavity through the sphenopalatine foramen, passes across the roof of the nasal cavity, then runs obliquely downward and forward in the nasal septum between the supporting bone and mucous membrane. It descends farther through the incisive canal and emerges into the anterior hard palate through the incisive foramen. Branches of the nasopalatine nerve anastomose with branches of the contralateral nasopalatine nerve and with the greater palatine nerve. Because the right and left nasopalatine nerves exit the incisive foramen in close proximity, one injection anesthetizes both sides of the anterior one third of the hard palate.

Injection Technique

- Using a cotton swab applicator, apply pressure close to the injection site to reduce the perception of pain. Insert the needle into the palatal mucosa lateral to the incisive papilla until bone is contacted (**Fig. A.9A** and **B**).

- After withdrawing the needle slightly and following a negative aspiration result, inject a very small volume of local anesthetic under minimal pressure. The tissue will be seen to blanch due to the vasoconstrictor in the local anesthetic solution.

Clinical Considerations

- This injection is used to supplement buccal infiltration injections for extraction of any of the maxillary anterior teeth.

- This injection is widely perceived to be the most painful variety of dental injection. It is particularly painful because the mucosa of the hard palate is tightly bound to the periosteum of the palate, allowing little space for the diffusion of local anesthetic.

Table A.8	**Anesthesia following a nasopalatine nerve block**
Area anesthetized (Fig. A.9C)	**Nerve (Fig. A.9B)**
The maxillary gingiva, mucosa, and supporting bone from the right maxillary canine to the left maxillary canine	Nasopalatine nerve

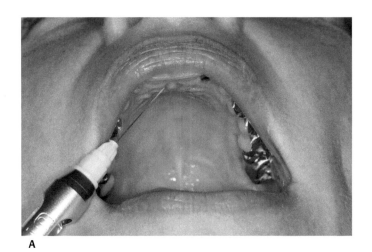

A

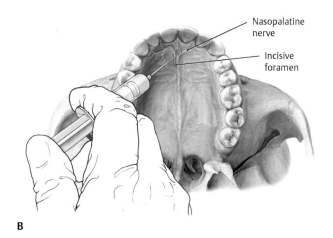

Nasopalatine nerve

Incisive foramen

B

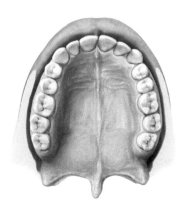

C

Fig. A.9 Nasopalatine nerve block
A Injection technique, inferior view.
B Nerves anesthetized, inferior view.
C Areas anesthetized, inferior view.

Greater Palatine Nerve Block

Anatomy

The greater palatine nerve is a branch of the maxillary nerve that passes through the greater palatine ganglion (**Table A.9**). It runs from the pterygopalatine fossa, down through the greater palatine canal, and through the greater palatine foramen to reach the hard palate. It then runs forward in a groove to a point just distal to the canine tooth.

Injection Technique

- The greater palatine foramen lies ~0.5 to 1.0 cm mesial to the margin of the gingiva at the distal border of the maxillary second molar (**Fig. A.10A** and **B**). It should be located by using a cotton swab applicator, which can be felt to sink slightly into the foramen. With the cotton swab applicator, apply pressure close to the injection site to reduce the perception of pain. Insert the needle until it contacts bone. Withdraw it slightly, then aspirate.

- Following a negative aspiration result, slowly inject around 0.1 mL of local anesthetic.

Clinical Considerations

- This injection is used to anesthetize palatal tissues for multiple extractions involving the maxillary premolars and molars on one side. It may also be useful for mucogingival surgical procedures.

- Bone contact prior to injection is necessary to ensure that the needle is not in the soft palate.

- The palate in the region of the greater palatine foramen is tightly bound to the supporting bone but less so than at the incisive foramen. Therefore, although still painful, this injection is less so than for the nasopalatine nerve block.

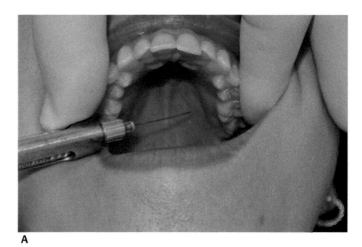

A

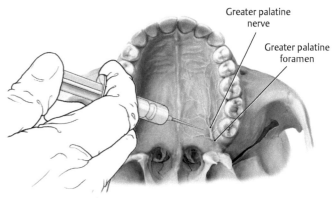

Greater palatine nerve

Greater palatine foramen

B

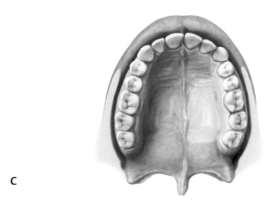

C

Table A.9	Anesthesia following a greater palatine nerve block	
Area anesthetized (Fig. A.10C)	**Nerve (Fig. A.10B)**	
The maxillary gingiva, mucosa, and supporting bone from the maxillary 1st premolar to the posterior hard palate to the midline of the hard palate	Greater palatine nerve	

Fig. A.10 **Greater palatine nerve block**
A Injection technique, inferior view.
B Nerves anesthetized, inferior view.
C Areas anesthetized, inferior view.

Supplementary Infiltration of the Palate

Anatomy

Supplementary infiltration of the palate may anesthetize fibers of the nasopalatine nerve and/or greater palatine nerve (depending on the site of the injection) (**Table A.10**).

Injection Technique

- Using a cotton swab applicator, apply pressure close to the injection site to reduce the perception of pain. Insert the needle into the palatal mucosa ~1 cm from the neck of the tooth to be anesthetized, until bone is contacted.

- Withdraw the needle slightly and aspirate.

- Following a negative aspiration result, inject ~0.1 mL of local anesthetic. The mucosa will be seen to blanch due to the vasoconstrictor in the local anesthetic.

Clinical Considerations

- This injection is used to supplement buccal infiltration, infraorbital, or posterior superior alveolar nerve blocks for extractions of the maxillary teeth. It is more commonly performed than a nasopalatine or greater palatine nerve block.

- The injection is painful.

Table A.10	Supplementary infiltration of the palate	
Areas anesthetized	**Nerve**	
Palatal gingival, mucosa, and supporting bone in the vicinity of the injection site	Fibers of the nasopalatine nerve and/or greater palatine nerve	

Mandibular Anesthesia

Mandibular Incisors and Canines

Anatomy

The incisors and canines are innervated by the incisive nerve, a terminal branch of the inferior alveolar nerve (**Table A.11**). Its course lies within bone, but it may be anesthetized by infiltration because the bone lamina in this area of the mandible is thin and porous. Because the bone around the canine teeth in adults may be denser, infiltration anesthesia may fail. In this case, a mental nerve block or inferior alveolar nerve block can be used to ensure sufficient anesthesia of a canine tooth.

The buccal soft tissues are innervated by the mental nerve, while the lingual gingiva and supporting bone are supplied by the sublingual nerve (a branch of the lingual nerve).

Injection Technique

The same infiltration technique is used as for the maxillary incisors and canines. Deposit around 1 mL of local anesthetic around the apices of the teeth (**Fig. A.11A** and **B**, **Table A.11**).

Clinical Considerations

- A mucobuccal fold injection is sufficient for cavity preparation and pulpal procedures of the mandibular incisors.
- Extractions require supplemental anesthesia of the lingual gingiva, mucosa, and supporting bone by sublingual infiltration (p. 515).

Table A.11	Anesthesia of mandibular incisors and canine
Areas anesthetized* (Fig. A.11C)	**Nerve (Fig. A.11B)**
Mandibular central and lateral incisors and canine (to a lesser extent)*	Incisive nerve
Periodontal ligaments, buccal gingiva, mucosa, and supporting bone associated with the incisors	Mental nerve
Lower lip	
Chin	
* This applies when the injection is placed at the mandibular lateral incisor.	

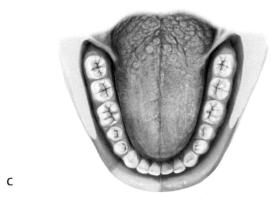

A

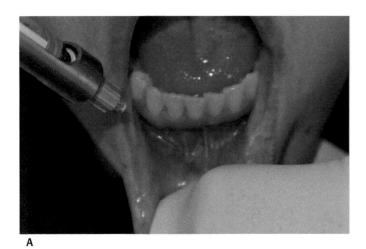

C

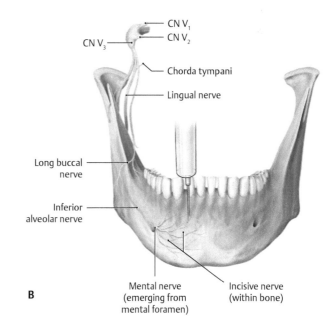

CN V$_3$ —
CN V$_1$
CN V$_2$
Chorda tympani
Lingual nerve
Long buccal nerve
Inferior alveolar nerve
Mental nerve (emerging from mental foramen)
Incisive nerve (within bone)

B

Fig. A.11 **Infiltration of the mandibular incisors**
A Injection technique, anterior view.
B Nerves anesthetized, anterior view.
C Areas anesthetized, superior view.

Mental Nerve Block

Anatomy

The mandibular first premolar is innervated by the incisive nerve (**Table A.12**). The mandibular second premolar is mainly innervated by the inferior alveolar nerve. The periodontal ligaments, buccal gingiva, mucosa, and supporting bone in the premolar area are innervated by the mental nerve, while the lingual gingiva is supplied by the sublingual nerve. The mental foramen lies between and inferior to the apices of the mandibular premolar teeth.

The thick, compact bone in the mandibular premolar region does not normally allow anesthesia of these teeth to be achieved by infiltration anesthesia; therefore, a mental nerve block or inferior alveolar nerve block is used. The exception to this is if articaine is used; in that case, infiltration anesthesia is effective (articaine can achieve anesthesia of all mandibular teeth with the exception of the second and third molars).

The anatomic direction of the canal that allows passage of the mental nerve is medial→anterior→caudal. The needle should not be oriented in this direction to prevent damage to the mental nerve and vessels within the canal.

Table A.12	Anesthesia following a mental nerve block
Areas anesthetized* (Fig. A.12C)	**Nerve (Fig. A.12B)**
Mandibular 1st premolar	Incisive nerve
Mandibular 2nd premolar**	Inferior alveolar nerve and perhaps some fibers from the mental nerve
Canine, lateral, and central incisor	Incisive nerve***
All periodontal ligaments, buccal gingiva, mucosa, and supporting bone from the 2nd premolar to the central incisor	Mental nerve
Lower lip and chin	Mental nerve

* On the same side as the injection.
** Unreliably anesthetized, as sufficient anesthetic has to diffuse through the mental foramen and spread proximally to anesthetize fibers of the inferior alveolar nerve, which innervates this tooth.
*** The incisive nerve is incidentally anesthetized by diffusion of local anesthetic during this block.

Injection Technique

- Locate the mental foramen by palpation or by referring to a radiograph.

- Insert the needle into the mucobuccal fold between the first and second mandibular premolar.

- Advance the needle until it is at the level of the mental foramen (**Fig. A.12A** and **B**).

- Following a negative aspiration result, slowly inject 1.0 to 1.5 mL of local anesthetic.

Clinical Considerations

- This injection is sufficient for cavity preparation and pulpal procedures on the mandibular 1st premolar. Cavity preparation may be able to be performed on the mandibular second premolar if anesthesia permits, but pulpal procedures and extensive cavity preparations are likely to require an inferior alveolar nerve block to be performed for adequate anesthesia.

- For extractions of the mandibular first premolar, a supplementary sublingual nerve infiltration is required. For extractions of the mandibular second premolar, an inferior alveolar nerve block is performed during which the lingual nerve is concurrently blocked.

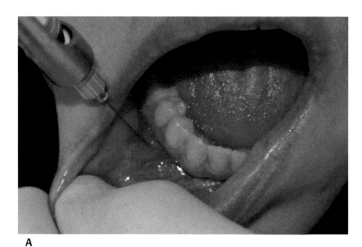

A

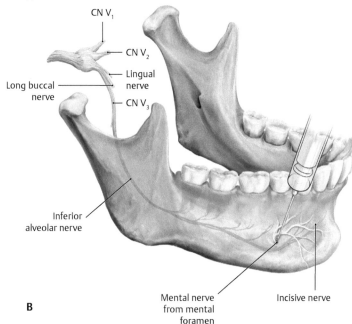

B

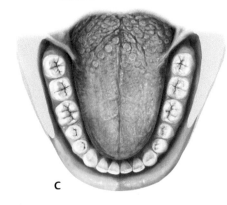

C

***Fig. A.12* Mental nerve block**
A Injection technique.
B Nerves anesthetized, right lateral view.
C Areas anesthetized, superior view.

Inferior Alveolar Nerve Block

Anatomy

All mandibular teeth are innervated by the inferior alveolar nerve (and its branches), which runs in the mandibular canal (**Table A.13**).

The thick, compact bone in the mandibular molar region often does not allow for infiltration anesthesia. Anesthesia of the mandibular molars therefore requires blockade of the inferior alveolar nerve before it enters the mandibular canal. However, an infiltration injection of articaine has been shown to be effective in anesthetizing all mandibular teeth except the second and third molars.

Injection Technique

- Instruct the patient to open widely to ensure good visualization of the anatomic landmarks.
- Palpate the coronoid notch of the mandible with the thumb of the supporting hand.
- The deepest part of the coronoid notch (about halfway up the thumb) generally corresponds to the level of the mandibular foramen.
- Move the thumb medially to palpate the internal oblique ridge and then the pterygomandibular space, lateral to the pterygomandibular raphe. The index and middle fingers lie at the ramus and angle of the mandible to support the mandible.
- Direct the needle from the contralateral premolar area into the pterygomandibular space at the level of the mandibular foramen, while keeping the needle parallel to the occlusal plane of the mandibular teeth on the injection side.
- Insert the needle 20 to 25 mm until bone is contacted (**Fig. A.13A** and **B**).
- Withdraw the needle slightly, then aspirate.
- Following a negative aspiration result, slowly inject ~1.5 mL of local anesthetic into the pterygomandibular space.
- The lingual nerve is concurrently blocked by withdrawing the needle about halfway (corresponding to the approximate level of the temporal crest), aspirating, and, if negative, slowly injecting the remaining 0.5 mL of local anesthetic.

Clinical Considerations

- This injection is sufficient for cavity preparations, pulpal procedures, and surgical procedures involving the lingual aspect of the mandibular teeth.
- Extractions of the mandibular molars require supplemental anesthesia of the long buccal nerve.
- The patient may describe an "electric shock" if the tip of the needle directly touches the inferior alveolar nerve. In this case, the needle should be withdrawn slightly, as the nerve may be damaged by intraneural injection, and the symptoms are often persistent.
- The mandibular foramen is not at the same level in all patients; therefore, this technique has to be modified accordingly. In children, it is located closer to the posterior border of the mandible until more bone is produced. In edentulous patients, alveolar bone resorption has occurred, making the deepest part of the coronoid notch lower than normal. To avoid making the block too low, direct the needle higher than the deepest part of the coronoid notch.
- In class II malocclusion, when the mandible is hypoplastic (underdeveloped), the mandibular foramen may be located more inferior than normal.
- In class III malocclusion, when the mandible is hyperplastic (overdeveloped) the mandibular foramen may be located more superior than normal.
- The medial pterygoid muscle is stretched and tense if the mouth is opened widely and may hinder proper placement of the needle. This can be overcome by slightly reducing mouth opening after the initial insertion of the needle.
- If the needle is angled too far mesially, the bone of the temporal crest is contacted almost immediately, and the needle should be repositioned laterally. If the needle is inserted too far posteriorly, then deposition of the local anesthetic solution may be made in the medial pterygoid muscle, causing postoperative muscle pain and trismus (muscle spasm). If the needle continues farther posteriorly, then it may penetrate the capsule of the parotid gland. If local anesthetic is deposited within the capsule, it causes a transient facial paralysis (Bell's palsy, see p. 499). Ensuring that the needle contacts bone at the appropriate depth ensures proper placement and mitigates the likelihood of any complications.

Table A.13	Anesthesia following an inferior alveolar nerve block
Areas anesthetized* (Fig. A.13C and D)	**Nerve (Fig. A.13B)**
All mandibular teeth	Inferior alveolar nerve
All buccal gingiva, mucosa, and supporting bone from the 2nd premolar to the central incisor	Mental nerve
Lower lip and chin	Mental nerve
All lingual gingiva, mucosa, and supporting bone	Lingual nerve (molar region) and its sublingual branch (premolar region to midline)
Anterior two thirds of the tongue	Lingual nerve
* On the same side as the injection.	

511

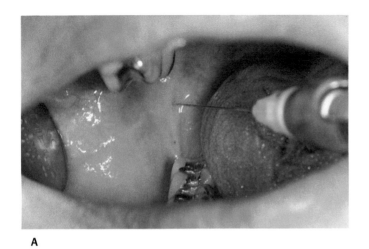

A

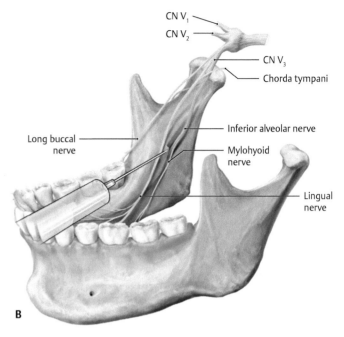

CN V$_1$

CN V$_2$

CN V$_3$

Chorda tympani

Long buccal nerve

Inferior alveolar nerve

Mylohyoid nerve

Lingual nerve

B

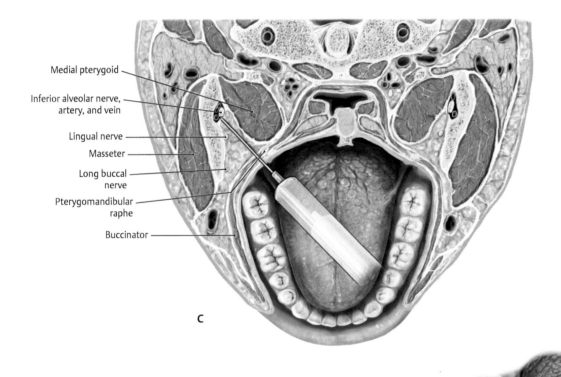

Medial pterygoid

Inferior alveolar nerve, artery, and vein

Lingual nerve

Masseter

Long buccal nerve

Pterygomandibular raphe

Buccinator

C

D

Fig. A.13 Inferior alveolar nerve block
A Injection technique.
B Nerves anesthetized, left lateral view.
C Transverse section just above the occlusal plane of the mandibular teeth, superior view.
D Areas anesthetized, superior view.

Gow–Gates Block

Anatomy

This block is a variation of the inferior alveolar nerve block. The aim is to anesthetize the inferior alveolar nerve at the level of the mandibular condyle but additional branches of CN V_3 are also anesthetized by at injection given at this level (**Table A.14**).

Injection Technique

- Instruct the patient to open as wide as possible.

- Direct the needle from the contralateral premolars and insert the needle high into the mucosa at the level of the maxillary second molar, just distal to the mesiolingual cusp (**Fig. A.14A** and **B**).

- Use the intertragic notch of the ear as an extraoral landmark to help reach the neck of the mandibular condyle.

- When contact with the neck of the condyle is made, withdraw the needle slightly and aspirate.

- Following a negative aspiration result, slowly inject 1.0 to 1.8 mL of local anesthetic.

Clinical Considerations

- This injection is useful for multiple procedures on mandibular teeth and buccal soft tissue.

- The rate of failure is lower and there are fewer aspiration issues than with the traditional inferior alveolar nerve block.

Table A.14	**Anesthesia following a Gow–Gates block**
Area anesthetized* (Fig. A.14C)	**Nerve (Fig. A.14B)**
All mandibular teeth	Inferior alveolar nerve
All periodontal ligaments, buccal gingiva, mucosa, and supporting alveolar bone from the 2nd premolar to the 3rd molar	Long buccal nerve
All periodontal ligaments, buccal gingiva, mucosa, and supporting alveolar bone from the 2nd premolar to the central incisor	Mental nerve
All lingual gingiva, supporting bone, and the mucosa of the floor of the mouth	Lingual nerve (molar region) and its sublingual branch (premolar to midline)
Anterior two thirds of the tongue	Lingual nerve
Lower lip	Mental nerve
Skin in the temple region and the skin anterior to the ear	Auriculotemporal nerve
Posterior part of the cheek	Long buccal nerve
* On the same side as the injection.	

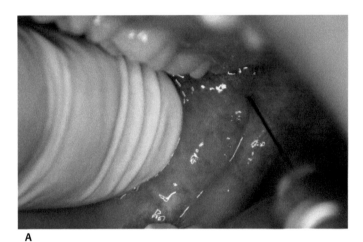

A

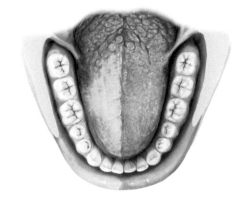

C

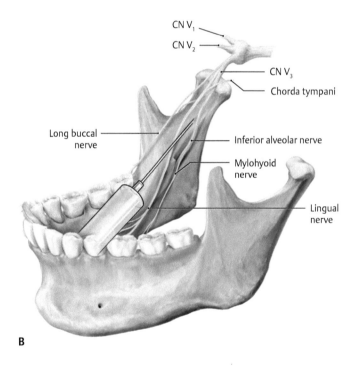

B

Fig. A.14 Gow–Gates block
A Injection technique.
B Nerves anesthetized, left lateral view.
C Areas anesthetized, superior view.

Akinosi Block

Anatomy

The Akinosi block is an alternative, closed-mouth method of performing an inferior alveolar nerve block (**Table A.15**). It is useful when the patient has a limited ability to open the mouth, or when the patient has a strong gag reflex that is elicited by conventional inferior alveolar nerve block.

Table A.15	Anesthesia following an Akinosi block
Areas anesthetized* (Fig. A.15D)	**Nerve (Fig. A.15B)**
All mandibular teeth	Inferior alveolar nerve
All buccal gingiva, mucosa, and supporting bone from the 2nd premolar to the central incisor	Mental nerve
All lingual gingiva, mucosa, and supporting bone	Lingual nerve
Anterior two-thirds of the tongue	Lingual nerve
Lower lip	Mental nerve
* On the same side as the injection.	

Injection Technique

- Instruct the patient to close his or her mouth.
- Insert the needle into the mucosa between the medial border of the mandibular ramus and the maxillary tuberosity at the level of the cervical margin of the maxillary molars.
- Advance the needle parallel to the maxillary occlusal plane ~20 to 25 mm. At this depth, the tip of the needle should be in the middle of the pterygomandibular space near the inferior alveolar and lingual nerves (**Fig. A.15A** and **B**).
- Following a negative aspiration result, slowly inject the full cartridge of local anesthetic (1.8 mL).

Clinical Considerations

- This injection is sufficient for cavity preparations, pulpal procedures, and surgical procedures involving the lingual aspect of the mandibular teeth.
- Extractions of the mandibular molars require supplemental anesthesia of the long buccal nerve.

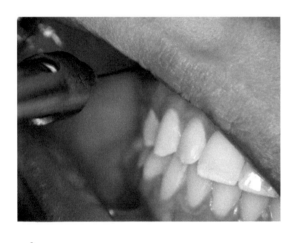

A

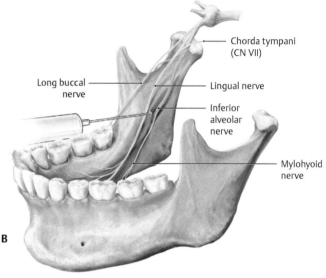

B

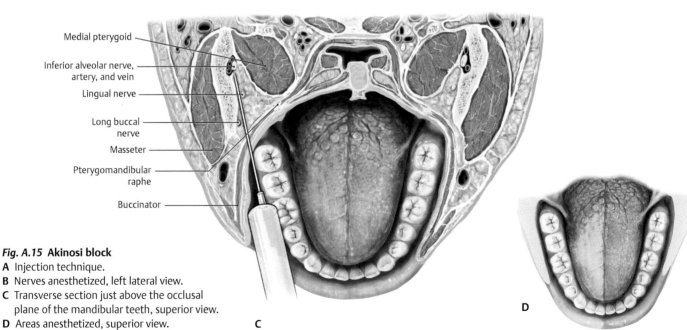

Fig. A.15 Akinosi block
A Injection technique.
B Nerves anesthetized, left lateral view.
C Transverse section just above the occlusal plane of the mandibular teeth, superior view.
D Areas anesthetized, superior view.

C

D

Long Buccal Nerve Block

Anatomy

The long buccal nerve is a branch of the inferior alveolar nerve (**Table A.16**). It passes along the medial side of the mandibular ramus anterior to the inferior alveolar nerve. It then crosses the anterior border of the mandibular ramus. Its branches innervate the buccal gingiva between the mandibular second premolar and molars, as well as the retromolar triangle

Table A.16	Anesthesia following a long buccal nerve block
Areas anesthetized* (Fig. A.16A)	**Nerve (Fig. A.16B)**
Buccal gingiva, mucosa, and supporting bone from the mandibular 2nd premolar to the last molar and retromolar trigone	Long buccal nerve (from CN V$_3$)
* On the same side as the injection.	

Injection Technique

- Insert the needle into the buccal mucosa posterior to the last molar. It will only penetrate ~2 mm (**Fig. A.16A** and **B**).

- Following a negative aspiration result, inject ~0.5 mL of local anesthetic.

Clinical Considerations

- This injection is used to supplement an inferior alveolar nerve block for extractions or surgical procedures involving the mandibular second premolars to molars.

Supplementary Sublingual Nerve Infiltration

Anatomy

The lingual nerve passes downward together with the inferior alveolar nerve and communicates with the chorda tympani of the facial nerve just before reaching the mandibular foramen. This connection gives off secretory fibers to the submandibular and sublingual glands via the submandibular ganglion and taste fibers to the anterior two-thirds of the tongue. The trunk of the lingual nerve gives off branches that innervate the lingual gingiva in the molar region. The lingual gingiva and mucosa of the floor of the mouth are innervated by the sublingual nerve, a branch of the lingual nerve (**Table A.17**).

Table A.17	Supplementary sublingual nerve infiltration
Areas anesthetized*	**Nerve**
Lingual gingiva and supporting bone, and the mucosa of the floor of the mouth in the vicinity of the infiltration	Sublingual nerve
* On the same side as the injection.	

Injection Technique

- Introduce the needle just below the attached gingiva on the lingual side of the tooth requiring lingual anesthesia.

- Following a negative aspiration result, slowly inject a small amount of local anesthetic.

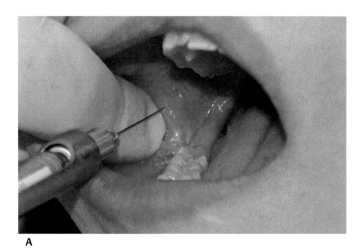

A

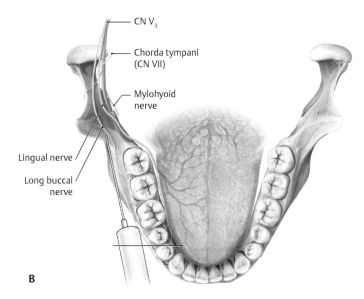

B

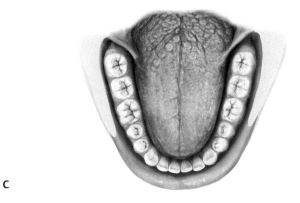

C

Fig. A.16 Long buccal nerve block
A Injection technique.
B Nerves anesthetized, superior view.
C Areas anesthetized, superior view.

Clinical Considerations

- This injection is used to supplement a mucobuccal fold infiltration or mental nerve block for extractions of the mandibular incisors, canine, and premolar teeth. It is not necessary for extraction of the mandibular molar teeth because the lingual nerve trunk is anesthetized as part of the inferior alveolar block given in these cases.

Factual Questions

The questions and answers from this section are available with the eBook edition on MedOne Education. They may also be accessed as part of MedOne's interactive "Questions and Answers" tab on the website.

Chapter 1 Embryology of the Head & Neck

1. The skeletal elements that develop within the 1st pharyngeal arch include the
   A. Hyoid bone
   B. Nasal bone
   C. Palatine bone
   D. Stapes
   E. Occipital bone

2. The incisive foramen is an anatomical landmark between the
   A. Hard and soft palates
   B. Primary and secondary palates
   C. Lateral palatine processes
   D. Palatine and maxillary bones
   E. Medial nasal prominences

3. The cranial nerves that carry sensory information from the part of the tongue derived from the hypopharyngeal eminence are the
   A. Glossopharyngeal and vagus nerves
   B. Trigeminal and facial nerves
   C. Vagus and hypoglossal nerves
   D. Facial and glossopharyngeal nerves
   E. Trigeminal and glossopharyngeal nerves

4. Secondary cleft palate, without primary cleft palate or cleft lip, results from the failure of fusion of the
   A. Maxillary prominence and medial nasal prominence
   B. Nasal septum and maxillary prominence
   C. Maxillary prominence and lateral palatine processes
   D. Left and right lateral palatine processes
   E. Intermaxillary segment

5. The intermaxillary segment of the developing face provides the alveolar sockets for the
   A. Mandibular molars
   B. Maxillary canines
   C. Deciduous teeth
   D. Mandibular premolars
   E. Maxillary incisors

6. A child presents with a midline swelling at the base of the tongue. Magnetic resonance imaging (MRI) shows a midsagittal growth referred to as a lingual cyst by the radiologist. The embryological origin of this lingual cyst is a
   A. Persistent 1st pharyngeal groove
   B. Nonmigrating thyroid gland
   C. Laryngeotracheal diverticulum
   D. 2nd pharyngeal pouch
   E. Metastasis of the lingual tonsil

Chapter 2 Cranial Bones

7. The hard palate has passages for branches of the maxillary division of the trigeminal nerve that include the incisive foramen for the nasopalatine nerve and the
   A. Greater palatine foramen for the greater palatine nerve
   B. Infraorbital foramen for the infraorbital nerve
   C. Mental foramen for the mental nerve
   D. Foramen rotundum for the maxillary nerve
   E. Sphenopalatine foramen for the nasopalatine nerve

8. The mandibular foramen of the ramus is protected by the bony _____ in a superoanterior position.
   A. Mental spine
   B. Pterygoid hamulus
   C. Coronoid process
   D. Lingula
   E. Condylar process

9. The anteromedial floor of the carotid canal in the petrous portion of the temporal bone is "open" to the nasopharynx through the
   A. Foramen ovale
   B. Foramen lacerum
   C. Jugular foramen
   D. Foramen spinosum
   E. Mastoid foramen

10. The anterior cranial fossa is separated from the middle cranial fossa by the
    A. Lateral pterygoid plate of the sphenoid bone
    B. Perpendicular plate of the ethmoid bone
    C. Lesser wing of the sphenoid bone
    D. Petrous part of the temporal bone
    E. Frontal crest of the frontal bone

11. What structure on the internal surface of the lateral wall of the cranial vault crosses over the area indicated by pterion?
    A. Groove for the middle meningeal artery
    B. Hypophyseal fossa
    C. Groove for the sigmoid sinus
    D. Internal acoustic meatus
    E. Crista galli of the ethmoid bone

12. The foramen rotundum exits the middle cranial fossa through which bone?
    A. Petrous temporal
    B. Ethmoid
    C. Occipital
    D. Mandibular
    E. Sphenoid

13. The majority of the hard palate of the oral cavity is formed from the union of the horizontal plate of the palatine bone with the
    A. Medial pterygoid plate of the sphenoid bone
    B. Perpendicular plate of the ethmoid bone
    C. Palatine process of the maxilla
    D. Squamous part of the temporal bone
    E. Alae of the vomer bone

14. With which of the following bones does the zygomatic bone NOT articulate?
    A. Maxilla
    B. Frontal
    C. Temporal
    D. Sphenoid

Chapter 3 Vasculature & Lymphatics of the Head & Neck

15. The branch of the mandibular part of the maxillary artery that passes through the foramen spinosum is the
    A. Middle meningeal artery
    B. Deep temporal artery
    C. Sphenopalatine artery
    D. Internal carotid artery
    E. Ophthalmic artery

16. The inferior alveolar artery, supplying blood to the mandibular molars, is a branch of which artery?
    A. Facial
    B. Maxillary
    C. Lingual
    D. Sphenopalatine
    E. Internal carotid

17. The vertebral artery is a branch of the
    A. External carotid artery
    B. Common carotid artery
    C. Subclavian artery
    D. Arch of the aorta
    E. Brachiocephalic trunk

18. The danger zone (triangle) of the face deals with venous drainage from superficial veins into deep veins and intracranial venous sinuses. The direct communication between the angular (facial) vein and the cavernous sinus is via the
    A. Pterygoid plexus
    B. Retromandibular vein
    C. Lingual vein
    D. Ophthalmic veins
    E. Brachiocephalic trunk

19. While weightlifting, a 22-year-old man attempting a personal record on the parallel back squat drops the barbell across his upper back. The compression from the barbell ruptures his left dorsal scapular artery, and immediately he starts to feel blood pooling deep to his trapezius and rhomboid muscles. Compression to the _____ will stop the bleeding.
    A. Brachiocephalic trunk
    B. Common carotid artery
    C. Thoracoacromial trunk
    D. Costocervical trunk
    E. Thyrocervical trunk

20. The middle cerebral artery is a direct branch of which artery?
    A. Common carotid
    B. External carotid
    C. Internal carotid
    D. Basilar
    E. Middle meningeal

21. Normal venous drainage of the cavernous venous dural sinus is directly through the
    A. Straight sinus
    B. Petrosal sinuses
    C. External jugular vein
    D. Basilar vein
    E. Maxillary sinus

22. The superficial parotid (preauricular) lymph nodes drain directly into the _____ lymph nodes as the lymph drains back toward the cardiovascular system through either the lymphatic (right) or thoracic (left) ducts.
    A. Occipital
    B. Facial
    C. Nuchal
    D. Laryngeotracheal
    E. Deep cervical (jugular)

23. An infection on the tip of the tongue would most likely be associated with the enlargement of which group of lymph nodes?
    A. Submental
    B. Buccal
    C. Superficial parotid
    D. Retropharyngeal
    E. Anterior jugular

Chapter 4 Neuroanatomy & Innervation of the Head & Neck

24. The passageway in the skull through which the abducent nerve passes is the
    A. Superior orbital fissure
    B. Foramen rotundum
    C. Foramen ovale
    D. Infraorbital foramen
    E. Foramen spinosum

25. Which nerve innervates the middle ear muscle that modulates the motion of the stapes?
    A. Optic
    B. Oculomotor
    C. Vestibulocochlear
    D. Trigeminal
    E. Facial

26. The extraocular muscle innervated by the trochlear nerve is the
    A. Lateral rectus
    B. Superior oblique
    C. Orbicularis oculi
    D. Rectus capitis lateralis
    E. Dilator pupillae

27. The vagus nerve exits the posterior cranial fossa at the
    A. Jugular foramen
    B. Internal auditory meatus
    C. Condylar canal
    D. Foramen magnum
    E. Foramen lacerum

28. The innervation for the hyoglossus muscle is the
    A. Ansa cervicalis
    B. Facial nerve
    C. Hypoglossal nerve
    D. Mylohyoid nerve
    E. Recurrent laryngeal nerve

29. The parasympathetic innervation to the parotid gland travels through the
    A. Chorda tympani
    B. Greater petrosal nerve
    C. Deep petrosal nerve
    D. Tympanic nerve
    E. Lingual nerve

30. The C8 spinal nerve exits the vertebral canal
    A. Above the C7 vertebra
    B. Below the C7 vertebra
    C. Below the C8 vertebra
    D. Through the C8 transverse foramen
    E. Never because there is no C8 spinal nerve

31. During a routine physical, a patient comments to his primary care physician that he has tingling and a sensation of cold that is focused on the top of his right shoulder. The likely cause of this condition is
    A. Osteophyte in the C1–C2 intervertebral foramen
    B. Compression of the axillary nerve
    C. C3–C4 slipped disk
    D. Referred pain from the spleen
    E. Avulsion of the C6 spinal nerve

32. The central nervous structure that develops from the embryological myelencephalon is the
    A. Cerebral peduncle
    B. Thalamus
    C. Pons
    D. Medulla oblongata
    E. Tectum

33. The voluntary motor cortex in the cerebral hemisphere is separated from the conscious body sensation cortex by the

    A. Calcarine sulcus
    B. Parieto-occipital sulcus
    C. Sylvian (lateral) sulcus
    D. Longitudinal fissure
    E. Central sulcus

34. The flow of cerebrospinal fluid (CSF) in an individual with noncommunicating hydrocephalus can be blocked by the choroid plexus in the

    A. Cerebral aqueduct
    B. Pontomedullary cistern
    C. Cerebellomedullary cistern
    D. Confluence of sinuses
    E. Arachnoid granulations

Chapter 5 Face & Scalp

35. Which facial muscle can act as an oral sphincter?

    A. Risorius
    B. Depressor labii inferioris
    C. Orbicularis oris
    D. Levator anguli oris
    E. Orbicularis oculi

36. Each of the following muscles is innervated by a branch of the facial nerve passing through the parotid gland except the

    A. Platysma
    B. Zygomaticus major
    C. Posterior auricular
    D. Risorius
    E. Buccinator

37. A facial muscle attached to the alveolar processes of the mandible and maxilla is the

    A. Depressor anguli oris
    B. Buccinator
    C. Levator labii superioris
    D. Zygomaticus minor
    E. Mentalis

38. Infections of the scalp are most likely to spread in which layer?

    A. Skin
    B. Connective tissue
    C. Epicranial aponeurosis
    D. Loose areolar connective tissue
    E. Pericranium

39. Which of the following arteries of the face is derived from the internal carotid artery?

    A. Supraorbital
    B. Facial
    C. Lateral nasal
    D. Superficial temporal
    E. Transverse facial

40. The nerve that supplies the skin of the posterior scalp (occiput) is the

    A. Maxillary
    B. Transverse cervical
    C. Great auricular
    D. Greater occipital
    E. Facial

41. The facial vein drains into the

    A. Angular vein
    B. Anterior jugular vein
    C. External jugular vein
    D. Common facial vein
    E. Deep facial vein

42. Which nerve carries sensory information from the upper lip?

    A. Anterior superior alveolar
    B. Buccal branch of the facial nerve
    C. Mental
    D. Supraorbital
    E. Infraorbital

Chapter 6 Temporal, Infratemporal, & Pterygopalatine Fossae

43. The insertion (posterior attachment) of the lateral pterygoid muscle is the

    A. Pterygoid rugosity on the medial angle of the mandible
    B. Medial side of the coronoid process of the mandible
    C. Medial side of the zygomatic process of the temporal bone
    D. Pterygoid fovea and the condylar process of the mandible
    E. Inferior temporal line of the frontal, temporal, and parietal bones

44. Much of the weight of the mandible is supported by the

    A. Mylohyoid muscle
    B. Sphenomandibular ligament
    C. Digastric muscle
    D. Pterygospinous ligament
    E. Buccinator

45. Which muscle of mastication is the primary retractor (retruder) of the mandible?

    A. Masseter
    B. Medial pterygoid
    C. Temporalis
    D. Lateral pterygoid
    E. Mylohyoid

46. The action of the lateral pterygoid muscle is to

    A. Protrude the mandible
    B. Tense the soft palate
    C. Depress the sphenoid bone
    D. Elevate the hyoid bone
    E. Retract the mandible

47. Which structure attaches to the lingula of the mandible?

    A. Masseter
    B. Sphenomandibular ligament
    C. Temporalis
    D. Stylomandibular ligament
    E. Pharyngotympanic tube

48. The nerve(s) that emerge from between the two heads of the lateral pterygoid muscle is/are the

    A. Inferior alveolar nerve
    B. Lingual nerve
    C. Deep temporal nerves
    D. Long buccal nerve
    E. Both A and B

49. Which of the following is not a branch of the maxillary artery?

    A. Middle meningeal artery
    B. Inferior tympanic artery
    C. Deep auricular artery
    D. Descending palatine artery
    E. Artery of the pterygoid canal

50. Sensation to the TMJ is provided by which of the following branches of the mandibular nerve?

    A. Inferior alveolar nerve
    B. Auriculotemporal nerve
    C. Lingual nerve
    D. Nerve to the lateral pterygoid
    E. Long buccal nerve

51. Through which opening does the pterygopalatine fossa communicate with the infratemporal fossa?

    A. Greater palatine canal
    B. Pterygoid canal
    C. Sphenopalatine foramen
    D. Foramen rotundum
    E. Pterygomaxillary fissure

52. The pterygopalatine ganglion receives preganglionic parasympathetic fibers traveling on which nerve?

    A. Maxillary nerve
    B. Chorda tympani
    C. Greater petrosal
    D. Lesser petrosal
    E. Deep petrosal

53. Which bone forms the superior boundary of the pterygopalatine fossa?

    A. Sphenoid
    B. Maxilla
    C. Palatine
    D. Temporal
    E. Vomer

Chapter 7 Nose & Nasal Cavity

54. The nasal cavity is enclosed by the ethmoid, vomer, maxillary, sphenoid, nasal, lacrimal, inferior nasal conchae, and which other bone?

    A. Palatine
    B. Zygomatic
    C. Mandibular
    D. Parietal
    E. Occipital

55. The frontal air sinus communicates with the _____ of the respiratory system.

    A. Inferior meatus
    B. Middle meatus
    C. Superior meatus
    D. Nasopharynx
    E. Sphenoethmoidal recess

56. Kiesselbach's area, the anastomosis of nasal septal arteries, links together branches of the superior labial, anterior ethmoidal, greater palatine, and _____ arteries.

    A. Superior posterior alveolar
    B. Middle meningeal
    C. Sphenopalatine
    D. Ascending pharyngeal
    E. Petrotympanic

57. Innervation to the mucosa covering the vomer bone is through which nerve?

    A. Olfactory
    B. Anterior ethmoidal
    C. Greater palatine
    D. Nasopalatine
    E. Posterior superior alveolar

58. A patient comes to the dentist's office complaining of pain from his left maxillary 2nd molar. The dentist examines the tooth and decides that it needs to be extracted. He knows that care needs to be taken to avoid introducing infection into the paranasal sinus just superior to the tooth. Which paranasal sinus can potentially be affected by this extraction?

    A. Frontal
    B. Ethmoid
    C. Mastoid
    D. Sphenoid
    E. Maxillary

59. A pituitary tumor (macroadenoma) causing headache and loss of peripheral vision for an individual needs to be surgically treated. The surgeon decides to access the tumor, for removal, through which air sinus separating the pituitary gland from the nasal cavity?

    A. Frontal
    B. Ethmoid
    C. Mastoid
    D. Sphenoid
    E. Maxillary

Chapter 8 Oral Cavity & Pharynx

60. Which suprahyoid muscle is innervated by the facial nerve?

    A. Mylohyoid
    B. Hyoglossus
    C. Posterior digastric
    D. Geniohyoid
    E. Stylopharyngeus

61. Taste information from the posterior one-third of the tongue travels along the glossopharyngeal nerve via the petrosal (inferior) ganglion to the nucleus of the solitary tract (gustatory part) in the open medullary part of the brainstem. From here it travels through the dorsal trigeminothalamic tract to reach the _____ nucleus of the thalamus. The final leg of the tract brings taste information to the insula and postcentral gyrus of the cerebral hemisphere.

    A. Ventral anterior
    B. Lateral dorsal
    C. Pulvinar
    D. Medial geniculate
    E. Ventral posteromedial

62. Which muscle of the soft palate is connected to the cartilaginous pharyngotympanic tube?

    A. Tensor veli palatini
    B. Palatoglossus
    C. Palatopharyngeus
    D. Tensor tympani
    E. Superior pharyngeal constrictor

63. The part of Waldeyer's (pharyngeal lymphatic) ring most closely associated with the epiglottis is the

    A. Tubal tonsil
    B. Lingual tonsil
    C. Pharyngeal tonsil
    D. Palatine tonsil
    E. Adenoid tonsil

64. The tooth layer immediately deep to the enamel is the

    A. Periodontal ligament
    B. Cementum
    C. Pulp
    D. Dentine
    E. Alveolar bone

65. Which of the following permanent teeth (secondary dentition) erupt at ~6 to 8 years of age?

    A. Canine
    B. 1st premolar
    C. 2nd premolar
    D. 1st molar
    E. 2nd molar

66. The sublingual salivary glands receive postganglionic parasympathetic innervation from which ganglion?

    A. Superior cervical
    B. Pterygopalatine
    C. Ciliary
    D. Otic
    E. Submandibular

67. The parotid gland produces which type of secretions?
    A. Mucous
    B. Serous
    C. Mixed mucous and serous

68. Infections from which teeth can spread to the peripharyngeal fascial spaces?
    A. Maxillary molars
    B. Maxillary canines
    C. Mandibular premolars
    D. Mandibular canines
    E. Mandibular incisors

69. Which potential space is located inferior to the mylohyoid line inferior and lateral to the mylohyoid muscle?
    A. Sublingual
    B. Submandibular
    C. Masticator
    D. Tonsillar
    E. Parotid

70. Which of the following structures pass through the 3rd pharyngeal gap?
    A. The pharyngotympanic tube and levator veli palatini muscle
    B. The tensor veli palatini muscle
    C. The internal laryngeal nerve and superior laryngeal artery
    D. The recurrent laryngeal nerve and inferior laryngeal artery
    E. The glossopharyngeal nerve and the stylopharyngeus muscle

Chapter 9 Orbit & Eye

71. The artery running through the optic canal to supply blood to the orbit is a branch of the
    A. Middle meningeal artery
    B. Deep temporal artery
    C. Sphenopalatine artery
    D. Internal carotid artery
    E. Ophthalmic artery

72. An extraocular muscle NOT innervated by the oculomotor nerve is the:
    A. Superior rectus
    B. Lateral rectus
    C. Medial rectus
    D. Inferior oblique
    E. Inferior rectus

73. Through which passageway in the skull does the superior branch of the oculomotor nerve pass?
    A. Superior orbital fissure
    B. Foramen rotundum
    C. Foramen ovale
    D. Infraorbital foramen
    E. Foramen spinosum

74. The quickest impulse conduction through the retina links the rod or cone photoreceptors to the retinal ganglion cells through the
    A. Horizontal cell
    B. Bipolar cell
    C. Amacrine cell
    D. Purkinje's cell
    E. Müller's cell

75. An individual complaining of tunnel vision (bitemporal hemianopia) asks her dentist to explain where the problem might be occurring. She also mentions that she is regularly experiencing headache, a change in her menstrual cycle, and significant weight gain. The dentist explains that there is a chance of a pituitary tumor (macroadenoma) creating pressure on the
    A. Optic nerve
    B. Optic tract
    C. Optic chiasm
    D. Retrolenticular internal capsule
    E. Splenium of the corpus callosum

Chapter 10 Ear

76. The blood supply to the external ear includes the posterior auricular artery and the
    A. Transverse facial artery
    B. Superficial temporal artery
    C. Sphenopalatine artery
    D. Internal carotid artery
    E. Occipital artery

77. Taste fibers traveling through the middle ear cavity are carried by a nerve that is a branch of the
    A. Trigeminal nerve
    B. Facial nerve
    C. Vestibulocochlear nerve
    D. Glossopharyngeal nerve
    E. Vagus nerve

78. The middle ear ossicle that fits into the oval window of the inner ear is the
    A. Malleus
    B. Pisiform
    C. Stapes
    D. Navicular
    E. Incus

79. The vestibulocochlear nerve exits the posterior cranial fossa to reach the inner ear of the temporal bone through the
    A. Petrosal hiatus
    B. External acoustic meatus
    C. Mastoid canaliculus
    D. Internal acoustic meatus
    E. Stylomastoid foramen

80. The right anterior semicircular canal of the vestibulocochlear apparatus of the petrous part of the temporal bone is at a parallel plane to the
    A. Right posterior semicircular canal
    B. Right lateral semicircular canal
    C. Left anterior semicircular canal
    D. Left lateral semicircular canal
    E. Left posterior semicircular canal

81. To detect sound, vibration of the hair cells is necessary. Movement at the oval window of the inner ear results in pressure waves that travel through the perilymph. Although the hair cells are not surrounded by perilymph, they are attached to a flexible structure separating perilymph from endolymph called the
    A. Basilar membrane
    B. Spiral ligament
    C. Vestibular membrane
    D. Tectorial membrane
    E. Helicotrema

82. The part of the auditory system that is critical for the localization of sound is the
    A. Vestibular nucleus
    B. Tensor tympani
    C. Spiral ganglion
    D. Lateral geniculate nucleus
    E. Medial lemniscus

Chapter 11 Bones, Ligaments, & Muscles of the Neck

83. Which muscle draws the hyoid bone forward and is innervated by the anterior ramus of the C1 spinal nerve?
    A. Mylohyoid
    B. Geniohyoid
    C. Stylohyoid
    D. Omohyoid
    E. Sternohyoid

84. The muscle of the neck that rotates the head to the contralateral side is the
    A. Rectus capitis posterior major
    B. Longissimus capitis
    C. Rectus capitis lateralis
    D. Splenius capitis
    E. Sternocleidomastoid

85. The origin (proximal attachment) of which back muscle includes the spinous process of the T6 vertebra?
    A. Splenius cervicis
    B. Levator costarum longus
    C. Serratus posterior superior
    D. Iliocostalis thoracis
    E. Longus colli

86. What is the innervation to the geniohyoid muscle?
    A. Mylohyoid nerve
    B. Facial nerve
    C. Anterior ramus of the C1 spinal nerve
    D. Inferior alveolar nerve
    E. Hypoglossal nerve

87. Which ligament attaches the C2 vertebra to the skull?
    A. Posterior atlanto-occipital membrane.
    B. Posterior longitudinal ligament
    C. Alar ligament
    D. Transverse ligament of the atlas
    E. Nuchal ligament

88. Which cervical vertebra has transverse foramina that do NOT contain a vertebral artery?
    A. Atlas (C1)
    B. Axis (C2)
    C. C6
    D. C7
    E. None of the above

Chapter 12 Neurovascular Topography of the Neck

89. Which pharyngeal space lies posterior to the tongue and lateral to the median glossoepiglottic fold?
    A. Vallecula
    B. Piriform recess
    C. Rima glottidis
    D. Foramen cecum
    E. Tonsillar fossa

90. The middle scalene muscle originates on the C1 and C2 transverse processes and the C3–C7 posterior tubercles, and it inserts into the
    A. Superomedial angle of the scapula
    B. 1st rib
    C. 2nd rib
    D. Basilar occipital bone
    E. Manubrium of the sternum

91. Name the neck triangle that provides the best access to the spinal accessory nerve.
    A. Submandibular
    B. Muscular
    C. Carotid
    D. Occipital
    E. Omoclavicular

92. Which cranial nerve travels from the base of the skull to the mediastinum in the carotid sheath?
    A. Facial
    B. Glossopharyngeal
    C. Vagus
    D. Spinal accessory
    E. Hypoglossal

93. Bacterial infection of the oral cavity may invade the parapharyngeal space and can easily spread inferiorly to the
    A. Cavernous sinus
    B. Lung
    C. Stomach
    D. Mediastinum
    E. Subarachnoid space

94. The superior root of the ansa cervicalis contains fibers from the
    A. Vagus nerve
    B. Hypoglossal nerve
    C. C3 anterior ramus
    D. C2 posterior ramus
    E. C1 anterior ramus

95. The external jugular vein collects blood directly from the posterior division of the retromandibular vein, posterior auricular vein, and
    A. Transverse cervical vein
    B. Inferior thyroid vein
    C. Pterygoid plexus
    D. Facial vein
    E. Lingual vein

Chapter 13 Larynx & Thyroid Gland

96. The epiglottic cartilage is attached to the _____ cartilage of the respiratory system.
    A. Thyroid
    B. Cricoid
    C. Arytenoid
    D. Corniculate
    E. Tracheal

97. The only laryngeal muscle that abducts the vocal cords and opens the rima glottidis is the
    A. Posterior cricoarytenoid
    B. Cricothyroid
    C. Lateral cricoarytenoid
    D. Transverse arytenoid
    E. Thyroarytenoid

98. The part of the thyroid gland that stretches anterior to the laryngeal prominence toward the foramen cecum of the tongue is the
    A. Lateral lobe
    B. Isthmus
    C. Pyramidal lobe
    D. Superior parathyroid
    E. Inferior parathyroid

99. A lesion of the recurrent laryngeal nerve could affect the function of each of the following laryngeal muscles except one. Which is the exception?
    A. Cricothyroid
    B. Posterior cricoarytenoid
    C. Thyroarytenoid
    D. Lateral cricoarytenoid
    E. Vocalis

100. Which nerve provides sensation to the laryngeal vestibule?
    A. Recurrent laryngeal nerve
    B. Internal laryngeal nerve
    C. External laryngeal nerve
    D. Inferior laryngeal nerve

101. The superior laryngeal artery enters the larynx by piercing the:

    A. Vestibular ligament
    B. Conus elasticus
    C. Cricothyroid membrane
    D. Vocal ligament
    E. Thyrohyoid membrane

102. The cricothyroid muscle

    A. Receives blood from the suprascapular artery
    B. Is supplied by the internal laryngeal nerve
    C. Inserts on the epiglottis
    D. Originates on the hyoid bone
    E. Lengthens and tenses the vocal folds

Chapter 14 Sectional Anatomy of the Head & Neck

103. What structure would you expect to find in a transverse section at the level of the C1 vertebra?

    A. Dens
    B. Pons
    C. Body of the mandible
    D. Common carotid artery
    E. Thyroid cartilage

104. What structure would you expect to find in a midsagittal section of the head?

    A. Internal carotid artery
    B. Hyoglossus muscle
    C. Pituitary gland
    D. Transverse sinus
    E. Ramus of the mandible

Chapter 15 Rest of Body Anatomy

105. Impingement of the suprascapular nerve as it runs inferior to the superior transverse ligament of the scapula can result in paralysis of the

    A. Infraspinatus
    B. Subclavius
    C. Teres major
    D. Rhomboid minor
    E. Deltoid

106. The brachial vein drains into the _____ to return blood to the heart.

    A. Cephalic vein
    B. Axillary vein
    C. Brachiocephalic vein
    D. Internal jugular vein
    E. Subclavian vein

107. The insertion/distal attachment of the biceps brachii is the

    A. Lateral intertubercular groove of the humerus
    B. Coracoid process of the scapula
    C. Ulnar tuberosity of the ulna
    D. Olecranon fossa of the humerus
    E. Radial tuberosity of the radius

108. The left 8th posterior intercostal vein drains directly into the

    A. Inferior vena cava
    B. Superior vena cava
    C. Hemiazygos vein
    D. Azygos vein
    E. Thoracic duct

109. The left (obtuse) marginal artery of the heart are branches off the

    A. Anterior interventricular (descending) artery
    B. Posterior interventricular artery
    C. Right coronary artery
    D. Circumflex artery
    E. Thebesian artery

110. An elderly man presents in the emergency department with sudden onset of breathlessness and chest pain along the superior posterolateral left chest wall. Imaging reveals a wedge-shaped opaque structure abutting the pleura, signifying a pulmonary infarction distal to a pulmonary embolism. The pulmonary lobe most likely affected is the

    A. Apicoposterior segment of the superior lobe of the left lung
    B. Apical segment of the superior lobe of the right lung
    C. Lateral segment of the middle lobe of the right lung
    D. Superior lingular segment of the superior lobe of the left lung
    E. Superior segment of the inferior lobe of the left lung

111. The spleen is normally located in which quadrant of the abdomen?

    A. Upper right
    B. Upper left
    C. Lower right
    D. Lower left
    E. More than one quadrant

112. Which of the following arteries is/are a direct branch of the celiac trunk (artery)?

    A. The splenic artery
    B. The left gastric artery
    C. The superior rectal artery
    D. Only A and B
    E. A, B, and C

113. Which of the following statements about the lungs is incorrect?

    A. The right lung is bigger than the left lung
    B. The left lung has an oblique fissure
    C. The right lung has a horizontal fissure
    D. The cardiac notch is on the right lung
    E. The lungs are covered by visceral pleura

114. Which of the following structures is intraperitoneal in adults?

    A. Spleen
    B. Kidney
    C. Pancreas
    D. Ascending colon
    E. Abdominal aorta

Appendix A Anatomy of Local Anesthesia for Dentistry

115. During the administration of an inferior alveolar nerve block, the needle passes through which structure?

    A. Medial pterygoid
    B. Lateral pterygoid
    C. Buccinator
    D. Pterygomandibular raphe
    E. Parotid capsule

116. Which maxillary tooth is used as a landmark for performing an infraorbital nerve block?

    A. Lateral incisor
    B. Canine
    C. 1st premolar
    D. 2nd premolar
    E. 1st molar

117. Which areas would be anesthetized following a Gow-Gates block?

    A. Ipsilateral mandibular teeth
    B. Ipsilateral anterior two thirds of the tongue
    C. Ipsilateral posterior one third of the tongue
    D. A and B
    E. A, B, and C

Answer Explanations

Chapter 1 Embryology of the Head & Neck

1. **C** The palatine bone develops from the midline fusion of the maxillary prominence of the 1st pharyngeal arch.

   A The lesser horn of the hyoid bone develops from the 2nd pharyngeal arch; the body and greater horn of the hyoid bone develop from the 3rd pharyngeal arch.
   B The nasal bones develop from the frontonasal prominence, a structure that is developmentally distinct from the pharyngeal arches.
   D The stapes, the most medial of the middle ear ossicles, develops from the posterior aspect of the 2nd pharyngeal arch.
   E The occipital bone develops from parachordal cartilage at the rostral end of the notochord and from occipital somites.

2. **B** The incisive foramen is a landmark between the primary and secondary palates.

   A The landmark between the hard and soft palates is the posterior edge of the horizontal plate of the palatine bone.
   C The landmark between the left and right lateral palatine processes is the intermaxillary suture of the hard palate.
   D The landmark between the palatine and maxillary bones is the transverse palatine (palatomaxillary) suture.
   E The landmark between the left and right medial nasal prominences is the nasal septum, the intermaxillary segment of the upper lip, and the philtrum.

3. **A** The hypopharyngeal eminence, which arises in the floor of the pharynx between the 3rd and 4th pharyngeal arches, gives rise to the posterior one-third of the tongue. It receives general (pain, touch) and special (taste) sensory innervation from both the glossopharyngeal and vagus cranial nerves (CN IX and X, respectively. The vagus nerve carries general and taste sensation from the root of the tongue and epiglottis, while the glossopharyngeal nerve receives general and taste sensation from the majority of the posterior one-third of the tongue).

   B The trigeminal nerve receives general sensory innervation, and the facial nerve receives special sensory innervation from the anterior two-thirds of the tongue, which develops in the floor of the pharynx between the 1st and 2nd pharyngeal arches.
   C Although the vagus nerve does carry sensory innervation from the region of the hypopharyngeal eminence, the hypoglossal nerve carries no sensory innervation. Instead, the hypoglossal nerve carries general somatic motor innervation to the tongue.
   D, E Although the facial, trigeminal, and glossopharyngeal nerves all carry sensory information from the tongue, only the glossopharyngeal nerve carries information from the hypopharyngeal eminence. The facial nerve carries special sensory information (taste) from the anterior two-thirds of the tongue; the trigeminal nerve carries general sensory information from the anterior two-thirds of the tongue.

4. **D** Failure of fusion of the left and right lateral palatine processes results in secondary cleft palate.

   A Failure of fusion of the maxillary prominence with the medial nasal prominence will result in a cleft lip, with no effect on the secondary palate, although it may affect the primary palate.
   B Failure of fusion of the nasal septum with the maxillary prominence will result in a persistent passage between the left and right nasal cavities but will have no effect on the hard palate of the oral cavity.
   C The lateral palatine processes are extensions of the maxillary prominence and begin as a single rostral part of the 1st pharyngeal arch and therefore never undergo fusion. They remain as a single bony structure throughout life.
   E Failure of fusion of the intermaxillary segment results from failure of fusion of the left and right medial nasal prominences. This would result in a midline cleft lip and a primary cleft palate.

5. **E** The maxillary incisors, both deciduous and secondary (therefore not answer choice C), are supported by the intermaxillary segment of the upper jaw.

   A, D The mandibular molars and premolars are supported by the caudal part of the 1st pharyngeal arch specifically, the mandibular prominence.
   B The maxillary canines are supported by the maxillary prominence, specifically, the lateral part of the lateral palatine processes.

6. **B** A nonmigrating thyroid gland would result in a lingual cyst presenting as a midline swelling at the base of the tongue in the region of foramen cecum. During normal development the thyroid gland passes from the oropharynx into the neck by invaginating the tongue through a path indicated by foramen cecum.

   A A persistent 1st pharyngeal groove would result in a deformed auricle of the ear, a surface defect (depression) in the cheek, and an enlarged mouth (macrostomia).
   C The laryngotracheal diverticulum is a normal embryological structure that gives rise to the connection between the respiratory and digestive systems. This persists in the adult as the laryngeal inlet and the rima glottidis.
   D The 2nd pharyngeal pouch becomes the sinus of the palatine tonsil. It is laterally located in the oropharynx, and it normally persists in the adult.
   E Metastasis of the lingual tonsil may present as a midline swelling of the root of the tongue, but it likely would first involve the surface of the tongue, and it would migrate laterally as well as deeper into the structure of the tongue. It is unlikely to remain solely at the midline. Such a metastasis would not be referred to as a lingual cyst.

Chapter 2 Cranial Bones

7. **A** The greater palatine foramen of the palatine bone at the posterior margin of the hard palate allows for passage for the greater palatine nerve (and artery), a branch of the maxillary nerve (and artery).

   B The infraorbital foramen allows for passage of the infraorbital nerve (and artery), a branch of the maxillary division of the trigeminal nerve, although these vessels do not supply the hard palate.
   C The mental foramen of the mandible allows passage for the terminal branches of the inferior alveolar nerve (and artery). The inferior alveolar nerve is a branch of the mandibular division of the trigeminal nerve, which innervates the inferior teeth. The inferior alveolar artery is a branch of the maxillary artery.
   D The foramen rotundum of the sphenoid bone is the passage for the unbranched (except middle meningeal nerve) maxillary division of the trigeminal nerve to exit the middle cranial fossa. From this point, it enters the pterygopalatine fossa and branches extensively. Some branches will innervate the hard palate (as the nasopalatine and greater palatine), but there are many other branches that provide no innervation to the hard palate.
   E The sphenopalatine foramen allows passage of the sphenopalatine artery (of the maxillary) and the nasopalatine, medial, and lateral posterior nasal nerves. Although the nasopalatine nerve innervates the hard palate, it enters the oral cavity via the incisive foramen.

8. **D** The mandibular foramen of the ramus is protected by the bony lingula in a superoanterior position. The lingula is an attachment site for the sphenomandibular ligament.

   A The mental spines (genial tubercles) are located in the internal genu of the mandible and are for the attachment of the geniohyoid and genioglossus muscles.

B The pterygoid hamulus is part of the medial pterygoid plate of the sphenoid bone and is used for a lever around which the tensor veli palatini muscle changes orientation from its vertical origin in the scaphoid fossa of the sphenoid bone to reach the horizontal palatine aponeurosis.

C The coronoid process of the mandible is located in the superoanterior ramus, but it is not associated with the mandibular foramen. Instead, it provides the attachment site for the insertion for the temporalis muscle.

E The condylar process of the mandible is located in the superoposterior ramus, but it is not associated with the mandibular foramen. Instead, it provides the mandibular articulation of the temporomandibular joint.

9. **B** The anteromedial floor of the carotid canal in the petrous portion of the temporal bone is "open" to the nasopharynx through the foramen lacerum, although it is typically filled with cartilage after birth.

    A The foramen ovale of the sphenoid bone provides passage from the middle cranial fossa to the infratemporal fossa for the mandibular division of the trigeminal nerve (CN V$_3$), the lesser petrosal nerve (CN IX), and the accessory meningeal artery.

    C The jugular foramen, located between the temporal and occipital bones, provides passage from the posterior cranial fossa to the deep prevertebral neck for the internal jugular vein and the glossopharyngeal, vagus, and spinal accessory nerves.

    D The foramen spinosum of the sphenoid bone provides passage from the infratemporal fossa to the middle cranial fossa for the middle meningeal artery, a branch of the maxillary artery, and the recurrent meningeal nerve (nervus spinosus).

    E The mastoid foramen is an inconsistent passage for emissary veins to pass through the temporal bone. When present, it provides communication between the sigmoid sinus and occipital veins.

10. **C** The anterior cranial fossa is separated from the middle cranial fossa by the posterior border of the lesser wing of the sphenoid bone.

    A The lateral pterygoid plate provides muscular attachment sites for both the medial and lateral pterygoid muscles of the infratemporal fossa. It is not located within the cranial vault.

    B The perpendicular plate of the ethmoid bone provides the superior half of the nasal septum and is in the nasal cavity, not the cranial vault.

    D The petrous part of the temporal bone separates the middle and posterior cranial fossae. It provides attachment for the cerebellar tentorium and houses the auditory and vestibular infrastructure.

    E The frontal crest of the frontal bone is in the anterior cranial fossa, but it provides an anterior anchor for the falx cerebri, in the midline. It is not in a lateral position to allow for separation between anterior and middle cranial fossae on both the right and left.

11. **A** The pterion, an H-shaped suture between the frontal, sphenoid, temporal, and parietal bones, marks the location of the groove for the middle meningeal artery on the internal surface of the lateral wall of the cranial vault.

    B The hypophyseal fossa, the central part of the sella turcica of the sphenoid bone, is a midline structure in the middle cranial fossa.

    C The groove for the sigmoid sinus begins just posterior to the mastoid process of the temporal bone, at the location of the asterion. It is in the internal lateral wall of the cranial vault, but posterior to the pterion.

    D The internal acoustic meatus is centrally located in the petrous part of the temporal bone, in the posterior cranial fossa.

    E The crista galli is a centrally located structure in the floor of the anterior cranial fossa.

12. **E** The foramen rotundum, a passageway for the maxillary division of the trigeminal nerve (CN V$_2$) to reach the pterygopalatine fossa, exits the middle cranial fossa through the sphenoid bone.

    A The petrous part of the temporal bone provides a posterolateral passage for the facial (CN VII) and vestibulocochlear (CN VIII) nerves via the internal acoustic meatus. It is located at the boundary between the middle and posterior cranial fossae.

    B The ethmoid bone provides passage for the anterior and posterior ethmoidal branches of the ophthalmic division of the trigeminal

nerve (CN V$_1$) via the anterior and posterior ethmoidal foramina on the medial wall of the orbit and passage of the olfactory nerves from the nasal cavity through the cribriform plate.

C The occipital bone provides anterolateral passage for the hypoglossal nerve (CN XII) via the hypoglossal (anterior condylar) canal. The hypoglossal canal is located in the anterolateral wall of foramen magnum of the posterior cranial fossa.

D The mandible provides internal passage of the inferior alveolar branch of the mandibular division of the trigeminal nerve (CN V$_3$) via the mandibular foramen and canal.

13. **C** The majority of the hard palate of the oral cavity is formed from the union of the horizontal plate of the palatine bone with the palatine process of the maxilla.

    A The medial pterygoid plate of the sphenoid bone forms the posterior lateral wall of the choana of the nasal cavity, superior to the hard palate. The pterygoid hamulus, the inferior anterior part of the medial pterygoid plate, forms a very small part of the posterolateral hard palate.

    B The perpendicular plate of the ethmoid bone forms the superior half of the nasal septum, inside the nasal cavity, above the hard palate. At no point does it touch the horizontal plate of the palatine bone, although posterolateral parts of the ethmoid bone will create suture joints with the vertical plates of the palatine bone.

    D The squamous part of the temporal bone is the lateral wall of the cranial vault. It is not associated with the hard palate in any way.

    E The alae of the vomer bone articulate with the horizontal plate of the palatine bone but do so in the floor of the nasal cavity as part of the nasal septum. They are not located in the oral cavity and do not contribute to the inferior surface of the hard palate.

14. **D** The zygomatic bone does not articulate with the sphenoid bone.

    A, B, C The maxillary, frontal, and temporal processes of the zygomatic bone articulate with the maxilla, frontal bone, and temporal bone, respectively.

Chapter 3 Vasculature & Lymphatics of the Head & Neck

15. **A** The middle meningeal artery is a branch of the mandibular part of the maxillary artery that enters the skull through the foramen spinosum of the sphenoid bone to supply blood to the lateral part of the internal cranial vault and meninges.

    B The deep temporal artery is a branch of the pterygoid part of the maxillary artery. It remains outside the skull between the external lateral cranial vault and the temporalis muscle and therefore does not traverse a foramen.

    C The sphenopalatine artery is a terminal branch of the maxillary artery. From the pterygopalatine fossa, it passes through the sphenopalatine foramen to enter the nasal cavity.

    D The internal carotid artery is not a branch of, and is substantially larger than, the maxillary artery. The internal carotid artery enters the skull through the carotid canal of the temporal bone to enter the middle cranial fossa.

    E The ophthalmic artery branches from the internal carotid artery within the middle cranial fossa. It runs anterior from the most rostral end of the internal carotid artery, through the optic canal, to reach the orbit.

16. **B** The mandibular (bony/1st) part of the maxillary artery gives rise to the inferior alveolar artery. It enters the ramus of the mandible at the mandibular foramen and subsequently gives off small branches that supply blood to the mandibular molars, premolars, canines, and incisors and ends on the face as the mental artery.

    A The facial artery is a direct branch of the external carotid artery, which wraps laterally around the body of the mandible but does not supply blood to any mandibular teeth. It does supply the cheeks, lips, nose, and anterior medial orbit.

    C The lingual artery is a direct branch of the external carotid artery, which is positioned medially to the mandible and does not supply any mandibular teeth. It supplies the tongue and floor of the oral cavity.

D The sphenopalatine artery is a branch of the pterygopalatine part of the maxillary artery. It supplies the posterior superior nasal cavity. Other branches of the pterygopalatine part of the maxillary artery are the posterior superior alveolar and infraorbital arteries. The posterior superior alveolar artery supplies the maxillary molars; the infraorbital artery gives off the middle superior alveolar artery to the maxillary premolars and the anterior superior alveolar artery to the maxillary incisors.

E The internal carotid artery does not have any branches external to the skull. It supplies blood to the anterior two-thirds of the brain and augments the blood supply to the posterior orbit.

17. **C** The vertebral artery is a major branch of the subclavian artery, along with the internal thoracic artery, thyrocervical trunk, and an inconsistent dorsal scapular artery and/or costocervical trunk. The vertebral artery supplies blood to the posterior one-third of the brain and the paravertebral musculature of the neck.

A The external carotid artery has eight branches that supply blood to the neck (superior thyroid), face (facial), tongue (lingual), upper and lower jaw (maxillary), lateral head (temporal), ear (posterior auricular), back of the head (occipital), and pharynx (ascending pharyngeal). It does not give rise to the vertebral artery.

B The common carotid artery has two major branches only, the internal and external carotid arteries.

D, E The arch of the aorta (D) gives rise to the brachiocephalic trunk (E) on the right and the left common carotid and left subclavian arteries. The brachiocephalic trunk subdivides into the right subclavian artery and the right common carotid artery. The subclavian arteries on each side branch to give rise to the vertebral arteries.

18. **D** The ophthalmic veins provide direct connections between the angular veins and the cavernous sinus via the orbit through the superior orbital fissure.

A The pterygoid plexus can serve as an intermediary between the angular vein and the cavernous sinus. To reach the pterygoid plexus, blood must first travel through the deep facial vein or the infraorbital vein to the pterygoid plexus, and subsequently through sphenoidal emissary veins to reach the cavernous sinus.

B The retromandibular vein has no direct connection to the cavernous sinus. It provides a connection between the facial (angular) vein and the maxillary and superficial temporal veins, but to reach the cavernous sinus, blood would once again need first to enter the pterygoid plexus.

C The lingual vein has no direct connection to the cavernous sinus. It drains into the retromandibular vein, but infection would have to traverse multiple additional veins to reach the cavernous sinus.

E The brachiocephalic trunk is an artery that supplies blood to the right side of the head and neck. Even the brachiocephalic vein, draining blood from the right (or left) side of the head and neck, does not provide direct a connection between the angular vein and the cavernous sinus.

19. **E** The thyrocervical trunk has four major branches: the inferior thyroid, suprascapular, transverse cervical, and ascending cervical arteries. The deep branch of the transverse cervical artery (also called the dorsal scapular artery) runs deep to the rhomboid muscles. The superficial branch of the transverse cervical artery runs deep to the trapezius.

A The brachiocephalic trunk is on the right side only. Compression of this structure, which is deep in the neck, is difficult; additionally, it would compromise the blood going to the right upper extremity, entire right side of the neck and face, and right side of the brain.

B The common carotid artery has only two branches, the internal and external carotid arteries, which supply blood to the neck and head only.

C The thoracoacromial trunk supplies blood in the anterior part of the shoulder. The four typical branches are the pectoral, deltoid, acromial, and clavicular branches. Although they may supply small amounts of blood to the superior edge of the trapezius, they do not run near the rhomboid muscles; therefore, compression will not arrest bleeding following this injury.

D The costocervical trunk supplies blood to the intercostal muscles between the first two ribs, in a more lateral than posterior position. The plane of the injury is superficial to where this artery runs.

20. **C** The middle cerebral artery is a direct branch of the internal carotid artery.

A The common carotid artery has only two major branches, the external carotid and internal carotid arteries.

B The external carotid artery has eight major branches: the superior thyroid, facial, lingual, maxillary, superficial temporal, posterior auricular, occipital, and ascending pharyngeal. These arteries and most of their branches stay external to the skull and do not supply any central nervous structures.

D The basilar artery forms from the union of the left and right vertebral arteries. It supplies blood to the brainstem and cerebellum. It terminally bifurcates into the two posterior cerebral arteries that supply blood to the inferior occipital lobe.

E The middle meningeal artery is a branch of the maxillary artery in the infratemporal fossa. It pierces the skull at the foramen spinosum and supplies blood to the dura in the lateral part of the skull.

21. **B** The petrosal sinuses (both superior and inferior) drain the cavernous sinuses . The superior petrosal sinus then drains into the sigmoid sinus; the inferior petrosal sinus drains into the internal jugular vein.

A The straight sinus drains the inferior sagittal sinus and internal and great cerebral veins posteriorly to the confluence of sinuses. There is no direct connection between the cavernous sinuses and the straight sinus.

C The external jugular vein drains the occipital vein, retromandibular vein (from the face and the lateral head via the superficial temporal), and posterior auricular veins. There is no direct connection between the cavernous sinuses and the external jugular vein.

D The basilar vein drains the inferior frontal lobe and infralateral diencephalon to the straight sinus. There is no direct connection between the cavernous sinuses and the basilar veins.

E The maxillary sinus is an air sinus, rather than a venous dural sinus. It is connected to the nasal cavity via the maxillary hiatus of the middle (semilunar) meatus.

22. **E** The deep cervical (jugular) lymph nodes drain lymph from the posterior (occipital), lateral (superficial parotid), and anterior (facial and submandibular) lymph nodes down to the jugulosubclavian venous junction, where the thoracic/lymphatic duct joins the cardiovascular system.

A The occipital lymph nodes drain lymph from the posterior head to the jugular (deep cervical) lymph nodes. They collect lymph from regions significantly posterior to the ear.

B The facial lymph nodes drain lymph from the anterior head into the submandibular lymph nodes. Subsequently, lymph drains into the jugular (deep cervical) nodes and from there to the cardiovascular system via the lymphatic/thoracic duct.

C The nuchal lymph nodes drain lymph from the posterior neck and posteroinferior head to the jugular (deep cervical) nodes and from there into the cardiovascular system via the lymphatic/thoracic duct.

D The laryngeotracheal lymph nodes drain lymph from the anterior neck and respiratory viscera to the jugular (deep cervical) nodes and from there to the cardiovascular system via the lymphatic/thoracic duct.

23. **A** The submental nodes receive lymph from the tip of the tongue.

B The buccal nodes receive lymph from the superficial face.

C The superficial parotid (preauricular) nodes receive lymph from the buccal mucosa, external acoustic meatus, and anterior external ear.

D The retropharyngeal nodes receive lymph from the nasal cavity, sinuses, soft palate, nasopharynx, and oropharynx.

E The anterior jugular nodes receive lymph from the skin and muscles of the anterior neck.

Chapter 4 Neuroanatomy & Innervation of the Head & Neck

24. **A** The abducent nerve (CN VI) passes through the superior orbital fissure.

    B The foramen rotundum is for passage of the maxillary division of the trigeminal nerve (CN V_2).
    C The foramen ovale is for passage of the mandibular division of the trigeminal nerve (CN V_3).
    D The infraorbital foramen is for passage of the infraorbital nerve (the largest branch of the maxillary division of the trigeminal nerve, CN V_2) to reach the surface of the face below the orbit.
    E The foramen spinosum is for passage of the middle meningeal artery to enter the middle cranial fossa of the skull.

25. **E** The facial nerve (CN VII) innervates the stapedius, the middle ear muscle that modulates the motion of the stapes.

    A The optic nerve (CN II) carries sensory innervation from the neural retina to the lateral geniculate nucleus of the thalamus.
    B The oculomotor nerve (CN III) innervates the superior, medial, and inferior rectus muscles, and the inferior oblique muscle (extraocular muscles), the sphincter pupillae and ciliary muscles (intrinsic eye muscles), and levator palpebrae superioris muscle of the eyelids.
    C The vestibulocochlear nerve (CN VIII) is responsible for transmitting sensory information for hearing and balance from the cochlea and vestibular apparatus, respectively, to the brain. It does not innervate any muscles.
    D The trigeminal nerve (CN V) innervates the tensor tympani, the middle ear muscle that is attached to the malleus, a 1st pharyngeal arch structure. Tensor tympani acts to dampen sound.

26. **B** The trochlear nerve innervates the superior oblique extraocular muscle.

    A The lateral rectus is innervated by the abducent nerve (CN VI).
    C The orbicularis oculi is innervated by the facial nerve (CN VII).
    D The rectus capitis lateralis is innervated by the anterior ramus of the C1 spinal nerve.
    E The dilator pupillae is innervated by the sympathetic root and the sympathetic components of the short and long ciliary nerves.

27. **A** The vagus nerve (CN X) exits the posterior cranial fossa at the jugular foramen.

    B The internal acoustic meatus is the posterior cranial fossa opening for the facial nerve (CN VII), vestibulocochlear nerve (CN VIII), and labyrinthine artery.
    C The condylar canal of the occipital bone is the posterior cranial fossa exit for an emissary vein connecting the sigmoid sinus to the occipital vein.
    D The foramen magnum is the posterior cranial fossa entry for the vertebral arteries, spinal component of the spinal accessory nerve (CN XI), medulla oblongata of the brainstem, and cranial meninges (pia, arachnoid, and dura).
    E The foramen lacerum is mostly closed by cartilage in a living body, but it is traversed by the internal carotid artery above and the pharyngotympanic tube below. The only structures passing through the foramen lacerum are the autonomics of the superior cervical ganglion that control vasoconstriction/vasodilation of the internal carotid artery.

28. **C** The hyoglossus is innervated by the hypoglossal nerve (CN XII), along with the genioglossus, styloglossus, and all intrinsic muscles of the tongue.

    A The ansa cervicalis, emerging from the anterior rami of the C1–C3 spinal nerves, innervates the sternohyoid, sternothyroid, and omohyoid muscles.
    B The facial nerve (CN VII) innervates the stapedius muscle of the middle ear, the stylohyoid and posterior digastric muscles, and the muscles of facial expression.
    D The mylohyoid nerve, a branch of the mandibular division of the trigeminal nerve (CN V_3), innervates the anterior digastric and mylohyoid muscles.

E The recurrent laryngeal nerve, a branch of the vagus nerve (CN X), controls the intrinsic muscles of the larynx, excluding the cricothyroid muscle.

29. **D** Preganglionic parasympathetic fibers travel to the parotid gland travels via the tympanic nerve, then the lesser petrosal nerves, both branches of the glossopharyngeal nerve (CN IX) to the otic ganglion. Postganglionic fibers then travel with the auriculotemporal nerve to the gland.

    A The chorda tympani, a branch of the facial nerve (CN VII), carries preganglionic parasympathetic innervation to the submandibular ganglion and subsequently to the submandibular and sublingual glands. It also carries taste innervation from the anterior two-thirds of the tongue.
    B The greater petrosal nerve, a branch of the facial nerve (CN VII), carries preganglionic parasympathetic innervation to the pterygopalatine ganglion . Branches of CN V_2 subsequently distribute postganglionic parasympathetic fibers to the lacrimal gland and small glands of the nasal cavity, palate, and nasopharynx.
    C The deep petrosal nerve arises from the internal carotid plexus and carries postganglionic sympathetic innervation to the lacrimal and small nasal glands, nasopharynx, and palate via branches of CN V_1 and CN V_2.
    E The lingual nerve, a branch of the mandibular division of the trigeminal nerve (CN V_3), carries hitchhiking pre- and postganglionic parasympathetic innervation to the submandibular and sublingual glands. It also carries hitchhiking taste innervation from the anterior two-thirds of the tongue to the chorda tympani, as well as general somatic (touch, pain, and proprioception) innervation from the anterior tongue back to the trigeminal nerve.

30. **B** The C8 spinal nerve exits the vertebral canal through the intervertebral foramen below the C7 vertebra (therefore not E).

    A The C7 spinal nerve exits the vertebral canal through the intervertebral foramen above the C7 vertebra.
    C, D There is no C8 vertebra in the human vertebral column and therefore no C8 transverse foramen.

31. **C** Slippage of the C3–C4 intervertebral disk to the right would result in compression of the C4 spinal nerve. This can present as changes in the C4 dermatome at the top of the shoulder.

    A An osteophyte in the C1–C2 intervertebral foramen would start to compress the C2 spinal nerve, which has a dermatome that correlates to the back of the head. Tingling and numbness here would be indicative of a problem at that level.
    B Compression of the axillary nerve would present with the patient complaining of an inability to abduct his arm and glenohumeral joint instability. Any cutaneous effects would relate to the superior lateral arm, not the top of the shoulder.
    D Referred pain from the spleen can travel through the phrenic nerve (C3–C5), but it normally would present as deep, throbbing or burning pain, rather than tingling or numbness, over the left shoulder.
    E Avulsion of the C6 spinal nerve would result in the patient's inability to move or feel his thenar (thumb) region of the hand.

32. **D** The medulla oblongata develops from the myelencephalon, the caudal end of the rhombencephalon.

    A The cerebral peduncle, for passage of the corticospinal, corticopontine, and corticobulbar tracts, is part of the mesencephalon, one of the primary vesicles of the developing brain.
    B The thalamus, a relay nucleus for most cortical input from subcortical regions, is part of the diencephalon. The diencephalon contains the thalamic structures, including the hypothalamus, epithalamus (pineal), subthalamus, and thalamus proper.
    C The pons is a synaptic and decussation site for the corticopontocerebellar tract. It is part of the metencephalon, which originally develops as the rostral end of the rhombencephalon.
    E The tectum, made from the superior and inferior colliculi, is closely associated with visual tracking and hearing. It originally develops as part of the midbrain, or mesencephalon.

33. **E** The central sulcus separates the voluntary motor cortex from the conscious body sensation cortex on the ipsilateral side.

    A The calcarine sulcus, located close to the cerebral falx, separates superior and inferior parts of the occipital lobe. This is the location of primary visual cortex. It is not associated with motor cortex.
    B The parieto-occipital sulcus separates the parietal lobe (conscious body sensation) from the occipital lobe (primary visual cortex). It is not associated with the motor cortex.
    C The lateral sulcus separates the voluntary motor cortex of the frontal lobe and the conscious body sensation cortex of the parietal lobe from the temporal lobe, which is the location of the primary auditory cortex and memory formation components of the limbic system.
    D The longitudinal fissure separates the right and left cerebral hemispheres.

34. **A** The cerebral aqueduct can be blocked by the choroid plexus of the 3rd ventricle; blockage results in noncommunicating hydrocephalus in an individual. There are no alternate CSF flow passages between the 3rd and 4th ventricles.

    B Blockage of CSF flow in the pontomedullary cistern in the subarachnoid space will not cause hydrocephalus. There are numerous alternate routes for the CSF to flow to reach the arachnoid granulations. For example, CSF could flow from the pontomedullary cistern to the cerebellomedullary cistern, then the vermian cistern, ambient cistern, and finally reach the arachnoid granulations.
    C Blockage of CSF flow in the cerebellomedullary cistern in the subarachnoid space will not cause hydrocephalus. There are numerous alternate routes for the CSF to flow to reach the arachnoid granulations. For example, CSF could flow from the cerebellomedullary cistern to the pontomedullary cistern, then the interpeduncular and chiasmatic (basal) cisterns, and finally reach the arachnoid granulations.
    D The confluence of sinuses is a dural venous sinus structure filled with deoxygenated blood. Blockage of this blood passage will not result in hydrocephalus.
    E The arachnoid granulations provide drainage of the CSF into the venous sinus system. Blockage here could result in a backup of CSF that may result in communicating hydrocephalus. However, all the internal CSF passages would remain open and unblocked.

Chapter 5 Face & Scalp

35. **C** The orbicularis oris acts as an oral sphincter.

    A The risorius retracts the corner of the mouth, pulling it posteriorly during grimacing and smiling.
    B The depressor labii inferioris pulls the lower lip inferolaterally during pouting.
    D The levator anguli oris raises the angle of the mouth during smirking and smiling, increasing the nasolabial furrow.
    E The orbital portion of the orbicularis oculi acts as an orbital sphincter to close the eyelids voluntarily; the palpebral portion closes the eyes involuntarily.

36. **C** The posterior auricular muscle is innervated by a branch of the posterior auricular nerve, which comes off the facial nerve before it enters the parotid gland.

    A The platysma is innervated by the cervical branch of the facial nerve.
    B The zygomaticus major is innervated by the zygomatic branch of the facial nerve.
    D, E The risorius and buccinator are innervated by the buccal branch of the facial nerve.

37. **B** The buccinator is attached to the alveolar processes of the mandible and maxilla, the pterygomandibular raphe, and the lips.

    A The depressor anguli oris is attached to the oblique line of the mandible and the skin at the corner of the mouth.
    C The levator labii superioris is attached to the frontal process and infraorbital margin of the maxilla and the skin of the upper lip.

    D The zygomaticus minor is attached to the zygomatic bone and the upper lip.
    E The mentalis is attached to the frenulum of the lower lip and the skin of the chin.

38. **D** Scalp infections can easily spread through the layer of loose areolar connective tissue.

    A–C, E Scalp infections are less likely to spread in the other four layers of the scalp.

39. **A** The supraorbital artery is a terminal branch of the ophthalmic artery, which arises from the internal carotid artery.

    B The facial artery is a branch of the external carotid artery.
    C The lateral nasal artery is a branch of the facial artery, which arises from the external carotid artery.
    D The superficial temporal artery is a branch of the external carotid artery.
    E The transverse facial artery is a branch of the superficial temporal artery, which arises from the external carotid artery.

40. **D** The greater occipital nerve (posterior ramus of C2) is sensory to the occiput.

    A The maxillary nerve (CN V_2) is sensory to the midface.
    B The transverse cervical nerve (anterior rami of C2–C3) is sensory to the anterior neck.
    C The great auricular nerve (anterior rami of C2–C3) is sensory to the lateral neck and earlobe.
    E The facial nerve (CN VII) is motor to muscles of facial expression stapedius, and posterior digastric and does not carry sensory information from the face or scalp.

41. **D** The facial vein joins the anterior division of the retromandibular vein to form the common facial vein.

    A The angular vein drains into the facial vein.
    B The anterior jugular vein originates from superficial veins in the neck and drains to the terminal end of the external jugular vein or the subclavian vein.
    C The external jugular vein is formed from the posterior division of the retromandibular vein and the posterior auricular vein and drains to the subclavian vein.
    E The deep facial vein connects the facial vein to the pterygoid plexus.

42. **E** Branches of the infraorbital nerve (a branch of the maxillary division of the trigeminal nerve) are sensory to the upper lip.

    A The anterior superior alveolar nerve (a branch of the infraorbital nerve [from CN V_2]) is sensory to the maxillary incisors and canines
    B The buccal branch of the facial nerve is motor to some of the muscles of facial expression.
    C The mental nerve (a branch of the mandibular division of the trigeminal nerve) is sensory to the lower lip and chin.
    D The supraorbital nerve (a branch of the ophthalmic division of the trigeminal nerve [CN V_1]) is sensory to the upper eyelid and skin of the forehead.

Chapter 6 Temporal, Infratemporal, & Pterygopalatine Fossae

43. **D** The insertion (posterior attachment) of the lateral pterygoid muscle is the pterygoid fovea and condylar process of the mandible and the temporomandibular joint (articular disk).

    A The medial pterygoid muscle inserts (inferiorly attaches) to the pterygoid rugosity of the mandible.
    B The temporalis muscle inserts (inferoanteriorly attaches) to the coronoid process of the mandible.
    C The masseter originates (superiorly attaches) from the body of the zygomatic bone and the zygomatic arch made from the temporal process of the zygomatic bone and the zygomatic process of the temporal bone.
    E The temporalis muscle originates (superiorly attaches) on the temporal lines of the lateral cranial vault.

44. **B** Much of the weight of the mandible is supported by the spheno-mandibular ligament.

    A The mylohyoid muscle is located inferior to the mandible and is attached to the body of the hyoid bone. It is not in a location where it can support the weight of the mandible in normal anatomical position.

    C The digastric muscle is located inferior to the mandible, but it is attached posteriorly to the mastoid notch of the temporal bone. Only during extreme mandibular dislocation would the digastric muscle play any role in supporting the weight of the mandible, after many other structures have been compromised.

    D The pterygospinous ligament stretches between the lateral pterygoid plate of the sphenoid bone and the spine of the sphenoid bone. The ligament, if it is present, spans the mandibular notch, but it does not attach to the mandible at any point and therefore cannot support its weight.

    E The buccinator muscle is attached to the alveolar processes of the mandible and maxilla. Its main function is to keep the cheek pressed against the teeth to avoid food accumulation in the oral vestibule. The muscle fibers are oriented anteroposterior to facilitate that action, not resist the vertical pull of the weight of the mandible.

45. **C** The location of temporalis, between the temporal lines of the frontal, parietal, and temporal bones and the coronoid process of the mandible places part of the muscle posterior to the temporomandibular joint (TMJ). This is the primary masticator that can retrude the mandible.

    A The location of the masseter muscle, between the zygomatic arch and the lateral ramus of the mandible, places the entire muscle anterior to the TMJ. It mainly elevates the mandible, although it assists with protraction, side-to-side motion, and some retraction (from its deep head).

    B The medial pterygoid muscle, located vertically in the infratemporal fossa between the medial side of the lateral pterygoid plate and the medial ramus of the mandible, is placed anterior to the TMJ. It mainly elevates the mandible.

    D The lateral pterygoid muscle, located horizontally in the infratemporal fossa between the lateral side of the lateral pterygoid plate and the neck and pterygoid fossa of the mandible, is placed anterior to the TMJ. Its main action is to protrude the mandible or assist in lateral motion for chewing.

    E The mylohyoid muscle is located in the floor of the oral cavity between the mylohyoid line of the mandible and the body of the hyoid and the mylohyoid raphe. The muscle is placed significantly anterior to the TMJ and is used to tighten the oral cavity floor and protract the hyoid bone.

46. **A** The lateral pterygoid protrudes the mandible and pulls it laterally for chewing.

    B Tensing the soft palate is performed by the tensor veli palatini and levator veli palatini.

    C Depression of the sphenoid bone is not possible.

    D Elevation of the hyoid bone is performed by the suprahyoid muscles—the digastric, geniohyoid, stylohyoid, and mylohyoid. The lateral pterygoid can only elevate the hyoid secondarily by first protruding the mandible.

    E Retraction of the mandible is performed by the temporalis muscle, assisted by the masseter.

47. **B** The sphenomandibular ligament runs between the base of the sphenoid bone and the lingula of the mandible. It supports the weight of the mandible and helps to prevent overprotraction of the mandible.

    A The masseter muscle has superior attachments on the body of the zygomatic bone and the anterior part of the zygomatic arch. The inferior attachment is the lateral ramus and the angle of the mandible.

    C The temporalis has superior attachment along the temporal lines of the frontal, parietal, and temporal bones and an inferior attachment on the coronoid process of the mandible.

    D The stylomandibular ligament runs between the styloid process of the temporal bone and the posterior ramus and angle of the mandible. Although it also prevents overprotraction, it does not attach to the lingula.

E The pharyngeotympanic tube has both bony and cartilaginous parts. The bony parts are supported within the petrous part of the temporal bone. The cartilaginous part is not supported by a bony structure within the nasopharynx but instead provides muscle attachment for some soft palate muscles.

48. **D** The long buccal nerve, a branch of the mandibular nerve, emerges between the two heads of the lateral pterygoid.

    A, B, E The inferior alveolar nerve and the lingual nerve emerge between the medial and lateral pterygoids.

    C The deep temporal nerves emerge superior to the superior head of the lateral pterygoid muscle.

49. **B** The inferior tympanic artery is a branch of the ascending pharyngeal artery.

    A, C The middle meningeal and deep auricular arteries are branches of the first (mandibular/bony) part of the maxillary artery.

    D, E The descending palatine artery and the artery of the pterygoid canal are branches of the third (pterygopalatine) part of the maxillary artery.

50. **B** The auriculotemporal nerve, along with the posterior deep temporal and the masseteric nerves, is sensory to the TMJ.

    A The inferior alveolar nerve is sensory to the mandibular teeth gingiva, and mucosa, as well as the chin and lower lip..

    C The lingual nerve is sensory to the tongue, floor of the mouth, and mandibular lingual gingiva.

    D The nerve to the lateral pterygoid is motor to the lateral pterygoid muscle.

    E The long buccal nerve is sensory to the mucosa on the inside of the cheek and the buccal gingiva and mucosa of the mandibular molars.

51. **E** The pterygomaxillary fissure connects the pterygopalatine fossa with the infratemporal fossa laterally. The maxillary artery and the posterior superior alveolar neurovascular bundle traverse this fissure.

    A The greater palatine canal connects the pterygopalatine fossa with the oral cavity inferiorly.

    B, D The pterygoid canal and foramen rotundum connect the pterygopalatine fossa with the middle cranial fossa posteriorly.

    C The sphenopalatine foramen connects the pterygopalatine fossa with the nasal cavity medially.

52. **C** The greater petrosal nerve is a branch of the facial nerve (CN VII) that carries preganglionic parasympathetic fibers to synapse in the pterygopalatine ganglion. Before reaching the ganglion, it joins with the deep petrosal nerve to form the nerve of the pterygoid canal (Vidian nerve).

    A The maxillary nerve (CN V_2) contains sensory fibers. Branches of the maxillary nerve carry hitchhiking postganglionic parasympathetic fibers from the pterygopalatine ganglion.

    B The chorda tympani is a branch of the facial nerve (CN VII) that carries preganglionic parasympathetic fibers to synapse in the submandibular ganglion.

    D The lesser petrosal nerve is a branch of the glossopharyngeal nerve (CN IX) that carries preganglionic parasympathetic fibers to synapse in the otic ganglion.

    E The deep petrosal nerve contains postsynaptic sympathetic fibers that join with the greater petrosal nerve to form the nerve of the pterygoid canal (vidian nerve).

53. **A** The greater wing of the sphenoid bone is the roof of the pterygopalatine fossa.

    B The posterior surface of the maxilla is the anterior wall of the pterygopalatine fossa.

    C The perpendicular plate of the palatine bone is the medial wall of the pterygopalatine fossa.

    D, E The temporal bone and vomer do not form boundaries of the pterygopalatine fossa.

Chapter 7 Nose & Nasal Cavity

54. **A** The palatine bone makes the posterior inferolateral walls and floor of the bony nasal cavity. It helps to separate the oral cavity from the nasal cavity, just anterior to the soft palate.

    B The zygomatic bone forms the cheek and the lateral wall of the maxillary air sinus, inferior to the orbit. It is located too laterally to help form the nasal cavity.
    C The mandible forms the lower jaw and the lateral walls of the oral cavity. Although it is a midline bone, it is too inferior to help form the nasal cavity.
    D The parietal bone forms the posterolateral walls of the neurocranium, supporting the brain. The left and right parietal bones reach the midline to create the sagittal suture but are not associated with the nasal cavity.
    E The occipital bone forms the bony roof of the nasopharynx, but not the nasal cavity.

55. **B** The middle meatus of the nasal cavity, superior to the inferior nasal concha, allows for drainage of the maxillary air sinus (via the semilunar hiatus), the anterior and middle ethmoid air cells, and the frontal sinus (via the frontonasal duct).

    A The inferior meatus of the nasal cavity, inferolateral to the inferior nasal concha, allows for drainage of the nasolacrimal duct from the orbit.
    C The superior meatus of the nasal cavity allows for drainage of the posterior ethmoid air cells.
    D The nasopharynx, posterior to the nasal cavity, allows for drainage of the pharyngotympanic tube from the middle ear.
    E The sphenoethmoidal recess, superior to the superior nasal concha, allows for drainage of the sphenoid air sinus into the most superior part of the nasal cavity.

56. **C** The sphenopalatine artery has posterior septal branches that anastomose with the anterior nasal septal arteries within Kiesselbach's area. It is a large branch of the maxillary artery that is found in the infratemporal fossa.

    A The superior posterior alveolar artery supplies blood to the upper molars, but it remains in a lateral position. It is a branch of the maxillary artery that stays within the maxillary bone. It does not anastomose with the anterior nasal septal arteries
    B The middle meningeal artery supplies blood to the lateral dura mater, inside the cranial vault. It is also a branch of the maxillary artery, but it does not supply the viscerocranium.
    D The ascending pharyngeal artery, a branch of the external carotid artery, supplies blood to the lateral pharynx and ascends toward the nasopharynx. It does not reach into the nasal cavity, nor does it anastomose with the anterior nasal sepal arteries.
    E The petrotympanic (anterior tympanic) artery, also a branch of the maxillary artery, supplies blood to the anterior part of the middle ear. It anastomoses with the posterior tympanic artery off the posterior auricular artery and pterygoid canal artery off the internal carotid artery.

57. **D** The nasopalatine nerve, a branch of the maxillary nerve (CN V_2), innervates the posterior nasal septum, including the vomer.

    A The olfactory nerve pierces the cribriform plate of the ethmoid bone and innervates the olfactory epithelium at the roof of the nasal cavity.
    B The anterior ethmoidal nerve, a branch of the ophthalmic nerve (CN V_1), innervates the anterior medial and lateral walls of the nasal cavity, including the anterior parts of the inferior nasal concha.
    C The greater palatine nerve, a branch of the maxillary nerve (CN V_2), innervates the hard palate of the oral cavity. It enters from a posterolateral position and runs anterior and medial.
    E The posterior superior alveolar nerve, a branch of the maxillary nerve (CN V_2), innervates the upper molars inside the maxillary bone. It remains quite lateral and never reaches the nasal cavity.

58. **E** The maxillary air sinus is located immediately superior to the upper molars. Complications with tooth extraction of the molars can result in problems within the maxillary air sinus.

    A The frontal air sinus is located superior to and between the orbits. No teeth are closely associated with this sinus.
    B The ethmoid air sinus (cells) are located superior to and between the orbits. This bone is not associated with any teeth.
    C The mastoid air sinus (cells) are located posterior and lateral to the middle ear. Although they are close to the temporomandibular joint, they are not closely associated with the superior molars.
    D The sphenoid air sinus is located posterior to the ethmoid air cells on the midline of the skull. The molars are not associated with midline bones.

59. **D** The sphenoid air sinus separates the nasal cavity from the hypophyseal fossa, the location of the pituitary gland. This route provides the most direct access to the macroadenoma.

    A The frontal sinus separates the nasal cavity from the cranial vault, but only for access to the frontal lobes of the cerebral hemispheres. The pituitary gland is located in the hypophyseal fossa (sella turcica) of the sphenoid bone, significantly posterior the frontal air sinus.
    B The ethmoid air sinus separates the nasal cavity from the orbit and the anterior cranial fossa. Access to this space will still require access into the cranial vault via the optic canal or superior orbital fissure (of the sphenoid bone).
    C The mastoid air sinus is only connected to the nasal cavity via the nasopharynx and pharyngotympanic tube. It would provide access from the middle or external ear to the posterior cranial vault, but it is exclusively contained within the temporal bone.
    E The maxillary air sinus separates the nasal cavity from the oral cavity below and orbit above. Neither of these spaces will provide direct access to the pituitary gland.

Chapter 8 Oral Cavity & Pharynx

60. **C** The posterior digastric is innervated by a small muscular branch of the facial nerve, just after it exits the stylomastoid foramen, before it enters the parotid gland to create the parotid plexus.

    A The mylohyoid is innervated by a branch of the mandibular division of the trigeminal nerve, specifically, the mylohyoid nerve.
    B The hyoglossus is innervated by a small muscular branch of the hypoglossal nerve.
    D The geniohyoid is innervated by a small contribution from the C1 anterior ramus that joins the hypoglossal nerve as it traverses the lateral neck. It breaks from the hypoglossal nerve as it approaches the posterior border of the mylohyoid.
    E The stylopharyngeus is not a true suprahyoid muscle. Furthermore, it is innervated by the glossopharyngeal nerve via a small muscular branch that breaks from the nerve along the superior border of the inferior pharyngeal constrictor.

61. **E** The ventral posteromedial nucleus receives somatosensory and special visceral sensory input from the head and neck. Input travels through the trigeminothalamic (central tegmental: taste) tract, spinothalamic tract (pain/temperature), and medial lemniscus (face), and output goes to the postcentral gyrus.

    A The ventral anterior nucleus of the thalamus receives input from the globus pallidus and deep cerebellar nuclei and sends output to the precentral gyrus of the cerebral hemispheres. It is a motor relay nucleus and is not associated with taste.
    B The lateral dorsal nucleus of the thalamus is closely associated with memory formation. It receives input from the hippocampus and sends output to the cingulate gyrus of the cerebral hemisphere.
    C The pulvinar nucleus of the thalamus receives input from the temporal, parietal, and occipital lobes of the association cortex and sends output back to the same association cortex. It is an intercortical relay nucleus that is partially obsolete due to the telencephalic cortical connections of the splenium of the corpus callosum.

D The medial geniculate nucleus deals with auditory information as a relay between the brainstem and the primary auditory cortex in the posterior superior temporal gyrus. Most of the input comes from the inferior colliculus, lateral lemniscus, or superior olivary nucleus, and the output goes through the acoustic radiations of the posterior limb of the internal capsule to the temporal lobe.

62. **A** The tensor veli palatini is connected to the anterolateral cartilaginous pharyngotympanic tube and the palatine aponeurosis via the pterygoid hamulus. It flattens the soft palate and opens the pharyngotympanic tube.

    B The palatoglossus is connected to the palatine aponeurosis and the lateral dorsal tongue (intrinsic muscles). It elevates the tongue and depresses the soft palate. It is not connected to the pharyngotympanic tube.
    C The palatopharyngeus is connected to the palatine aponeurosis and the lateral pharynx and thyroid cartilage. It elevates the pharynx and depresses the soft palate. It is also not connected to the pharyngotympanic tube.
    D The tensor tympani is connected to the pharyngotympanic tube within the petrous part of the temporal bone. It runs posterolaterally to insert into the malleus. It stiffens the tympanic membrane to reduce the transmission of sound. It is not associated with the soft palate.
    E The superior pharyngeal constrictor has a variety of attachments, including both bony and fibrous, but no cartilaginous attachments. It originates on the pterygoid hamulus and mylohyoid line (bony) and the pterygomandibular raphe and lateral tongue (fibrous). It inserts into the pharyngeal tubercle of the basilar part of the occipital bone. It is not associated with the soft palate.

63. **B** The lingual tonsil is located on the dorsal root of the tongue, closely associated with the epiglottis of the larynx. This midline tonsil completes the inferior extent of the pharyngeal lymphatic ring.

    A The tubal tonsils are associated with the pharyngotympanic tube of the nasopharynx. They are located posterolateral within the space and are not closely related to the midline epiglottis.
    C The pharyngeal tonsil is a midline structure located between the right and left pharyngeotympanic tubes of the nasopharynx. It is adjacent to the left and right tubal tonsils and completes the superior extent of the pharyngeal lymphatic ring, but it is not closely associated with the epiglottis.
    D The palatine tonsils are located between the palatoglossal (anterior) and palatopharyngeal (posterior) arches of the oropharynx. These two laterally located lymph structures are closely associated with the lateral tongue, close to but not immediately adjacent to the epiglottis.
    E The adenoid tonsil is another name for the pharyngeal tonsil of the nasopharynx. It is the superiormost part of the pharyngeal lymphatic ring.

64. **D** Dentine makes up the majority of the tooth volume. It is deep to the enamel and cementum and surrounds the pulp chamber.

    A The periodontal ligament connects the cementum to the alveolar bone.
    B Cementum covers the roots of the teeth (enamel covers the crowns). The cementum and enamel meet at the cementoenamel junction, located at the cervical margin of the tooth.
    C The pulp is located in the pulp chamber at the center of the tooth. The pulp chamber is surrounded by dentine, enamel, and cementum.
    E The roots of the teeth are embedded in the alveolar bone of the mandible and maxilla.

65. **D** The 1st molars erupt at 6 to 8 years of age and are commonly called the "6-year molars."

    A The canines erupt at 9 to 14 years of age.
    B The 1st premolars erupt at 9 to 13 years of age.
    C The 2nd premolars erupt at 11 to 14 years of age.
    E The 2nd molars erupt at 10 to 14 years of age.

66. **E** The submandibular ganglion provides postganglionic parasympathetic fibers for the submandibular and sublingual glands.

    A The superior cervical ganglion provides postganglionic sympathetic fibers (not parasympathetic) for the head.
    B The pterygopalatine ganglion provides postganglionic parasympathetic fibers for the palate, nasal mucosa, and lacrimal glands.
    C The ciliary ganglion provides postganglionic parasympathetic fibers for the eye.
    D The otic ganglion provides postganglionic parasympathetic fibers for the parotid gland.

67. **B** The parotid is a serous gland.

    A, C The parotid gland does not produce mucous secretions. The submandibular gland produces both mucous and serous secretions. The sublingual gland is a mixed gland with predominantly mucous secretions.

68. **A** Infections from the maxillary and mandibular molars can spread to the peripharyngeal (retropharyngeal and parapharyngeal) spaces. They can also spread to the buccal space or submandibular, sublingual, or masticator spaces (mandibular molars only).

    B Infections from the maxillary canines can spread to the infraorbital space.
    C Infections from the mandibular premolars can spread to the buccal and sublingual spaces.
    D, E Infections from the mandibular canines and incisors can spread to the submental space.

69. **B** The submandibular space is inferior to the mylohyoid line, superior to the hyoid bone, inferior and lateral to the mylohyoid, and medial to the superficial fascia and skin.

    A The sublingual space is inferior to the mucosa of the oral floor, superior to the mylohyoid, lateral to the tongue, and medial to the mandible.
    C The masticator space is anterior to the stylomandibular ligament, medial to the cervical fascia, and inferior to the roof of the infratemporal fossa and the origin of the temporalis.
    D The tonsillar space is posterior to the palatoglossus, anterior to the palatopharyngeus, lateral to the mucosa of the oropharynx, and medial to the pharyngobasilar fascia.
    E The parotid space is posterior to the ramus of the mandible and stylomandibular ligament, anterior to the sternocleidomastoid, lateral to the styloid process and attaching muscles, and medial to the skin.

70. **C** The internal laryngeal nerve and superior laryngeal artery pass through the 3rd pharyngeal gap, between the middle and inferior pharyngeal constrictors.

    A The pharyngotympanic tube and levator veli palatini pass through the 1st pharyngeal gap, superior to the superior pharyngeal constrictor.
    B The tensor veli palatini does not pass through a pharyngeal gap.
    D The recurrent laryngeal nerve and inferior laryngeal artery pass through the 4th pharyngeal gap, inferior to the inferior pharyngeal constrictor.
    E The glossopharyngeal nerve and the stylopharyngeus muscle pass through the 2nd pharyngeal gap between the superior and middle pharyngeal constrictors.

Chapter 9 Orbit & Eye

71. **D** The ophthalmic artery (E) runs through the optic canal and supplies blood to the orbit; it is a branch of the internal carotid artery after it has entered the middle cranial fossa.

    A The middle meningeal artery is a superior branch of the mandibular (bony/1st) part of the maxillary artery that enters the skull through the foramen spinosum of the sphenoid bone to supply blood to the lateral part of the internal cranial vault.

B The deep temporal artery stays outside the skull and runs between the external lateral cranial vault and the temporalis muscle. It is a branch of the pterygoid (muscular/2nd) part of the maxillary artery that never runs through a foramen.

C The sphenopalatine artery is the anteromedial terminal branch of the maxillary artery that enters the skull at the pterygomaxillary fissure to access the posterolateral nasal cavity. It runs medially through the sphenopalatine foramen to reach the nasal cavity.

72. **B** The lateral rectus is innervated by the abducent nerve (CN VI).

A, C, D, E These rectus muscles (and levator palpebrae superioris) are innervated by the oculomotor nerve (CN III). The remaining extraocular muscle, the superior oblique, is innervated by the trochlear nerve (CN IV).

73. **A** The superior orbital fissure is for the passage of the superior and inferior parts of the oculomotor nerve (CN III), in addition to all parts of the ophthalmic division of the trigeminal nerve (CN V_1), trochlear nerve (CN IV), abducent nerve (CN VI), and superior ophthalmic vein.

B The foramen rotundum is for passage of the maxillary division of the trigeminal nerve (CN V_2).
C The foramen ovale is for passage of the mandibular division of the trigeminal nerve (CN V_3).
D The infraorbital foramen is for passage of the largest branch of the maxillary division of the trigeminal nerve (CN V_2) to reach the surface of the skull in the upper jaw.
E The foramen spinosum is for passage of the middle meningeal artery to enter the middle cranial fossa of the skull.

74. **B** The bipolar cell, located in the inner nuclear layer, is the intermediate neuron (sensory) between the photoreceptor cells and the retinal ganglion cells.

A The horizontal cell, located in the outer region of the inner nuclear layer, interconnects the photoreceptors to spread or collect visual signals. It does not connect to the retinal ganglion cells.
C The amacrine cell, located in the inner region of the inner nuclear layer, interconnects the bipolar cells and the retinal ganglion cells to start to process visual signals. It does not connect to the photoreceptor cells.
D The Purkinje cell, located in the cortical layer of the cerebellum, is the output neuron that connects the cerebellar cortex to the deep cerebellar nuclei. It is not associated with the retina.
E The Müller's cell, located in the inner nuclear layer, is the main glial support cell of the retina. Although its cell body is located in this layer, its peripheral and central processes make the inner and outer limiting membranes. It does not connect to either photoreceptor cells or retinal ganglion cells.

75. **C** The optic chiasm is where nasal retinal information (from the temporal field) from both eyes crosses to the contralateral side. It is located anterosuperior to the pituitary gland. A problem here would produce tunnel vision; it also can be associated with pituitary problems such as weight gain and reproductive cycle changes.

A The optic nerve sends information from a single eyeball to both right and left lateral geniculate nuclei. A problem here would likely present with orbital problems, such as blindness in one eye, paralysis of the extraocular muscles, and dry eye. It would not be associated with weight gain or a change in the menstrual cycle.
B The optic track sends information from both eyes, from a single visual field (right or left) to the ipsilateral lateral geniculate nucleus. A problem here would present with blindness in either the right or left visual field (contralateral homonymus hemianopia). It would not be associated with weight gain or a change in the menstrual cycle.
D The retrolenticular limb of the internal capsule is the location of the optic radiations that send information from the lateral geniculate nucleus to the primary visual cortex (in the calcarine sulcus of the occipital lobe). A problem here would result in a modified form of hemianopia that has a specific subquadrant missing from the patient's visual space (contralateral homonymus quadrantanopia). It would not be associated with weight gain or a change in the menstrual cycle.

E The splenium of the corpus callosum interconnects the right and left posterior parietal, posterior temporal, and occipital lobes. It allows for cortical communication between the two hemispheres. Problems here would be auditory, visual, memory, and somatosensory. It would not be associated with weight gain or a change in the menstrual cycle.

Chapter 10 Ear

76. **B** The superficial temporal artery has anterior auricular branches that supply blood to the anterior external ear.

A The transverse facial artery runs anterior, immediately inferior to the zygomatic arch. It supplies blood to the deep facial muscles and the lateral cheek. It does not run posteriorly toward the ear.
C The sphenopalatine artery is a terminal branch of the maxillary artery that supplies blood to the medial and lateral part of the nasal cavity. It does not run posteriorly or superficially toward the ear.
D The internal carotid artery enters the skull through the carotid canal of the temporal bone to access the middle cranial fossa from below. It supplies blood to the anterior brain and has no branches that supply the external ear.
E The occipital artery is a posterior branch of the external carotid artery. It runs deep to the sternocleidomastoid muscle and supplies blood to the posterior scalp and occipitalis muscle.

77. **B** The facial nerve carries taste fibers in its chorda tympani branch. This branch of the facial nerve traverses the middle ear cavity, just medial to the neck of the malleus and the tympanic membrane.

A The trigeminal nerve only carries hitchhiking taste fibers that originate in the facial nerve. The branch that carries these taste fibers is the lingual nerve, which is joined by the chorda tympani inferior to the skull as they both approach the oral cavity from a posterior direction.
C The vestibulocochlear nerve does not carry any taste fibers. It carries other special somatic sensory fibers to the cochlea and vestibular apparatus, but these terminate at the inner ear and do not enter the middle ear cavity.
D The glossopharyngeal nerve carries taste fibers, but they reside within the pharyngeal branches that join the main trunk of the nerve and enter the skull through the jugular foramen. The tympanic nerve, which also traverses the air space of the middle ear cavity, is a branch of the glossopharyngeal nerve, but it only carries general somatic afferent (pain, touch, and proprioception) from the middle ear and visceromotor fibers to the otic ganglion to drive secretion in the parotid gland.
E The vagus nerve carries taste fibers from the root of the tongue, epiglottis, and pharynx, but they reside in pharyngeal branches that join the main trunk of the nerve and enter the skull through the jugular foramen.

78. **C** The stapes of the middle ear cavity has a footplate that fits neatly into the oval window of the medial wall of the middle ear cavity. It is used to transmit sound waves, detected by the tympanic membrane, to the inner ear.

A The malleus of the middle ear cavity is attached to the tympanic membrane via its handle. Although it is in the middle ear cavity, it is not physically attached to the medial wall or the inner ear.
B The pisiform is a carpal bone located in the proximal anteromedial wrist, adjacent to the head of the ulna. It is not located in the middle ear region of the temporal bone of the skull.
D The navicular bone of the foot supports the medial side of the talus and transmits forces into the three cuneiform bones of the foot. It is not located in the middle ear.
E The incus of the middle ear cavity is supported between the malleus and stapes (and by other ligaments of the middle ear cavity). It is not physically attached to the medial wall or the inner ear.

79. **D** The internal acoustic meatus provides a passage for the vestibulocochlear nerve to exit the posterior cranial fossa and reach the inner ear. The internal acoustic meatus also transmits the facial nerve and the labyrinthine artery.

    A The greater petrosal hiatus provides a passage for the greater petrosal nerve (a branch of the facial nerve) and the superficial petrosal artery to exit the petrous part of the temporal bone and enter the middle cranial fossa as they course toward the foramen lacerum.
    B The external acoustic meatus provides a passage for sound waves to enter the skull and reach the tympanic membrane, located within the temporal bone. It does not provide access to the posterior cranial fossa.
    C The mastoid canaliculus provides passage for the auricular branch of the vagus nerve to enter the external auditory canal from an inferior direction. It does not provide access to the posterior cranial fossa.
    E The stylomastoid foramen provides passage for the facial nerve and stylomastoid artery to exit the petrous part of the temporal bone on the inferior aspect of the skull.

80. **E** The left posterior semicircular canal aligns with a 45-degree plane offset from the median (posterior-anterior) axis of the head. It lies in a plane parallel to the right anterior semicircular canal.

    A The right posterior semicircular canal aligns with a 45-degree plane offset from the median (anterior-posterior) axis of the head. It lies in a plane parallel to the left anterior semicircular canal.
    B The right lateral semicircular canal aligns with a 30-degree plane offset from the horizontal axis of the head. It lies in the exact same (parallel) plane as the left lateral semicircular canal.
    C The left anterior semicircular canal aligns with a 45-degree plane offset from the median (anterior-posterior) axis of the head. It lies in a plane parallel to the right posterior semicircular canal.
    D The left lateral semicircular canal aligns with a 30-degree plane offset from the horizontal axis of the head. It lies in the exact same (parallel) plane as the right lateral semicircular canal.

81. **A** The basilar membrane stretches between the modiolus and spiral ligament and therefore lies between the endolymph and perilymph. It physically supports the hair cells of the cochlear.

    B The spiral ligament underlies the stria vascularis of the cochlear duct. It supports the secretory stria, but it is not physically attached to the hair cells and does not come into contact with perilymph.
    C The vestibular membrane stretches between the modiolus and the spiral ligament and also separates endolymph and perilymph. However, it is not a support structure of the hair cells and is not closely associated with sound detection.
    D The tectorial membrane covers (supports) the stereocilia of the hair cells of the cochlear duct. It is completely enclosed within the cochlear duct and does not separate perilymph from endolymph.
    E The helicotrema is a perilymphatic passage between the scala vestibuli and scala tympani. It does not separate endolymph from perilymph and is not associated with the hair cells.

82. **C** The spiral ganglion contains the cell bodies whose peripheral processes synapse with the inner hair cells and whose central processes are the main synaptic input for the cochlear nuclei. Without this input, no sound perception can be detected, so no sound could be localized.

    A The vestibular nuclei are critical for the perception of linear or angular acceleration changes of the head due to motion. None of these systems are critical for the localization of sound in auditory space (anterior, posterior, right, or left), which can be accomplished in a stationary head.
    B The tensor tympani muscle contracts to change the tuning of the tympanic membrane. Although it can be used to augment (or depress) the perception of sound, it is not used to localize sound.
    D The lateral geniculate nucleus is one of the synaptic targets of the optic tract. It deals exclusively with visual information, which is not necessary for the localization of sound.
    E The medial lemniscus is the midbrain tegmental pathway connecting the posterior column nuclei (gracilis and cuneatus) to the ventroposterolateral and ventroposteromedial nuclei of the thalamus. This pathway is for perception of touch and conscious proprioception and is not necessary for the localization of sound.

Chapter 11 Bones, Ligaments, & Muscles of the Neck

83. **B** The geniohyoid draws the hyoid bone anteriorly and is innervated by the anterior ramus of the C1 spinal nerve carried by the hypoglossal nerve.

    A The mylohyoid draws the hyoid bone anteriorly, but it is innervated by the mylohyoid nerve, a branch of the mandibular division of the trigeminal nerve (CN V_3).
    C The stylohyoid elevates the hyoid (and helps with posterior motion) and is innervated by the facial nerve (CN VII).
    D The omohyoid depresses the hyoid and fixes it in place. It is innervated by the ansa cervicalis, the C1–C3 anterior rami that innervate most infrahyoid muscles in the anterior neck.
    E The sternohyoid depresses the hyoid and fixes it in place. It is also innervated by the ansa cervicalis, the C1–C3 anterior rami.

84. **E** The sternocleidomastoid muscle of the neck rotates the head to the contralateral (opposite) side.

    A, B The rectus capitis posterior major and longissimus capitis extend the head and rotate it to the ipsilateral (same) side.
    C The rectus capitis lateralis flexes the head at the atlanto-occipital joint anteriorly and laterally to the ipsilateral side.
    D The splenius capitis extends the cervical spine and head, as well as flexes and rotates the head to the ipsilateral side.

85. **A** The splenius cervicis originates (proximally attaches) to the spinous process of T3–T6.

    B The levator costarum longii muscles originate (inferiorly attach) to the transverse processes of the C7–T11 vertebrae.
    C The serratus posterior superior originates (proximally attaches) on the nuchal ligament and the spines of the C7–T3 vertebrae. It does not extend as inferior as the T6 vertebra.
    D The iliocostalis thoracis originates (proximally attaches) on the iliac crest, sacrum, thoracolumbar fascia, and inferior ribs.
    E The longus colli originates (inferiorly attaches) to the anterior surfaces of the T1–T3 vertebrae in the prevertebral space.

86. **C** The geniohyoid muscle of the suprahyoid group is innervated by the anterior ramus of the C1 spinal nerve.

    A The mylohyoid nerve, a branch of the mandibular division of the trigeminal nerve (CN V_3), innervates the mylohyoid and anterior digastric muscles of the suprahyoid group, but it does not reach deeper than the mylohyoid.
    B The facial nerve (CN VII) innervates the muscles of facial expression, the posterior digastric and stylohyoid muscle of the suprahyoid group, and the stapedius muscle. The branches that reach far enough anterior (marginal mandibular and cervical) do not reach deeper than the thin facial muscles.
    D The inferior alveolar nerve (of CN V_3) is a purely sensory nerve that travels the length of the body of the mandible to reach the mental foramen and provide sensory perception from the mandibular teeth and the mental region of the face. It does not innervate any muscles.
    E The hypoglossal nerve (CN XII) carries innervation to the intrinsic and most extrinsic muscles of the tongue (genioglossus, hyoglossus, and styloglossus, not palatoglossus). It provides a route for the ventral ramus of the C1 spinal nerve to reach the geniohyoid but does not innervate any of the suprahyoid muscles.

87. **C** The alar ligaments connect the dens of C2 to the medial aspect of the occipital condyles of the occipital bone.

    A The posterior atlanto-occipital membrane attaches the atlas (C1) to the occipital bone.
    B The posterior longitudinal ligament runs posterior to vertebral bodies. It is continuous with the tectorial membrane which connects the body of C2 to the anterior border of the foramen magnum.
    D The transverse ligament of the atlas is part of the cruciate ligament, holding the dens (C2) to the anterior arch of the atlas (C1).
    E The nuchal ligament is an expansion of the supraspinous ligament, extending from the spinous processes of cervical vertebrae to the occipital bone.

88. **D** The C7 vertebra has transverse foramina for the passage of vertebral veins. The vertebral arteries typically enter the transverse foramina at C6.

   A, B, C, E The vertebral arteries run in the transverse foramina of vertebrae C6 to C1, before entering the foramen magnum.

Chapter 12 Neurovascular Topography of the Neck

89. **A** The valleculae are the spaces between the tongue and the epiglottis that allow nursing infants to be able to breathe (through their nose) and nurse simultaneously. They are at the superior end of a gutter that extends through the piriform recesses to reach the laryngopharynx and the esophagus.

   B The piriform recesses are lateral to the epiglottis, superior and lateral to the cricoid cartilage. They are continuous with the valleculae superiorly and the esophagus inferiorly.
   C The rima glottidis is the aperture between the left and right vocal ligaments and cords. This is a midline structure that lies posterior and inferior to the epiglottis.
   D The foramen cecum is a small pit at the boundary of the anterior and posterior tongue that is the embryological remnant of the thyroglossal duct. It is located on the midline, posterior to the vallate papilla.
   E The tonsillar fossa is occupied by the palatine tonsil, located between the palatoglossal and palatopharyngeal arches. This lies anterior to the epiglottis, lateral to the tongue.

90. **B** The middle scalene muscle inserts (distally attaches) into the 1st rib posterior to the groove for the subclavian artery.

   A The superomedial angle of the scapula provides the insertion (distal attachment) for the levator scapulae. Lateral to this position on the scapula, the omohyoid muscle has an origin (proximal attachment). The middle scalene is not connected to the scapula.
   C The 2nd rib provides the insertion (distal attachment) for the posterior scalene muscle, which shares some of the same origin (proximal attachment) as the middle scalene muscle, but the muscle fibers run in a slightly different direction. The middle scalene is not connected to the 2nd rib.
   D The basilar occipital bone provides the insertion (distal attachment) for a variety of prevertebral muscles, including the longus capitis, rectus capitis anterior, rectus capitis lateralis, and superior pharyngeal constrictor. Although some of these muscles share the same origin (proximal attachment) as the middle scalene, they run in completely different directions. The middle scalene is not connected to the basal skull.
   E The manubrium of the sternum is the origin (proximal attachment) of the sternocleidomastoid and pectoralis major muscles. Although the sternocleidomastoid is very close and runs in a similar direction to the middle scalene, they have very different functions. The middle scalene is not attached to the manubrium.

91. **D** The occipital triangle provides the best access to the spinal accessory nerve as it travels superficial to the levator scapulae as it crosses the sternocleidomastoid and trapezius muscles in the posterior triangle of the neck. It also contains some of the supraclavicular nerves and the occipital nerves of the neck.

   A The submandibular triangle of the anterior neck contains the hypoglossal nerve, branches of the C1 anterior ramus, and branches of the mandibular division of the trigeminal nerve. It is located too far anterior to provide access to the spinal accessory nerve.
   B The muscular triangle of the anterior neck contains laryngeal branches of the vagus nerve and most of the ansa cervicalis (C1–C3 anterior rami). It is located too far anterior to provide access to the spinal accessory nerve.

   C The carotid triangle of the anterior neck lies just anterior to the middle part of the sternocleidomastoid. In this triangle, the ansa cervicalis and vagus nerves are the most prominent nervous structures. There are carotid branches of the glossopharyngeal nerve as well, but these are usually quite small.
   E The omoclavicular triangle, located in the posterior triangle of the neck, has no nervous structures located in it. Deep to the triangle, it is possible to access the brachial plexus, but not the spinal accessory nerve.

92. **C** The vagus nerve travels the entire length of the carotid sheath, running parallel to the common and internal carotid arteries and the internal jugular vein.

   A The facial nerve and its branches remain in the head for the most part. There is a cervical branch of the facial nerve that drops into the neck to innervate the platysma, superficial to the carotid sheath. No other branches come close to the carotid sheath.
   B, D, E The glossopharyngeal, spinal accessory, and hypoglossal nerves pass tangentially (anteroinferior) through the most superior part of the carotid sheath. The glossopharyngeal nerve contributes to the pharyngeal plexus and has branches innervating the stylopharyngeus and the carotid body. The spinal accessory nerve innervates the sternocleidomastoid and trapezius muscles. The hypoglossal nerve innervates the intrinsic and extrinsic tongue muscles (except the palatoglossus).

93. **D** The parapharyngeal space will allow infections from the oral cavity to drain, via gravitational abscess, into the mediastinum, causing mediastinitis.

   A The cavernous sinus is accessible from the parapharyngeal space, but it lies superior to the parapharyngeal space associated with the oral cavity. An inferior bacterial spread (gravitational abscess) would not move to this location.
   B The lung is somewhat isolated from the parapharyngeal space due to the nature of the pleura of the thoracic cavity. Bacterial infection would need to traverse this barrier to spread to the lungs.
   C The stomach is isolated from the parapharyngeal space due to the nature of the peritoneum of the abdominal cavity. Bacterial infections would need to traverse this barrier to spread to the stomach.
   E The subarachnoid space is accessible from the parapharyngeal space, but it lies superior to the parapharyngeal space associated with the oral cavity. An inferior bacterial spread (gravitational abscess) would not move to this location.

94. **E** The C1 anterior ramus is the main contributor to the superior root of the ansa cervicalis. It breaks away from the hypoglossal nerve, where it is temporarily carried, in such a way as it appears that the superior root of the ansa cervicalis is a large branch of the hypoglossal nerve.

   A The vagus nerve has branches that contribute to the pharyngeal plexus, superior laryngeal nerve, and recurrent laryngeal nerve. All of these branches are significantly deeper than the ansa cervicalis.
   B The hypoglossal nerve seems to have a large contribution to the superior root of the ansa cervicalis, but it is really just the anterior ramus of the C1 spinal nerve that breaks away to create the superior root. The branches of the hypoglossal nerve innervate the muscles of the tongue only.
   C The C3 anterior ramus contributes to the inferior root of the ansa cervicalis, as well as the phrenic, supraclavicular, transverse cervical, and great auricular nerves. Most branches run either significantly inferior or posterior to the ansa cervicalis.
   D The C2 posterior ramus contributes to the innervation of the muscles of the posterior cervical region and the greater occipital nerve. It is a posterior nerve that has no branches that run anteriorly toward the ansa cervicalis.

95. **A** The transverse cervical vein drains anteriorly in the occipital triangle to reach the external jugular vein. It collects blood from the retroauricular vein and occipital veins as it moves across the lateral neck.

    B The inferior thyroid vein drains inferiorly directly into to the brachiocephalic veins. It can be accompanied by a small thyroidea ima artery, but it is not associated with the external jugular vein.
    C The pterygoid plexus drains blood from the infratemporal fossa through the maxillary vein to reach the retromandibular vein. From here, blood can flow anterior into a common facial vein (facial and anterior division of the retromandibular) or posteriorly into the external jugular vein. There are no direct connections between the pterygoid plexus and the external jugular vein.
    D The facial vein drains posteroinferiorly along the body of the mandible and meets the anterior division of the retromandibular vein. From here, blood drains through a common facial vein to reach the internal jugular vein. It is only through increased venous pressure that blood might flow superiorly through the retromandibular vein to the external jugular vein.
    E The lingual vein drains blood from the floor of the oral cavity and meets the facial vein just prior to becoming the common facial vein. From here, blood typically drains into the internal jugular vein.

Chapter 13 Larynx & Thyroid Gland

96. **A** The base of the thyroid cartilage provides an attachment for the midline of the epiglottic cartilage via the thyroepiglottic ligament. It is at the posterior union of the two thyroid plates that this ligament attaches.

    B The cricoid cartilage physically supports the two arytenoid cartilages and maintains two cricothyroid joints in a posterolateral position with the inferior horn of the thyroid cartilage. There are no direct connections between the cricoid cartilage and the epiglottis.
    C The arytenoid cartilages rest on the arytenoid articular facets in a lateral position on the superior posterior surface of the cricoid cartilage. The arytenoid cartilages physically support the corniculate cartilages at their apex.
    D The corniculate cartilages rest on the superior medial apex of the arytenoid cartilages, in a slightly lateral and posterior position within the larynx. The epiglottis is attached at an anterior inferior position, diagonally opposite the position of these cartilages.
    E The tracheal cartilage rings occupy anterior and lateral positions inferior to the larynx. They reside inferior to the cricoid and thyroid cartilages, significantly inferior to the anterior midline attachment of the epiglottic cartilage.

97. **A** The posterior cricoarytenoid rotates the arytenoid cartilage outward and toward the side to abduct the vocal cords and open the rima glottidis.

    B The cricothyroid changes the angle between the thyroid and cricoid cartilages to increase tension on the vocal cords but does not necessarily change their position in the larynx.
    C The lateral cricoarytenoid rotates the arytenoid cartilage inward, which adducts the vocal cords and closes the rima glottidis.
    D The transverse arytenoid moves the two arytenoid cartilages toward each other, adducts the vocal cords, and closes the rima glottidis.
    E The thyroarytenoid and its inferior fibers (vocalis) rotate the arytenoid cartilage anteriorly, which relaxes (the vocalis tightens) the vocal cords and closes (or has no effect on) the rima glottidis.

98. **C** The pyramidal lobe of the thyroid gland is the embryological remnant of the thyroglossal duct indicating the origin of the thyroid gland at the root of the tongue. It typically runs anterior to the laryngeal prominence of the thyroid cartilage.

    A The lateral lobes of the thyroid gland reside lateral to the cricoid cartilage and inferolateral to the thyroid cartilage. They do not approach the midline (except at the isthmus) of the neck.

    B The isthmus of the thyroid gland joins the left and right lateral lobes, anterior to the anterior arch of the cricoid cartilage. It is a midline structure, but it is not as superiorly located as the laryngeal prominence.
    D The superior parathyroid gland, a separate embryological structure (4th pharyngeal pouch) from the thyroid gland (thyroid diverticulum), resides deep to the lateral lobe of the thyroid gland. It maintains this lateral position and does not shift toward the midline.
    E The inferior parathyroid gland, a separate embryological structure (3rd pharyngeal pouch) from the thyroid gland (thyroid diverticulum), resides medial to the lateral lobe of the thyroid gland. It maintains this lateral position and does not shift toward the midline.

99. **A** The cricothyroid muscle is innervated by the external laryngeal nerve, not the recurrent laryngeal nerve.

    B, C, D, E The remaining intrinsic laryngeal muscles are all innervated by the recurrent laryngeal nerve.

100. **B** The vestibule is superior to the vocal folds; therefore, its mucosa is innervated by the internal laryngeal nerve, a branch of the superior laryngeal nerve. The internal laryngeal nerve provides sensation to all of the mucosa of the larynx above the vocal folds, as well as the mucosa covering the epiglottis, in the vallecula, and a small area at the base of the tongue.

     A The recurrent laryngeal nerve is a mixed nerve that provides sensation to mucosa below the vocal folds.
     C The external laryngeal nerve is the motor branch of the superior laryngeal nerve.
     D The terminal branch of the recurrent laryngeal nerve is sometimes called the inferior laryngeal nerve.

101. **E** The thyrohyoid membrane spans the gap between the hyoid bone and the thyroid cartilage. It is pierced by the superior laryngeal artery and vein and the internal laryngeal nerve.

     A, B, C, D The vestibular ligament, conus elasticus, cricothyroid membrane, and vocal ligament are all ligaments of the larynx, but are not pierced by the superior laryngeal artery.

102. **E** When the cricothyroid muscle contracts, it pulls the thyroid cartilage anteriorly relative to the cricoid cartilage, lengthening and tensing the vocal folds, resulting in a higher pitched phonation.

     A The cricothyroid muscle receives blood from the superior laryngeal artery.
     B The cricothyroid muscle is innervated by the external laryngeal nerve.
     C, D The cricothyroid muscle originates from the cricoid cartilage and inserts on the thyroid cartilage.

Chapter 14 Sectional Anatomy of the Head & Neck

103. **A** A section through C1 would run through the median atlantoaxial joint, where the dens and the anterior arch of the atlas articulate.

     B The pons is in the cranial cavity, superior to C1.
     C The body of the mandible is inferior to C1.
     D The common carotid artery divides more inferiorly, typically at the superior edge of the thyroid cartilage. The internal carotid artery would be visible in a transverse section at C1.
     E The thyroid cartilage is inferior to C1.

104. **C** The pituitary gland is a midline structure, and would therefore be found in a midsagittal section.

     A, B, D, E The internal carotid artery, hyoglossus muscle, transverse sinus, and ramus of the mandible are bilateral structures and therefore are not located in the midline.

Chapter 15 Rest of Body Anatomy

105. **A** The infraspinatus is innervated by the suprascapular nerve (C4–C6) after it passes through the suprascapular notch, covered by the superior transverse ligament of the scapula.

   B The subclavius is innervated by the nerve to the subclavius (C5–C6), which passes inferior to the medial end of the clavicle. The nerve to the subclavius does not approach the scapula.
   C The teres major is innervated by the lower subscapular nerve (C5–C6), which passes anterior to the subscapularis muscle in the axilla. The lower subscapular nerve reaches only the posterior lateral edge of the scapula, not in a superior position.
   D The rhomboid minor is innervated by the dorsal scapular nerve (C4–C5), which passes posterior and medial to the medial border of the scapula. The dorsal scapular nerve never reaches the superior lateral edge of the scapula, where the supra scapular notch is located.
   E The deltoid is innervated by the axillary nerve (C5–C6), which passes through the quadrangular space to reach the posterior undersurface of the deltoid. The axillary nerve passes anterior to the superior edge of the subscapularis, then passes posterior along the lateral edge of the scapula.

106. **B** The brachial (and cephalic) veins drain into the distal (and proximal) end of the axillary vein. From here, blood flows sequentially into the subclavian vein, brachiocephalic vein, and superior vena cava before reaching the heart.

   A The cephalic vein is not directly connected to the brachial vein. There are connections through the median cubital vein, but valves prevent back (peripheral) flow from the brachial vein to the cephalic vein.
   C The brachiocephalic vein is not directly connected to the brachial vein. Between the two are both the axillary vein and the subclavian vein. The brachiocephalic vein is necessary to drain brachial vein blood back to the heart.
   D The internal jugular vein is not directly connected to the brachial vein. Blood from the brachial vein eventually drains through the subclavian vein, which joins with the internal jugular vein, but there are valves in both the subclavian vein and the internal jugular vein that prevent back (peripheral) flow between them.
   E The subclavian vein drains blood from the axillary vein and some smaller veins, but it has no other major contributors from the arm. It runs inferior to the clavicle, whereas the brachial vein ends at the distal extent of the axilla.

107. **E** The radial tuberosity of the radius is the insertion/distal attachment of the biceps brachii tendon, which provides both forearm flexion and supination at the radioulnar joint.

   A The lateral intertubercular groove is the insertion of the pectoralis major.
   B The coracoid process of the scapula is the insertion of the pectoralis minor and the origin/proximal attachment for the coracobrachialis and biceps brachii, short head.
   C The ulnar tuberosity of the ulna is the insertion/distal attachment for the brachialis, another flexor of the forearm.
   D The olecranon fossa of the humerus is the space in which the olecranon of the ulna fits during forearm extension. No muscles attach in this space.

108. **C** The left 8th posterior intercostal vein drains into the hemiazygos vein. Communications from this vein drain to the right to reach the azygos vein and subsequently the superior vena cava prior to returning blood to the heart.

   A The inferior vena cava is not directly connected to the posterior intercostal veins. To reach the inferior vena cava, blood would have to drain from the posterior intercostal veins to the azygos (right) or hemiazygos (left) veins and then drain inferiorly to reach the ascending lumbar veins. From here, blood could drain through the lumbar veins to reach the inferior vena cava.

   B The superior vena cava is not directly connected to the posterior intercostal veins. To reach the superior vena cava, blood would have to drain from the posterior intercostal veins to the hemiazygos (left) or azygos (right) veins. The hemiazygos vein drains to the azygos vein, which in turn drains to the superior vena cava.
   D The azygos vein drains the posterior intercostal veins on the right, not the left, side of the thorax. It collects blood from the hemiazygos and accessory hemiazygos veins and drains into the superior vena cava, but there are typically no direct connections between the left posterior intercostal veins and the azygos vein.
   E The thoracic duct is a lymphatic passage that drains lymph from the lower extremities, pelvis, and abdomen. No veins drain directly into this lymphatic structure.

109. **D** The circumflex artery is one of two major branches of the left coronary artery. It wraps around the heart from anterior to posterior in the left atrioventricular sulcus, giving rise to one or more obtuse (left) marginal arteries that supply blood to the left side of the left ventricle. It is paralleled by the great cardiac vein.

   A The anterior interventricular artery is a branch of the left coronary artery that descends between the right and left ventricles on the anterior heart. Its branches are the diagonal (left) and septal (internal) branches that supply blood to the anterior left ventricle and interventricular septum. The anterior interventricular artery is paralleled by the great cardiac vein before it turns into the left atrioventricular sulcus and starts to parallel the circumflex artery.
   B The posterior interventricular vessels are typically terminal branches of the right coronary artery and the middle cardiac vein. These vessels run between the right and left ventricles on the posterior aspect of the heart. Occasionally, the posterior interventricular vessels arise from the circumflex branch of the left coronary artery (left dominant heart).
   C The right coronary vessels follow the right atrioventricular sulcus from the anterior aspect of the heart to the posterior interventricular sulcus. The right coronary artery has the acute (right) marginal artery branches, but it does not supply blood to the left side of the heart. The small cardiac vein typically parallels the right coronary artery but still would not reach the left side of the heart before it drained into the coronary sinus.
   E Thebesian vessels are veins that drain blood from the right ventricle directly into the right atrium, bypassing the small cardiac vein and the coronary sinus. There are no thebesian arteries. Because these vessels are restricted to the right side of the heart, there is no way for these small vessels to reach the left (obtuse) margin of the heart.

110. **A** A pulmonary embolism in the apicoposterior segment of the superior lobe of the left lung would result in breathlessness and chest wall pain along the posterior superior lateral margin of the left thorax.

   B A pulmonary embolism in the apical segment of the superior lobe of the right lung would result in breathlessness and chest wall pain along the superior margin of the right thorax.
   C A pulmonary embolism in the lateral segment of the middle lobe of the right lung would result in breathlessness and chest wall pain along the lateral margin of the right thorax.
   D A pulmonary embolism in the superior lingular segment of the superior lobe of the left lung would result in breathlessness and chest wall pain along the midlateral margin of the left thorax.
   E A pulmonary embolism in the superior segment of the inferior lobe of the left lung would result in breathlessness and chest wall pain along the posterior and lateral margin of the left thorax.

111. **B** The spleen is usually found in the upper left quadrant - to the left of the stomach, just under the diaphragm.

   A, C, D, E The spleen is small enough and lateral enough that it does not extend into any other abdominal quadrants.

112. **D** The splenic and left gastric arteries are both direct branches of the celiac trunk, along with the common hepatic artery.

> A The splenic artery is a direct branch off of the celiac trunk, but this is not the most complete answer to the question.
> B The left gastric artery is a direct branch off of the celiac trunk, but this is not the most complete answer to the question.
> C, E The superior rectal artery is a branch of the inferior mesenteric artery.

113. **D** The cardiac notch is on the left lung, not the right lung.

> A It is true that the right lung is usually larger than the left lung, both in volume and in number of lobes.
> B, C Both lungs have an oblique fissure, but only the right lung also has a horizontal fissure.
> E The lungs are covered by a layer of visceral pleura. The pleura that lines other structures in the thorax is called parietal pleura.

114. **A** The spleen is an intraperitoneal organ, as it has a mesentery and is almost completely covered by visceral peritoneum.

> B, E The kidneys and abdominal aorta are both examples of primary retroperitoneal organs.
> C, D The pancreas and ascending colon (along with the descending colon, most of the duodenum and part of the rectum) are secondary retroperitoneal organs.

Appendix A Anatomy of Local Anesthesia for Dentistry

115. **C** The needle passes through the buccinator muscle during an inferior alveolar nerve block. The fact that the needle passes through muscle accounts for the particularly painful nature of this injection.

> A The needle passes into the pterygomandibular space lateral to the medial pterygoid muscle during an inferior alveolar injection. If the needle is mistakenly aimed too far medially, the injection will be given into the medial pterygoid muscle, causing failure of anesthesia and trimus (muscle spasm) of this muscle.

> B An inferior alveolar nerve block is given anteriorly to the lateral pterygoid muscle, so this muscle is not affected by this injection (intentionally or otherwise).
> D An inferior alveolar nerve block is given just laterally to the pterygomandibular raphe, a landmark structure for this injection.
> E If an inferior alveolar nerve block is aimed too posterolaterally, and bone is not contacted before the injection is given, then the needle is likely to have pierced the capsule of the parotid gland. This will cause anesthesia of the branches of the facial nerve that run through the gland, leading to a temporary facial paralysis (Bell's palsy).

116. **C** When administering an infraorbital nerve block, the needle is inserted at the mucobuccal fold superior to the 1st maxillary premolar.

> A, B The maxillary incisors and canines are positioned medial to the infraorbital foramen,
> D, E The 2nd maxillary premolar and the maxillary molars are positioned lateral to the infraorbital foramen.

117. **D** A Gow-Gates block is similar to an inferior alveolar nerve block, but also anesthetizes additional branches of CN V_3. This procedure would anesthetize the mandibular teeth (innervated by the inferior alveolar nerve) and the anterior two thirds of the tongue (innervated by the lingual nerve), as well as other structures such as mandibular gingiva and some regions of skin and mucosa.

> A A Gow-Gates block would anesthetize the ipsilateral mandibular teeth, but this is not the most complete answer to the question.
> B A Gow-Gates block would anesthetize the ipsilateral anterior two thirds of the tongue, but this is not the most complete answer to the question.
> C, E Sensation from the posterior one third of the tongue travels on the glossopharyngeal nerve and would not be anesthetized following a Gow-Gates block.

Clinical Questions

The questions and answers from this section are available with the eBook edition on MedOne Education. They may also be accessed as part of MedOne's interactive "Questions and Answers" tab on the website.

For Questions **1 to 3**:

Mark has been experiencing a troubling series of symptoms involving his right upper limb. These symptoms have become exacerbated over the past few months. They include intermittent periods of intense pain in various areas of the limb and a tingling sensation (paresthesia) in others. He is also now experiencing various motor difficulties. He is sent for tests that include magnetic resonance imaging (MRI). It is discovered that he has a slipped disk that is impinging on spinal nerve C5.

1. To which of the following areas of the upper limb would his pain and/or paresthesia be primarily localized?
   A. Superolateral aspect of the arm extending inferior to the lateral aspect of the midpoint of the forearm
   B. Axillary fold extending into the medial aspect of the arm
   C. Medial aspect of the arm and forearm
   D. Medial aspect of the forearm extending into the hypothenar eminence of the hand
   E. Lateral aspect of the forearm extending into the thenar eminence of the hand

2. Which of the following nerves would be totally dysfunctional as a result of a compression of C5?
   A. Axillary
   B. Thoracodorsal
   C. Long thoracic
   D. Dorsal scapular
   E. Lateral pectoral

3. Which of the following actions would be least affected as a result of compression of C5?
   A. Abduction and adduction of the fingers
   B. Flexion at the elbow
   C. Abduction at the glenohumeral joint
   D. Lateral rotation at the glenohumeral joint
   E. Extension at the glenohumeral joint

For Questions **4 to 7**:

Your friend William is walking down the street when he stares upward, then crumples to the ground. He lies there unconscious as you call for an ambulance. His wife arrives at the hospital, and after he becomes conscious, it is clear from his symptoms that he had an occlusion of the left middle cerebral artery.

4. One of the most obvious and prominent symptoms exhibited by William is almost total paralysis of his upper and lower limbs on the right side of his body. This occurred because of lack of blood flow to which of the following parts of the brain?
   A. Left internal capsule
   B. Left putamen
   C. Right precentral gyrus
   D. Right premotor cortex
   E. Left postcentral gyrus

5. Assuming that William is left brain dominant, in addition to the difficulty mentioned previously, all of the following symptoms are consistent with an occlusion of the middle cerebral artery, except for
   A. Apraxia (inability to perform a movement correctly in response to a verbal or written request)
   B. Alexia (inability to read)
   C. Agraphia (inability to write)
   D. Right-sided paralysis
   E. Anosognosia (inability to recognize disease or debilitation in oneself)

6. It is clear from William's interactions with those around him that he understands what is being said about him and what is being asked of him. However, when he is asked to respond to a question or speak in general, he can only respond with grunts and garbled utterances. It is clear that this is very frustrating to him. Based on this specific symptom, which of the following areas of his cerebrum is damaged?
   A. Posterior aspect of the superior temporal gyrus
   B. Supramarginal gyrus
   C. Lingual gyrus
   D. Inferior frontal cortex
   E. Inferior aspect of the precentral gyrus

7. If, for the sake of argument, the right middle cerebral artery was occluded rather than the left middle cerebral artery in a left brain–dominant individual, which of the following symptoms would be apparent?
   A. Inability to move his right hand
   B. Inability to move the muscles of facial expression on the right side of his face
   C. Inability to appreciate tonality in speech or in music
   D. Inability to calculate figures on a check during dinner
   E. Inability to understand what is spoken to him and responding with clearly enunciated but nonsense sentences

For Questions **8 to 11**:

Max is a 65-year-old patient of long standing, but you have not seen him for over a year. His primary complaint is that things "don't feel right" when he chews, specifically, on the left side of his mouth. He has the sensation that he just cannot seem to put his teeth into the correct position. The initial examination reveals a carious lesion of the 2nd maxillary molar on the left side. Also, wear patterns and abfraction (pathological loss of tooth structure attributed to biomechanical forces or chemical degradation) on the left maxillary teeth are noted.

8. The initial thought was that Max was favoring his left side due to the pain associated with the carious tooth. To painlessly remove the decay, which of the following nerves need to be anesthetized?
   A. Posterior superior alveolar
   B. Long buccal nerve
   C. Middle superior alveolar
   D. Greater palatine
   E. Lesser palatine

9. Two weeks after the decay was removed, Max returns to the office with the same complaint. Now not only do things not "feel right," but he is also in pain. The pain at times radiates throughout his entire maxillary arch. Before you can explore the region, Max states that he wants all of the teeth anesthetized. You explain that this is not necessary and that the procedure for anesthetizing the entire maxillary nerve is complex and potentially problematic. The most conventional form of this procedure would involve which of the following?
   A. Inserting a needle extraorally into the infratemporal fossa and the foramen ovale. Fluid would then enter into the most inferior aspect of the cranium at the point of exit of the maxillary nerve.
   B. Inserting a needle intraorally through the buccinator muscle into the infratemporal fossa, then placement of the needle adjacent to the foramen rotundum. Fluid would gain access to the inferior aspect of the cranium at the point of exit of the maxillary nerve.
   C. Inserting a needle extraorally into the infratemporal fossa and approximating the pterygomaxillary fissure. Fluid would then gain access to the pterygopalatine fossa, and the maxillary nerve would be anesthetized.
   D. Inserting a needle intraorally into the greater palatine foramen. Fluid would then travel up the greater palatine canal into the pterygopalatine fossa, and the maxillary nerve would be anesthetized.
   E. Inserting a needle into the infraorbital foramen. Fluid would then be placed into the foramen and would travel posteriorly to the pterygopalatine fossa, and the maxillary nerve would be anesthetized.

537

10. Max returns 3 weeks later. He is clearly agitated and states that things still do not "feel right." You carefully palpate the external aspect of his jaw and infratemporal region and discover the muscles that elevate the mandible on the left side of his head seem to be slightly hypertrophied and spasmodic as compared with the same muscles on the opposite side. The muscles that you were able to palpate include the

A. Temporalis only
B. Temporalis and masseter
C. Temporalis, masseter, and buccinator
D. Temporalis, masseter, and zygomaticus major
E. Temporalis, masseter, and lateral pterygoid

11. As a result of the previous examination, you suggest that Max use a bite splint at night. He does as requested, but 1 month later, rather enraged, he returns with the same complaint i.e., that things do not "feel right" when he chews. You now ask him if there was any major health event or emergency that occurred during the year before the first examination. He states that he had a minor stroke from which he believes he has fully recovered. You contact the neurologist and discover that it was a brainstem stroke involving the pons. After a consultation with the neurologist, you tell Max that, unfortunately, there is very little that you can do to ameliorate his discomfort. Your rationale for this statement is the following.

A. The motor nucleus of cranial nerve (CN) V was damaged on the right side of the brainstem. This would explain the abnormal activity of the muscles of mastication on the right side of the jaw.
B. The mesencephalic nucleus of CN V was damaged on the left side of the brainstem. This would explain the report of "things not feeling right," as this nucleus is responsible for proprioception impulses that travel to nerves of the mandibular and maxillary molars and sensory fibers associated with the temporomandibular joint (TMJ).
C. The principal sensory nucleus of CN V was damaged on the left side of the brainstem. This would explain the intense pain experienced.
D. The nucleus caudalis was damaged on the right side of the brainstem. This would explain the uneven wear patterns seen, as this nucleus helps to control the coordination of muscles of the TMJ on the left and right sides of the jaw.
E. The nucleus interpolaris was damaged on the right side of the brainstem. This would explain the uneven wear patterns, as this nucleus is specifically responsible for fine touch and would come into play when Max tries to approximate his maxillary teeth to his mandibular teeth.

For Questions 12 and 13:

Your friend is lying in a hospital bed after being in a head-on automobile collision. Unfortunately, his classic car had neither seatbelts nor an airbag, so upon colliding with the other car, he catapulted forward, with his head violently hitting the windshield. Upon awaking, it was discovered that he was suffering with both anosmia (loss of olfaction) and bilateral total anopsia (total blindness in both eyes).

12. His anosmia possibly resulted from damage to fibers that run through the

A. Inferior orbital fissure
B. Foramen rotundum
C. Foramen ovale
D. Cribriform plate
E. Foramen spinosum

13. The bilateral anopsia possibly resulted from damage to the optic chiasm because it was severed by which of the following broken shards of bone?

A. Ethmoid
B. Frontal
C. Lesser wing of the sphenoid bone
D. Petrosal portion of the temporal bone
E. Clivus

For Questions 14 to 16:

A restoration needs to be performed on a carious lesion on a maxillary 2nd molar. An anesthetic procedure takes place to numb the tooth. Unfortunately, sufficient care is not taken to ensure that the needle is sterile. In addition, when the needle is placed into the tissue, it is not withdrawn to discern whether or not it was inadvertently placed into a blood vessel.

Three days after the procedure, the patient is rushed to an emergency room with a fever of 104°F (40°C). The patient is dizzy, disoriented, and nauseated. He is also experiencing acute exophthalmia (marked protrusion of the eyeball) of his left eye and difficulty moving his left eye laterally.

14. The anesthetic procedure was to anesthetize which of the following nerves?

A. Middle superior alveolar
B. Anterior superior alveolar
C. Posterior superior alveolar
D. Greater palatine
E. Lesser palatine

15. The symptoms he is experiencing are a result of bacteria being introduced into the _____, which then traveled into the _____.

A. External carotid artery, middle meningeal artery
B. Ophthalmic vein, cavernous sinus
C. Maxillary vein, retromandibular vein
D. Pterygoid plexus, cavernous sinus
E. Infraorbital vein, cavernous sinus

16. The difficulty the patient has in moving his eye laterally is directly related to irritation of the _____ nerve, resulting in dysfunction of the _____ muscle.

A. Abducens, inferior oblique
B. Oculomotor, superior rectus
C. Oculomotor, inferior rectus
D. Abducens, lateral rectus
E. Trochlear, superior oblique

For question 17 to 20:

Your patient has arrived with a carious lesion of his right 2nd mandibular molar. You attempt an inferior alveolar nerve anesthetic procedure. Initially, all appears to be proceeding as planned. However, ~5 minutes after the injection, the patient reports no lower lip anesthesia and a symptom that is quite worrisome. Based on this symptom, you realize that you have injected anesthetic fluid into the parotid capsule.

17. What is the symptom that is causing you concern?

A. Difficulty depressing the mandible on the side of the injection
B. Inability to close the palpebral fissure on the side of the injection
C. Inability to open the palpebral fissure on the side opposite the injection
D. Difficulty with swallowing
E. Inability to raise the mandible on the side opposite the injection

18. Which of these structures is found in the parotid space?

A. Retromandibular vein
B. Internal carotid artery
C. Internal jugular vein
D. Masseteric branch of the maxillary artery
E. Buccal branch of the maxillary artery

19. These symptoms probably occurred as a result of the needle placement that is

A. Too far superior and anterior
B. Too far posterior and inferior
C. Too far anterior and inferior
D. Too far medial and inferior
E. Too far medial and superior

20. A second injection was then performed to anesthetize the mandibular tooth. This did not provide the necessary anesthesia, and again it was assumed that the anesthetic fluid did not properly approximate the inferior alveolar nerve. However, the lack of anesthesia might not have been due to the procedure but because there are accessory sensory fibers that sometimes supply the roots of the mandibular molars. These fibers travel on or with the

    A. Lingual nerve
    B. Long buccal nerve
    C. Nerve to the mylohyoid
    D. Marginal mandibular nerve
    E. Buccal branch of CN VII

For Questions **21 to 24**:

A 35-year old man presents to the physician's office with a report of shooting, excruciating pain on the left side of his face. This is episodic pain that is described as being jabbed by an electrified pin every 10 seconds or so. The pain radiates down the external aspect of the mandible and includes the skin over the mandible, the general area of the lower extent of the infratemporal fossa, and the mucosa of the tongue and internal aspect of the mouth. The pain is only on the left side. In addition, when asked to open his mouth, the patient cannot fully do so without experiencing the same excruciating pain. Furthermore, as he opens his mouth, the muscles that oppose this motion become spasmodic.

21. Based on the symptoms, it is determined that he is suffering from

    A. Bell's palsy
    B. Trigeminal neuralgia
    C. Geniculate neuralgia
    D. Glossopharyngeal neuralgia
    E. Temporal arteritis

22. A compression of which of the following nerves might be responsible for the aforementioned syndrome and the symptoms described in the scenario?

    A. Trigeminal
    B. Mandibular branch of the trigeminal
    C. Maxillary branch of the trigeminal
    D. Inferior alveolar nerve
    E. Lingual nerve

23. As stated, when asked to open his mouth, the patient experiences great difficulty as the muscles that oppose this action go into spasm. The muscles that are becoming spasmodic include the

    A. Buccinator
    B. Lateral pterygoid
    C. Temporalis
    D. Mylohyoid
    E. Anterior digastric

24. In a person facing this degree of pain, it is sometimes necessary to take rather extreme measures. One of these measures is to ablate the ganglion involved with the transmission of pain impulses back to the central nervous system. This procedure is known as percutaneous needle rhizotomy. In this case, to alleviate the pain, the ganglion that would need to be ablated is the

    A. Geniculate ganglion
    B. Semilunar ganglion
    C. Superior ganglion of CN IX
    D. Pterygopalatine ganglion
    E. Superior ganglion of CN X

For Questions **25 to 28**:

A 25-year old male patient sits in your dental chair with an obvious disparity in the appearance of the right and left sides of his face. The entire left side of his face is drooping. This includes his lips and the muscles above and below his oral cavity. He is also wearing an eye patch over his left eye. He tells you that the symptoms appeared "out of nowhere." He went to bed one night feeling normal and awoke the next morning with the symptoms you are observing. He states that there was no other precipitating factor that would account for what occurred. He also states that there is apparently nothing else that ails him, and he is not experiencing muscle paralysis in any other area of his face or body. It is now 1 month to the day since the symptoms first manifested themselves.

25. Based on his appearance and the onset of his problems, even before you discuss the matter with him, you conclude that he is suffering from

    A. A left-sided cerebral stroke
    B. A right-sided cerebral stroke
    C. Trigeminal neuralgia
    D. Bell's palsy
    E. Glossopharyngeal neuralgia

26. On the other hand, it might be a compression of the facial nerve that is unrelated to any of the syndromes or diseases related above. Based on these symptoms, and these symptoms only, it could be a compression of the facial nerve

    A. As it travels through the parotid gland
    B. Just distal to the point at which it exits through the stylomastoid foramen
    C. Just proximal to the point at which it exits through the stylomastoid foramen
    D. Just proximal to the point at which the chorda tympani branches
    E. Just distal to the point at which the chorda tympani branches

27. Before you relate your thoughts to your patient, he tells you that he is also suffering from diminished taste. He further informs you that he is wearing the eye patch so that the fluid (artificial tears) he is placing onto his cornea will not escape. This is necessary because he is not lacrimating in his left eye. Finally, he tells you he is experiencing anesthesia of a portion of the skin on the external auditory meatus. Based on this additional information, your analysis of where the compression of the facial nerve has occurred has now changed. You now believe that the compression of the facial nerve has occurred

    A. As it travels through the parotid gland
    B. Just proximal to the point at which the chorda tympani branches
    C. Just proximal to the point at which the greater petrosal nerve branches
    D. Just distal to the point at which the greater petrosal nerve branches
    E. Just distal to the point at which the chorda tympani branches

28. You ask your patient to briefly remove his eye patch and notice that the upper eyelid is abnormally elevated. This is because the _____ muscle that is innervated by the _____ nerve is unopposed in its action.

    A. Orbicularis oculi, zygomatic branch of CN VII
    B. Orbicularis oculi, temporal branch of CN VII
    C. Levator palpebrae superioris, temporal branch of CN VII
    D. Levator palpebrae superioris, oculomotor nerve
    E. Corrugator supercilii and frontalis working as a unit, temporal branch of CN VII

539

For Question **29**:

A patient presents himself to his physician with a persistent left-sided throat "tickle" and a nonproductive cough. He also says that as of late he has experienced an intermittent hoarse voice. The initial treatment is palliative with a course of throat lozenges, inhalants, and basic antiinflammatory drugs that are purchased over the counter. However, the patient returns in 2 weeks with the same complaint, and an X-ray of the thorax is ordered. Even though the X-ray results are speculative at best, because of the persistence of the symptoms, a computed tomography (CT) scan with contrast is ordered. As a result of the CT scan, an aneurysm of the arch of the aorta is clearly visible.

29. Based on this, it is clear that the symptoms are a result of a compression of the
   - A. Left vagus nerve
   - B. Left external laryngeal nerve
   - C. Left recurrent laryngeal nerve
   - D. Left superior laryngeal nerve
   - E. Left internal laryngeal nerve

For Questions **30 to 32**:

A 35-year-old man presents with what he believes to be pain associated with "a left upper tooth." The pain seems to be rather diffuse, so he cannot be more specific. After a full set of dental X-rays and a thorough intraoral examination, no lesion is found to be associated with any of his maxillary or mandibular teeth. Furthermore, the gingiva appears to be essentially normal. Upon further questioning of the patient, he tells you the pain tends to recur and is worst during the spring and the fall.

30. Based on the patient's clinical presentation, even before you proceed with a full set of X-rays and other clinical tests, you suspect that his pain is associated with which of the following?
   - A. Trigeminal neuralgia
   - B. Masseteric spasms
   - C. Maxillary sinusitis
   - D. Middle ear infection
   - E. Temporomandibular dysfunction

31. One of the difficulties in determining the exact location of pain emanating in the head is that there are many structures found in a confined area. All of these structures send neuronal impulses to the structure in the brain responsible for determining which impulses are originating from which area. This structure is the
   - A. Superior colliculus
   - B. Inferior colliculus
   - C. Thalamus
   - D. Hypothalamus
   - E. Globus pallidus

32. Although the structure in question 31 is responsible for locating pain, the actual perception of pain is associated with a different area of the brain. This area is the
   - A. Postcentral gyrus
   - B. Precentral gyrus
   - C. Superior temporal gyrus
   - D. Lingual gyrus
   - E. Cingulate gyrus

For Questions **33 to 35**:

A 58-year-old man presents to the clinic complaining of pain that prevents him from fully opening his mouth. He has a lump over the angle of the mandible on the left side of his jaw that he says has been slowly getting bigger over the past 18 months but that it has not hurt until recently, so he was not worried about it. Because the patient has a limited opening, you decide that a panoramic radiograph is in order. Based on further testing and a biopsy, it is discovered that the lump is an ameloblastoma that originated within the mandible.

33. The insertions (distal attachments) of what two muscles of mastication may be displaced as this tumor continues to disrupt the angle of the mandible?
   - A. Medial and lateral pterygoids
   - B. Medial pterygoid and masseter
   - C. Masseter and temporalis
   - D. Temporalis and medial pterygoid
   - E. Temporalis and lateral pterygoid

34. From which branchial arch do the muscles of mastication develop?
   - A. 1st branchial arch
   - B. 2nd branchial arch
   - C. 3rd branchial arch
   - D. 4th branchial arch
   - E. 5th branchial arch

35. Which of the following nerves is most likely to be initially displaced by this tumor?
   - A. Long buccal nerve
   - B. Lingual nerve
   - C. Deep temporal nerve
   - D. Nerve to the lateral pterygoid
   - E. Inferior alveolar nerve

For Questions **36 to 39**:

A 73-year-old man complains that things are "tasting funny" and that this difficulty with taste has existed for the past few months. He says that he does not have a fever and has not suffered with a cold or virus in the past 3 months. He does not smoke cigarettes, a pipe, or cigars, nor does he chew tobacco.

36. You initially examine his tongue to discern whether there is any damage that might affect the taste buds on his tongue. You do this based on the knowledge that taste to the anterior two-thirds of the tongue initially runs in the
   - A. Glossopharyngeal nerve
   - B. Inferior alveolar branch of the trigeminal nerve
   - C. Chorda tympani branch of the facial nerve
   - D. Greater petrosal branch of the facial nerve
   - E. Lesser petrosal branch of the glossopharyngeal nerve

37. Taste buds are primarily associated with which of the following papillae of the tongue?
   - A. Filiform
   - B. Fungiform
   - C. Circumvallate
   - D. Foliate
   - E. Taste buds are found in abundance on all of the aforementioned papillae.

38. Another problem that can affect taste, especially in older individuals, is a decline in salivary fluid production. Parasympathetic fibers that stimulate salivary output run with which of the following nerves?
   - A. Greater petrosal nerve
   - B. Lesser petrosal nerve
   - C. Deep petrosal nerve
   - D. A and B only
   - E. A, B, and C

39. Ganglia involved with fibers that stimulate salivary output from the major salivary glands include which of the following?
   - A. Ciliary
   - B. Superior cervical
   - C. Middle cervical
   - D. Submandibular
   - E. Pterygopalatine

For Questions **40 to 42**:

A man is rushed into the emergency room displaying exaggerated swelling in the submandibular area. The patient is clearly having difficulty breathing, has a fever of 103°F (39.4°C), tachycardia, and tachypnea. He has a hard swelling in the floor of the mouth resulting in superoposterior displacement of the tongue, which is interfering with the airway. The patient is presumed to be suffering with Ludwig's angina. As treatment begins, the medical staff works to maintain the airway, administers antibiotics, and makes an external incision in the submandibular area to begin drainage.

40. The infection is found in which of the following spaces?

    A. Submandibular only
    B. Sublingual only
    C. Submandibular and sublingual
    D. Submandibular and submental
    E. Submandibular, sublingual, and submental

41. The infection can originate from which of the following teeth?

    A. Mandibular molars only
    B. Mandibular incisors, canines, and premolars only
    C. Any mandibular tooth
    D. Maxillary molars
    E. Any maxillary tooth

42. If it is necessary to insert an intraoral drain, the mucosa of the floor of the mouth will need to be incised. Which of the following structures will be the first to be encountered?

    A. Submandibular duct
    B. Lingual nerve
    C. Lingual artery
    D. Hypoglossal nerve
    E. Glossopharyngeal nerve

For Questions **43 to 45**:

A 50-year-old woman arrives in your office with a painless mass in the floor of her mouth. She reports that the mass first appeared 2 years ago, but it remained small and painless, so she never bothered seeing a clinician. Recently, the mass has begun to grow at a faster pace. The patient also reports a history of tobacco and alcohol use, including smoking four packs of cigarettes a week since her early 20s. Upon examination you find a nonulcerated, red-purple mass in the floor of her mouth just lingual to the patient's right mandibular posterior teeth. External palpation of the submandibular triangle reveals an enlarged, slightly tender submandibular gland that feels fixated to the surrounding tissue. A CT scan confirms an enlarged submandibular gland. You decide to perform an excisional biopsy.

43. When performing the extraoral excisional biopsy, one must be careful when resecting the submandibular gland not to damage the following structure that runs through the gland?

    A. Facial vein
    B. Facial artery
    C. Lingual artery
    D. Hypoglossal nerve
    E. Anterior division of the retromandibular vein

44. Likewise, during resection one must be very careful not to damage the following structure that runs on the superficial surface of the gland?

    A. Cervical branch of the facial nerve
    B. Marginal mandibular branch of the facial nerve
    C. Mental branch of the trigeminal nerve
    D. Inferior fibers of the long buccal branch of the trigeminal nerve
    E. Inferior fibers of the buccal branch of the facial nerve

45. Once the gland is exposed, it is clear that a portion of the submandibular gland wraps around the

    A. Hyoglossus
    B. Anterior belly of the digastric
    C. Posterior belly of the digastric
    D. Genioglossus
    E. Mylohyoid

For Questions **46 to 48**:

A 55-year-old male patient called your office with a complaint that his right rear lower tooth really hurt. You suggested he come see you so that you could take a look at the tooth and the structures that surrounded it. Five days later, he called back happily proclaiming that he was no longer in pain. You suggested that he should see you anyway. Your concern was that if it was an infection in the tooth, it could have now progressed from the tooth into a fascial space. Three days after his second call to you, the patient appears in an emergency room with the following symptoms:

- Temperature of 101.3°F (38.5°C)
- Elevated white blood cell count
- Reddened and flushed appearance on both sides of the neck
- Pain upon movement of the neck
- Great difficulty swallowing and breathing

Dental examination and subsequent X-rays revealed that the apparent infection probably emanated in the second mandibular molar and spread to the retropharyngeal space and the danger space.

46. In this case, it is irrelevant whether the infection is in the retropharyngeal space and/or danger space because the fascia between the two has degenerated. This fascia is the

    A. Prevertebral fascia
    B. Pretracheal fascia
    C. Buccopharyngeal fascia
    D. Medial aspect of the carotid sheath
    E. Alar fascia

47. One of the primary concerns of infections that gain access to the retropharyngeal space is that they can then spread to the

    A. Maxillary sinus
    B. Cavernous sinus
    C. Mediastinum
    D. Peritoneal cavity
    E. Orbit

48. Because of the marked difficulty in breathing, it is decided that an emergency tracheostomy must be performed. Sometimes, in performing a tracheostomy, the thyroid gland must be cut vertically at its isthmus. Why is this not a problem with respect to the health of the patient?

    A. As humans age, the thyroid gland markedly regresses, and by the age of 55, it has little or no functional significance.
    B. The thyroid gland is an exocrine gland, and its ducts are located inferolaterally. Thus, a vertical incision through the midline of the gland will not affect its ability to send substances to the remainder of the body.
    C. The thyroid is an exocrine gland, and its ducts are located superolaterally. Thus, a vertical incision through the midline of the gland will not affect its ability to send substances to the remainder of the body.
    D. The thyroid is an endocrine gland that secretes copious amounts of angiogenic factors. Thus, even with damage to the midline venous and arterial structures, once it is placed back into position, additional arteries and veins grow to take their place.
    E. The thyroid is an endocrine gland, and its hormones are secreted into veins that are found on the lateral aspect of the gland. These veins are normally not harmed when a midline vertical incision is performed.

For Questions **49 to 51**:

Tim Brody, a quarterback for the champion Northwest Coffee Grinders, is viciously slammed to the ground in the semifinals. The training staff rushes onto the field, where he lies semiconscious. They immediately shine a light in his left eye, and as they do so, they check the response of the pupils in the left and right eyes. Based on what they see, they are relatively pleased, and as Tim begins to become alert, they raise him to his feet. He staggers to the sidelines, where the trainers sit him down for further assessment.

49. By shining the light in one eye, then looking at both eyes, the training staff is testing for which of the following reflexes?

    A. Corneal
    B. Pupillary dilator
    C. Vestibulo-ocular
    D. Consensual light
    E. Accommodation

50. All of the following structures are involved in the aforementioned reflex, except for the

    A. Medial geniculate body
    B. Ciliary ganglion
    C. Edinger–Westphal nucleus
    D. Posterior commissure
    E. Optic nerve

51. This test is performed, at least in part, to try to determine if which of the following occurred?

    A. Tear of the lining of the lateral ventricle
    B. Epidural hematoma
    C. Subdural hematoma
    D. Occlusion of the anterior cerebral artery
    E. Occlusion of the posterior cerebral artery

For Questions **52 to 54**:

A middle-aged female dental patient returned for a prosthodontic evaluation after undergoing a radical neck dissection, mandibular reconstruction, and bone grafting following removal of a tumor on the right side of her neck and face. The evaluation occurred 8 weeks after the operation, and the healing was for all intents and purposes complete. The patient experienced difficulty rotating her head. It was necessary for her to rotate her trunk to face the assistant. The patient also experienced difficulty elevating her shoulder on her right side. She reported sporadically experiencing muscle spasms and pain in the neck. Additionally, when asked to protrude her tongue, it was noted that the patient's tongue deviated to the right (see photograph).

52. The diminished ability to rotate her head is most likely due to

    A. Idiopathic spasmodic torticollis (abnormal wrenching of the neck)
    B. Damage to the accessory nerve on the right side as a result of a surgical complication
    C. Damage to the vagus nerve on the right side as a result of a surgical complication
    D. Damage to the ansa cervicalis on the right side as a result of a surgical complication
    E. Damage to the phrenic nerve on the right side as a result of a surgical complication

53. Based on the movement of the tongue seen in the patient, which of the following nerves was probably damaged while surgically removing the tumor in the mandible?

    A. Inferior alveolar
    B. Chorda tympani
    C. Hypoglossal
    D. Mandibular
    E. Glossopharyngeal

54. As stated previously, when asked to stick out her tongue, what occurred is what is shown in the photo below. Based on this, which of the following muscles is not functioning properly?

    A. Right hyoglossus
    B. Left hyoglossus
    C. Right genioglossus
    D. Left genioglossus
    E. Neither the left genioglossus nor the left hyoglossus is properly functioning.

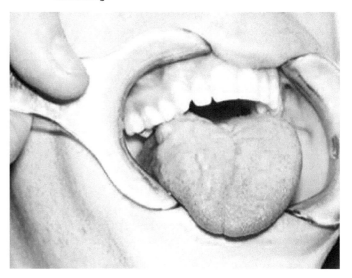

For Questions **55 to 58**:

A.J., a 35-year-old female patient, tells you that she has been diagnosed with breast cancer and is considering a modified radical mastectomy. She has had extensive discussions with her primary physician and an oncologist. It is feared that the cancer is in the first stages of possibly spreading through her lymphatic system to the axillary nodes.

55. All of the following are considered to be part of the axillary nodes except for the

    A. Pectoral nodes
    B. Lateral nodes
    C. Subscapular nodes
    D. Infraclavicular nodes
    E. Apical nodes

56. A modified radical mastectomy is being considered rather than a full radical mastectomy. In a modified radical mastectomy, the pectoralis major is spared. This not only provides mass on the anterior chest wall, thus aiding with a possible breast reconstruction procedure, but also spares which of the following motions performed by the pectoralis major?

    A. Inferior rotation of the scapula
    B. Superior rotation of the scapula
    C. Medial rotation of the humerus
    D. Abduction of the humerus
    E. Extension of the humerus

57. In a radical mastectomy, the lymph nodes and adipose tissue in the area of the chest and axilla are removed. Because of its placement on the superficial surface of the muscle that it innervates, as well as its proximity to the axilla, one of the following nerves is sometimes severed in the procedure. This nerve is the

    A. Long thoracic
    B. Medial pectoral
    C. Lateral pectoral
    D. Thoracodorsal
    E. Axillary

58. When the nerve mentioned in question 56 is severed, the muscles that retract the scapulae are basically unopposed in their action, resulting in "winged scapulae." Muscles that retract the scapulae include the

    A. Rhomboid major
    B. Teres major
    C. Teres minor
    D. Latissimus dorsi
    E. Longissimus

For Questions **59 to 62**:

A 55-year-old rock star is preparing for a concert at the Palladium in London when he experiences intense midsternal pain. He is rushed to the hospital and submitted to a series of blood tests and an electrocardiogram (ECG). Neither the blood tests nor the ECG indicate he has had a heart attack. He feels somewhat relieved with the news, but the chest pains, though not as pronounced, still remain. Because of the unrelenting pain, it is decided that he should undergo an angiography. The results of the angiography are also negative.

59. The arteries that were visualized using the angiography, as well as with the arteries from which they branch, are the

    A. Left coronary artery that branches from the arch of the aorta
    B. Anterior interventricular artery that branches from the right coronary artery
    C. Sinoatrial artery that branches from the right coronary artery
    D. Posterior interventricular artery that branches from the left coronary
    E. Right marginal artery that branches from the anterior interventricular artery

60. Pain from the heart can be referred to areas other than the midsternal region. These areas normally include all of the following except for the

    A. Left shoulder
    B. Posterior neck
    C. Midline of the mandible
    D. Anterior aspect of the neck
    E. Right hypogastrium

61. The pain could be referred from areas or organs other than the heart. These organs include the

    A. Esophagus
    B. Stomach
    C. Pancreas
    D. A and B only
    E. A, B, and C

62. After further testing, it is determined that the star is suffering with pericarditis, and an appropriate treatment is begun. One of the necessary steps is to drain excess pericardial fluid from the pericardial space. This space is found between which of the following two layers?

    A. Fibrous pericardium and outer pericardial fat
    B. Fibrous pericardium and the parietal layer of the serous pericardium
    C. Parietal layer of the serous pericardium and the visceral layer of the serous pericardium
    D. Serous layer of the visceral pericardium and the myocardium
    E. Myocardium and endocardium

For Questions **63 to 65**:

A 25-year-old woman is riding her bicycle on a busy street in Boston. As she rides past a row of cars, one of the drivers opens the door without looking. She does not have time to stop and catapults over the door. As she lands, she attempts to break her fall by throwing her right hand forward. The palm of her hand hits the ground, with the force of the fall being sent up through her wrist, forearm, and arm. Initially, her hand and wrist are sore, but over the next couple of hours, the soreness seems to subside. However, upon looking at her wrist, she sees a pronounced black-and-blue mark forming over the ventral aspect of her wrist and the extreme distal portion of her forearm. She goes to her primary physician, who expresses some alarm and informs her that her wrist may be broken and that she may be suffering from anterior compartment syndrome. Her physician makes an immediate appointment for her to see an orthopedist specializing in the upper limb. The orthopedist takes immediate action to drain the blood from the anterior compartment and repair the fracture.

63. Which of the following nerves is found in the anterior compartment of the forearm and also passes through the carpal tunnel with the long digital flexor tendons?

    A. Deep branch of the radial
    B. Superficial branch of the radial
    C. Lateral cutaneous nerve of the forearm
    D. Ulnar
    E. Median

64. If left unabated, the accumulation of blood could compress the nerve and cause permanent dysfunction of which of the following muscles?

    A. Flexor pollicis longus
    B. Flexor pollicis brevis
    C. Flexor digitorum superficialis
    D. Flexor carpi radialis
    E. All of the above

65. If this compression did occur, which of the following actions would be most affected?

    A. Fine motor movements of the thumb
    B. Adduction of the thumb
    C. Flexion of the fingers
    D. Extension at the carpometacarpal joints
    E. All of the above

For Questions **66 to 67**:

A 26-year-old man was in car accident while driving a car with a malfunctioning air bag. His face hit the steering wheel at a high velocity. Imaging showed symmetrical fractures along the zygomaticomaxillary and nasofrontal sutures as well as the pterygoid process of the sphenoid.

66. How would you classify this injury?

    A. Le Fort I
    B. Le Fort II
    C. Le Fort III
    D. Le Fort IV

67. Which of the following structures would also have fracture lines?

    A. Hard palate
    B. Zygomatic arch
    C. Ethmoid bone
    D. Lateral wall of orbit

For Questions **68 to 69**:

Patient
59 year old man
Chief Complaint
"My tongue moves funny."
Background and/or Patient History
High blood pressure currently treated with medication Recent history of neck surgery for an internal carotid artery dissection
Current Findings
When asked to stick out his tongue, the patient's tongue moves to the left.

68. Which structures would have been at risk of injury during the patient's surgery?
    A. Submandibular gland and facial artery on the left.
    B. Internal jugular vein and vagus nerve on the left.
    C. Hypoglossal nerve and accessory nerve on the right.
    D. Anterior jugular vein and omohyoid muscle on the right.

69. Which muscle is paralyzed, causing the tongue to deviate to the left?
    A. Right geniohyoid
    B. Left palatoglossus
    C. Left genioglossus
    D. Right styloglossus
    E. Left superior longitudinal muscle

For Questions **70 to 72**:

Patient
28 year old man
Chief Complaint
"The side of my jaw hurts. It gets really bad when I'm eating."
Background and/or Patient History
No significant history
Current Findings
You diagnose a salivary stone blocking the right submandibular duct.

70. The duct with the blockage crosses _____ to the _____ nerve.
    A. Superior; glossopharyngeal
    B. Superior; lingual
    C. Superior; hypoglossal
    D. Inferior; glossopharyngeal
    E. Inferior; lingual

71. The gland that empties into the blocked duct is stimulated to secrete saliva by postganglionic parasympathetic neurons with cell bodies located in the _____.
    A. Superior salivatory nucleus
    B. Pterygopalatine ganglion
    C. Superior cervical ganglion
    D. Inferior salivatory nucleus
    E. Submandibular ganglion

72. The pain felt by the patient could be transmitted by which nerve?
    A. Mandibular
    B. Facial
    C. C1
    D. Hypoglossal
    E. Maxillary

For Questions **73 to 75**:

Patient
19 year old woman
Chief Complaint
"The back of my mouth hurts."
Background and/or Patient History
No significant history
Current Findings
Tooth #32 (right mandibular third molar) is impacted. You extract the tooth.

73. While extracting the tooth, the bone on the lingual surface of the tooth was fractured. This injury damaged the lingual nerve. What symptom(s) would you expect to appear in this patient?
    A. Numbness of the anterior two-thirds of the tongue on the right side
    B. Loss of taste on the anterior two-thirds of the tongue on the right side
    C. Paralysis of the right side of the tongue
    D. A and B
    E. A, B, and C

74. The extracted tooth receives blood from which of the following arteries?
    A. Posterior superior alveolar
    B. Mental
    C. Lingual
    D. Facial
    E. Inferior alveolar

75. If the surgical site becomes infected, to which area is the infection most likely to spread first?
    A. Submandibular space
    B. Submental space
    C. Sublingual space
    D. Retropharyngeal space
    E. Canine space

Answer Explanations

1. **A** The dermatomal distribution for C5 is the superolateral aspect of the arm extending inferior to the lateral aspect of the midpoint of the forearm; therefore, pain and/or paresthesia would be localized to these areas.

    B The axillary fold extending into the medial aspect of the arm is the dermatomal distribution for T1 or T2.
    C The medial aspect of the arm and forearm is the dermatomal distribution that encompasses portions of T1 and C8.
    D The medial aspect of the forearm extending into the hypothenar eminence is the dermatomal distribution for C8.
    E The lateral aspect of the forearm extending into the thenar eminence of the hand is the dermatomal distribution for C6.

2. **D** The dorsal scapular nerve contains fibers from C5 only, so it would be totally dysfunctional.

    A The axillary nerve contains fibers from both C5 and C6, so it would not be totally dysfunctional.
    B The thoracodorsal nerve contains fibers from both C6–C8, so it would be completely functional.
    C, E The long thoracic and lateral pectoral nerves contains fibers from C5–C7, so they would not be totally dysfunctional.

3. **A** Abduction and adduction of the fingers are accomplished through the actions of the interossei, which are innervated by the ulnar nerve. The ulnar nerve is composed of fibers from C7 to T1, so it would be totally unaffected by compression of C5.

    B Flexion at the elbow is primarily, although not exclusively, accomplished through the action of the brachialis and biceps brachii. These muscles are innervated by the musculocutaneous nerve, which contains neuronal fibers from C5 to C7. There would be a slight diminishment in this action. It should be remembered that the brachioradialis also participates in flexion at the elbow. The brachioradialis is innervated by the radial nerve, which receives neuronal fibers from C5 to T1. The radial nerve would probably be almost thoroughly functional, as would the brachioradialis.
    C Abduction at the glenohumeral joint is accomplished through the actions of the supraspinatus and medial fibers of the deltoid. The supraspinatus is innervated by the suprascapular nerve, which receives neuronal fibers from C5 and C6. The deltoid is innervated by the axillary nerve, which receives fibers from C5 and C6. Thus, these nerves, muscles, and actions would be affected as a result of compression of C5.
    D Lateral rotation at the glenohumeral joint is accomplished through the actions of the teres minor, infraspinatus, and posterior fibers of the deltoid muscle. The teres minor and deltoid are innervated by the axillary nerve (described in answer explanation C). The infraspinatus is innervated by the suprascapular nerve (described in answer explanation C).
    E Extension at the glenohumeral joint is accomplished through the actions of the posterior fibers of the deltoid, teres major, and latissimus dorsi. The teres major is innervated by the lower subscapular nerve, which receives fibers from C5 and C6. The posterior fibers of the deltoid are innervated by the axillary nerve, which receives fibers from C5 and C6. The latissimus dorsi is innervated by the thoracodorsal nerve, which receives fibers from C6 through C8.

4. **A** Motor fibers that synapse on anterior horn cells of the spinal cord originate in the contralateral motor and premotor cortices as part of the pyramidal tract, specifically, the corticospinal tracts (lateral and anterior). Prior to decussating, these fibers travel in the internal capsule. Thus, damage to the left internal capsule, which is supplied via branches of the middle cerebral artery (specifically, the lenticulostriate branches), would result in contralateral paralysis. Therefore, in William, damage to the left internal capsule would result in paralysis of the right upper and lower limbs.

    B The putamen, left or right, is involved in modulation, not initiation, of motion. Damage to the putamen, such as in Huntington's disease, would result in a multiplicity of motor symptoms, including ballismus, but not paralysis.
    C, D Motor fibers that originate in the motor and premotor cortices travel to contralateral anterior horn cells. Thus, damage to the right precentral gyrus and/or right premotor cortices would result in paralysis of the left limbs, not the right.
    E The postcentral gyrus is involved with interpretation of sensory input, not motor output.

5. **E** Anosognosia is associated with damage to the right cerebral hemisphere in a left brain–dominant individual.

    A–C Apraxia, alexia, and agraphia are associated with damage to the left cerebral hemisphere of a left brain–dominant individual.
    D Right-sided paralysis will occur because the left precentral gyrus and premotor cortex are supplied by branches of the left middle cerebral artery. Also, the left lenticulostriate artery is a branch of the left middle cerebral artery, and lack of blood flow to the lenticulostriate artery can result in damage to the left internal capsule, left putamen, left globus pallidus, and left caudate nucleus. This will also result in paralysis of the right side of the body.

6. **D** The inferior frontal cortex contains Broca's area. It is in this area that motor impulses from the precentral gyrus and premotor cortices, among other areas, cascade. These are then coordinated so the muscle groups needed to articulate speech can work as a unit. Damage to Broca's area results in William's symptoms.

    A Wernicke's area is found in the posterior aspect of the superior temporal gyrus. Damage to this area results in an individual who is often fluent in language, but the conversation makes no sense in context.
    B Damage to the supramarginal gyrus can result in anomia (a problem with word finding or recall) or alexia (inability to read), among other problems. However, it does not result in the symptoms associated with William.
    C The lingual gyrus, located in the occipital lobe, is involved with sight, not speech.
    E The precentral gyrus is involved with sensory perception and coordination of sensory information from various areas of the cerebrum. Damage to the precentral gyrus produces numerous sensory deficits but not the symptom listed above.

7. **C** Prosody, or the ability to recognize tonality in speech or music, is associated with the right cerebral hemisphere of a left brain–dominant individual. Thus, this would be affected in an individual with an occlusion of the right middle cerebral artery.

    A Occlusion of the middle cerebral artery results in contralateral, not ipsilateral, paralysis of the trunk and limbs.
    B Occlusion of the middle cerebral artery results in contralateral paralysis of the muscles of facial expression inferior to the zygomatic arch, not total ipsilateral paralysis of the muscles of facial expression.
    D Acalculia, or the inability to perform mathematical calculations, is associated with the left cerebral hemisphere of a left brain–dominant individual. It would be unaffected in an occlusion of the right middle cerebral artery.
    E Inability to speak sentences that make sense in response to a verbal or written request is associated with damage to Wernicke's area, which is found in the left cerebral hemisphere of a left brain–dominant individual. This would not occur in an individual with an occlusion of the right middle cerebral artery.

8. **A** The posterior superior alveolar nerve on each side innervates the maxillary molars and their associated buccal gingiva, mucosa, and periosteum.

> B The long buccal nerve on each side innervates the mucosa of the cheek and the gingiva between the mandibular 2nd premolar and molars, as well as the retromolar triangle. It does not innervate any teeth.
> C The middle superior alveolar nerve on each side (when present) innervates the roots of the 1st and 2nd premolars and the mesiobuccal root of the 1st molar.
> D The greater palatine nerve innervates the palatal gingiva, mucosa, and periosteum from the maxillary 1st premolar to the posterior hard palate to the midline of the hard palate on the same side as the injection, that is, the posterior two-thirds of the hard palate. The anterior two-thirds of the hard palate is supplied by the nasopalatine nerve.
> E The lesser palatine nerve supplies the mucosa of the soft palate.

9. **D** The greater palatine foramen and canal are sufficiently large so that a small-bore needle can be placed within the foramen and fluid expressed that can gain access to the pterygopalatine fossa. The maxillary nerve lies within the fossa.

> A, B Under no circumstances would anesthetic fluid, by any direction or means, be intentionally placed into the cranial vault. This could have disastrous effects on the brain.
> C Under extreme circumstances, fluid could be injected into the pterygopalatine fossa via the extraoral route. However, this is extremely dangerous, as the needle could damage any number of structures in the infratemporal fossa, including the mandibular nerve and its two major branches (inferior alveolar and lingual), maxillary artery, and pterygoid plexus of veins. Also, bacteria from the skin or superficial fascia could enter the fossa via this route.
> E In theory, anesthetic fluid could be placed into the infraorbital foramen and expressed through the canal into the pterygopalatine canal. However, because of the force needed, there are several side effects that could occur, including temporary paralysis of the extraocular muscles and temporary blindness. These side effects are a result of anesthetic fluid traveling from the infraorbital canal into the orbit.

10. **B** Both the temporalis and masseter elevate the mandible, and both can be externally palpated (therefore not answer choice A). The temporalis participates in elevation, retrusion, and lateral excursion of the mandible. The masseter participates in elevation, protrusion, retrusion, and lateral excursion of the mandible.

> C The buccinator does not elevate the mandible; rather, it presses the cheek against the molar teeth, working with the tongue to keep food between the occlusal surfaces and out of the oral vestibule.
> D The zygomaticus major does not elevate the mandible but rather pulls the corner of the mouth superiorly and laterally.
> E The lateral pterygoid functions in depressing, protruding, and medially excursing the mandible (inferior head). It also functions in stabilizing the mandible during retrusion (superior head). In addition, this muscle cannot be palpated externally.

11. **B** The mesencephalic nucleus of CN V is specifically associated with proprioception from the TMJ, the muscles that act upon it, and the teeth that directly surround it. Damage to the ipsilateral mesencephalic nucleus of CN V would result in the symptoms described.

> A Damage to the motor nucleus of CN V, and or hyperactivity associated with the motor nucleus of V, could result in the hyperactivity associated with muscles, but the damage would need to be ipsilateral to the effect. Thus, it is the left motor nucleus of CN V that would need to be damaged, not the right.
> C The principal sensory nucleus of CN V is responsible for proprioception in the majority of the areas of the head and fine touch. However, the specific areas described in the question are served by the mesencephalic nucleus of CN V.
> D The nucleus caudalis of the spinal nucleus of CN V is involved with pain, temperature, pressure, and crude touch. It is not involved with coordinating muscle activity.

> E The function of the nucleus interpolaris is still a matter of conjecture, but it is definitely not involved with fine touch. Also, if it were to be involved, it would need to be located on the left side of the brainstem, not the right.

12. **D** Fibers of the olfactory nerve travel through the cribriform plate of the ethmoid bone. The force of the collision as it was transmitted posteriorly could break through this rather tenuous bone.

> A The infraorbital nerve and vessels travel through the inferior orbital fissure.
> B The maxillary branch of the trigeminal nerve (CN V) travels through the foramen rotundum.
> C The mandibular branch of the trigeminal nerve and the lesser petrosal branch of the glossopharyngeal nerve travel through the foramen ovale.
> E The middle meningeal artery and nerve (nervus spinosus) travel through the foramen spinosum.

13. **C** The force of his head hitting the windshield during the collision was transmitted back through the frontal bone to the suture between the frontal bone and lesser wing of the sphenoid bone, causing breakage of the lesser wing and a severing of the optic chiasm.

> A As stated in Q12, fibers of the olfactory, not the optic, nerve travel through the cribriform plate of the ethmoid bone.
> B The frontal bone is sufficiently massive, so that it probably would not break and cause the damage as described.
> D, E The petrosal portion of the temporal bone and the clivus lie posterior to all of the structures listed in the scenario.

14. **C** The posterior superior alveolar nerve carries sensory fibers to the maxillary molars, a portion of the mucosa of the maxillary sinus, a portion of the buccal gingiva of the maxillary molars, and a portion of the cheek. It is the nerve that is anesthetized in this procedure.

> A The middle superior alveolar nerve carries sensory fibers to the premolar teeth and associated buccal gingiva and possibly the mesiobuccal root of the 1st molar.
> B The anterior superior alveolar nerve carries sensory fibers to the central and lateral incisors, the canines, the mucosa of the maxillary sinus, the labial gingiva associated with the incisors and maxillary canines, and various nasal branches to the mucosa of a portion of the nasal septum, wall, and floor of the nasal cavity.
> D The greater palatine nerve supplies the palatine gingiva and mucosa from the maxillary premolars posteriorly.
> E The lesser palatine nerve supplies sensory innervation to the mucosa of the soft palate.

15. Overall, the symptoms described are indicative of a cavernous sinus thrombosis. The most common organism introduced into the sinus to cause the thrombosis is Staphylococcus aureus, with streptococci and pneumococci being less common (Andreoli et al., Cecil Essentials of Medicine, 6th ed. Elsevier, 2004). This question relates to the manner by which the organisms were introduced into the sinus.
D Small tributaries of the pterygoid plexus can be punctured in an attempt to anesthetize the posterior superior alveolar nerve. The pterygoid plexus communicates with the cavernous sinus via a system of emissary veins.

> A The middle meningeal artery is a branch of the external carotid artery, but neither connects to the cavernous sinus.
> B The ophthalmic vein does drain into the cavernous sinus. However, in a procedure to anesthetize the maxillary molars, the needle should not be in the vicinity of the ophthalmic vein.
> C The maxillary vein does drain into the retromandibular vein. However, the retromandibular vein does not drain into the cavernous sinus.
> E The infraorbital vein drains into the pterygoid plexus. However, in a procedure to anesthetize the maxillary molars, the needle should not be in the vicinity of the infraorbital vein.

16. **D** The oculomotor, trochlear, and abducent nerves all travel through the cavernous sinus. However, the oculomotor and trochlear nerves travel in its lateral aspect and are wrapped in, and protected by, the dura mater. In contrast, the abducent nerve runs through the center of the sinus and is unprotected. Thus, in a cavernous sinus thrombosis, symptoms involving the abducent nerve are seen before those associated with either the trochlear or oculomotor nerve. The lateral rectus muscle, innervated by the abducent nerve, moves the eyeball laterally.

    A The inferior oblique primarily acts in elevation of the eyeball. It is innervated via fibers of the oculomotor, not the abducent, nerve.
    B The superior rectus is innervated via fibers of the oculomotor nerve, but its primary action is elevation of the eyeball. It plays a minor role in adduction of the eyeball.
    C The inferior rectus is innervated via fibers of the oculomotor nerve, but its primary action is depression of the eyeball. It plays a minor role in adduction of the eyeball.
    E The superior oblique muscle primarily acts in depression of the eyeball. It is innervated via branches of the trochlear nerve. It plays a minor role in abduction of the eyeball, but damage to it, in and of itself, would not cause major difficulty in moving the eyeball laterally.

17. **B** Lowering the eyelid is achieved via the orbicularis oculi, which is innervated by branches of the facial nerve (CN VII). The facial nerve runs through the parotid space and thus would be anesthetized on the side of the injection as a result of the procedure described.

    A Depressing the mandible is accomplished through the action of the lateral pterygoid, suprahyoid, and infrahyoid muscles. The lateral pterygoid, mylohyoid, and anterior digastric muscles are innervated by branches of the mandibular division of the trigeminal nerve (CN V$_3$). The posterior digastric and stylohyoid are innervated by branches of the facial nerve (CN VII). The geniohyoid and thyrohyoid are innervated by fibers of C1, and the remainder of the infrahyoid muscles are innervated by branches of the ansa cervicalis. None of these nerves run through the parotid space.
    C Raising the upper eyelid is achieved via the levator palpebrae superioris, which is innervated by the oculomotor nerve. This also would be unaffected, as it is on the opposite side of the injection.
    D Swallowing is achieved via branches of the glossopharyngeal (CN IX), vagus (CN X), and accessory (CN XI) nerves.
    E Raising the mandible is accomplished via the temporalis, masseter, and medial pterygoid muscles, which are innervated by branches of the mandibular division of the trigeminal nerve (CN V$_3$). They would also be unaffected on the opposite side of the injection.

18. **A** The retromandibular vein runs through the parotid space.

    B, C The internal carotid artery and the internal jugular vein travel medial to the parotid space.
    D The masseteric branch of the maxillary artery branches from the maxillary artery medial and internal to the parotid space.
    E The buccal branch of the maxillary artery branches from the maxillary artery medial and internal to the parotid space.

19. **B** If the injection was too far posterior and inferior, there would be penetration into the parotid space with probable anesthesia of branches of the facial nerve. There would be no anesthesia of the inferior alveolar nerve, as evidenced by failure to numb the lower lip (no lower lip sign).

    A, C, E If the injection was too far superior and anterior, too far anterior and inferior, or too far medial and superior, there would only be anesthesia at the injection site and no anesthesia of the inferior alveolar nerve, as evidenced by failure to numb the lower lip (no lower lip sign). There also would be no penetration into the parotid space.
    D If the injection was too far medial and inferior, there would be possible anesthesia of the lingual nerve. More likely, there would only be anesthesia at the injection site and no anesthesia of the inferior alveolar nerve, as evidenced by failure to numb the lower lip (no lower lip sign). There also would be no penetration into the parotid space.

20. **C** There are sensory fibers that sometimes travel on the nerve to the mylohyoid. These sensory fibers may provide innervation to the mandibular teeth.

    A The lingual nerve carries sensory fibers to the anterior two-thirds of the tongue and the lingual gingiva of the mandibular molars, but not to the teeth themselves.
    B The long buccal nerve provides sensory fibers to the mucosa and skin of the cheek and to the buccal gingiva of the mandibular molars, but not to the teeth themselves.
    D The marginal mandibular nerve is a motor branch of the facial nerve.
    E The buccal branch of CN VII is a motor branch of the facial nerve.

21. **B** Trigeminal neuralgia affects the branches of the trigeminal nerve, typically in the following order: V$_2$ > V$_3$ > V$_1$. More often than not, it only affects the maxillary nerve and mandibular nerve and their branches. As described in this scenario, it is affecting branches of the mandibular nerve, with the associated pattern of pain.

    A Bell's palsy affects the facial nerve and the muscles of facial expression, not the muscles of mastication.
    C Geniculate neuralgia involves similar pain patterns as trigeminal neuralgia but deals with the pain areas of the facial, not the trigeminal, nerve. This may include pain associated with the external auditory meatus or even pain felt deep within the ear. It is sometimes associated with herpes zoster and can result in vesicular eruptions on the eardrum and external auditory canal.
    D Glossopharyngeal neuralgia involves similar pain patterns as trigeminal neuralgia but deals with the pain areas of the glossopharyngeal, not the trigeminal, nerve. This may include pain associated with the tongue, pharynx, throat, ear, and tonsils.
    E Temporal arteritis is pain associated with areas overlying, or adjacent to, the superior temporal artery, although it can be other arteries in the head. Severe headaches can result from temporal arteritis.

22. **B** The areas of pain associated with the scenario include regions of the inferior alveolar nerve (the mandible, skin over the mandible, and skin over the inferior aspect of the infratemporal fossa, as well as a portion of the internal aspect of the mouth) and the lingual nerve (mucosa of the anterior two-thirds of the tongue and a portion of the internal aspect of the mouth).

    A Pain associated with the trigeminal nerve would be all of the pain domains of the ophthalmic, maxillary, and mandibular branches, which include the entire side of the face from the upper frontal regions down to the neck. This is not what occurred in the scenario.
    C The sensory distribution areas of the maxillary nerve are the more superior aspect of the infratemporal fossa, the skin overlying the maxilla and a portion of the nasal area, the maxillary teeth, and the mucosa and gingiva of the maxillary region. Pain was not described in these regions.
    D Areas of pain associated with the inferior alveolar nerve were reported, but pain associated with areas of the lingual nerve was also reported.
    E Areas of pain associated with the lingual nerve were reported, but pain associated with areas of the inferior alveolar nerve was also reported.

23. **C** The temporalis is one of the major elevators of the mandible. The other two are the masseter and medial pterygoid.

    A The buccinator is a muscle of facial expression and does not move the mandible.
    B Actions of the lateral pterygoid include protrusion, depression, and medial excursion of the mandible. The upper head of the lateral pterygoid also stabilizes the mandibular condyle during retrusion. The lateral pterygoid does not function in elevation of the mandible.
    D, E The mylohyoid and anterior digastric play a role in depression of the mandible.

547

24. **B** The semilunar ganglion, otherwise known as the Gasserian or trigeminal ganglion, would be ablated in this procedure.

   A The geniculate ganglion is associated with the facial nerve (CN VII). As previously stated, the facial nerve would not be involved in this syndrome.
   C The inferior (not superior) ganglion of CN IX is the general sensory ganglion of the glossopharyngeal nerve and thus would not be involved with pain patterns associated with the trigeminal nerve (CN V).
   D The pterygopalatine ganglion is one of the parasympathetic motor ganglia of the head. It is associated with the facial nerve.
   E The superior ganglion of CN X is the general sensory ganglion of the vagus nerve and thus would not be involved with pain patterns associated with the trigeminal nerve.

25. **D** Bell's palsy involves dysfunction of the facial nerve. This is normally of unknown etiology. It can involve all of the functions associated with the facial nerve but most often involves only ipsilateral paralysis of all of the muscles of facial expression.

   A A left-sided cerebral stroke produces paralysis of all of the muscles of the right side of the body, not just the face.
   B A right-sided cerebral stroke produces paralysis of all of the muscles on the left side of the body, not just the face.
   C, E Trigeminal neuralgia and glossopharyngeal neuralgia produce tremendous pain, but not muscle paralysis.

26. **A** As initially stated, the symptoms involve only the muscles of facial expression. This is consistent with damage to the facial nerve at a spot where only branchial efferent impulses are carried. This spot is either just proximal to or within the parotid gland.

   B There are motor fibers of the facial nerve that supply the occipitalis and small muscles of the skin around the ear (auriculares). These muscles would be affected if the damage to the facial nerve was just distal to its exit from the stylomastoid foramen. In addition, the stylohyoid and posterior belly of the digastric would be denervated.
   C The same caveat as for answer choice B applies for this answer. In addition, depending on where the compression occurred, there may be disruption of sensory impulses to the auricular branch of CN VII.
   D If the compression was just proximal to the branching of the chorda tympani, not only would all of the aforementioned symptoms occur, but symptoms involving the chorda tympani would also be witnessed. These include difficulties with taste and a possible perception of lessened salivation.
   E If the compression was just distal to the branching of the chorda tympani, the symptoms would be the same as described in answer choice C.

27. **C** If the compression was just proximal to the point at which the greater petrosal nerve branches, the symptoms would include ipsilateral paralysis of the muscles of facial expression and the occipitalis and small muscles of the external ear. In addition, the stylohyoid and posterior belly of the digastric would also be denervated. Symptoms would include a lack of sensation associated with the auricular branch of CN VII, diminished taste, and a possible perception of lessened salivation. Functions associated with the greater petrosal nerve would be disrupted, including loss of parasympathetic output from the pterygopalatine ganglion to glands in the nasal cavity, pharynx, and mucosa of the palate, as well as to the lacrimal gland, resulting in lack of lacrimation. In addition, there would be lack of taste from scattered taste buds on the soft palate, although this would be barely perceptible by the patient. Finally, there might be a perception of increased "noise" on the side of the injury due to lack of function of the nerve to the stapedius.

   A Only the muscles of facial expression, ipsilateral to the damage, would be affected as a result of compression of the facial nerve as it travels through the parotid gland.
   B If the compression was just proximal to the branching of the chorda tympani, the symptoms would include ipsilateral paralysis of the muscles of facial expression, the occipitalis, and small muscles of the external ear. In addition, the stylohyoid and posterior belly of the digastric would be denervated. Symptoms would include a lack of sensation associated with the auricular branch of CN VII, diminished taste, and a possible perception of lessened salivation.

D The symptoms would include all those stated in answer choice B if the compression was just distal to where the greater petrosal nerve branches. In addition, there might be a perception of increased "noise" on the side of the injury due to a lack of function of the nerve to the stapedius.
E If the compression was just distal to the point at which the chorda tympani branches, symptoms would include ipsilateral paralysis of the muscles of facial expression, ipsilateral paralysis of the small muscles of the external ear and occipitalis, denervation of the stylohyoid and posterior belly of the digastric, and loss of sensation associated with the auricular branch of CN VII.

28. **D** The levator palpebrae superioris is innervated by the oculomotor nerve and acts in elevating the eyelid. It is unopposed in facial nerve (CN VII) paralysis, causing the eyelid to be abnormally elevated.

   A, B The orbicularis oculi is innervated by the zygomatic and temporal branches of CN VII. However, these nerves act to depress the eyelid, not elevate it.
   C The levator palpebrae superioris does elevate the eyelid. However, it is innervated by a branch of the oculomotor nerve, not the temporal branch of CN VII.
   E The corrugator supercilii and frontalis are innervated by branches of the temporal branch of CN VII. However, neither acts to elevate the eyelid.

29. **C** Fibers of the left recurrent laryngeal nerve supply the majority of intrinsic muscles of the larynx. They also supply the mucosa of the larynx from the vocal folds and below. It is this nerve that would be constricted as it loops around the arch of the aorta.

   A Symptoms due to damage to the vagus nerve, depending on the location of the damage, would include those described for all of the nerves listed in the question. In addition, there might be changes in heart rate and in muscle tone associated with the gastrointestinal tract.
   B Fibers from the external laryngeal nerve innervate only the cricothyroid muscle of the larynx and sometimes the cricopharyngeus muscle of the pharynx. The symptoms described above would not result from compression of this nerve, nor does it loop around the aorta.
   D The external and internal laryngeal nerves are branches of the superior laryngeal nerve. The function of the external laryngeal nerve has already been described.
   E The internal laryngeal nerve supplies sensory fibers to the mucosa of the larynx above the vocal folds. This might produce some of the same symptoms; however, because the nerve does not loop around the aorta, it would not be constricted in this scenario.

30. **C** Maxillary sinusitis can be interpreted as pain associated with the maxillary molars. In many patients, this pain is exacerbated because of allergies associated with flowering plants in the spring and rotting leaves in the fall.

   A Pain associated with trigeminal neuralgia is episodic and extreme. It also does not occur on a seasonal basis.
   B, D, E Masseteric spasms, middle ear infection, and temporomandibular dysfunction can be interpreted as pain associated with the maxillary molars. However, the pain would not occur on a seasonal basis.

31. **C** Sensory impulses to the cerebrum are relayed through the thalamus. The thalamus is involved in localizing sensory impulses to areas in the body.

   A The superior colliculus is involved with sight and the coordination of the muscles that move the eyeballs.
   B The inferior colliculus is involved with hearing.
   D The hypothalamus, among other things, is involved with hunger, thirst, memory, and sexuality. It is not involved with the localization of sensory impulses.
   E The globus pallidus is part of the basal ganglia. Its primary function is modulation of motor impulses.

32. **A** Perception of pain, along with perception of most other sensations, is associated with the postcentral gyrus of the parietal lobe.

> B Initiation of motor impulses is associated with the precentral gyrus of the frontal lobe.
> C The superior temporal gyrus is associated with hearing, both perception and memory.
> D The lingual gyrus of the occipital lobe is involved with sight.
> E The cingulate gyrus is involved with memory, primarily long-term retrograde.

33. **B** The medial pterygoid inserts on the internal aspect of the angle of the mandible, and the masseter inserts on the external aspect of the angle of the mandible. These two form the pterygomasseteric sling.

> A The medial pterygoid inserts on the internal aspect of the angle of the mandible; the lateral pterygoid inserts onto the condyle of the mandible, the meniscus, and the pterygoid fovea of the mandible.
> C The masseter inserts on the external aspect of the angle of the mandible; the temporalis inserts on the coronoid process of the mandible and the internal aspect of the superior portion of the ramus of the mandible.
> D, E The insertions of the temporalis, medial pterygoid, and lateral pterygoid have already been described.

34. **A** The muscles of mastication, anterior digastric, mylohyoid, tensor tympani, and tensor veli palatini develop from the 1st branchial arch.

> B The muscles of facial expression, occipitalis, auricular muscles, posterior digastric, stylohyoid, and stapedius develop from the 2nd branchial arch.
> C The stylopharyngeus develops from the 3rd branchial arch.
> D Muscles of the soft palate, pharynx, and larynx develop from the 4th branchial arch.
> E The 5th branchial arch degenerates; nothing develops from it.

35. **E** The ameloblastoma develops within the mandible. It can break out from the mandible, but it would first affect nerves that travel through the mandible, and the only nerve listed that fulfills that criterion is the inferior alveolar nerve. The inferior alveolar nerve originates in the infratemporal fossa and travels through the mandibular foramen to gain access to the internal aspect of the mandible.

> A The long buccal nerve runs on the lateral aspect of the maxilla down to the external aspect of the mandible and the gingiva of the internal aspect of the mandible.
> B The lingual nerve originates in the infratemporal fossa and enters into the oral cavity deep to the mylohyoid and hyoglossus.
> C The deep temporal nerve originates in the infratemporal fossa and travels to the temporal fossa to innervate the temporalis.
> D The nerve to the lateral pterygoid originates in the infratemporal fossa and terminates in the deep aspect of the two heads of the lateral pterygoid.

36. **C** The chorda tympani carries taste fibers from the facial nerve. These taste fibers then travel from the chorda tympani to the lingual nerve.

> A Taste does hitchhike in the lingual branch of the trigeminal nerve to the anterior two-thirds of the tongue, but not initially.
> B The inferior alveolar branch of the trigeminal nerve carries branchial efferent fibers and general sensory fibers, not taste fibers.
> D The greater petrosal branch of the facial nerve carries parasympathetic and taste fibers. However, the taste fibers go to scattered taste buds associated with the soft palate, not the tongue. Also, there are so few taste buds associated with these fibers, that their dysfunction would be barely noticeable.
> E The lesser petrosal branch of the glossopharyngeal nerve carries preganglionic parasympathetic fibers that synapse in the otic ganglion.

37. **C** The majority of taste buds are found on the circumvallate papillae.

> A There are no taste buds on filiform papillae.
> B There are a minimal number of taste buds on fungiform papillae.
> D There are a few scattered taste buds associated with the foliate papillae.
> E Taste buds are primarily associated with the circumvallate (vallate) papillae.

38. **D** The greater and lesser petrosal nerves both contain fibers that stimulate salivation (therefore not A or B alone). The greater petrosal nerve carries preganglionic parasympathetic fibers from the facial nerve that synapse in the pterygopalatine ganglion. Some postganglionic parasympathetic fibers travel to scattered salivary glands in the mucosa of the soft palate. The lesser petrosal nerve carries preganglionic parasympathetic fibers from the glossopharyngeal nerve that synapse in the otic ganglion. Postganglionic parasympathetic fibers travel in the auriculotemporal nerve to the parotid salivary gland.

> C The deep petrosal nerve carries postganglionic sympathetic fibers that originate in the superior cervical ganglion. These fibers are not involved with stimulation of salivation. Salivation is predominantly under parasympathetic control but sympathetic stimulation may result in a small flow of saliva that is rich in protein.
> E Incorrect.

39. **D** Preganglionic parasympathetic fibers originate in the facial nerve, travel to the chorda tympani, and synapse in the submandibular ganglion. Postganglionic fibers travel to the submandibular and sublingual glands and small salivary groups found in the tongue and oral mucosa.

> A The ciliary ganglion is a parasympathetic ganglion associated with the oculomotor nerve (CN III). Postganglionic fibers from the ganglion carry impulses that cause constriction of the pupil as they innervate the pupillary constrictor muscle and accommodation via ciliary muscle contraction.
> B The superior cervical ganglion is a sympathetic ganglion that provides postganglionic fibers for the head and neck.
> C The middle cervical ganglion is a sympathetic ganglion that provides postganglionic fibers to the heart and thyroid gland.
> E Preganglionic parasympathetic fibers originate in the facial nerve, travel to the greater petrosal nerve and the nerve of the pterygoid canal, then synapse in the pterygopalatine ganglion. Postganglionic fibers go to very minor salivary glands found in the soft palate and mucosa of the oral cavity. They also travel to the lacrimal gland.

40. **E** In Ludwig's angina, infection is found bilaterally in the submandibular and sublingual spaces and in the submental space.

> A–D In Ludwig's angina, infection is found in these spaces, but not exclusively.

41. **C** Ludwig's angina results from an infection of a root of a tooth that impinges into either the submandibular or the sublingual space; therefore, it can emanate from any of the mandibular teeth.

> A The inferior aspects of the mandibular molars are found in the submandibular space, but they do not exclusively lead to Ludwig's angina.
> B The inferior aspects of the roots of the mandibular incisors and canines are found in the sublingual space, but they do not exclusively lead to Ludwig's angina. .
> D, E Roots of the maxillary teeth do not gain access to the submandibular or sublingual spaces.

42. **A** Because the most superior structure is the submandibular duct, it will be encountered first.

> B The lingual nerve is found just inferior to the submandibular duct.
> C The lingual artery is the most inferior of the structures listed.
> D The hypoglossal nerve runs between the lingual nerve and the lingual artery.
> E The glossopharyngeal nerve is not found in the floor of the oral cavity. It enters the tongue on its posterior aspect.

43. **B** The facial artery runs through the submandibular gland.

> A The facial vein runs superficial to the submandibular gland.
> C The lingual artery runs deep to the submandibular gland.
> D The hypoglossal nerve runs deep to the submandibular gland.
> E The anterior division of the retromandibular vein runs superior to the submandibular gland.

549

44. **B** The marginal mandibular branch of the facial nerve runs on the superficial surface of the submandibular gland.

> A The cervical branch of the facial nerve runs posterior to the submandibular gland.
> C The mental branch of the trigeminal nerve runs on the anteromedial surface of the mandible and is superior and anterior to the submandibular gland.
> D The fibers of the long buccal branch of the trigeminal nerve run on the superficial aspect of the cheek and into the gingiva of the mandible, not onto the submandibular gland.
> E The inferior fibers of the buccal branch of the facial nerve travel on the lateral aspect of the cheek and are superior to the submandibular gland.

45. **E** The submandibular gland sits on the anterior surface of the mylohyoid muscle, and a portion of the posterior aspect of the gland, as well as the submandibular duct, wraps around the muscle to its inferior aspect.

> A The hyoglossus is deep to both the submandibular gland and the mylohyoid muscle.
> B The anterior belly of the digastric is the anterior border of the submandibular triangle, and the submandibular gland sits within the triangle. The submandibular gland is posterior, and superficial, to much of the anterior belly. It does not wrap around it.
> C The posterior belly of the digastric is the posterior border of the submandibular triangle. The submandibular gland sits anterior to the posterior digastric.
> D The genioglossus muscle essentially sits within the oral cavity and is deep to the submandibular triangle. It is also anterior to the submandibular gland.

46. **E** The alar fascia (anterior layer of the prevertebral fascia) is the border between the danger space and the retropharyngeal space.

> A The posterior layer of the prevertebral fascia is the posterior border of the danger space.
> B The pretracheal fascia is the anterior border of the retropharyngeal space.
> C In this case, the buccopharyngeal fascia is synonymous with the pretracheal fascial; that is, they are continuous.
> D The medial aspect of the carotid sheath is the lateral border of the retropharyngeal space.

47. **C** Infections from the retropharyngeal space and/or danger space travel into the mediastinum and can then spread to the heart, resulting in pericarditis (inflammation of the pericardium [outer layer] of the heart).

> A Infections from the roots of the maxillary teeth, nasal cavity, or orbit may travel into the maxillary sinus with a resulting maxillary sinus infection.
> B Infections from the periorbital and infraorbital space, the supraorbital area, and the veins of the face, specifically, the pterygoid plexus of veins, may travel into the cavernous sinus. This can result in a cavernous sinus infection and/or thrombosis, which can be fatal in a matter of days.
> D Infections from the head normally do not gain access to the peritoneal cavity.
> E Infections from the supraorbital and infraorbital areas, as well as the nasal cavity and maxillary sinus, can gain access to the orbit. Symptoms associated with infections in the orbit include exophthalmos (bulging eyes) and diplopia (double vision).

48. **E** The thyroid gland is an endocrine gland and secretes into veins that are located on its lateral aspect. A vertical midline incision does not harm these vessels.

> A The thymus regresses as we age, not the thyroid gland.
> B, C The thyroid gland is an endocrine not an exocrine, gland.
> D The thyroid gland does not secrete angiogenic factors. Vessels cannot grow back to the thyroid gland once they are severed.

49. **D** The consensual light reflex occurs when a light is shined in one pupil, resulting in both pupils constricting.

> A The corneal reflex involves brushing the cornea and watching for the eyelid to shut.
> B The pupillary dilator reflex is an involuntary reflex involving dilation of the pupil.
> C The vestibulo-ocular reflex occurs when the head is moved, but the image viewed remains in a constant point on the retina.
> E The accommodation reflex is the adjustment of the shape of the lens to keep objects in focus when focal lengths change. This was not being tested.

50. **A** The medial geniculate body is involved with hearing. It is part of the auditory pathway. Fibers from the inferior colliculus travel to, and synapse in, the medial geniculate body. Fibers from the medial geniculate body travel to the auditory cortex of the temporal lobe. It is therefore not involved in the consensual light reflex.

> B–E In the consensual light reflex, sensory impulses from the retina travel to the pretectal nuclei via the optic nerve (E). Fibers from the pretectal nuclei communicate with each other via the posterior commissure (D). Fibers from the pretectal nuclei travel to the Edinger–Westphal nucleus. Preganglionic fibers from the Edinger–Westphal (C) nucleus travel to the ciliary ganglion (B). Postganglionic fibers from the ciliary ganglion travel to the pupillary constrictor muscle and cause the pupil to constrict.

51. **B** The middle meningeal artery is found in the epidural space. A sudden tear of the artery would enlarge the space and potentially compress structures found on the dorsal aspect of the midbrain, including the pretectal nucleus and posterior commissure. This could result in disruption of the consensual light reflex.

> A A tear of the lining of a ventricle could cause leakage of cerebrospinal fluid (CSF). However, this could not be tested through the consensual light reflex. A small tear of the ventricle would gradually leak CSF, but under most circumstances, there is no way to directly test for this.
> C Meningeal and cerebral veins are found in the subdural space; in some rare cases, when they rip, pooling of blood can compress neuronal structures. However, in most cases, these tears result in a slow bleed that is not detected for a matter of hours or days, whereas the testing was to determine if a neuronal difficulty had occurred immediately. Testing for tears of these veins would only occur after symptoms, such as dizziness or semiconsciousness, had manifested themselves. The testing would involve CT scans or MRI with contrast.
> D, E An occlusion of a cerebral artery would not be tested via the consensual light reflex. An angiography of the cerebral vessels would determine if this occlusion occurred.

52. **B** The accessory nerve can be damaged in a radical neck dissection. The accessory nerve innervates the sternocleidomastoid, which participates in rotation of the head. It also innervates the trapezius, which participates in elevation of the shoulder (scapula).

> A Idiopathic spasmodic torticollis is normally inherited and not due to acute damage to a nerve.
> C The vagus nerve lies in the carotid sheath and is normally not damaged in a radical neck dissection.
> D Branches of the ansa cervicalis could be injured in a radical neck dissection, but the muscles it innervates (inferior belly of the omohyoid, superior belly of the omohyoid, sternohyoid, and sternothyroid) are not involved in rotation of the head.
> E The phrenic nerve could conceivably be damaged in a radical neck dissection; however, it does not innervate muscles involved with rotation of the head, but rather innervates the diaphragm.

53. **C** The hypoglossal nerve (CN XII) innervates all of the intrinsic muscles of the tongue and all extrinsic muscles of the tongue (genioglossus, hyoglossus, and styloglossus) except the palatoglossus, which is innervated by the vagus nerve (CN X).

A The inferior alveolar nerve supplies sensory fibers to the mandibular teeth and the skin overlying a portion of the mandible.
B The chorda tympani carries preganglionic parasympathetic fibers and taste fibers.
D The mandibular branch of the trigeminal nerve supplies sensory fibers to the majority of the head and motor fibers to the muscles of mastication, the mylohyoid, the anterior digastric, the tensor tympani, and the tensor veli palatini.
E The glossopharyngeal nerve supplies taste to the posterior one-third of the tongue, sensory from the upper portion of the pharynx, general sensory to the posterior one-third of the tongue, sensory from the external auditory meatus, and motor to the stylopharyngeus. It does not supply muscles of the tongue.

54. **C** Damage to the right hypoglossal nerve results in the right genioglossus not working properly. The right genioglossus protrudes the tongue toward the left. Thus, the left genioglossus would work unopposed, and the tongue, upon protrusion, deviates to the right. That is what is demonstrated in the photo.

A, B The hyoglossus depresses and retrudes the tongue. Protrusion is demonstrated in the photo.
B, D Damage to the left genioglossus results in the tongue deviating toward the left.
E Damage to the left genioglossus results in the tongue deviating toward the left. Damage to the left hyoglossus results in difficulties with depressing and retruding the tongue.

55. **D** The infraclavicular nodes are not part of the axillary group of nodes. Lymph from the axillary group drains to the infraclavicular and supraclavicular nodes.

A The pectoral nodes are part of the axillary group of nodes. Lymph from the anterior chest wall and mammary glands drains to the pectoral nodes.
B The lateral nodes are part of the axillary group of nodes. Lymph from the upper limb drains to the lateral nodes.
C The subscapular nodes are part of the axillary group of nodes. Lymph from the neck, back, and posterior aspect of the thoracic wall drains to the subscapular nodes.
E The apical nodes are part of the axillary group of nodes. Lymph from the lateral nodes drains to the apical nodes.

56. **C** Medial rotation of the humerus is accomplished through the actions of the pectoralis major, teres major, latissimus dorsi, and subscapularis.

A Inferior rotation of the scapula is accomplished through the actions of the rhomboid major, rhomboid minor, levator scapulae, and pectoralis minor.
B Superior rotation of the scapula is accomplished through the actions of the trapezius and serratus anterior.
D Abduction of the humerus is accomplished through the action of the medial fibers of the deltoid, supraspinatus and serratus anterior.
E Extension of the humerus is accomplished through the actions of the latissimus dorsi and posterior fibers of the deltoid.

57. **A** The long thoracic nerve is found on the lateral chest wall. A portion of it is found within the confines of the axilla. As the long thoracic nerve travels on the superficial aspect of the serratus anterior, fibers from the nerve gain access to individual parts of the muscle. Because of its placement on the superficial aspect of the muscle, it is sometimes damaged as lymph and adipose tissue are removed during a radical mastectomy.

B The medial pectoral nerve innervates the pectoralis minor, but fibers from the nerve enter it from its deep aspect. The nerve then travels to the deep surface of the pectoralis major, which it also innervates.
C The lateral pectoral nerve innervates the pectoralis major muscle. It gains access to the muscle from its deep aspect.

D The thoracodorsal nerve innervates the latissimus dorsi and gains access to it from its deep aspect.
E The axillary nerve innervates the deltoid and teres minor. In both cases, as it travels through the quadrangular space, it gains access to the deep aspects of the muscles.

58. **A** The rhomboid major participates in retraction, elevation, and inferior rotation of the scapulae.

B The teres major participates in medial rotation, extension, and adduction of the humerus.
C The teres minor participates in lateral rotation of the humerus.
D The latissimus dorsi participates in medial rotation, extension, and adduction of the humerus.
E The longissimus participates in extension and stabilization of the vertebral column.

59. **C** The sinoatrial artery is a branch of the right coronary artery.

A The left coronary artery branches at the most proximal portion of the ascending portion of the aorta.
B The anterior ventricular artery is a branch of the left coronary artery.
D The posterior interventricular artery is a branch of the right coronary artery.
E The right marginal artery branches from the right coronary artery.

60. **E** Referred pain from the heart is normally not referred to the right hypogastrium. Some of the structures found in the right hypogastrium are the cecum, appendix, and ascending colon.

A–D Pain associated with angina is classically referred to the left shoulder and left upper limb (A). It can also be referred to the posterior shoulder and back, although the pain associated with aortic dissection is more commonly felt in the back between the shoulder blades. (B), to the midline of the mandible (C), and to the anterior aspect of the neck (D).

61. **E** Referred pain from the esophagus, as in esophagitis or gastric reflux, can be referred to the midsternal region (A), as can pain from the stomach (B) and the pancreas, as in pancreatitis or pancreatic cancer (C).

D Not applicable.

62. **C** The pericardial space (or cavity), with pericardial fluid, is found between the parietal layers of the serous pericardium and the visceral layer of the serous pericardium. Fluid is drained from the pericardial space by needle aspiration in a procedure known as pericardiocentesis.

A The pericardial fat lies on the superficial aspect of the fibrous pericardium. There is no discernible space between the two layers.
B There is a small bit of nonspecific lymphatic-type fluid between the parietal layer of the serous pericardium and fibrous pericardium, but there is no discernible space.
D The serous layer of the pericardium is superficial to the myocardium; there is no potential, or actual, space between them.
E The myocardium is superficial to the endocardium; there is no potential, or actual, space between them.

63. **E** The median nerve is found in the forearm and runs deep to the flexor retinaculum of the wrist and travels through the carpal tunnel.

A The deep branch of the radial nerve is found in the posterior compartment of the forearm.
B The superficial branch of the radial nerve is found in the superficial fascia of the posterior compartment.
C The lateral cutaneous nerve of the forearm is found in the superficial fascia of the anterolateral aspect of the forearm.
D The ulnar nerve is found in the proximal portion of the anterior compartment of the forearm but is superficial to the investing fascia in the distal portion of the forearm and superficial to the flexor retinaculum of the wrist. The ulnar nerve does not run through the carpal tunnel.

551

64. **B** The flexor pollicis brevis is innervated by the recurrent branch of the median nerve. If the median nerve was compressed in the distal aspect of the forearm or in the carpal tunnel, the recurrent branch would be dysfunctional.

    A, C, D The flexor pollicis longus, flexor digitorum superficialis, and flexor carpi radialis are innervated by the median nerve, but the nerve enters into these muscles in the proximal portion of the forearm and thus should not be affected in the scenario presented.
    E Not applicable.

65. **A** Fine motor movements of the thumb are achieved through the action of the flexor pollicis brevis, abductor pollicis brevis, and opponens brevis. All of these muscles are innervated by the recurrent branch of the median nerve, which may be affected in anterior compartment syndrome.

    B Adduction of the thumb is via the adductor pollicis, which is innervated by the ulnar nerve.
    C Flexion of the fingers is accomplished via the flexor digitorum superficialis, which is innervated by the median nerve, but the median nerve enters the muscle proximal to where the blood would pool. The flexor digitorum profundus is innervated by the median nerve (same caveat applies) and the ulnar nerve.
    D Extension at the carpometacarpal joints is accomplished through the action of the extensor digitorum and extensor indicis. Both muscles are innervated by the radial nerve.
    E Not applicable.

66. **B** The injuries described are characteristic of a Le Fort II fracture. The midface is fractured in a pyramidal shape, with the maxillary dentition at the base, and the nasofrontal suture at the apex.

    A Le Fort I fractures are horizontal fractures of the maxilla that separate the hard palate and dentition from the rest of the midface.
    C Le Fort III fractures are fractures in which the face separates from the cranial base. It can involve a fracture at the nasofrontal suture, but necessitates a fracture of the lateral wall of the orbit.
    D There is no Le Fort IV in the Le Fort classification system.

67. **C** The medial wall of the orbit, including the ethmoid bone, would also be fractured.

    A The hard palate stays intact in all Le Fort fractures.
    B The zygomatic arch may be fractured in a Le Fort III fracture.
    D The lateral orbital walls are fractured in a Le Fort III fracture.

68. **B** The internal carotid artery is found in the carotid triangle of the neck. The internal jugular vein and the vagus nerve are also found in the carotid triangle (and are, in fact, with the internal carotid artery within the carotid sheath), so are therefore at risk of injury.
    The deviation of the tongue to the left indicates that there is an injury to the *left* hypoglossal nerve (the hypoglossal nerve can also be found in the carotid triangle). Therefore, the left side of the patient's neck must have been the side that underwent surgery.

    A The submandibular gland and facial artery are found in the submandibular triangle.
    C The hypoglossal nerve is found in the carotid triangle, but as discussed above, the left side of the neck had the surgery, not the right side. The accessory nerve is found in the occipital triangle.
    D The anterior jugular vein and omohyoid muscle are found in the muscular triangle.

69. **C** As discussed in the explanation to question 68, the patient's left hypoglossal nerve was damaged. This paralyzed the muscles of the tongue on the left side (the intrinsic muscles and the extrinsic muscles except for the palatoglossus). When the patient tries to protrude his tongue using the genioglossus muscles, only the right genioglossus is functional, and the tongue deviates to the left.

    A, D The injury is on the left, not the right. Furthermore, neither muscle protrudes the tongue: geniohyoid raises the hyoid bone, and the styloglossus retracts and elevates the tongue.
    B, E Neither muscle protrudes the tongue: the palatoglossus elevates the tongue, and the superior longitudinal muscle shortens the tongue.

70. **B** The submandibular duct crosses superior to the lingual nerve.

    A, C, D The submandibular duct does not contact the glossopharyngeal or hypoglossal nerves.
    E The submandibular duct is superior, not inferior, to the lingual nerve.

71. **E** The postganglionic parasympathetic neurons to the submandibular gland are located in the submandibular ganglion.

    A The superior salivatory nucleus contains preganglionic, not postganglionic, parasympathetic cell bodies.
    B The pterygopalatine ganglion contains postganglionic parasympathetic cell bodies that supply glands accessed via branches of the maxillary nerve, as well as the lacrimal gland, but not the submandibular gland.
    C The superior cervical ganglion contains postganglionic sympathetic, not parasympathetic cell bodies.
    D The inferior salivatory nucleus contains preganglionic, not postganglionic, parasympathetic cell bodies. These neurons will synapse in the otic ganglion and will not supply the submandibular gland.

72. **A** The mandibular nerve is sensory to the structures adjacent to the mandible.

    B The facial nerve is not sensory to this region of the face.
    C C1 is not sensory to the neck or the face.
    D The hypoglossal nerve is motor, not sensory.
    E The maxillary nerve is sensory to the face, but supplies a region superior to the submandibular gland.

73. **D** The lingual nerve (CN V3) carries general sensation to the anterior two-thirds of the tongue. It also carries special taste fibers to the same region via the chorda tympani (CN VII). Damage to the lingual nerve would result in the loss of these functions on the ipsilateral side.

    A, B Both of these symptoms would appear in this patient, not just one of them.
    C, E The tongue receives its motor supply from the hypoglossal, not the lingual, nerve, so damage to the lingual nerve would not result in paralysis.

74. **E** All mandibular dentition receive blood from the inferior alveolar artery.

    A The posterior superior alveolar artery supplies the maxillary molars, not the mandibular molars.
    B The mental artery is a branch of the inferior alveolar artery that does not supply any teeth.
    C, D The lingual and facial arteries are branches of the external carotid artery that do not supply any teeth.

75. **A** Infections form mandibular third molars can spread to the submandibular, buccal, masseteric, or pterygomandibular spaces.

    B Infections from anterior mandibular teeth, not the molars, are likely to spread first to the submental space.
    C Infections from the first and second mandibular molars are likely to spread first to the sublingual space.
    D An infection can spread from the submandibular to the retropharyngeal space, but would not spread to the retropharyngeal space directly.
    E The most likely origin of odontogenic infection in the canine space would be a maxillary tooth.

Index